P⁓ ⸚ks ar

Oxford Medical Publications

Tobacco control in developing countries

D1549659

This volume is dedicated to the approximately 100 million people who have died in the twentieth century as a result of smoking. It is our hope that lessons learned from their deaths will help to avoid many of the 1 billion deaths expected to occur in the twenty-first century, on current smoking patterns.

Tobacco control in developing countries

Editors

Prabhat Jha and Frank J. Chaloupka

Published by Oxford University Press on behalf of The Human
Development Network, the World Bank, and The Economics
Advisory Service, World Health Organization

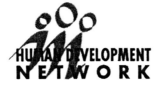

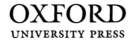

OXFORD

UNIVERSITY PRESS

This book has been printed digitally and produced in a standard specification
in order to ensure its continuing availability

OXFORD
UNIVERSITY PRESS

Great Clarendon Street, Oxford OX2 6DP

Oxford University Press is a department of the University of Oxford.
It furthers the University's objective of excellence in research, scholarship,
and education by publishing worldwide in

Oxford New York

Auckland Cape Town Dar es Salaam Hong Kong Karachi
Kuala Lumpur Madrid Melbourne Mexico City Nairobi
New Delhi Shanghai Taipei Toronto
With offices in
Argentina Austria Brazil Chile Czech Republic France Greece
Guatemala Hungary Italy Japan South Korea Poland Portugal
Singapore Switzerland Thailand Turkey Ukraine Vietnam

Oxford is a registered trade mark of Oxford University Press
in the UK and in certain other countries

Published in the United States
by Oxford University Press Inc., New York

© The World Bank, 2000

ISBN 978-0-19-263246-3

Contents

Section I Tobacco use and its consequences

Section II Analytics of tobacco use

Section III Demand for tobacco

Section IV Supply of tobacco

Contents

Section V Policy directions

Contributors

Editors

Prabhat Jha

Prabhat Jha is a Senior Health Specialist at the World Bank, Washington, DC. He is currently on special assignment to the World Health Organization, where he is Senior Scientist in the Economics Advisory Service, Cluster on Evidence Information and Policy. Email: Pjha@worldbank.org or Jhap@who.ch

Frank J. Chaloupka

Frank J. Chaloupka is Professor of Economics, University of Illinois at Chicago (UIC) and Research Associate, Health Economics Program, National Bureau of Economic Research. Professor Chaloupka is also Director of ImpacTeen: a Policy Research Partnership to Reduce Youth Substance Abuse, UIC Health Research and Policy Centers. Email: Fjc@uic.edu

Authors

Samira Asma: *Senior Service Fellow/Visiting Scientist, Office on Smoking and Health, Centers for Disease Control and Prevention, Atlanta, Georgia, United States. Email: Sea5@cdc.gov*

Martin Bobak: *Senior Lecturer, Department of Epidemiology and Public Health, University College, London, London, United Kingdom. Email: Martinb@public-health.ucl.ac.uk*

Phyllida Brown: *Scientific Editor, London, United Kingdom. Email: Pbrown@brixworks.freeserve.co.uk*

Thomas C. Capehart: *Economist, Economic Research Service, United States Department of Agriculture, Washington, DC, United States. Email: Thomasc@econ.ag.gov*

Likwang Chen: *Assistant Investigator, Division of Health Policy Research, National Health Research Institutes, Taipei, Taiwan. Email: Likwang@nhri.org.tw*

Jillian Clare Cohen: *World Bank-PAHO Pharmaceuticals Liaison Officer, The World Bank, Washington, DC, United States. Email: Jcohen@worldbank.org*

David Collins: *Adjunct Professor of Economics, Division of Economic and Financial Studies, Macquarie University, Sydney, Australia. Email: Dcollins@efs.mq.edu.au*

Michaelyn Corbett: *Ph.D. candidate, Department of Economics, University of Illinois-Chicago, Chicago, Illinois, United States. Email: Mcorbe1@uic.edu*

Joy de Beyer: *Economist, Health, Nutrition, and Population, The World Bank, Washington, DC, United States. Email: Jdebeyer@worldbank.org*

C. K. Gajalakshmi: *Head, Division of Epidemiology and Cancer Registry, Cancer Institute, Tamil Nadu, India. Email: Gaja_1@hotmail.com*

H. Frederick Gale: *Economist, Economic Research Service, United States Department of Agriculture, Washington, DC, United States. Email: Fgale@econ.ag.gov*

Michael Grossman: *Director, Health Economics Research Program, National Bureau of Economic Research, New York, New York, United States. Email: mgrossman@gc.cuny.edu*

Emmanuel Guindon: *Economist, Tobacco Free Initiative, World Health Organization, Geneva, Switzerland. Email: Guindone@who.ch*

Teh-Wei Hu: *Professor of Economics, Department of Health Economics, University of California-Berkeley, Berkeley, California, United States. Email: Thu@uclink2.berkeley.edu*

Rowena Jacobs: *Research Fellow, Centre for Health Economics, University of York, Heslington, York, United Kingdom. Email: Rj3@york.ac.uk*

Martin Jarvis: *Professor of Epidemiology, Department of Epidemiology and Public Health, University College, London, London, United Kingdom. Email: Martin.jarvis@ucl.ac.uk*

Luk Joossens: *Consultant, International Union Against Cancer, Brussels, Belgium. Email: Joossens@globalink.org*

Donald Kenkel: *Associate Professor, Department of Policy Analysis and Management, Cornell University, Ithaca, New York, United States. Email: Dsk10@cornell.edu*

Helen Lapsley: *Senior Lecturer, School of Health Service Management, University of New South Wales, Sydney, Australia. Email: H.Lapsley@unsw.edu.au*

James Lightwood: *Assistant Adjunct Professor of Economics, Department of Clinical Pharmacy, School of Pharmacy, University of California San Francisco, San Francisco, California, United States. Email: Lightwo@itsa.ucsf.edu*

David Merriman: *Associate Professor of Economics, Department of Economics, Loyola University, Chicago, Chicago, Illinois, United States. Email: Dmerrim@luc.edu*

Philip Musgrove: *Principal Economist, Health, Nutrition and Population, The World Bank, Washington, DC, United States. Email: Pmusgrove@worldbank.org*

Son Nguyen: *Young Professional, The World Bank, Washington DC, United States. Email: Snguyen@worldbank.org*

Thomas E. Novotny: *Deputy Assistant Secretary for International and Refugee Health, United States Department of Health and Human Services, Rockville, Maryland, United States. Email: Tnovotny@osophs.dhhs.gov*

Fred Paccaud: *Professor, Institute of Social and Preventive Medicine, School of Medicine, University of Lausanne, Lausanne, Switzerland. Email: Fred.Paccaud@inst.hospvd.ch*

Richard Peck: *Associate Professor of Economics, Department of Economics, University of Illinois-Chicago, Chicago, Illinois, United States. Email: Rmpeck@uic.edu*

Kent Ranson: *Ph.D. Candidate, Health Policy Unit, London School of Hygiene and Tropical Medicine, London, United Kingdom. Email: K.ranson@lshtm.ac.uk*

Henry Saffer: *Research Associate, National Bureau of Economic Research, New York, New York, United States. Email: Hsaffer@gc.cuny.edu*

Donald Sharp: *Senior Medical Officer, Office on Smoking and Health, Atlanta, Georgia, United States. Email: Das8@cdc.gov*

Emil M. Sunley: *Assistant Director, Fiscal Affairs Department, International Monetary Fund, Washington, DC, United States. Email: Esunley@imf.org*

David Sweanor: *Senior Legal Counsel, Non-Smokers' Rights Association, Ottawa, Ontario, Canada. Email: Dsweanor@nsra-adnf.ca*

John A. Tauras: *Post-Doctoral Research Fellow, Department of Health Management and Policy, University of Michigan, Ann Arbor, Michigan, United States. Email: tauras@sph.umich.edu*

Allyn Taylor: *Advisor, Tobacco Free Initiative, World Health Organization, Geneva, Switzerland; Adjunct Professor, Johns Hopkins School of Hygiene and Public Health, Baltimore, Maryland, United States. Email: altaylor@jhsph.edu*

Kenneth E. Warner: *Professor of Economics, Director of University of Michigan Tobacco Research Network, Department of Health Management and Policy, School of Public Health, University of Michigan, Ann Arbor, Michigan, United States. Email: Kwarner@umich.edu*

Trevor Woollery: *Economist, Office on Smoking and Health, Centers for Disease Control and Prevention, Atlanta, Georgia, United States. Email: Tgw2@cdc.gov*

Ayda Yurekli: *Economist, Health, Nutrition and Population, The World Bank, Washington, DC, United States. Email: Ayurekli@worldbank.org*

Ping Zhang: *Assistant Professor of Economics, Department of Agricultural Economics, Kansas State University, Manhattan, Kansas, United States. Email: Pzhang@loki.agecon.ksu.edu*

Foreword

Tobacco is rapidly becoming one of the single biggest causes of death worldwide, and by 2030 it is expected kill about 10 million people per year. Until recently, this epidemic of chronic disease and premature death mainly affected rich countries. But by 2030, some 70% of tobacco deaths will be in low-income and middle-income countries. And in rich countries, smoking is increasingly concentrated among the poor, and is responsible for much of their ill health and premature mortality.

For both the World Health Organization (WHO) and the World Bank, increased action to reduce this burden is a priority, as part of their missions to improve health and reduce poverty. Such action must clearly take place within countries, involving governments and civil society. As knowledge-based institutions, the World Bank and the WHO can enable action at local levels by providing sound evidence for policy-makers. This book is the result of a partnership between the two organizations.

Tobacco is different from many other health challenges. Cigarettes are demanded by consumers and form part of the social custom of many societies. Cigarettes are extensively traded and profitable commodities, whose production and consumption are part of the economies of developed and developing countries alike. The economic aspects of tobacco use are, therefore, critical to the debate on its control. However, until recently, these economic aspects have received little global attention.

This book is intended primarily to fill that gap. It covers key, and often complex, economic issues that most societies and policy-makers face when they think about tobacco or its control.

The world saw unprecedented health gains in the twentieth century. As we enter the twenty-first, both our organizations are committed to helping governments to sustain these gains and to extend good health to the poorest of the world. It is our hope that the impressive evidence base presented in this book will enable early action with control policies that are simple, cost-effective, and available now. Without such action, the world can expect about 1 billion people to be killed by tobacco in the twenty-first century.

James D. Wolfensohn, President, the World Bank
Gro Harlem Brundtland, Director General, World Health Organization
May 2000

James D. Wolfensohn	Gro Harlem Brundtland
President	Director General
The World Bank	World Health Organization

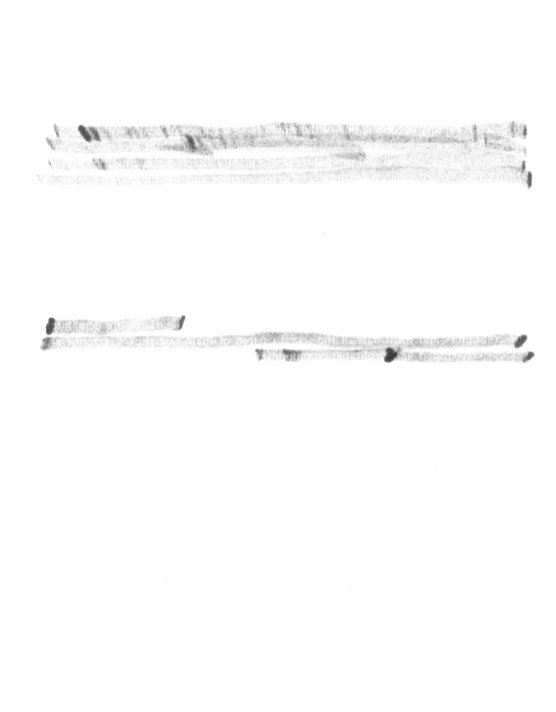

Preface

More than 40 years' worth of epidemiological studies in high-income countries, and a growing number in developing countries, have removed any doubt that smoking is damaging global health on an unprecedented scale.

In contrast, there is continuing debate on the economics of tobacco control, including the costs and consequences of tobacco-control policies. In the 1950s, the British Chancellor of the Exchequer (Pollock 1996) warned of:

... the enormous contribution to the Exchequer from tobacco duties and the serious effect on the Commonwealth.... that a campaign against smoking would have.

Forty years later, an Asian health minister made similar claims (*Australian Financial Review* 1996) in stating that:

... cigarette producers are making large contributions to our economy.... We have to think about workers and tobacco farmers.

This volume aims to fill the analytic gap around the economics of tobacco control. Its aim is to address key questions such as: What is the economic nature of addiction? What is the rationale for governments to intervene in the tobacco market? Which interventions are effective and which are not? Does tobacco control harm the economy? What are the costs and cost-effectiveness of tobacco-control policies? The book is primarily intended for technical staff within governments and international agencies, and academic economists and epidemiologists.

We made a deliberate decision to recruit as many economists working on tobacco as possible for this volume. At the outset we sought to ensure that analyses were robust and critical. The volume builds on earlier analytic work, including an international conference on the economics of tobacco control held in Cape Town, South Africa in February 1998. The proceedings of this conference, the first of its kind, have been published elsewhere (Abedian *et al.* 1998).

To help meet the needs of our audience, we have aimed to provide a high level of critical peer review. There have been four types of review. First, a panel of external, anonymous, peers reviewed nearly every chapter at least twice. Second, authors, selected experts and potential users reviewed each chapter at Technical Review Meetings in November 1998 in Lausanne, Switzerland and in June 1999 in Antalya, Turkey. Third, a panel convened by the US Centers for Disease Control and Prevention provided anonymous reviews of most chapters prior to the Lausanne meeting. Finally, the key messages from most chapters were reviewed in the World Bank on three occasions. Earlier drafts of the papers in this volume formed the basis for a World Bank summary report (Jha and Chaloupka 1999). This report aims mainly to meet the needs of policy makers. The Bank report has been disseminated widely, and has been translated into about a dozen languages.[1]

The evidence base on the economics of tobacco control is nascent. Yet, even at this early stage, economics provides a powerful tool for tobacco control. We hope that this volume will help to increase the numbers of countries who apply economics to tobacco control, to improve the quality of the economic analyses in all countries, and to spur further research. It is our firm belief that on-going analytic work is the basis for public health action worldwide.

PJ

FJC

April 2000

References

Abedian, I., van der Merwe, R., Wilkins, N., and Jha, P. (1998). *The Economics of Tobacco Control: Towards an Optimal Policy Mix*. University of Cape Town, South Africa.

Australian Financial Review June 3, 1996, cited in Anon. (1997). Play it again. *Tobacco Control* 6, 56–58.

Pollock, D. (1996). Forty years on: a war to recognise and win. How the tobacco industry has survived the revelations on smoking and health. *British Medical Bulletin*, **52**, 174–82.

Jha P. and Chaloupka, F. J. (1999). *Curbing the Epidemic: Governments and the Economics of Tobacco Control:* Development in Practice, World Bank, Washington DC.

[1] This volume does not represent official views of the World Bank or the World Health Organization. Authors of individual chapters take responsibility for factual content.

Acknowledgments

This volume benefited greatly from many collaborators and supporters. We are grateful to Phyllida Brown, in particular, for her editing of this volume, and also for the drafting of the World Bank summary report. The wide impact of that report owes much to the clarity of Phyllida's writing. Her patience, high-standards, and dedication were crucial to both the report and this volume. We also wish to thank Son Nguyen for his perseverance, dedication, and energy, which enabled this volume to come into reality.

We thank Christopher Lovelace, Helen Saxenian, Ayda Yurekli and Joy de Beyer, at the World Bank for enabling the happy marriage of this volume with the World Bank report. We also wish to thank Dean Jamison, Derek Yach, and Jonas Store at the World Health Organization for their encouragement in completing this collaborative volume. We are indebted to the considerable number of reviewers who read and re-read drafts and provided invaluable comments, criticisms, and suggestions. We appreciate Fred Paccaud at the University of Lausanne for his assistance and for so capably organizing and co-chairing the Technical Review Meetings. We are grateful to Michael Eriksen at the US Centers for Disease Control and Prevention for his tireless support of the volume, including organizing anonymous reviews of the chapters. Helen Liepman's support from Oxford University Press was extremely helpful throughout. At the risk of excluding others who made substantial contributions, we wish to acknowledge major contributions from Iraj Abedian, Gunal Akbay, Howard Barnum, Richard Feachem, Peter Heller, Paul Isenman, Maureen Law, Judith Mackay, Thomas Novotny, Richard Peto, and Kenneth Warner.

Support for this volume came from the Human Development Network of the World Bank, the Economics Advisory Service of the World Health Organization, the Institute for Social and Preventive Medicine, University of Lausanne, and the Office on Smoking and Health at the US Centers for Disease Control and Prevention. Their assistance is warmly acknowledged.

Finally, we thank our spouses, Varsha Malhotra and Eshell Chaloupka. For their patient support and understanding, as we (but perhaps more they) endured long hours, we are forever grateful.

1
Overview

Prabhat Jha, Frank J. Chaloupka, and Phyllida Brown

This book brings together a set of critical reviews of the current status of knowledge on tobacco control. It is intended to provide a sound and comprehensive evidence-base for the design of effective tobacco control policies in any country, with an emphasis on the needs of the low-income and middle-income countries where most smokers live.

The book at a glance

The structure of the book is as follows. Following the Overview, there are six sections. Section I provides brief descriptive overviews of global trends in smoking and the impact of tobacco on health, as well as a discussion of the costs of tobacco use. Section II provides an economic analysis of tobacco use, focusing on three key issues: tobacco addiction, the costs and benefits of tobacco use, and the economic rationale for government intervention in the tobacco market. Section III reviews the effectiveness of policies intended to reduce *demand* for tobacco: the provision of consumer information about tobacco; the impact of advertising and promotion; the taxation of tobacco products; clean indoor-air policies and other regulatory measures; and smoking cessation therapies. Section IV examines issues affecting the *supply* of tobacco, including a review of the impact of tobacco-control policies on national economies and employment. Section V addresses questions about the design of effective policies, and models the impact of various different control measures on tobacco-related mortality. In this section, there is also a discussion of strategic priorities for international organizations in responding to the global tobacco epidemic. Finally, there are statistical appendices and directions to electronic sources of data on tobacco.

Summaries of the chapters

Section I Tobacco use and its consequences

Chapter 2 Global patterns of smoking and smoking-attributable mortality

Gajalakshmi *et al.* review global data on the prevalence of smoking, trends in tobacco consumption, and smoking-related deaths. They find that eight out of ten smokers now live in developing countries, and that, while the prevalence of smoking has fallen overall in the past two decades in the high-income countries, it has been rising in most low-income and middle-income countries. Most smokers start early in life and the number of young people who take up regular smoking is estimated to be about 100 000 per day. The addictive nature of nicotine is discussed. Data from the high-income countries, where the tobacco epidemic is well established, suggest that about half of long-term regular smokers are killed by tobacco, and of these, about half die in middle age. Currently, worldwide, about 4 million people die of tobacco-related disease every year. This figure is expected to rise to 10 million by 2030, with seven out of ten deaths being in developing countries. Estimates from the high-income countries indicate that, worldwide, the number of people killed by tobacco through the whole of the twentieth century was about 0.1 billion; for the twenty-first century, the cumulative number could be 1 billion if current smoking patterns continue. Many of the deaths expected in coming decades could be averted if people alive today quit smoking, but in low-income and middle-income countries, quitters are rare.

Chapter 3 Poverty and smoking

Bobak *et al.* examine the available data on the prevalence of smoking in different socio-economic groups, and on socio-economic differences in tobacco-related mortality. They find that, in almost all countries studied, smoking is more common among men of low socio-economic status. For women, who have been smoking in large numbers for a shorter period, the relationship between smoking and socio-economic status is more variable. Where mortality data can be reliably measured, in the high-income countries and the former socialist countries of Europe, it appears that much of the excess mortality of poor and less-educated men can be attributed to smoking.

Chapter 4 Estimating the costs of tobacco use

Lightwood *et al.* review studies that attempt to estimate the costs of tobacco use, focusing on the costs for health systems. Since the methods for these estimates are complex and subject to debate, the authors first review the various methods and their strengths and weaknesses. They show that estimates of the *gross* costs of healthcare related to tobacco use—that is, all care costs in any given year that can be attributed to the extra health needs of smokers—range from 0.1 to 1.1% of gross domestic product in the high-income countries. In low-income countries, there are fewer studies, but those that exist indicate that the gross healthcare costs may be proportionately as high as in high-income countries. Studies of the *net* healthcare costs, which are usually assessed over a lifetime and take account of the fact that smokers' lives tend to be shorter than non-smokers', reach more heterogeneous conclusions because of the different approaches they take. However, the studies that the authors consider to be most robust do conclude that there are net healthcare costs from smoking.

Section II Analytics of tobacco use

Chapter 5 The economics of addiction

Chaloupka *et al.* review economic approaches to addiction and consumer choice, including a discussion of recent work on new economic models of addiction. Having summarized existing knowledge on the addictive potential of tobacco, the authors discuss economic models of addictive behavior. In the past, economists largely ignored addiction, viewing it as an irrational behavior for which basic economic principles did not apply. Only in recent years have there been attempts to model addiction. Economic models hypothesize that, for addictive behavior, past consumption choices determine current consumption choices because, by definition, a consumer who is addicted to something must have consumed it in the past and will need to maintain, or increase, past consumption levels to service the addiction. This hypothesis is supported by the findings of empirical research. However, empirical applications of the models clearly indicate that increases in cigarette prices and other costs of smoking will reduce cigarette consumption, with the effects of price increases being greater in the long-run than in the short-run. Recent extensions to these models emphasize particular aspects of addictive behavior, including the youth of most 'beginner' smokers and the inadequate level of consumer information available to them. These newer models also discuss the adjustment costs of quitting for adult smokers. Most of these newer models have yet to be tested empirically.

Chapter 6 *A welfare analysis of tobacco use*

Peck *et al.* provide a novel approach to assessing the costs and benefits of tobacco use. First, the authors estimate the benefits of smoking to smokers and producers, using the relationship of price and expenditure to the demand and supply curve, respectively. Estimating costs is more difficult, as the authors discuss. Traditional cost–benefit analysis assumes that smokers take into account the costs to themselves when they buy cigarettes, and that these costs should therefore be excluded from the analysis. However, the authors argue that smokers may not be aware of some of the costs of their choice for themselves, such as health damage. Most smokers start young and quickly become addicted, and, in high-income countries where health information is widely available, most adult smokers say that they regret starting. Existing research suggests that people are willing to pay to avoid the costs of lost health and life. In the context of tobacco, the authors argue that uninformed smokers would be willing to pay to avoid premature death or disability, or to avoid the costs of trying to quit. Using a conservative value of the willingness to pay to avoid such costs, the authors then calculate what percentage of the smoking population would have to be unaware of the health risks of smoking for the net benefits from smoking to be zero. Their calculations indicate that if up to 23% of smokers underestimate the health costs of tobacco, then the net benefits of smoking are zero. While higher prices would cause smokers a loss of satisfaction from having to reduce their consumption or quit, the extra health gains from a price increase of 10% globally would outweigh the losses if as few as 3% of smokers are uninformed.

Chapter 7 *The economic rationale for intervention in the tobacco market*

Economic theory suggests that, if consumers know all the risks and bear all the costs of their choices, there is no justification, on efficiency grounds, for governments to intervene in a market. Jha *et al.* discuss three key inefficiencies in the tobacco market, or market failures: inadequate information about the health risks of tobacco; inadequate information about the risks of addicton; and physical or financial costs imposed on non-smokers. They conclude that there are clear economic grounds for intervening, particularly to protect young people and non-smokers. The authors identify the ideal responses to these failures and the most effective responses, pointing out that these are not always the same. They conclude that taxation is the most effective measure for correcting several of these market failures, although taxation imposes costs on all smokers. The authors also discuss government intervention on the grounds of reducing inequality between poor and non-poor groups.

Section III Demand for tobacco

Chapter 8 Consumer information and tobacco use

Kenkel and Chen address two questions: first, whether consumers are well informed about the consequences of smoking; and second, whether public policies to improve consumer information about smoking can reduce tobacco consumption. The review finds that there is widespread general awareness of the risks of smoking in high-income countries. However, in low-income and middle-income countries this general awareness of the risks may be more limited. Moreover, even among people who are generally aware of the health risks of tobacco, many underestimate these risks relative to other health risks, and many fail to apply the knowledge to themselves personally. Young people, it appears, underestimate the addictive potential of cigarettes. In some countries, improvements in the quality and extent of information to consumers are still possible; in others, most of the potential improvements in consumer awareness have probably already been achieved. Reviews of the impact of specific types of information (such as 'information shocks'—the publication of new evidence on the health consequences of smoking—and warnings on cigarette packs) indicate that these can effectively reduce the prevalence of smoking in a population. The evidence suggests that government policies to increase consumer information about the health consequences of smoking can form part of an effective tobacco-control program.

Chapter 9 Tobacco advertising and promotion

Although public health advocates argue that tobacco advertising affects the number of people who smoke and the amount of tobacco they consume, the existing empirical literature concludes that advertising has little or no such impact. Here, Saffer examines the empirical studies more closely, and offers important insight into their limitations. The chapter discusses an alternative approach, based on studying the effects of bans on advertising and promotion. The primary conclusion is that comprehensive bans on tobacco advertising and promotion do reduce cigarette consumption, whereas partial bans have little or no effect. Counter-advertising, the provision of health information about smoking, is also found to be effective.

Chapter 10 The taxation of tobacco products

Chaloupka *et al.* review a significant body of research from high-income countries on the impact of tax increases on cigarette consumption. The studies consistently show that higher tobacco prices significantly reduce tobacco use. The majority conclude that an increase in price of 10% would reduce demand by about 4% in these countries. A small but growing body of research indicates that smokers in low-income and middle-income countries are more responsive to price changes than those in high-income countries. Most estimates suggest that a price increase of 10% in these countries would reduce demand by about 8%. In most studies, about half of the reduced demand takes the form of quitting, and about half takes the form of reduced consumption. The evidence indicates that young people are more responsive to price changes than adults. Further studies indicate that people on low incomes and people with lower levels of education are also more responsive to price changes than wealthier, highly-educated people. Because of the addictive nature of tobacco use, the authors find, the impact of price rises on tobacco consumption will be greater in the long-run than in the short-run. The authors discuss the various reasons that governments might choose to increase tobacco taxes, including the generation of revenue, the desire to correct economic inefficiencies, or the desire to improve public health.

Chapter 11 Clean indoor-air laws and youth access restrictions

In this short chapter Woollery *et al.* review the evidence, mainly from the United States, of the impact of policies designed to prevent smoking in public places, work-places, and other facilities. The authors also assess the evidence on the effectiveness of policies to restrict young people's access to purchasing cigarettes. They find that comprehensive clean-air laws can reduce cigarette consumption, but that such policies work best when there is a strong social consensus against smoking in public places and therefore self-enforcement of the restrictions. Clean-air laws do impose costs on smokers who want to continue to smoke, but claims that they reduce revenues for business, tourism, and the leisure sector are not supported by data. The evidence for the effectiveness of youth access restrictions is more mixed. Some show a promising effect, while others show little or no effect. The importance of enforcing such restrictions is discussed.

Chapter 12 Smoking cessation and nicotine-replacement therapies

In this chapter, Novotny *et al.* briefly review the evidence for the effectiveness of cessation programs and, in particular, of nicotine-replacement therapies (NRTs) of various types. They find that NRTs and other pharmacological quitting aides can approximately double the chances that an individual will succeed in quitting compared with unaided attempts. The authors compare the small and highly regulated market for NRTs with the large and unregulated market for cigarettes, against which NRTs compete. The NRT market is limited by several factors including, at present, high costs in some areas, a relatively low global demand for quitting, and complex regulatory issues. Where there have been studies, these have found that NRTs can be a cost-effective component of tobacco-control programs. The policy implications for governments, such as options for deregulating the NRT market, or financing NRTs for poorer smokers, are discussed.

Section IV Supply of tobacco

Chapter 13 *The supply-side effects of tobacco-control policies*

Jacobs *et al.* describe the size and nature of the tobacco industry, both farming and manufacturing. They then examine the impact of tobacco control measures on countries' economies, in particular on employment. They find that, if tobacco consumption were to fall because of control policies, the impact on total employment would be minimal or zero in most countries, since the money consumers once spent on tobacco would be spent instead on other goods and services, hence generating jobs. For a small number of tobacco-producing countries that are heavily dependent on this crop, however, there would be net job losses. Reductions in jobs and other adjustments in the economy that result from demand-side measures would be spread over decades or longer. The authors also discuss the effects on cigarette consumption of supply-side policies, such as price supports and quotas, that provide incentives to grow tobacco. They conclude that the net impact of these policies on retail price, and hence on consumption, is small. Attempts to reduce tobacco consumption by reducing the tobacco supply are unlikely to succeed. Given high demand and the presence of alternative suppliers, policies such as crop diversification or buy-outs are largely ineffective. However, diversification, placed within broader rural development programs, can help meet the transition costs of the poorest farmers.

Chapter 14 *The impact of trade liberalization on tobacco consumption*

Recent trends in global trade, and their impact on tobacco markets and tobacco consumption, are discussed by Taylor *et al.* The authors find that a variety of trade agreements in recent years have significantly reduced the barriers to trade in tobacco products. Economic theory suggests that the reductions in these barriers will increase competition within tobacco markets, reduce prices, and increase marketing efforts, as well as raise incomes. As a result, tobacco use is likely to increase, particularly in low-income and middle-income countries. The limited empirical literature confirms this hypothesis. The authors' new empirical analysis provides additional evidence that cigarette consumption is rising because of freer trade, with the biggest impact on low-income and middle-income countries. The policy implications are briefly discussed.

Chapter 15 *How big is the worldwide cigarette-smuggling problem?*

In this chapter Merriman *et al.* review the economic theory and empirical literature on cigarette smuggling and provide new estimates of the extent of this illicit trade. By examining the difference between recorded cigarette exports and imports, the authors estimate that about one-third of cigarettes are lost in transit. If these are smuggled, the implication is that about 6% of the total number of cigarettes consumed worldwide is smuggled. A second analysis uses country-level data to examine the key determinants of smuggling. The risk of smuggling is often cited as a counter-argument to the policy or raising cigarette taxes, because large tax differentials between nearby legislatures provide an obvious motive for smuggling. However, Merriman *et al.* conclude that corruption within countries is a stronger predictor of smuggling than price. The authors also analyze data from European countries to estimate the extent of bootlegging in response to inter-country price differentials. They find that bootlegged tobacco products account for about 8.5% of consumption. Based on simulations from this European analysis, the authors conclude that a unilateral tax increase by one country would lead to increased tax revenues, even after the likely impact of increasing smuggling is taken into account. Coordinated tax increases between neighboring legislatures would increase tax revenues by greater amounts. The authors conclude that the problem of smuggling should not be seen as an insurmountable obstacle to increasing taxes. Higher cigarette taxes will both reduce cigarette smoking and increase government revenues, even in the presence of smuggling.

Chapter 16 Issues in the smuggling of tobacco products

Joossens *et al.* describe the different types of legal, quasi-legal, and illegal activities that are variously described as cross-border shopping and smuggling, and discuss their determinants. The impact of tax increases on smuggling is examined in more detail, with particular reference to the experiences of Canada and Sweden, where taxes were cut because of a perceived problem with smuggling. In each case, as a result of the cut, cigarette consumption climbed and revenue fell. The authors conclude, like the authors of Chapter 15, that higher taxes do lead to reduced consumption and increased revenues. Evidence for the tobacco industry's involvement in smuggling is reviewed. The policy options for dealing with smuggling are briefly discussed.

Section V Policy directions

Chapter 17 The design, administration, and potential revenue of tobacco excises

This chapter discusses the practical and policy issues in designing tobacco excise taxes in low-income and middle-income countries. Sunley *et al.* provide estimates of the revenue-generating potential of tax increases based on existing empirical evidence on price, tax and demand elasticity for 70 countries. The authors conclude that an increase of 10% in the tax on cigarettes in each of these countries would raise government revenues by nearly 7% on average. The increase in revenues would be somewhat larger in high-income countries, where demand is more inelastic and taxes account for a larger share of pack price. However, in low-income countries, the increased revenues, though smaller, would still be considerable.

Chapter 18 The effectiveness and cost-effectiveness of price increases and other tobacco-control policies

Ranson *et al.* examine the global impact of various tobacco-control measures on cigarette consumption and tobacco-attributable deaths, for the cohort of smokers alive in 1995. Based on deliberately conservative assumptions, they find that tax increases that would raise the real price of cigarettes by about 10% worldwide could cause about 42 million smokers alive in 1995 to quit, and could prevent a minimum of 10 million premature tobacco-related deaths. A set of 'non-price' measures, including information campaigns, comprehensive bans on advertising and promotion, prominent warning labels, and clean-air restrictions, could persuade 23 million smokers alive in 1995 to quit and could avert 5 million deaths. A third measure, the widely increased use of nicotine-replacement therapies, could persuade 6 million to quit and could avert 1 million deaths. By weighing the public-sector costs of implementing these interventions against their expected health gains (measured in disability-adjusted life years), and based on various assumptions, the researchers conclude that all three types of intervention could be cost-effective compared with many other health interventions. However, given substantial variation in implementation costs and likely effectiveness in different contexts, local cost-effectiveness estimates would be useful for the design of policies.

Chapter 19 Strategic priorities in tobacco control for governments and international agencies

This final chapter discusses some of the issues facing governments and international agencies when developing policies. Jha *et al.* first review national comprehensive control programs, including their goals, targets, and instruments. They find that for short-term progress in reducing tobacco mortality, programs need to focus on preventing the uptake of smoking by children, and persuading adults to quit. Most tobacco-control programs will use a mix of price, information, and regulation interventions, although the exact mix will vary across countries. The evidence from countries where comprehensive tobacco-control programs have been evaluated suggests that they can significantly reduce cigarette consumption. To be effective, control programs need to use a broad mix of policy instruments, involving finance and commerce ministries, as well as health ministries. Given the global nature of trade, some aspects of tobacco control require international or cross-border action. The WHO's *Framework Convention on Tobacco Control* is a promising vehicle for such action. Finally, the authors argue, research on the causes and consequences of tobacco use—including the costs of smoking—is a high priority and an international public good. Most importantly, middle-income and low-income countries require detailed ongoing studies of the impact of tobacco on population health, including studies of the impact of quitting.

Appendices

The statistical appendices provide information for readers about other sources of information on the tobacco epidemic that are updated periodically. For example, we provide information on the epidemiology of tobacco-attributable diseases, the prevalence of tobacco use, taxes, prices, smuggling, agricultural and industrial issues, spending on tobacco control, and the extent of existing tobacco-control programs. The reader is referred to web sites and other sources where information can be presented in much greater detail than is possible in book form. Appendix 3 provides important information about the classification of countries by World Bank definitions of income and by World Bank regions. This information is key to an understanding of many of the tables and figures in the chapters.

Section I
Tobacco use and its consequences

2

Global patterns of smoking and smoking-attributable mortality

C. K. Gajalakshmi, Prabhat Jha, Kent Ranson, and Son Nguyen

This chapter reviews the global data on the prevalence of smoking and its incidence (or uptake), on consumption trends, and on smoking-attributable deaths. The vast majority of the world's 1.1 billion smokers in 1995 lived in low-income and middle-income countries. Cigarette consumption has risen over the past two decades in these countries, in contrast to declines in overall consumption in high-income countries. Most smokers start in youth, and there is some evidence that the average age of smoking uptake is falling. Because of the long delay between the age at which people take up smoking and their death from tobacco-related disease, current mortality patterns largely reflect past smoking patterns, and future mortality depends on current and future smoking. Currently, tobacco deaths number about 4 million per year worldwide, about one in ten of all adult deaths. For the twentieth century, the cumulative number of tobacco deaths is estimated to have been about 100 million, with about 60 million of these in the high-income countries and the former socialist countries. Projections are difficult to make with precision, but on current smoking trends it is plausible that there will be 10 million tobacco deaths per year, about one in six of all adult deaths, by 2030. About seven in ten of these deaths will be in low-income countries. The variations in the tobacco epidemic over time, sex, age group, and region, attest to the importance of conducting further reliable long-term epidemiological studies. If current patterns of smoking continue, about 0.5 billion of the world's population alive today will be killed by smoking, half of them in middle age (defined as ages 35–69). Over the twenty-first century as a whole, about 1 billion tobacco deaths are projected. Much of the projected mortality increase over the next fifty years could be avoided if adults quit smoking. However, quitting remains rare in low-income and middle-income countries.

numbers

2.1 Introduction

The use of non-manufactured tobacco is a habit of antiquity. The Chinese record that they cultivated and smoked it before the first millennium, and it can be reliably traced to at least the Middle Ages among native populations of the Americas. When Columbus landed in the New World on 11 October 1492, he was offered dried tobacco leaves at the House of the Arawaks. In the middle of the sixteenth century, tobacco was introduced into Europe and subsequently brought to Africa and Asia (Corti 1931). The use of manufactured tobacco is much more recent: the first manufactured cigarette appeared in the mid-nineteenth century. Today, cigarettes, both manufactured and various hand-rolled forms, including *bidis*—popular in India and South-east Asia—and clove cigarettes, account for about 65–85% of all tobacco produced worldwide. (WHO 1997). This review will focus on the use of manufactured cigarettes and, to a lesser extent, on the use of *bidis* (see Box 2.1). These forms of tobacco appear to pose the greatest health risks, since their combustion products are absorbed though the pulmonary and vascular systems. Manufactured cigarettes are gradually replacing other forms of tobacco.

This chapter is in six sections. First, we describe regional patterns of smoking in 1995.[1] Second, we discuss trends in cigarette consumption over recent decades. Third, we summarize the evidence on current and projected smoking-attributable mortality. The reader may find more detailed reviews elsewhere on mortality patterns and on other aspects of health and smoking, and these reviews are cited in the appropriate section of the chapter. Fourth, we describe the patterns of smoking cessation and its health consequences. Fifth, we briefly discuss research priorities for monitoring smoking and smoking-attributable disease. Finally, we summarize the key findings.

> **Box 2.1** Types of tobacco use other than manufactured cigarettes
>
> In addition to cigarettes, various other types of tobacco use are common, but their health impacts and economics are poorly studied. The *bidi* is a hand-rolled cigarette common to South-east Asia and India. A *bidi* consists of 0.2–0.3 g of sun-cured tobacco loosely packed and rolled in a rectangular piece of dried leaf and tied with cotton thread. *Bidis* may allow two or three times as many puffs as an ordinary cigarette. Because of the low porosity of their wrappers and their poor combustibility, *bidis* must be puffed continuously to be kept alight and so they probably deliver a relatively higher dose of tar to the smoker (IARC 1986).
>
> Other cigarettes include clove cigarettes, made from shredded clove buds and tobacco, which are manufactured in Indonesia, and herbal cigarettes, which consist of tobacco blended with herbs, and are common in China.
>
> The oldest recorded form of smoking is probably pipe smoking: the habit has different names in different regions. In South-east Asia, clay pipes known as *sulpa*, *chilum*, and *hookli* are used. In Asia, Egypt, and other middle-eastern countries, water-pipe smoking is common. The tobacco is covered with pieces of

[1] The World Bank regions are as defined in World Development Indicators (1999) and are reproduced in Appendix 3. High-income countries are those with a 1995 gross national product (GNP) per capita of $9386 or more. Low-income and middle-income countries (which are sometimes referred to as developing countries) have 1995 GNPs per capita of $765 or less, and $766–$9385, respectively. Low-income and middle-income countries are further divided by geographic region: East Asia and Pacific (EAP), Europe and Central Asia (ECA), Latin America and Caribbean (LAC), Middle East and North Africa (MNA), South Asia (SSA), and Sub-Saharan Africa (SSA).
Note that wherever possible we present data by World Bank region. However, some data are presented according to an earlier classification used by some sources. This classification, based on regional groupings, is as follows: China (CHN), Established Market Economies (EME), Former Socialist Economies of Europe (FSE), India (IND), Latin America and Caribbean (LAC), Middle East Crescent (MEC), Other Asia and Islands (OAI) and Sub-Saharan Africa (SSA).

glowing charcoal and kept burning on the head of the pipe, and the smoke is drawn through a long tube; smoke bubbles through water before reaching the mouth. The tobacco is cured or fermented in molasses, honey, or fruit juices. In Bangladesh in the 1970s, the majority of smokers used water pipes; today, they are more likely to smoke *bidis*.

Smokeless tobacco is most common in the United States and South Asia. In India, tobacco-chewing is picked up as a traditional habit from parents and at work. Tobacco is chewed alone or with *quid*, which consists of betel leaf, a leaf of the vine *Piper betel* (*Piperaceae*), small pieces of areca nut of the tree *Areca catechu* (*Palmaceae*), and a pinch of aqueous lime (calcium hydroxide). Throughout South-east Asia and in many North African and Eastern Mediterranean countries, tobacco is chewed with flavorings. Among other forms of smokeless tobacco, nasal snuff is a dry finely powdered tobacco that is inhaled through nostrils. Oral snuff is a moist coarsely ground tobacco that is applied to the gums.

2.2 Smoking patterns worldwide

2.2.1 Smoking prevalence

We provide estimates of the numbers of smokers, and cigarettes consumed, for each of the seven different World Bank regions. The estimates were made by following the steps described below.

Methodology

Step 1. Population by region, gender, and age category

World Bank population figures for each of the Bank's seven regions were used as defined in Appendix 3. Population figures for 1995 were used throughout the analysis. Age categories (ages 15–19, 20–29, 30–39, 40–49, 50–59, 60+) were chosen to coincide with the categories most commonly used in smoking prevalence studies.

Step 2. Smoking prevalence by region and gender

The results of 89 studies were used to estimate smoking prevalence, by gender, for each of the seven regions (see Appendix 2). Most of these studies were compiled by the World Health Organization (WHO), and were judged to be 'methodologically sound and to provide reasonably reliable and comparable results' (WHO 1997). Other studies were found from literature searches. Most countries that carried out prevalence surveys reported daily smoking and this is the basic prevalence indicator that has been used here. Country-specific data are combined to estimate regional prevalence values by weighting country estimates by the adult population (>15 years of age) of those countries. Country-specific population figures for 1995 are drawn from a World Bank database (World Bank 1999). The resulting weighted average smoking prevalences are assumed to apply to the entire region, including those countries for which smoking prevalence is not known.

Step 3. *Prevalence of cigarette versus* bidi *smoking in South Asia*

In all regions, with the exception of South Asia, cigarettes constitute the major form of smoked tobacco. In the countries of South Asia, however, many people smoke *bidis*. All calculations for South Asia are conducted separately for cigarettes and *bidis*. Data from three studies (two from India and one from Sri Lanka) suggest that 47–51% of male smokers and 52–95% of female smokers smoke *bidis* (Gupta 1996; Venkat Narayan 1996; WHO 1997, p. 427). In this analysis, it is assumed that 50% of male and 80% of female smokers smoke *bidis*, with the remainder smoking cigarettes.

Step 4. *Smoking prevalence by age category*

An attempt has been made to find one large-scale study of smoking prevalence by age category for each of the seven regions. China is used as the model country for East Asia and Pacific (Gong 1995), Hungary for Europe and Central Asia (Hungary Central Statistics Office 1994), Argentina for Latin America and the Caribbean (Pan American Health Organization 1992, p. 17), India for South Asia (Goa Cancer Society 1992), and Germany for high-income countries (MarketFile 1998). Data for Sub-Saharan Africa (SSA), the Middle East and North Africa (MNA) were particularly scarce. For SSA, the age distribution amongst 'Africans' in South Africa (i.e. excluding white, Asian, and mixed-race populations) was extrapolated to the entire region (Yach *et al.* 1992). For MNA, the age distribution amongst a group of male Egyptians was extrapolated to both males and females throughout the region (Hassan, personal communication). The age categories used in some of the primary studies do not correspond to the categories being used in this analysis (for example, the study in Argentina provided prevalence values by 10-year age categories starting 15–24, 25–34, etc.). Prevalence values are estimated for the age categories being used in this analysis based on the assumption that the prevalence of smoking is uniform within each age category used in the primary studies (for example, it was assumed that in Argentina, the prevalence of smoking amongst the 1.2 million men of ages 25–29 is the same as amongst the 1.1 million men of ages 30–34, at 57%). Ratios of smoking prevalence amongst older age categories compared to 15–19 year-olds were calculated. These ratios were applied to the entire region, including those countries for which the age ratios of smoking prevalence are not known. A simplified example is shown below.

Argentina is used as the model country for Latin America and the Caribbean. The primary study, which finds an age-weighted male prevalence of smoking of 43% (PAHO 1992) provides the following age breakdown:

Age category	Prevalence (%)	Prevalence ratio
15–19	31	1.0
20–59	49	1.6
60+	16	0.5

From the data collected in steps 1 and 2, the total number of male smokers in Latin America and the Caribbean is estimated to be 62 million (a prevalence of

40% in a population of 156 million). Given the total population for each age category, the age-specific prevalence of 15–19 year-olds for this region can be calculated as follows:

1. $Prev_{15-19} \times Pop_{15-19} + Prev_{20-59} \times Pop_{20-59} + Prev_{60+} \times Pop_{60+} = \text{total smokers.}$

2. $Prev_{15-19} \times 25\,m + Prev_{20-59} \times 114\,m + Prev_{60+} \times 17\,m = 62\,m.$

3. $Prev_{15-19} \times 25\,m + 1.6/(Prev_{15-19}) \times 114\,m + 0.5/(Prev_{15-19}) + \times 17\,m = 62\,m.$

4. $Prev_{15-19} = 62\,m/(25\,m + 1.6 \times 114\,m + 0.5 \times 17\,m).$

5. $Prev_{15-19} = 29\%.$

   Prevalence values for the other age categories are calculated by multiplying $Prev_{15-19}$ by the appropriate prevalence ratio.

Step 5. Total number of smokers by region, gender, and age

Number of smokers is calculated by multiplying 'population' by 'smoking prevalence'.

Step 6. Number of cigarettes smoked per day per smoker by region and gender

From the WHO database (WHO 1997), and published epidemiological studies, data were collected on the number of cigarettes smoked per smoker per day. For many countries, gender-specific values are not available. For these countries, it was assumed that the number is the same for male and female smokers. For many countries, more than one estimate of the number of cigarettes smoked per smoker per day was available; in these cases, the flat average of available values was used. National-level estimates are weighted by the adult population (defined as those over 15 years of age) of those countries to estimate regional values. The resulting weighted averages were then assumed to apply to the entire region, including those countries for which data are not available.

Step 7. Number of cigarettes smoked per day per smoker by age category

National data on the number of cigarettes smoked per day per smoker by age category (gender-specific) are available for a number of high-income countries (Nicolaides-Bouman *et al.* 1993); similar data for low-income countries are scarce. In this analysis, national-level data were combined by weighting national estimates by the adult population (>15 years of age) of those countries. Age-specific values were then adjusted to correspond to the age-categories being used in this analysis. Finally, the ratios of cigarettes smoked per smoker per day amongst older age categories relative to 15–19 year-olds were calculated. These ratios were applied to all regions, including those for which no data are available.

Step 8. Total number of cigarettes smoked per year by gender, age, and region

For each region, the total number of cigarettes smoked by each age and gender category was calculated by multiplying 'population' by 'smoking prevalence' by 'number of cigarettes smoked per day per smoker' by 365.25 (assuming that a year has 365 whole days and one quarter day).

Results

Our estimates reveal variations in smoking prevalence across regions, gender and age, and variations in smoking amount. First, globally in 1995, 29% of the population aged 15 years and over smoked daily (Table 2.1). Low-income and middle-income countries, whose populations account for four-fifths of the global adult population, accounted for

Table 2.1 Prevalence of smoking among adults aged 15 and over, by World Bank region, 1995

World Bank region	Smoking prevalence (%)			Total smokers	
	Males	Females	Overall	(millions)	(% of all smokers)
East Asia and Pacific	61	4	33	413	36
Europe and Central Asia	57	26	40	145	13
Latin America and Caribbean	40	21	30	95	8
Middle East and North Africa	44	5	25	40	3
South Asia (cigarettes)	21	1	11	88	8
South Asia (*bidis*)	21	4	13	99	9
Sub-Saharan Africa	29	9	18	59	5
Low-income & Middle-income	49	9	29	939	82
High-income	38	21	29	205	18
World	47	11	29	1143	100

Source: authors' calculations.

Table 2.2 Global prevalence of smoking, by age, 1995

Age categories	Males		Females		Total		
	Prevalence (%)	Number of smokers (millions)	Prevalence (%)	Number of smokers (millions)	Prevalence (%)	Number of smokers (millions)	% Total
15–19	33	86	5	12	19	98	9
20–29	42	213	11	54	27	267	23
30–39	57	235	15	58	36	293	26
40–49	58	182	14	44	37	225	20
50–59	51	108	11	23	31	131	11
60+	41	101	9	28	24	129	11
TOTAL	47	925	11	218	29	1143	100
% of total		81		19		100	

Source: authors' calculations.

82% of the world's smokers. East Asia and the Pacific, which includes China, accounted for 36% (413 million) of all smokers, but only 32% of the population aged 15 years and over. Overall, smoking prevalence was highest in Europe and Central Asia at 40%, and lowest in Sub-Saharan Africa at 18%.

For both males and females, there was wide variation in smoking prevalence between regions. The prevalence of smoking amongst males was highest in East Asia and the Pacific, and in Europe and Central Asia, at about 60% in each case, and lowest in Sub-Saharan Africa at 29%. Among females, the prevalence of smoking was highest in Europe and Central Asia at 26% and lowest in South Asia at 5% (for cigarettes and *bidis* combined) and Middle East and North Africa at 6%.

Second, the prevalence of daily smoking was higher overall for men (47%) than for women (11%). WHO data at country level suggest that the proportion of men who smoke is well above 50% in many low-income and middle-income countries: 82% in Indonesia, 78% in the Philippines, 75% in Cuba, 72% in Colombia, 70% in Bangladesh, 68% in Romania and Poland, and 62% in China (WHO 1997). Globally, males account for four in five of all smokers (Table 2.2).

Third, the prevalence of smoking is highest for people aged 30–49 years (36–37%, Table 2.2). The prevalence of daily smoking is lowest amongst youth aged 15–19 years (19%), and is also relatively low among people aged 60 and older (24%). These trends in age-specific smoking prevalence are similar for both males and females.

2.2.2 Cigarette and *bidi* consumption levels

On average, the world's smokers consume 14 cigarettes (or *bidis*) each per day (Fig. 2.1). Daily consumption per smoker is highest in high-income countries, where both males and females smoke on average 20 cigarettes a day, and lowest in Latin America and the Caribbean.

Almost 6 trillion units (cigarettes and *bidis*) were smoked in 1995. Three-quarters of these were consumed in low-income countries, with one-third consumed in East Asia and the Pacific alone (Table 2.3).

The limitations of these estimates are obvious. First, definitions of current smoking vary across the 89 studies on which we based our estimates. Second, we assumed that the smoking pattern for a country did not change between the year of the survey and 1995. Thus recent increases in smoking may not be captured in our estimates. Recent decreases are unlikely, given that rates of quitting are low in developing countries. Third, while the overall smoking prevalence data are likely to be plausible, given that they are derived from direct studies in various countries, our indirect estimates of age- and gender-specific patterns are less likely to be robust. Finally, there is great variation in smoking prevalence even within countries. For example, the prevalence among males in cities usually exceeds that of rural males (WHO 1997). Despite these limitations, the prevalence estimates are internally consistent because the totals do not exceed total global smoking prevalence. These estimates are also consistent with other reports of smoking prevalence (WHO 1997), manufacturing reports (Marketfile 1998), and agricultural, import, and export data (USDA 1998).

Some points are noteworthy. Low-income and middle-income countries have a similar aggregate smoking prevalence to that of high-income countries; they account

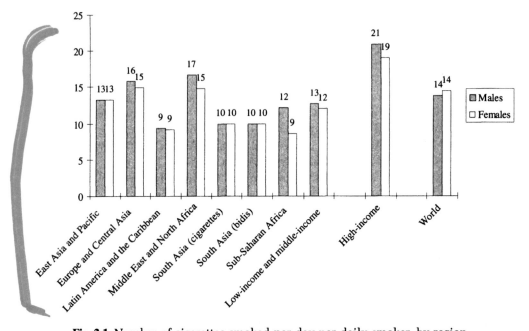

Fig. 2.1 Number of cigarettes smoked per day per daily smoker, by region.

Table 2.3 Estimated number of cigarettes and *bidis* smoked per year, by World Bank region, 1995

World Bank Region	Number (billions)	% Total
East Asia and Pacific	2003	34
Europe and Central Asia	822	14
Latin America and Caribbean	325	6
Middle East and North Africa	242	4
South Asia (cigarettes)	323	6
South Asia (*bidis*)	361	6
Sub-Saharan Africa	244	4
Low-income & middle-income	4319	74
High-income	1508	26
World	5827	100

Source: authors' calculations.

for the majority (82%) of the world's smokers; and they consume three-quarters of the cigarettes and *bidis* smoked worldwide. Males in low-income countries have a higher prevalence of daily smoking (49%) than do males in high-income countries (38%), while the reverse is true for females (9% in low-income countries and 21% in high-income countries).

2.2.3 Smoking incidence

The majority of epidemiological studies suggest that individuals who avoid starting to smoke in adolescence or young adulthood are unlikely ever to become smokers. Nowadays, most smokers start before age 25, often in childhood or adolescence (see Fig. 2.2). In the high-income countries, eight out of ten begin in their teens. In middle-income and low-income countries, for which data are available, it appears that most smokers start by their early twenties, but the trend is towards younger ages. For example, in China between 1984 and 1996, there was a significant increase in the number of young men aged between 15 and 19 years who took up smoking. This resulted in the average age of initiation dropping from 23 in 1984 to 20 by 1996 (Chinese Academy of Preventive Medicine 1997). A similar decline in the average age of starting has been observed over this century in the United States (USDHHS 1989; and Fig. 2.2).

In order to obtain a broad estimate of the number of young people who take up smoking every day worldwide, the following method was used. We used:

(1) World Bank data on the number of young people, male and female, who reached age 20 in 1995, for each World Bank region; and
(2) the above prevalence estimates based on WHO data to estimate the number of smokers in all age groups up to age30 in each of these regions.

For an upper estimate, we assumed that the number of young people who take up smoking every day is a product of (1) multiplied by (2) per region, for each gender.

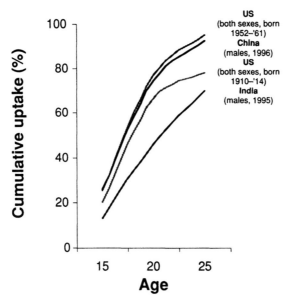

Fig. 2.2 Smoking initiation age in China, India and the United States. Source: Gupta 1996; USDHHS 1989 and 1994; Chinese Academy of Preventive Medicine 1997.

Table 2.4 Estimated number of 20-year-olds who become long-term smokers each day, by World Bank Region, 1995

	Number per day (in thousands)	
	Lower estimate	Upper estimate
East Asia Pacific	29	31
Eastern Europe and Central Asia	9	12
Latin America	9	11
Middle East and North Africa	4	6
South Asia	11	17
Sub-Saharan Africa	7	8
Low-income & middle-income	68	84
High-income	13	14
World total	81	98

Source: authors' calculations.

For a lower estimate, we reduced the prevalence value used by region-specific estimates for the proportion of smokers who start after the age of 30. We added three conservative assumptions. First, that there have been minimal changes over time in the average age of uptake. In fact, as we have shown, there have been recent downward trends in the age of uptake in young Chinese men, but our assumption of little change means that, if anything, our figures are underestimates. Second, we focused on regular smokers, excluding the much larger number of children who would try smoking but not become regular smokers. Third, we assumed that, among more established adolescent smokers, quitting before adulthood is rare. In high-income countries, quitting is common, but in low-income and middle-income countries it is currently very rare.

With these assumptions, we calculated that the number of children and young people taking up smoking ranges from 13 000 to 14 000 per day in the high-income countries as a whole. For middle-income and low-income countries, the estimated numbers range from 68 000 to 84 000 (Table 2.4). This means that every day worldwide there are between 81 000 and 98 000 young people becoming long-term smokers. These figures are consistent with existing estimates for individual high-income countries, such as for the United States (Pierce *et al.* 1989).

2.2.4 Past trends in smoking patterns

Smoking patterns vary over time according to income level, population size, age, gender, and the presence of control policies. In this section, we briefly review trends in consumption over the past few decades and attempt to project patterns for the next few decades. Detailed age- and sex-specific trends data are not available. Thus we concentrate on aggregate smoking trends at the level of countries.

From about 1970 to the mid-1990s, annual world cigarette and *bidi* consumption increased from about 3 trillion to 6 trillion sticks However, consumption per capita has remained flat since about 1970, stabilizing at about 1650 cigarettes per adult annually from 1980–82 to 1990–92 (Fig. 2.3). This is because developed countries are consuming less, and developing countries are consuming more.

Tobacco consumption fell over the past 20 years in most high-income countries, such as Australia, Britain, Canada, New Zealand, the United States, and most northern European countries. Consumption among men peaked around 1970 in many countries but patterns among women are more uncertain. In the United States, about 55% of males smoked at the peak of consumption in the 1950s, but the proportion had fallen to 28% by the mid-1990s. However, among certain groups, such as teenagers and young women, the proportion of those who smoke increased in the 1990s.

In contrast to overall declines in the high-income countries, tobacco consumption increased in middle-income and low-income countries by about 3.4% per annum between 1970 and 1990 (Fig. 2.3 and Table 2.5).

Overall, the ratio of average cigarette consumption per adult between developed and developing countries has narrowed from 3.3 in the early 1970s to 1.8 in the early 1990s. According to WHO data for 111 countries, there are 30 countries where annual cigarette consumption per capita has increased by at least one tertile from 1970 to 1990. Of these 30 countries, 25 are low-income and middle-income countries.

In China, among men, the new popularity of smoking appears to be particularly pronounced. The first national smoking survey of more than half a million individuals was conducted in China in 1984 (Weng 1988). The results of the survey showed that 61% of males older than age 15 in China smoked, and the prevalence of smoking in

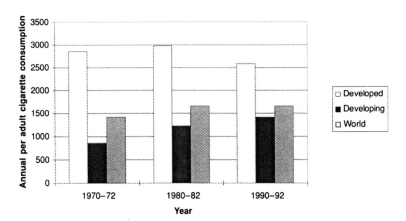

Fig. 2.3 Trends in per capita cigarette consumption in developed and developing countries. Source: WHO 1997.

Table 2.5 Cigarette consumption per adult aged 15 years and over: selected countries 1970–72 to 1990–92

Income group	Country	Cigarette consumption per adult 1970–90	
		Relative increase over 1970–72 levels (%)	Absolute Increase since 1970–72 (sticks)
Low-income	Nepal	241	410
	Haiti	241	410
	Cameroon	174	470
	China	160	1170
	Senegal	144	620
	Bangladesh	94	480
	Sierra Leone	76	350
	Yemen, Rep.	72	340
	Madagascar	70	190
	Myanmar	67	60
	Malawi	65	130
	Niger	55	60
	Ethiopia	50	30
	India	36	360
	Cambodia	30	280
Lower-middle	Indonesia	136	680
	Syria	111	1050
	Algeria	68	650
	Egypt, Arab Rep.	66	480
	Jordan	65	660
	Suriname	61	710
	Fiji	38	440
	Morocco	35	240
	Ecuador	34	220
	Thailand	30	240
Upper-middle	Saudi Arabia	75	910
	Mauritius	40	520
High-income	Cyprus	41	890
	Portugal	40	570
	Greece	36	950

Source: WHO 1997.

all occupational groups was higher than for the corresponding groups in the United States. By 1996 the prevalence of smoking in Chinese men had risen further, to 63% (Chinese Academy of Preventive Medicine 1997). The average consumption of cigarettes per Chinese man per day was 1 in 1952, 4 in 1972, 10 in 1992, and 11 in 1996 (Weng 1988, 1990; Mackay 1995; Chinese Academy of Preventive Medicine 1997; WHO 1997).

2.3 Smoking-attributable mortality

It is well established that prolonged smoking is an important cause of chronic disease. Here we summarize the literature on mortality from chronic diseases attributable to smoking. We begin by discussing the long delay between the onset of smoking and chronic disease, given that this key feature of smoking is important to individual choices and the perception of risk, and to public policy. We then describe current smoking mortality in developed and developing populations, including differences by gender, duration of exposure, and age. Finally, we review projections of tobacco deaths into the twenty-first century.

Tobacco contains nicotine, a substance that is recognized to be addictive by WHO and several other international medical organizations (see, for example: USDHHS 1988; WHO 1992). There is increasing evidence that nicotine addiction is central to consumer choices (see Chapter 5, for a discussion of the economics of addiction, and Chapter 12, for a discussion on nicotine replacement therapies). We refer the reader to several key references for a more comprehensive discussion on smoking and addiction (USDHHS 1988, 1994). Similarly, we refer the reader elsewhere for comprehensive reviews of maternal smoking (Naeye 1980; Taylor 1989; Groff *et al.* 1997; Horta *et al.* 1997; Eriksson *et al.* 1998; Ventura *et al.* 1998) or environmental tobacco smoke (Trichopoulos 1981, 1983; Hirayama 1983, 1984; USDHHS 1986; Glantz and Parmley 1991; EPA 1992; OEHHA 1997).

2.3.1 The long delay between the onset of smoking and death

There is no longer doubt about the causal connection between tobacco use and chronic disease. Prolonged smoking causes many diseases in addition to lung cancer, notably other cancers and chronic respiratory and cardiovascular diseases. Smokers are at greater risk than non-smokers for malignancies, both of organs that are in direct contact with smoke, such as the oral cavity, oropharynx, esophagus, larynx, and lung, and in organs and tissues not in direct contact with smoke, such as the pancreas, urinary track, kidney, stomach, and hemotopoietic tissues.

Past and current misunderstandings about the hazards of smoking are due in large part to the long delay between the onset of smoking and the occurrence of tobacco-related disease in individuals, and to the long delay between an increase in smoking rates within a population and a full increase in that population's death rates from tobacco-related diseases. For example, in the United States, per capita tobacco consumption increased 44% between 1920 and 1950, mostly due to smoking by young men. Lung cancer rates increased three-fold during that time. After 1950, per capita tobacco consumption stabilized but lung cancer rates increased by greater than 11-fold (Peto *et al.* 1992; USDA 1998; Table 2.6). The stabilization of lung cancer rates in men in the United States since about 1985 reflects a decline in the prevalence of smoking in males over the past few decades.

Similar evidence of the long delay between an increase in smoking and an increase in death rates is found in other countries with reliable ascertainment of both consumption and deaths, such as Japan, Finland, Norway, and the United Kingdom (Peto and Zaridze 1986). In Japan, smoking markedly increased in males after the Second

Table 2.6 Trends in tobacco consumption and lung cancer in the United States

Year	Percentage increase in per capita tobacco consumption in pounds weight (increase over 1920–29 average baseline)	Percentage increase in age-adjusted lung cancer rates per 100 000 (average of 1930–34 as baseline)
1940–45	19	104
1950–55	42	300
1960–65	34	528
1970–75	9	837
1980–85	−16	1103

Source: USDA 1998; Doll and Peto 1981.

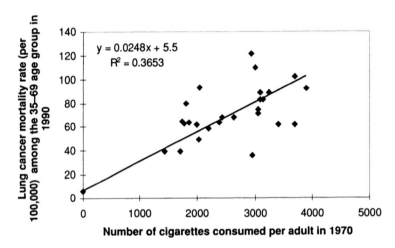

Fig. 2.4 Cigarette smoking in 1970 and lung cancer in 1990. Source: author's calculations, based on Peto *et al.* 1994 and USDA 1998.

World War, peaked in the 1960s, and then started to decline. However, tobacco-attributable mortality continues to increase to this day. Moreover, sub-populations without marked increases in smoking, such as young males living in Japan during the Second World War, do not have marked increases in lung cancer rates 20 years later (Tominaga 1986). Across the populations of the industrialized countries with a history of prolonged smoking, past consumption predicts current tobacco-attributable mortality remarkably with a lag of about 20 years (Fig. 2.4).

The long delay between smoking and disease has several implications, the most important of which is to lead smokers to underestimate their risk of disease (see Chapter 8). Smokers may be aware of the findings of epidemiological studies, but such studies conducted at the earlier stages of a tobacco epidemic may seriously mislead or underestimate the true long-term hazards from tobacco use. In the British Doctors'

Table 2.7 Annual deaths by cause in smokers and non-smokers: British Doctors' Study 1951–91

Cause of death	Annual death rate per 100000 men			
	1951–71		1971–91	
	Non-smokers	Cigarette smokers	Non-smokers	Cigarette smokers
All neoplastic causes	382	743	394	993
Lung cancer	17	264	17	314
All respiratory causes	165	384	121	466
Chronic obstructive lung disease	7	151	15	208
Other respiratory diseases	156	253	106	258
All vascular causes	1626	2416	1153	2003
Cerebrovascular disease	401	516	276	501
Cardiovascular disease	1225	1900	857	1502
Other diseases	258	370	198	388
Trauma and poisoning	94	119	74	156
All causes	2523	4077	1954	4026

Source: Doll *et al.* 1994. Reproduced with permission of the BMJ Publishing Group.

Table 2.8 Lung cancer deaths, United States: two million-person prospective studies

Period	Males		Females	
	Death rate /100000 Non-smokers	Death rate ratios Smoker:non-smoker	Death rate /100000 Non-smokers	Death rate ratios Smoker:non-smoker
1960s	6	12	4	3
1980s	6	22	5	11

Source: Peto *et al.* 1994; USDHHS 1989.

study (Doll *et al.* 1994), the mortality among middle-aged smokers was two times that of non-smokers during the first 20-year follow-up period, and three times that of non-smokers during the second 20-year follow-up period. This implies that half of deaths in middle age among the smokers in the first 20-year follow-up period, and two-thirds of those deaths in the second 20-year period, were caused by tobacco. Thus, in the British Doctors' study, the excess mortality among middle-aged smokers was substantially higher during the second follow-up period than it was during the first (Table 2.7).

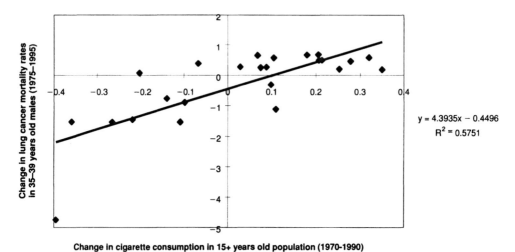

Change in cigarette consumption in 15+ years old population (1970-1990)

Fig. 2.5 Changes in cigarette consumption and changes in lung cancer mortality rates in 35–39 year-old males (1975–95), selected countries. Source: authors' calculations from Peto *et al.* 1994 and WHO 1997.

A comparable pattern has emerged in the United States. Table 2.8 shows change over time in the ratio of deaths from lung cancer for smokers versus non-smokers. The death rate from this disease among non-smokers did not change appreciably in 20 years, whereas the death rate among smokers increased substantially in in both sexes between the 1960s and the 1980s (Peto *et al.* 1994).

Despite the long lag between smoking and its full impact, *recent* changes in lung cancer rates in *young* men and women are a very sensitive indicator of recent changes in tobacco consumption. This is because lung cancer in young adults is easier to diagnose than at older ages. Across high-income countries, changes in total cigarette consumption in the past 20 years have predicted changes in lung cancer rates in young males (Figure 2.5).

2.3.2 Current estimates of tobacco-attributable mortality worldwide

The WHO has produced estimates of global mortality from smoking (WHO 1999),[2] using a method known as the *smoking impact ratio*, which indexes various causes of death to lung cancer (Peto *et al.* 1994). The method has been applied to low-income and middle-income countries. The results are shown in Table 2.9.

How plausible are these estimates? Given the long delay between onset of smoking and disease, the most reliable estimates are for men in the established market economies and the former socialist economies. In these countries, men took up

---

[2] WHO also provide estimates of the disability-adjusted life years (DALYs) attributable to tobacco. For a full explanation of how this measure of disease burden is calculated see Murray and Lopez (1996). In brief, total DALYs from tobacco in 1998 were 49 288 000 or about 3.6% of all DALYs.

Table 2.9 Estimates of tobacco-attributable mortality, by region, in thousands, during 1998

Region or country	Males	Females	Total
Established market economies	840	400	1240
China	783	130	913
Formerly socialist economies of Europe	595	88	683
India	332	51	383
Other Asia and islands	242	34	276
Middle Eastern Crescent	210	28	238
Latin America	130	38	168
Sub-Saharan Africa	109	13	122
World	3241	782	4023
% of worldwide deaths	11.4	3.1	7.5

Source: WHO (1999) with adaptation to the regional classification used in Murray and Lopez (1996).

Table 2.10 Smoking and death among males aged 35–69 in the United States

Cause of death	Mean[a] annual mortality rate per 100 000 males aged 35–69		
	Nonsmokers	Current cigarette smokers	Excess rate in smokers
Lung cancer	8	196	441
Upper aerodigestive cancer[b]	5	28	23
Other cancers	109	188	79
Respiratory	9	62	53
Vascular	176	446	270
Cirrhosis	5	19	14
Other medical	39	81	42
Non-medical (suicide, homicide, accident, etc.)	31	62	31
All causes	382	1083	701

[a] Average of rates by each cause for seven age groups: 35–39, 40–44, 45–49, 50–54, 55–59, 60–64, and 65–69.
[b] Cancers of the mouth, oesophagus, pharynx and larynx.
Source: Peto *et al.* 1994.

smoking in large numbers 30–60 years ago and deaths today from various causes are reliably measured, as shown, for example, in the American Cancer Society's Cancer Prevention Study (CPS-II) (USDHHS 1990) (Table 2.10).

Based on the CPS-II, Peto and colleagues have derived a novel approach of using the absolute age- and sex-specific lung cancer rates, minus USA non-smoker lung cancer rates from the CPS-II, to approximate the proportions of deaths from various other diseases that can be attributed to tobacco. This methodology was applied to routinely collected mortality data in high-income western countries and former socialist countries (Peto *et al.* 1994). It indicated that in 1990, tobacco was responsible for 17% of total deaths or 2.1 million deaths per year in these countries (Table 2.11). Throughout Europe in 1990, tobacco smoking caused three-quarters of a million deaths in middle age. In the countries of Central and Eastern Europe, including the former Soviet Union, there were 441 200 deaths in middle-aged men and 42 100 deaths in women. The highest burdens of tobacco-attributable mortality were in Eastern Europe. Retrospective application of this method indicates that tobacco-attributable mortality has risen in most developed countries over the past 40 years, but that non-tobacco-attributable mortality is generally falling. From 1950 to 2000, according to this method, tobacco caused about 60 million deaths in developed countries, or 20% of total male deaths and 4% of total female deaths. Of these 60 million deaths, about 40 million were in middle age and 20 million in old age. On the basis of newer data from China and India (see below), it is plausible that between 20 million and 30 million tobacco deaths have occurred since 1950 in low-income and middle-income countries. These deaths, combined with an estimated several million deaths between 1900 and 1950, suggest that the twentieth century has seen a total of about 100 million tobacco deaths (Peto and Lopez in press).

Cardiovascular disease—in particular ischemic heart disease—is the most common smoking-related cause of death in developed countries. By calculating the smoking impact ratio, researchers have attributed a significant proportion of deaths from cancer, vascular disease, and chronic obstructive pulmonary disease to tobacco (Table 2.11; Peto *et al.* 1994; WHO 1997).

The strengths and weaknesses of this indirect methodology have been reviewed previously (Peto *et al.* 1994). Most importantly, these methods are indirect and may under- or over-estimate smoking-attributable mortality. The method may be less reliable in estimating deaths from cardiovascular disease in Eastern Europe (Murray and Bobadilla 1997). Ongoing epidemiological studies in Poland and Russia should help to validate these indirect estimates, particularly for Eastern European populations.

Countries in South and East Asia, Africa and Latin America are at earlier stages in

Table 2.11 Percentage of deaths in middle age attributed to smoking, by cause, in high-income countries and former socialist countries during 1995

Sex	All causes	All cancer	Lung cancer	Upper aerodigestive cancer	Chronic obstructive pulmonary disease	Vascular disease
Males	36	50	94	70	82	35
Females	13	13	71	34	55	12
Both sexes	28	35	89	65	73	28

Source: Peto *et al.* 1994.

the pattern of cigarette consumption seen in developed countries. Because it is only those who start smoking in early adult life who are at really high risk of death from tobacco in middle and old age, there will generally be a delay of about half a century between the time of the main increase in smoking by young adults and the time of main increase in death from tobacco in later life. Hence, the peak of the epidemic of tobacco-related morbidity and mortality is yet to be seen in many developing countries. In addition, these countries have few direct or indirect studies of tobacco-attributable mortality. One important exception, however, is China. A large retrospective Chinese study, conducted in 98 geographically defined areas, revealed that one smoker in four has already been killed by tobacco. However, the proportion of all deaths caused by tobacco is currently lower than that in the West (Table 2.12; Liu *et al.* 1998), partly because the full effects of the large recent increases in male cigarette consumption are not yet evident. Even at this early stage, however, China has more tobacco deaths than the USA or Russia. In 1990, tobacco-attributed deaths numbered 0.6 million (0.5 million males and 0.1 million females). By 2000, tobacco deaths are expected to reach at least 0.8 million (0.7 million of them in males). Half of these deaths will occur in middle age (defined as ages 35–69) and half in old age.

The Chinese data also reveal that the causes of tobacco-attributable death may differ between developing and developed countries. Chronic obstructive pulmonary disease (COPD) accounted for almost half the tobacco-attributed deaths in China (three times as great a proportion as in the USA), while ischaemic heart disease accounted for only a relatively small percentage. Smoking appeared to cause about as many deaths from tuberculosis as from ischaemic heart disease in China. In India, earlier studies have shown that the use of tobacco increases the risk of developing lung cancer among tuberculosis patients (Willcox *et al.* 1982). In Egypt, a higher risk of bladder cancer has been seen among smokers infected with the pathogen *Schistosoma haematobium* than among non-smokers (Makhyoun 1974). Moreover, various populations have high underlying vascular mortality, such as India, Malaysia, Mauritius, and Sri Lanka (WHO 1997), and smoking may exacerbate this pattern in the future.

Reliable evidence of tobacco-attributable mortality in other large developing

Table 2.12 Percentage of deaths in middle age attributed to smoking, by cause, in China during 1986–88

Sex	All causes	All cancer	Lung cancer	Oesophagus cancer	Stomach cancer	Chronic obstructive pulmonary disease	Respiratory tuberculosis	Vascular disease
Males	13	24	52	28	18	23	11	9
Females	3	4	19	3	2	9	3	0.2
Both sexes	9	17	42	19	13	17	8	9

Source: Liu *et al.* 1998. Reproduced with permission from the BMJ Publishing Group.

countries is lacking, although several studies are ongoing. In India, 48% of male
cancers and 20% of female cancers are tobacco-related (Gajalakshmi *et al.* 1996). Preliminary results from a large retrospective study in Chennai of the smoking habits of
48,000 adults who died recently and of 48,000 live controls suggest that, in middle age,
smokers have about twice the age-standardized death rate of non-smokers, i.e., that
half of all the male smokers who die in middle age would not have done so at non-
smoker death rates. A substantial minority of these tobacco-attributed deaths involve
tuberculosis (Gajalakshmi and Peto 1999). If, eventually, the twofold difference in male
death rates between smokers and non-smokers at ages 25–69 observed in Chennai is
found in many parts of urban and rural India, then about 30% of the male deaths in
middle age and about 10% of the male deaths in old age will be attributable to smoking
in India.

In all attempts to estimate the burden of tobacco-attributable disease, a major area
of uncertainty is the impact of prolonged smoking on women. Table 2.9 notes that less
than one in five of all current tobacco deaths are among women. Patterns of tobacco-
attributable mortality among men are well established from observations over the past
40 years in populations where mass smoking in men started at various times between
1920 and 1960. In contrast, the pattern for women is less well established, because
women took up smoking in mass numbers more recently. If women's smoking patterns
approached those of men, then the number of female deaths from tobacco would be
expected to rise as high as as those seen among males. In the United States, smoking-
attributable mortality in females aged 35–69 has increased from 5% in 1965 to 31% in
1995. In many developed countries, lung cancer had equalled breast cancer, the leading
cause of cancer deaths in women, by the mid-1980s (USDHHS 1986). On current
smoking patterns, death rates from lung cancer and other tobacco-attributable diseases
among women will rise continuously in the twenty-first century.

Another important factor in assessments of the burden of tobacco-attributable
disease is the effect of early initiation to smoking. In assessing the risk of disease, the
total amount of tobacco smoked appears to be less important than the age of onset
and the duration of smoking. The risks are notably higher in individuals who start
smoking early and continue for prolonged periods. Starting at age 15 and smoking
10–20 cigarettes a day for 45 years, increases the risk of lung cancer about twice as
much as does smoking 21–39 cigarettes per day starting at age 25 (Peto 1986). Differences in the relative hazards of smoking with age have only recently emerged. A
large retrospective study of 14 000 myocardial infarction survivors and 32 000 controls
found non-fatal myocardial infarction rates are five times as common in smokers as in
non-smokers aged 30–49, three times as great at ages 50–59, and twice as great at ages
60–79 (Parish *et al.* 1995). In addition, the risks of tobacco use are more extreme in
middle age than in old age. Both the British Doctors' study and studies in the United
States showed higher death rates among smokers in middle age compared to those in
old age.

2.3.3 Future mortality from smoking

Policy-makers must be concerned not so much by the current mortality from past
smoking patterns, but by the much larger death rates that are projected in coming

decades as a result of current smoking, especially for low-income and middle-income countries.

Smoking-attributable deaths are projected to increase for two reasons: first, increases in the susceptible population size; and second, increases in age-specific disease rates. For example, in China, male per capita consumption of manufactured cigarettes rose 10-fold between 1952 and 1992. The incidence of lung cancer in China has increased more than six-fold during the period 1970 to 1980 (Sidel and Sidel 1982), and is likely to increase 7.5-fold in the near future. During the same period, the population that will contract lung cancer will increase four-fold. The net result is that 30 000 lung cancer deaths per year in 1975 will increase to 900 000 per year by 2025 (i.e. 30 000 × 7.5 × 4).

Using data on previous smoking and mortality patterns, Peto *et al.* (1994) have estimated the magnitude of the tobacco epidemic in developing countries during the next few decades. They conclude that tobacco will cause about 0.5 billion deaths among smokers alive today. At some point in the second decade of the twenty-first century, annual deaths from tobacco will average 10 million a year. This total may appear earlier or later, the researchers conclude, depending on smoking patterns and background rates of tobacco-attributable diseases. On current smoking patterns, there will be about 450 million tobacco deaths between 2000 and 2050 (Peto *et al.* 1999). Projections beyond 2050 are more uncertain. If the proportion of people taking up smoking continues, as at present, to be between one-quarter and one-third of young adults, then, given population growth, an additional 500 billion tobacco deaths are expected in the second half of the twenty-first century. Thus, in the twenty-first century overall, tobacco would be expected, on current patterns, to kill about a billion people, or ten times as many people as in the twentieth century (Peto and Lopez in press).

Direct estimates for China based on retrospective and prospective studies (Liu *et al.* 1998; Niu *et al.* 1998) suggest that, on current patterns, smoking may account for one in three of all adult male deaths in China, or about 100 million of the 300 million Chinese males now aged 0–29. Annual tobacco deaths will rise to 1 million before 2010 and 2 million by 2025, when young adults of today reach old age. Similar preliminary estimates for India based on large retrospective and prospective studies suggest that about 30% of male deaths in middle age are attributable to smoking and about 80 million Indian males currently aged 0–34 years will eventually be killed by tobacco.

Projections of tobacco mortality based on econometric models by Murray and Lopez suggest that there will be 8.3 million tobacco-attributable deaths per year in 2020 (Table 2.13). These researchers have predicted elsewhere that global deaths attributed to tobacco would rise from 6% of all deaths in 1990 to about 12% in 2020 (Murray and Lopez 1997).

2.4 Smoking cessation: patterns and consequences

It is clear that, worldwide, most smoking begins in youth. However, the percentage of adult smokers who quit varies greatly between high-income countries and the rest of the world. The prevalence of ex-smokers is the most reliable estimate of levels of

Table 2.13 Econometric model projections of deaths and disease burden attributable to tobacco, estimates for 1990 and projections for 2020

Region	Total deaths (thousands)		Deaths (% of total)	
	1990	2020	1990	2020
Established market economies	1063	1286	15	15
Former socialist economies	515	1101	14	23
Demographically developing countries[a]	1460	5996	4	11
World	3038	8383	6	12

[a] Other than a few exceptions, low-income and middle-income economies make up the grouping of demographically developing countries in this table. For the listing of countries in this grouping, please see appendix C of WHO (1996).

Source: WHO 1996.

Table 2.14 Prevalence of ex-smokers in selected countries, ranked by per capita GDP

	Prevalence (%)	
Country	Time period 1	Time period 2
High-income		
United States	20 (1965)	30 (1991)
Australia	28 (1986)	32 (1992)
Italy	22 (1990)	28 (1995)
Sweden	20 (1963)	41 (1994)
Spain	17 (1989)	19 (1992)
Middle-income		
South Africa	N/A	06 (1996)
Hungary	15 (1986)	14 (1994)
Poland	18 (1974)	21 (1997)
Low-income		
China	N/A	02 (1993)
India	N/A	05 (1992–94)
Vietnam	N/A	10 (1997)

Sources: Giovino *et al.* 1994; Hill and White 1995; Hill 1998; La Vecchia *et al.* 1994; Pagano *et al.* 1998; Wersall and Eklund 1998; del Rio and Alvarez 1994; Reddy 1999 (unpublished data); Hungary Central Statistics Office 1994; Zatonski 1996; Gong *et al.* 1995; Gupta 1996; Jenkins *et al.* 1997.

quitting within a population. In high-income countries, ex-smoker rates have increased over the past two to three decades, and today about 30% of the male population are former smokers (Table 2.14). In contrast, only 2% of Chinese men surveyed in 1993 had quit; only 5% of Indian men had done so at around the same period; and only 10% of Vietnamese men had quit in 1997. Even these low figures may be misleadingly high because they include those people who quit because of illness.

There is considerable evidence that smoking cessation reduces the risk of death from tobacco-related diseases. A reduction in the risk of lung cancer after smoking cessation has been observed in the United States, Canada, Europe, United Kingdom, Canada, Asia, Latin America, and Sweden. There has been some marked reduction in tobacco-attributable mortality in some countries, largely due to quitting. For example, male deaths in middle age from tobacco-related disease in the United Kingdom have fallen from 69 000 to 28 000 during the period 1965–95 (Peto *et al.* 1994). Around 1970, British men had the worst death rate in the world from tobacco, but with adults quitting, Britain has the world's biggest decrease in tobacco deaths. Data presented by Bobak *et al.* (Chapter 3) also reveal that declines in tobacco-attributable mortality differ by socio-economic group within countries, largely reflecting differences in quitting.

There is as yet unclear evidence from epidemiological studies about the rate at which the risks of morbidity and mortality decline after an individual quits. Former smokers face a lower risk of tobacco-related diseases than current smokers, but their risks remain higher than those of non-smokers. As the time since quitting increases, the risks to former smokers of tobacco-related diseases falls. In studies in the United Kingdom, those who quit smoking before the onset of major disease avoided most of the excess hazard of smoking (Doll *et al.* 1994). The benefits of quitting were largest in those who quit early (between ages 35 and 44) but still significant in those who quit later (between ages 45 and 54). In the United States, former smokers who have quit for 15 years or more have lung cancer mortality rates twice those of non-smokers. This compares with rates 15 times greater than those of non-smokers among continuing smokers who started in their early teens (USDHHS 1983). In Sweden, it was found that men who had ceased smoking for 10 years had no significant excess risk of coronary heart disease over non-smokers, and the results for women were consistent with those for men (Rosenberg *et al.* 1990). In Britain, the relative risk of coronary heart disease among men aged between 30 and 54 years compared to non-smokers was 1.9 for those who had discontinued smoking for less than 5 years, 1.3 for those who had discontinued for between 15 and 5 years, and among men who had quit for more than 15 years, the risks were virtually identical to those of non-smokers (USDHHS 1983).

2.5 Directions for research

The smoking epidemic is not uniform. There is considerable variation in mortality across age groups, by gender, over time, by geography, and by socio-economic group (see Chapter 3). Thus, while the hazards of smoking appear well documented, at least in high-income countries, the importance of monitoring the epidemic is clear. Three types of key data would be required for an overall strategy for research on tobacco (see Chapter 19 and Baris 1999). First, epidemiologists would need reliable estimates of smoking prevalence and incidence across different populations. Standardized methods of measuring smoking prevalence, akin to the National Health Interview Survey (US National Center for Health Statistics 1999) are required in all countries to monitor the smoking epidemic, as well as the success of interventions and control programs. Second, reliable data on absolute numbers of cigarettes sold in any country would be needed as a proxy indicator of the overall levels of future disease in a population. Third, retrospective 'proportional mortality' studies, which compare the proportions of smokers and non-smokers who have died of tobacco-attributable diseases to calculate the excess in smokers, and 'case-control' studies, which use deceased persons as cases and their surviving spouses/close relatives as controls, would be required to project future mortality patterns. Both proportional mortality and case-control studies involve simple ascertainment by an interviewer of the cause of death, along with a measure of past smoking gathered from living household members. Experience from China (Liu *et al.* 1998) suggest that simple information on death certificates about whether or not the deceased person smoked would permit a robust analysis of proportional mortality. Such an analysis compares the tobacco habits of adults who died of cancers, vascular and respiratory diseases, to those who died of other causes as 'reference groups'. For example, the excess of lung cancer deaths among smokers can be inferred from the excess of smokers among lung cancer deaths. Proportional mortality results in China are comparable to those from an early prospective study (Niu *et al.* 1998). In Chennai, India, a retrospective case-control study to assess the health effects of tobacco use is under way; the smoking and tobacco-chewing habits of those who died in Chennai during 1995–97 are being analyzed by interviewing the surviving spouse/close relatives (Gajalakshmi and Peto 1999). Living women are compared to dead women for the magnitude of risk from exposure to tobacco, and living men are compared to dead men. In this study design, the data on both cases and controls are obtained at the same time. South Africa now obtains past smoking status on all death certificates, and a review of early implementation is under way (Sitas *et al.* 1998). By January 2000, India began to record past tobacco use on all death certificates. Similar efforts are required in other countries to enable effective monitoring of the smoking epidemic.

2.6 Conclusions

The majority of smokers today live in low-income and middle-income countries, where consumption has risen over the last two decades. Most smokers worldwide start their addiction as children, and there is some evidence from China that the average age of smoking onset is falling. Current tobacco-attributable mortality is about 4 million deaths per year, with half of these deaths in low- and middle-income countries. Current risks for prolonged smoking are considerable: one in two long-term smokers will be killed by tobacco, half of these in middle age. On current smoking trends, there will be 10 million annual deaths (about one in six of all adult deaths) by 2030. About seven in ten of these deaths will be in low-income countries. All told, on current smoking patterns, about 0.5 billion of the world's population alive today will be killed by smoking, half of them in middle age, and the twenty-first century is likely to see about 1 billion tobacco deaths. Evidence from developed countries suggests that quitting can avoid much of the excess risk from smoking, but quitting remains rare in low-income and middle-income countries. Alongside specific action to reduce mortality, further specific research is required to monitor the great epidemic of the twenty-first century.

References

Baris, E. (1999). *Confronting the Epidemic: A Global Agenda for Tobacco Control Research*. Geneva: World Health Organization and Research for International Tobacco Control.

Chinese Academy of Preventive Medicine (1997). *Smoking in China: 1996 National Prevalence Survey of Smoking Pattern*. Beijing: China Science and Technology Press.

Corti, C. (1931). *A History of Smoking*, pp. 27–33, 39, 53–66. London, Backen Books (edition 1996).

del Rio, M. C. and Alvarez, F. J. (1994). Patterns of smoking in Spain. Results from a regional general population survey. *Eur. J. Epidemiol.*, **10**(5), 595–8.

Doll, R. and Peto, R. (1981). The causes of cancer: quantitative estimates of avoidable risks of cancer in the United States today. *Journal of National Cancer Institute*, **66**, 1191–308.

Doll, R., Peto, R., Wheatley, K., Gray, R., and Sutherland, I. (1994). Mortality in relation to smoking: 40 years' observations on male British doctors. *BMJ*, **309**, 901–11.

EPA (United States Environmental Protection Agency) (1992). *Respiratory Health Effects of Passive Smoking: Lung cancer and other disorders*. EPA, Office of Research and Development, Office of Air and Radiation. EPA/600/6–90/006F. Washington DC.

Eriksson, K. M., Haug, K., Salvesen, K. A., Nesheim, B. I., Nylander, G., Rasmussen, S. (1998). Smoking habits among pregnant women in Norway 1994–95. *Acta Obstet. Gynecol. Scand.*, **77**, 159–64.

Gajalakshmi, C. K., Ravichandran, K., and Shanta, V. (1996). Tobacco-related cancers in Madras, India. *E. J. Cancer*, **5**, 63–8.

Gajalakshmi, C. K. and Peto, R. (1997). *Studies on Tobacco in Chennai, India*. Presented at the 10th World Conference on Tobacco or Health, Chinese Medical Association, Beijing.

Gajalakshmi, C.K. and Peto, R. (1999). *Tobacco epidemiology in the state of Tamil Nadu, India*. The Proceedings of the XV Asia Pacific Cancer Conference, Chennai, 1999 (in press).

Giovino, G. A., Schooley, M. W., Zhu, B. P., Chrismon, J. H., Tomar, S. L., Peddicord, J. P. *et al.* (1994). Surveillance for selected tobacco-use behaviors—United States, 1900–1994. *Mor. Mortal. Wkly Rep. CDC Surveill. Summ.*, **43**(3), 1–43.

Glantz, S. A. and Parmley, W. W. (1991). Passive smoking and heart disease. Epidemilogy, physiology and biochemistry. *Circulation*, **83**, 1–12.

Goa Cancer Society (1992). *Assessment of the Efficacy of Anti-tobacco Community Education Program*. Dona Paula, Goa.

Gong, Y. L., Koplan, J. P., Feng, W., Chen, C. H., Zheng, P., and Harris, J. R. (1995). Cigarette smoking in China. Prevalence, characteristics, and attitudes in Minhang District. *JAMA*, **274**(15), 1232–4.

Groff, J. Y., Mullen, P. D., Mongoven, M., and Burau, K. (1997). Prenatal weight gain patterns and infant birthweight associated with maternal smoking. *Birth*, **24**, 234–9.

Gupta, P. C. (1996). Socio-demographic characterstics of tobacco use among 99 598 individuals in Bombay, India using hand-held computers. *Tobacco Control*, **5**(2), 114–20.

Hill, D. J. (1988). Australian patterns of tobacco smoking in 1986. *Med. J. Aust.*, **149**(1), 6–10.

Hill, D. J. and White, V. M. (1995). Australian adult smoking prevalence in 1992. *Aust. J. Public Health*, **19**(3), 305–8.

Hirayama, T. (1983). Passive smoking and lung cancer: consistency of association. *Lancet*, **2**(8364), 1425–6.

Hirayama, T. (1984). Cancer mortality in nonsmoking women with smoking husbands based on a large-scale cohort study in Japan. *Prev. Med.*, **13**(6), 680–90.

Horta, B. L., Victora, C. G., Menezes, A. M., Halpern, R., and Barros, F. C. (1997). Low birthweight, preterm births and intrauterine growth retardation in relation to maternal smoking. *Paediatr. Perinat. Epidemiol.*, **11**(2), 140–51.

Hungary Central Statistics Office (1994). *Hungary Health Behaviour Survey*. Budapest.

IARC, International Agency for Research on Cancer (1986). *IARC Monograph on the Evaluation of Carcinogenic Risk of Chemicals to Humans—Tobacco Smoking*. Switzerland: World Health Organization.

Japanese Public Welfare Ministry (1993). *Smoking Problems and Health II*. Health and Medical Foundation, Tokyo.

Jenkins, C. N., Dai, P. X., Ngoc, D. H., Kinh, H. V., Hoang, T. T., Bales, S. *et al.* (1997). Tobacco use in Vietnam. Prevalence, predictors, and the role of the transnational tobacco corporations. *JAMA*, **277**(21), 1726–31.

La Vecchia, C., Pagano, R., Decarli, A., and Ferraroni, M. (1994). Smoking in Italy, 1990–1991. *Tumori*, **80**(3), 175–80.

Liu, B. Q., Peto, R., Chen, Z. M., Boreham, J., Wu, Y. P., Li, J. Y. *et al.* (1998). Emerging tobacco hazards in China: 1, Retrospective proportional mortality study of one million deaths. *BMJ*, **317**(7170), 1411–22.

Mackay, J. (1995). Transnational tobacco companies versus state monopolies in Asia. In *Tobacco and Health*. Proceedings of the Ninth World Conference on Tobacco and Health, (ed. K. Slama), pp. 61–66. Plenum Press, New York.

Makhyoun, N. A. (1974). Smoking and bladder cancer in Egypt. *Br. J. Cancer*, **30**, 577–81.

Marketfile (1998). *Online tobacco database*.
http://www.marketfile.com/market/tobacco/index.htm

Murray, C. J. L. and Lopez, A. D. (ed.) (1996). *The Global Burden of Disease*. Cambridge, MA: Harvard University Press.

Murray, C. J. L. and Bobadilla, J. L. (1997). Epidemiological transition in the formerly socialist economies: divergent patterns of mortality and causes of death. In *Premature Death in the New Independent States* (ed. J. L. Bobadilla, C. A. Costello and F. Mitchell), pp. 184–214. National Research Council, Washington DC.

Murray, C. J. L. and Lopez, A. D. (1997). Global mortality, disability, and the contribution of risk factors: Global Burden of Disease Study. *Lancet*, **349**, 1436–42.

Naeye, R. L. (1980). Abruptio placentae and placenta previa; frequency, perinatal mortality, and cigarette smoking. *Obstet. Gynecol.*, **55**, 701–4.

Nicolaides-Bouman, A., Wald, N., Forey, B., and Lee, P. (1993). *International Smoking Statistics: a Collection of Historical Data from 22 Economically Developed Countries*. New York: Oxford University Press.

Niu, S. R., Yang, G. H., Chen, Z. M., Wang, J. L., Wang, G. H., He, X. Z. *et al.* (1998). Emerging tobacco hazards in China 2. Early mortality results from a prospective study. *BMJ*, **317**(7170), 1423–4.

Office of Environmental Health Hazard Assessment (OEHHA) (1997). *Health Effects of Exposure to Environmental Tobacco Smoke: Final Report*. California Environmental Protection Agency.

Pagano, R., La Vecchia, C., and Decarli, A. (1998). Smoking in Italy, 1995. *Tumori*, **84**(4), 456–9.

Pan American Health Organization (1992). *Tobacco or health: Status in the Americas*. Scientific Publication No. 536. Washington, D.C.

Parish, S., Collins, R., Peto, R., Youngman, L., Barton, J., Jayne, K., *et al.* (1995). Cigarette smoking, tar yields, and non-fatal myocardial infarction: 14000 cases and 32000 controls in the United Kingdom. The International Studies of Infarct Survival (ISIS) Collaborators. *BMJ*, **311**, 471–7.

Peto, R. (1986). Influence of dose and duration of smoking on lung cancer rates. In *Tobacco: a Major International Health Hazard*, (ed. D. Zaridze and R. Peto), pp. 23–34. Lyon, International Agency for Research on Cancer, IARC Scientific Publication 74.

Peto, R. (1994). Smoking and death: the past 40 years and the next 40. *BMJ*, **309**, 937–9.

Peto, R. and Zaridze, D. (ed.) (1986). *Tobacco: a Major International Health Hazard*. *Lyon, International Agency for Research on Cancer*. IARC Scientific Publications, no. 74.

Peto, R., Lopez, A. D., Boreham, J., Thun, M., and Heath, C. Jr. (1992). Mortality from tobacco in developed countries: indirect estimation from national vital statistics. *Lancet*, **339**, 1268–78.

Peto, R., Lopez, A. D., Boreham, J., Thun, M., and Heath, C. Jr. (1994). *Mortality from Smoking in Developed Countries, 1950–2000*. Oxford, Oxford University Press.

Peto, R., Chen, Z. M., and Boreham, J. (1999). Tobacco: the growing epidemic. *Nature Medicine*, **5** (1), 15–7.

Peto, R. and Lopez, A. D. (in press). The future worldwide health effects of current smoking patterns. In *Global Health in the 21st Century*, (ed. Koop E.C., Pearson C.E. and Schwarz R.M. Jossey-Bass), New York, 2000.

Pierce, J. P., Fiore, M. C., Novotny, T. E., Hatziandreu, E. J., and Davis, R. M. (1989). Trends in cigarette smoking in the United States. Projections to the year 2000. *JAMA*, **261**(1), 61–5.

Rosenberg, L., Palmer, J. R., and Shapiro, S. (1990). Decline in the risk of myocardial infarction among women who stop smoking. *New Engl J. Med.*, **322**, 213–7.

Sidel, R. and Sidel, V. W. (1982). *The Health of China*. Boston: Beacon Press.

Sitas, F., Pacella-Norman, R., Peto, R., Collins, R., Bradshaw, D., Kleinschmidt, I. *et al.* (1998). Why do we need a large study on tobacco-attributed mortality in South Africa? *S. Afr. Med. J.*, **88**(8), 925–6.

Taylor, S. A. (1989). Tobacco and economic growth in developing nations. *Business in the Contemporary World*, Winter, 55–70.

Tominaga, S. (1986). Smoking and cancer patterns and trends in Japan. In *Tobacco. A Major International Health Hazard*, (ed. D. Zaridze and R. Peto), pp. 103–113. Lyon. International Agency for Research on Cancer, 1986, IARC Scientific Publication 74.

Trichopoulos, D., Kalandidi, A., Sparros, L., and MacMahon, B. (1981). Lung cancer and passive smoking. *Int. J. Cancer*, **27**, 1–4.

Trichopoulos, D., Kalandidi, A., and Sparros, L. (1983). Lung cancer and passive smoking: conclusion of Greek study. *Lancet*, **2**(8351), 677–8.

USDA (US Department of Agriculture) (1998). US Department of Agriculture Database, USDA: Washington DC, USA.

US Department of Health and Human Services (1983). *The Health Consequences of Smoking:*

Cardiovascular Disease. US Department of Health and Human Services, Washington, DC: Govt. Printing Office. DHHS publication No (PHS) 84–50204.

US Department of Health and Human Services (1986). *The Health Consequences of Smoking For Women*. US Department of Health and Human Services, Public Health Service, Office of the Assistant Secretary for Health, Office on Smoking and Health. Rockville, Maryland.

US Department of Health and Human Services (1988). *The Health Consequences of Smoking–Nicotine Addiction: A Report of the Surgeon General*. Rockville, Maryland: US Dept of Health and Human Services, Public Health Service, Centers for Disease Control, Center for Health Promotion and Disease Prevention, Office on Smoking and Health. DHHS publication no. (CDC)88–8406.

US Department of Health and Human Services (1989). *Reducing the Health Consequences of Smoking–25 Years of Progress: a Report of the Surgeon General*. Rockville, Maryland: US Dept of Health and Human Services, Public Health Service, Centers for Disease Control, Center for Chronic Disease Prevention and Health Promotion, Office on Smoking and Health. DHHS publication no. (CDC)89–8411.

US Department of Health and Human Services (1990). *The health benefits of smoking cessation*. US Department of Health and Human Services, Public Health Service, Centers for Disease Control, Center for Chronic Disease Prevention and Health Promotion, Office on Smoking and Health. DHHS Publication No. (CDC) 90-8416, 1990.

US Department of Health and Human Services (1994). *Preventing Tobacco Use Among Young People. A Report of the Surgeon Genera*. Atlanta, Georgia: US Dept of Health and Human Services, Public Health Service, Centers for Disease Control, Center for Chronic Disease Prevention and Health Promotion, Office on Smoking and Health.

US National Center for Health Satistics (1999). Website on National Health Interview Survey. http://www.cdc.gov/nchs/about/major/nhis/nhis.htm

Venkat Narayan, K. M., Chadha, S. L., Hanson, R. L., Tandon, R., Shekhawat, S., Fernandes, R. J. *et al.* (1996). Prevalence and patterns of smoking in Delhi: cross sectional study. *BMJ*, **312**(7046), 1576–9.

Ventura, S. J., Martin, J. A., Curtin, S. C., and Mathews, T. J. (1998). Report of final natality statistics, 1996. *Mon. Vital Stat. Rep.*, **46**(Supplement 11), 1–99.

Weng, X. Z. (ed) (1988). *Report on the 1984 Chinese National Smoking Prevalence Survey*. People's Medical Publishing House, Beijing.

Weng, X. Z. (1990). The anti-smoking campaign in China. In *Tobacco and Health 1990— The Global War* (ed. B. Dunstan and K. Jamrozik), pp. 131–2. Proceedings of the Seventh World Conference on Tobacco and Health. Health Department of Western Australia, Perth.

Wersall, J. P. and Eklund, G. (1997). The decline of smoking among Swedish men. *Int. J. Epidemiol.*, **27**(1), 20–6.

Willcox, P. A., Benatar, S. R., and Potgieter, P. D. (1982). Use of the fexible fibreoptic bronchoscope in diagnosis of sputum-negative pulmonary tuberculosis. *Thorax*, **37**, 598–601.

World Bank (1999). World Development Indicators: database. Washington, D.C.

World Health Organization (1992). *International Statistical Classification of Diseases and Related Health Problems* (10th revision). Geneva, World Health Organization.

World Health Organisation (1996). *Investing in Health Research and Development*. Report of the Ad Hoc Committee on Health Research Relating to Future Intervention Options (Document TDR/Gen/96.1). Geneva, World Health Organization.

World Health Organization (1997). *Tobacco or Health: a global status report*. Geneva, World Health Organization.

World Health Organization (1999). World Health Report: Making a Difference. Geneva, World Health Organization.

Zatonski, W. (1996). *Evolution of Health in Poland since 1988*. Maria Sklodowska-Curie Cancer Center and Institute of Oncology. Warsaw.

Yach, D., McIntyre, D., and Saloojee, Y. (1992). Smoking in South Africa: the health and economic impact. *Tobacco Control*, **1**, 272–80.

3
Poverty and smoking

Martin Bobak, Prabhat Jha, Son Nguyen, and Martin Jarvis

This chapter examines the association between poverty and tobacco use. It provides a comprehensive review of the data on smoking prevalence and consumption levels in different socio-economic groups, both within individual countries and internationally. It finds that smoking is more common among poor men (variously defined by income, education, occupation, or social class) than rich men in nearly all countries. In high-income countries, the social gradients of smoking are clearly established for men: smoking has been widespread for several decades, and smoking-attributable mortality can be measured reliably. Analyses of smoking-attributable mortality in middle age (defined as ages 35–69) in Canada, England and Wales, Poland, and the United States reveal that smoking is responsible for most of the excess mortality of poor men in these countries. For women, the situation is more variable, partly reflecting the more recent onset of mass smoking by women in certain parts of the world. Why poor people smoke more remains a complex question that requires further research.

3.1 Introduction

Poverty is a major determinant of premature mortality and ill health. International comparisons show a strong association between economic indicators such as gross domestic product (GDP) and life expectancy (World Bank 1993). Within individual countries for which data exist, lower socio-economic groups experience higher rates of death from most diseases, at any given age, than affluent groups. Poverty affects health through numerous intermediate factors. Most of the major proximal causes of ill health (such as poor water and sanitation, certain sexual behaviors, or poor nutrition) are strongly related to poverty (Marmot and Bobak, in press).

In addition to absolute poverty, seen in most low-income countries and in some middle-income countries, we consider relative poverty—often called relative deprivation—in which an individual is poorer than others in the social hierarchy. Relative poverty is also strongly associated with mortality and other adverse health outcomes in middle-income and high-income countries. For example, in a study of British civil servants, the risk of death gradually increases with decreasing employment grade, despite the fact that no civil servants live in poverty (Rose and Marmot 1981). In high-income countries where absolute poverty is not common, relative poverty is thought to contribute to the social gradient in health (Wilkinson 1996).

An important goal of health policy for many governments in developing and developed countries, and for international agencies, is to reduce inequalities in health between the rich and the poor (World Bank 1997). In this volume (Chapter 2), Gajalakshmi *et al.* describe trends in tobacco use and tobacco-related disease and death worldwide. Here, we consider the consequences of tobacco use specifically on the poor, focusing on the adverse health effects. There are also many economic consequences of smoking on the poor, such as reduced production and earnings, and effects on investment and consumption, insurance, and labour, but data on these are scantier than even the limited data on health effects reviewed here. The reader is referred to a general discussion on the economic consequences of adult health and disease(Over *et al.*1992) The chapter reviews the data on smoking prevalence by socio-economic group, between and within countries and over time. Differences in tobacco consumption levels between socio-economic groups are also discussed. The review then examines the evidence from developed countries that tobacco is responsible for much of the excess risk of premature death in lower socio-economic groups. It closes with a short discussion of the possible reasons why the poor smoke more than the rich. It concludes that the adverse health consequences of tobacco use are concentrated more heavily on the poor, and that smoking may be contributing to the widening mortality gap between the rich and the poor in developed countries. The policy implications are complex and are discussed in more detail by Jha *et al.* in Chapter 7.

3.2 Data sources and definitions

Standardized data on smoking prevalence, smoking-attributable mortality, and tobacco expenditure do not exist for all countries. Data for this review were obtained from various sources, often with non-comparable measures for smoking, mortality, or socio-economic class.

3.2.1 Data for smoking prevalence and consumption levels

These data were derived from 89 studies compiled by the World Health Organization (WHO 1997) and others, and used to estimate smoking prevalence, by gender, for each of the seven World Bank regions for 1995 (see Appendix 2 for a list of these regions and Appendix 3 for definitions). In most of these studies, the assessments of smoking prevalence were based on the number of people who reported smoking daily, and excluded others such as occasional smokers. Wherever possible this review, likewise, refers to daily smokers. The definitions of socio-economic class vary between studies: some used education levels, others used occupation, and still others used income levels. These definitions are not comparable in every country, but are correlated with each other and have been used interchangeably in previous studies of poverty and health. For the purposes of this review such data were used to assess the prevalence of smoking in rich and poor groups within countries, and the relative differences between these groups. Additional data on smoking prevalence were obtained from literature searches and contact with researchers. Many of these additional data were restricted to selected groups within populations, such as the poor.

3.2.2 Data on smoking and mortality

These were obtained largely from a review of smoking-attributable mortality in Canada, England and Wales, Poland, and the United States (Jha *et al.*, in press). Data on mortality by socio-economic class, age, and gender were obtained for these countries. Estimates of the overall risk of death due to smoking in middle age (defined as ages 35–69) were derived using a measure known as the smoking impact ratio (Peto *et al.* 1992, 1994). This method first calculates absolute lung cancer rates (excluding lung cancer not caused by smoking) in any one population, such as Canadian males. The absolute lung cancer rates are used to approximate the proportion due to tobacco of deaths from various other diseases, such as cancers other than lung cancer, vascular and respiratory disease, and othe causes. The proportions are estimated from a prospective study of 1 million Americans conducted in the 1980s (Garfinkel 1985).

3.3 Findings

In this section, we discuss the distribution of smoking across socio-economic groups.

3.3.1 Smoking prevalence in men with low incomes

Gajalakshmi *et al.* (Chapter 2) describe smoking prevalence in men and women by region, and note that the rates among men in low-income and middle-income countries are higher than in high-income countries. The overall smoking prevalence among men in 1995 was 49% in low-income and middle-income countries, while it was 38% in high-income countries. Further data support these findings and show in greater detail the strong inverse relationship between socio-economic status and male smoking prevalence: in 29 countries with data on smoking prevalence, 50% or more of men smoked in 1995. Of these, 22 are low-income or middle-income countries (Table 3.1). Other studies confirm the finding for males. In the WHO MONICA Project (WHO 1989), which collected data on cardiovascular risk factors in 27 populations, mainly in high-income and middle-income countries, the prevalence of smoking among men was higher in the middle-income, former socialist economies of Europe than in the high-income countries. However, this pattern was apparent only for male smoking. In 1995, smoking prevalence among women was 10% in low-income and middle-income countries overall, and 22% in high-income countries. But, while female smoking has remained comparatively rare outside the high-income countries, levels vary sharply between regions. In Latin America and the Caribbean, and Eastern Europe and Central Asia, female smoking prevalence, at 21% and 26%, respectively, was similar to that in high-income countries.

3.3.2 International comparisons of the smoking prevalence 'gradient' between socio-economic groups

Figure 3.1 describes the ratio of smoking prevalence between the lowest and highest socio-economic groups in an analysis of 74 studies from 41 countries. A total of 13, 25, and 36 studies were included for low-income, middle-income, and high-income countries, respectively. Socio-economic group was variously defined on the basis of either income, education, or profession. In total, the studies reveal that differences in smoking

Table 3.1 Estimated smoking prevalence among men, selected countries

Income group	Country	Smoking prevalence (%)
Low-income	Cambodia	80
	Vietnam	73
	China	63
	Bangladesh	60
	Sri Lanka	55
Lower-middle income	Latvia	67
	Russian Federation	67
	Dominican Republic	66
	Tonga	65
	Turkey	63
	Fiji	59
	Tunisia	58
	Panama	56
	Algeria	53
	Indonesia	53
	Samoa	53
	Estonia	52
	Lithuania	52
	Bolivia	50
Upper- middle income	Saudi Arabia	53
	South Africa	52
	Seychelles	51
	Poland	51
High-income	Korea, Rep.	68
	Japan	59
	Kuwait	52

Sources: WHO 1997; Jenkins *et al.* 1997; Chinese Academy of Preventive Medicine 1997.

prevalence between poor and rich groups are greater in low-income countries than those in high-income countries. Using education as a marker for socio-economic status, a regression of this ratio of smoking prevalence between high- and low-education groups to a log of 1994 gross domestic product (GDP) per capita (in constant 1987 dollars) is significant ($y = -0.4177x + 5.4931$, R squared of 0.348).

As Kenkel and Chen (Chapter 8) discuss, levels of information on the hazards of smoking are highest in rich countries. Moreover, several studies indicate that the rich in any country are more likely to make use of health-related information than the poor. Thus our finding that there are greater differences in smoking prevalence between rich and poor groups in low-income countries than in high-income countries is unexpected. The results could represent bias, since studies among low-income countries are fewer and may not be based on representative samples.

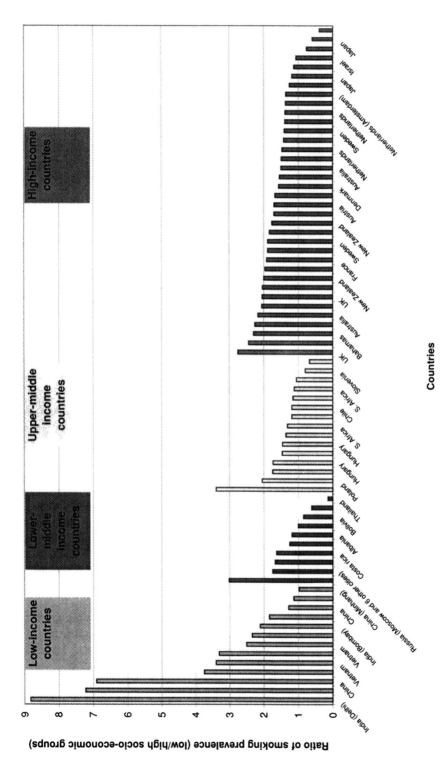

Countries

Fig. 3.1 Smoking prevalence in the highest and lowest socio-economic groups, expressed as a ratio, in various countries during the 1980s to 1990s. Source: authors' calculations, based on WHO's unpublished data; Gupta 1996; Narayan et al. 1996; Chinese Academy of Preventive Medicine 1997; Gong et al. 1995; Zatonski 1996; Hungary Central Statistics Office 1994; Yach et al. 1992; European Commission 1996; MarketFile 1998; CDC 1997.

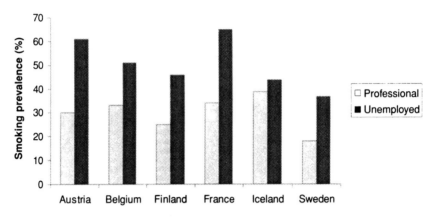

Fig. 3.2 Smoking prevalence among professional and unemployed males in six European
countries in the 1990s. Source: European Commission 1994.

3.3.3 Smoking prevalence by socio-economic group within countries

Given the great variation in smoking prevalence between countries, closer scrutiny of
studies *within* countries is likely to be informative.

Current prevalence patterns in high-income countries

In high-income countries, the prevalence of smoking is closely and inversely associated with socio-economic status. In the United Kingdom, for instance, only 10% of
women and 12% of men in the highest socio-economic group are smokers; in the lowest
socio-economic groups the corresponding figures are three-fold greater: 35% and 40%
(UK Department of Health 1998). The same inverse relationship is found between education levels and smoking. The pattern and magnitude of the differences was identical
in men and women (Wardle *et al.* 1998). A striking feature is that smoking prevalence
follows a continuous upward gradient from high to low socio-economic groups. Among
British civil servants, the prevalence of smoking falls with each successive employment
grade (Marmot *et al.* 1991). The situation is similar in most high-income countries.
Figures 3.2 and 3.3 show that the prevalence of smoking is consistently higher in unemployed people than among professionals, in both men and women, in several European countries.

The same relationship is found between education levels and smoking. In the United
States, educational status also predicts differences in smoking prevalence more consistently than income, sex, or race (Pamuk *et al.* 1998).

Current smoking patterns in the former socialist economies

The association between socio-economic status and tobacco in the former socialist
economies is more complex than in western countries. This may be due to different
development in the post-war period and, to a smaller extent, the recent economic

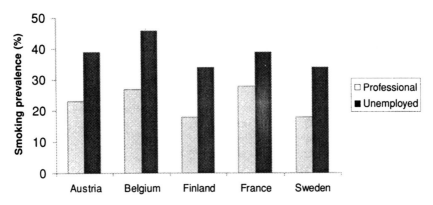

Fig. 3.3 Smoking prevalence among professional and unemployed females in five Euro pean countries in the 1990s. Source: European Commission 1994.

Table 3.2 Smoking prevalence by education level in four Central and Eastern European countries in men during the late 1980s

Age group	Education	Czech	Hungary	Poland: Warsaw (urban)	Poland Tarnobrzeg (rural)	Lithuania
35–44	Primary	51	49	71	66	50
	Secondary	44	35	61	55	56
	University	44	36	49	21	33
45–54.	Primary	47	37	61	62	49
	Secondary	34	22	54	72	37
	University	32	33	33	41	26

Source: WHO 1989.

upheaval in these countries. An analysis of data from Poland, Hungary, the Czech Republic, and Lithuania, collected by the WHO MONICA Project in the late 1980s, shows that the prevalence of smoking was higher among men with lower levels of education than with higher levels of education (Table 3.2). Among women, however, the educational gradient differed by age group. Among younger women, the prevalence of smoking was higher in those with lower education. By contrast, in older age groups, the prevalence increased with higher education (Table 3.3). It is interesting that during the economic transition, differences in smoking prevalence according to educational level increased in the Czech Republic (Bobak *et al.* 1997). This trend was particularly pronounced among women, where an increase in smoking prevalence was recorded among those with the lowest education. In multi-factorial analysis, education was the most prominent predictor of smoking, while material circumstances were less important (Bobak *et al.* 1999).

Table 3.3 Smoking prevalence (%) by education level in four Central and Eastern European countries in women during the late 1980s

Age group	Education	Czech Rep.	Hungary	Poland Warsaw (urban)	Poland Tarnobrzeg (rural)	Lithuania
35–44	Primary	37	42	60	11	<1
	Secondary	30	42	54	35	8
	University	22	28	41	30	8
45–54	Primary	17	19	34	6	5
	Secondary	25	29	36	23	5
	University	57	33	21	14	5

Source: WHO 1989.

The situation is different in Russia. A survey in a national sample of the Russian population in 1996 (McKee *et al.* 1998) showed that there was no apparent association between smoking and either education or income among men. Interestingly, material deprivation (measured as not having enough money to buy food, clothes, or fuel) was positively related to smoking prevalence. Intriguing and potentially important are the differences between men and women. First, smoking prevalence was generally lower in women than in men. The same was found in the Lithuanian MONICA study. Second, there was a strong age effect, possibly a cohort effect. Smoking prevalence was five times higher in young women than in those aged over 55 years. Third, smoking prevalence was three times higher in urban than in rural women.

Current patterns in other middle-income and low-income countries

Studies of smoking prevalence in developing countries are fewer and their results are more often mixed, depending on the type of population studied. In some low-income and middle-income countries, smoking was reported to be more prevalent among the more affluent (Gunther *et al.* 1988; Strebel *et al.* 1989; Taylor *et al.* 1996); this contrasts with the gradient seen in high-income countries. On the other hand, many studies in low-income countries, particularly in more recent years, found a social gradient similar to that of Western countries (Siegrist *et al.* 1990; Chung *et al.* 1993; Duncan *et al.* 1993; Gupta *et al.* 1994). Tobacco use is now more prevalent among the poor in India, China, Brazil, Mexico, Vietnam, Guatemala, Poland, Hungary, South Africa, and Costa Rica (Table 3.4). Figure 3.4, for example, shows education level to be a strong determinant of smoking in Chennai, India (Gajalaksmi and Peto 1997). Much depends on the study population used. A collaborative study by the International Clinical Epidemiology Network (INCLEN) examined prevalence of risk factors by socio-economic status in 12 centers in seven middle-income and low-income income countries (Noguiera *et al.* 1994). In each center, the study population was 200 middle-aged men drawn at random within the locality (not designed to be necessarily representative of the general population). Smoking prevalence was positively (but not significantly) related to education in three populations: Sao Paulo, Brazil; and Santiago and Temuco, both in Chile.

Table 3.4 Gradient in smoking prevalence between high and low socio-economic groups, various countries

Place (reference)	Difference in smoking prevalence	Comparisons
India (Delhi) (Narayan *et al.* 1996)	8.8-fold	Skilled and unskilled workers vs. professionals, supervisors and officers.
India (Bombay) (Gupta 1996)	7.2-fold	Illiterate vs. college.
China (Chinese Academy of Preventive Medicine 1997)	6.9	No schooling vs. college and above (females).
Brazil (World Bank 1990)	5.0-fold	Uneducated vs. secondary schooled adults.
Mexico (WHO unpublished data)	3.4-fold	Workers vs. professionals.
Vietnam (Jenkins *et al.* 1997)	3.4-fold	Less than 5 years vs. more than 16 years of schooling.
Guatemala (WHO unpublished data)	3.0-fold	Unskilled worker vs. skilled worker.
Vietnam (Jenkins *et al.* 1997)	2.5-fold	Peasant vs. white collar.
Poland (Zatonski 1996)	2.1-fold	Unskilled workers vs. white collar.
Cuba (WHO unpublished data)	1.7-fold	Agriculture and industrial worker vs. professional.
South Africa (Yach *et al.* 1992)	1.7-fold	Completed 6 years of schooling vs. completed 6 years of university.
Hungary (Hungary Central Statistics Office 1994)	1.7-fold	High school vs. college and university education.
Costa Rica (WHO unpublished data)	1.6-fold	Technical worker vs. professional.

Source: authors' calculations from various studies.

It was inversely related to education (the so-called 'Western pattern') in five populations: Bogota, Colombia; Chengdu and Shanghai, both in China; and Khon Kaen and Sonkia, both in Thailand. The relationship was flat in the remaining four centers: Rio de Janeiro, Brazil; Bangkok, Thailand; Manila, Philippines; and Yogyakarta, Indonesia. Smoking tends to be more common in urban areas (Strebel *et al.* 1989; Swai *et al.* 1993),

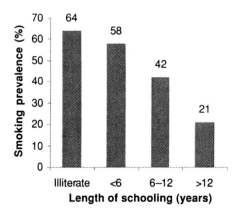

Fig. 3.4 Smoking prevalence among men in Chennai, India, by educational level. Source: Gajalakshmi and Peto 1997.

partly because of higher income levels and higher levels of tobacco promotion. Finally, when several indicators of social position are available, the inverse gradient is often pronounced along the educational axis, but less closely related to material deprivation (Chung *et al.* 1993; Duncan *et al.* 1993).

3.3.4 Trends over time

Reliable data on trends in smoking prevalence in different socio-economic groups are available only for high-income countries. In most of these countries, socio-economic differences in smoking have been increasing in recent decades. In Norway, smoking prevalence among high-income and low-income men, respectively, was 75% and 60% in 1955; by 1990, the rates had fallen to 28% and 40%, respectively (Lund *et al.* 1995) (Fig. 3.5), and smoking had become more prevalent among poorer men than among richer men. Thus the rich were the first to pick up the smoking habit and they were also the first to quit. Similarly, men were the first to start smoking, and may also be quitting sooner than women. In the United Kingdom in 1973, the absolute differences in smoking prevalence between the least and most deprived groups were about 33% and 31% in men and women, respectively. By 1996, those absolute differences increased to 46% and 44%, mainly because the decline in smoking was much slower among the more deprived (Wardle *et al.* 1998) (Table 3.5). In the United States, smoking prevalence declined between 1974 and 1987 nine times faster in the most educated group than in the least educated group(USDHHS 1989). It is clear that public health efforts to educate the public about the ill-health effects of smoking are not reaching all socio-economic groups equally and that higher socio-economic groups benefit more from information.

Changes over time, such as those described above, may help to explain the different smoking patterns in different countries seen at any one point in time. The smoking epidemic goes through different stages. Initially, smoking is more common among the more affluent groups and rarer among the poor. This pattern appears to reverse over

Table 3.5 Trends in smoking prevalence (%) by social class in the United Kingdom, 1974–94

Year	Social class I (men)	Social class V (men)	Social class I (women)	Social class V (women)
1974	29	61	25	43
1976	25	58	28	38
1978	25	60	23	41
1980	21	57	21	41
1982	20	49	21	41
1984	17	49	15	36
1986	18	43	19	33
1988	16	43	17	39
1990	16	48	16	36
1992	14	42	13	35
1994	16	40	12	34

Source: Wardle *et al.* 1998.

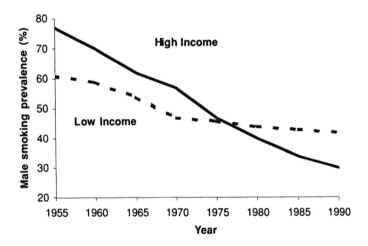

Fig. 3.5 Smoking trends in Norwegian men by income group, 1955–90. Source: Lund *et al.* 1995.

time, at least in countries for which data are available. The 'switch-over', which emerged first in Western countries, is well illustrated by the data from Norway. It is likely that the switch-over is also at least partly responsible for a similar change in the socio-economic gradient in coronary heart disease in these countries (Marmot *et al.* 1978; Morgenstern 1980; Mackenbach *et al.* 1989). In some low-income countries a higher prevalence of smoking is still seen in higher socio-economic groups. (Sarvoyatham and Berry 1968; Shaper 1973; Vaughan 1978; Chadha *et al.* 1992). Some middle-income and low-income countries, including the former socialist economies, may have been undergoing this change of social gradient more recently. Women have taken up smoking in mass numbers more recently and thus changes in the links between tobacco consumption and socio-economic status are still evolving. For example, Russian women may be undergoing the transition at present, and at a more rapid speed, than in Western countries.

3.3.5 Comparisons of cigarette consumption levels between and within countries

Cigarette consumption per capita is still higher in high-income countries, at 20 cigarettes a day, than in low-income and middle-income countries, at 13 per day (Chapter 2). However, with consumption falling in high-income countries and rising in low-income countries, the gap is narrowing quickly. Within the past 20 years, the ratio of cigarette consumption between developed and developing countries has fallen from 3.3 to 1.8 (Chapter 2).

Within individual countries there are few data on the number of cigarettes smoked daily by different socio-economic groups. In high-income countries, with some exceptions, the poor and less educated smoke more cigarettes per day than the richer and more educated. For example, Australian adult smokers with fewer than 9 years of education consume 22% more cigarettes, respectively, than those with university degrees (Hill and White 1995). Similarly, in the United States, daily cigarette consumption is 14% higher in smokers with a high-school education, or less, than in those with more than 17 years of schooling (Rogers *et al.* 1995). Chinese male smokers with a college education or above consume 15% fewer cigarettes than those with primary or middle-school education (Chinese Academy of Preventive Medicine 1997). In India, not surprisingly, smokers with college-level education tend to consume more cigarettes, which are relatively more expensive, while smokers with low levels of education consume larger numbers of the inexpensive *bidis*. Nevertheless, when both *bidis* and cigarettes are combined in the calculation of consumption, smokers with college education smoke much less than those with secondary education or less (Gupta and Mehta, in press).

3.4 Smoking and the excess mortality of the poor in developed countries

Since the poorer groups in developed countries appear to smoke more than the rich, tobacco-related deaths would be expected to be more common among them than among the rich. Smoking is, therefore, a powerful mediator of the association between poverty and mortality. For the purposes of this review, new analyses were commissioned of smoking-attributable mortality by socio-economic group (Jha *et al.* in press), in order to estimate what fraction of the mortality difference between rich and poor group can be explained by smoking. Such analyses are most reliable among males in developed countries, where smoking has been common for a long time and where reliable statistics exist on causes of death by socio-economic group. Analyses were commissioned for Canada, England and Wales, Poland, and the United States (see Figs 3.6–3.9).

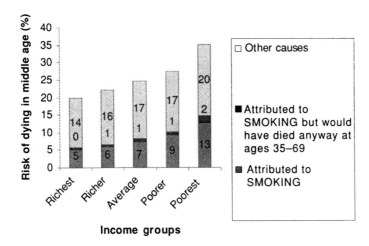

Fig. 3.6 The contribution of smoking to the risk of premature death among males at ages 35–69, by income group, Canada, 1991. Source: Jha *et al.*, in press.

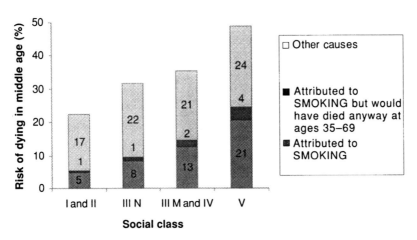

Fig. 3.7 The contribution of smoking to the risk of premature death among males at ages 35–69, by social class, England and Wales, 1991. Source: Jha *et al.*, in press. Note: In the UK, at the time of the study, socio-economic status was categorized into five groups from I (the highest) to V (the lowest). N represents nonmanual workers and M represents manual workers.

Figure 3.6 shows results for urban areas in Canada in 1991, using income as the indicator of socio-economic status. Overall, urban Canadian males in the richest quintile of income had a 19% risk of death between ages 35 and 69, whereas those in the poorest quintile had a 35% risk. The risks of death attributable to smoking were 5% and 15%, respectively (risk ratio 3). Avoiding deaths caused by smoking would thus

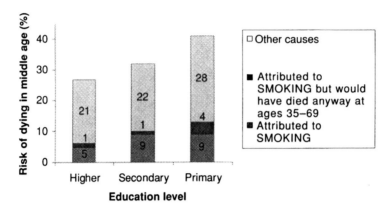

Fig. 3.8 The contribution of smoking to the risk of premature death among males at ages 35–69, by education level, Poland, 1996. Source: Jha *et al.*, in press.

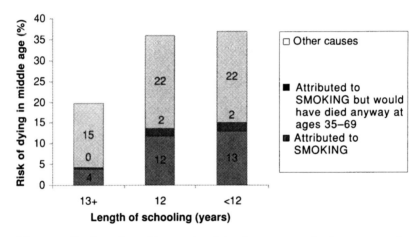

Fig. 3.9 The contribution of smoking to the risk of premature death among males at ages 35–69, by education level, United States, 1996. Source: Jha *et al.*, in press.

reduce the risks of death to 14% and 20%, respectively, and the ratio of risk in the lowest versus the highest educational groups to 1.4.

The calculations are virtually identical for Poland, where education is the available indicator of socio-economic status (see Fig. 3.8). The overall risk of death in 1996 between ages 35 and 69 for a male with university education was 27%. For a man with primary education it was 51%, about twice as great. The risks of death attributable to smoking were 6% and 23%, respectively; thus the risk ratio is 3.8, almost the same as in England and Wales. Avoiding deaths caused by smoking would reduce the risks of death to 21% and 28%, respectively. The ratio of risks between the lowest and highest education groups would fall to 1.3.

In the United States, where education is the available indicator of socio-economic status, the results are similar (see Fig. 3.9). The overall risk of death in 1996 between ages 35 and 69 for a man with 13 or more years of education was 19%. For a man with less than 12 years of education, it was 37%, a risk ratio of 1.9. The risks of death attributable to smoking are 4% and 15%, respectively, a risk ratio of 3.8. Avoiding deaths caused by smoking would reduce the risks of death to 15% and 22%, respectively. The ratio of risk between the lowest and the highest education groups would be reduced from 1.9 to 1.5.

Data on women from Canada, Poland, and the United States suggest a similar profile, although the effects are somewhat smaller, probably because the female population started smoking more recently than the male population, with the result that the risks may currently be underestimated. In the United States, if smoking-attributable disease could be eliminated, the ratio of risk for death between the highest and lowest socio-economic groups of middle-aged women would fall from 1.7 to 1.5. For Canada, it would fall from 1. 5 to 1.3, and in Poland, from 1.8 to 1.6. Data on social class for women in England and Wales are not shown because they are less reliable, as women were at that time classified by their husband's social class.

In addition to cross-sectional differences in mortality, smoking is also partly responsible for the widening of socio-economic differences over time. In Canada, the risk of death in middle age for men in the poorest income group fell from 46% in 1971 to 35% in 1996—a decline of about 24%. The risk of death from smoking-attributable causes fell from 17% in 1971 to 15% in 1996—a decline of only 12%. In contrast, in the richest income group, the risk of death in men fell from 32% to 20%, a decline of 38%; and the risk of death from smoking-attributable disease fell from 9% to 6%, a decline of about one-third. In Canada, in relative terms, the gap in mortality risk between poorest and richest income group increased from 1.4 for total risk and 1.9 for smoking-attributable risk in 1971, to 1.8 for total risk and 3 for smoking-attributable risk in 1991.

In England and Wales, the risk of death in middle age for men in the lowest socio-economic group marginally increased between 1970–72 and 1990–92, from 47% to 49%. (Note that the numbers of people in the lowest social classes changed over time, so the two time periods are not directly comparable.) The risk attributed to smoking also rose marginally from 24% to 25%. In contrast, for men in social classes I or II, the total risk of death in middle age fell from 30% in 1970–72 to 23% in 1990–92, a 36% decline. The risk of death attributable to smoking fell from 13% to 6%, a 54% decline. In relative terms the gap between mortality in lowest and highest social classes increased from 1.6 for total risk and 1.8 for smoking-attributable risk in 1970–72, to 2.1 for total risk and 4.2 for smoking-attributable risk in 1990–92. In England and Wales, if the lowest social class had had the same rate of decline in smoking-attributable mortality, the total risk in the lowest social class would have been 34% in 1991. The relative gap between the lowest and the highest social classes in 1990–92 would have narrowed from 2.1 to 1.5. In the absence of smoking, relative differences in total risk between low and high social classes would have narrowed even further to 1.4 in 1991.

Thus, in Canada, England and Wales, Poland, and the United States, smoking is responsible for much of the socio-economic gradient in male mortality. Eliminating smoking-attributable differences would approximately halve the social gradients in mortality among men in these four countries. The apparently smaller effects among women can be explained by the fact that the female tobacco epidemic is at an earlier stage.

The results from this analysis—which used an indirect measure to assess tobacco-attributable deaths—are consistent with studies where the effects of smoking are directly observed, for example, in cohort and case-control studies. Such studies find that adjusting for smoking typically reduces, but does not eliminate, the differences in mortality rates between socio-economic groups (Novotny *et al.* 1993). Other data also point to similar conclusions. Lung cancer incidence rates decrease as educational status increases. In one study in the United States, lung cancer incidence was 78% higher for whites with fewer than 12 years of education, than for whites who were college graduates; for African Americans, lung cancer incidence was 38% higher for persons with fewer than 12 years of education compared to college graduates. People with an annual income of less than $15 000 were 70–80% more likely to develop lung cancer than persons with annual incomes of more than $30 000 (Baquet *et al.* 1991). Lung cancer also shows a strong trend of decreasing risk with increasing income for white men; the rate in the lowest income group was 50% higher than that for the highest income group. Similar patterns were noted for black men; the rate in the lowest income group was 20% higher than that of the highest income group (Devesa and Diamond 1983). Low socio-economic status, as measured by employment status, family income, or education, is also strongly related to increased mortality from chronic obstructive pulmonary disease (Higgins 1992).

These results are based on data from industrialized countries and may, therefore, not apply in low-income countries where the tobacco epidemic is less advanced. Unfortunately, reliable data by socio-economic status are not available in low-income countries, and corresponding calculations cannot, therefore, be done. However, as the tobacco epidemic in low-income and middle-income countries matures, it is plausible that social patterns and impacts of smoking will be similar to those in high-income countries.

3.5 Why is smoking more prevalent among poor people?

As we have seen, smoking tends to be more prevalent among the poor than the rich in most settings; but the reasons for this are unclear. The success of strategies intended to reduce smoking will depend in part on a better explanation of this phenomenon. Poverty itself is not a cause of smoking. Indeed, the fact that tobacco is consumed more by groups for which it is, in relative terms, more expensive, is paradoxical. It is important to note that the poor do not smoke more than the rich in every country, and that education may be a more important predictor of smoking than material circumstances.

Several hypotheses have been put forward to explain the socio-economic gradient in smoking. These hypotheses relate mostly to Western countries, but may well apply to other populations. First, it is argued that the poor and less educated are less aware of the health hazards of smoking and thus more likely to adopt this harmful practice. Second, it is argued that smoking may be a self-medication used to regulate mood, manage stress, and to cope with the strains of material deprivation (Graham 1987, 1994). However, this self-medication hypothesis is not very tenable due to the lack of sedative or anxiolytic effects of nicotine. Third, it is argued that the adoption of

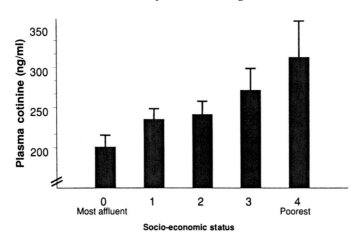

Fig. 3.10 Plasma cotinine in adult smokers by socio-economic status. Source: Wardle *et al.* 1999

smoking may be a replacement reward, as smoking is often described as one of the few things a poor person can do for himself or herself (Graham 1994). Fourth, economic hypotheses suggest that, given the same perceived benefits from smoking, a person whose income is low would have less to lose from future health problems than a person with a higher income. Finally, there is some evidence to suggest that the extent of nicotine dependence in poor smokers may be greater, although this observation cannot alone explain why poor people smoke more in the first place.

Data from the United Kingdom show that across increasing levels of social disadvantage there is a gradient in nicotine dependence as indicated by markers such as the time between waking and smoking the first cigarette of the day, or perceived difficulty in abstaining from cigarettes (Jarvis 1998; Wardle *et al.* 1998). Plasma cotinine concentrations measured in representative population samples in the Health Survey for England, which provide an objective measure of total nicotine intake over time and hence of nicotine dependence, show a similar picture, being lowest in the most affluent and highest in the poorest smokers (see Fig. 3.10). Data from the United States comparing cotinine levels in black and white smokers support these observations. Higher cotinine concentrations and higher nicotine intakes per cigarette smoked are seen in black than white smokers (Wagenknecht *et al.* 1990; English *et al.* 1994; Caraballo *et al.* 1998; Perez-Stable *et al.* 1998). Thus, in addition to any barriers to cessation due to factors such as lower awareness and concern about health risks, and a less supportive social environment, poor smokers face further difficulties through higher levels of addiction to nicotine, through both higher cigarette consumption and higher intake of nicotine per cigarette.

It is likely that deprivation affects the risk of smoking at different stages:

(1) by increasing the risk of starting to smoke;
(2) by increasing the risk of higher degree of dependence, and
(3) by reducing the chance of successful quitting.

Indeed, data from the United States and the United Kingdom suggest that not only are the poor and the less educated less likely to attempt to quit smoking, but their chances of becoming successful quitters are also lower (Jones 1994).

3.6 Conclusions

Although more research is still needed, there is little doubt that the poorest socio-economic groups suffer the consequences of tobacco use more than the richest. Analyses presented here suggest that smoking prevalence in most developing countries is already highest among the poor, and that if these countries experience a similar pattern to the high-income countries, the gap in smoking between rich and poor groups will widen over time. The implications for poor adults in middle age are considerable. In Canada, England and Wales, Poland, and the United States, middle-age mortality differences between rich and poor would fall by between one-half and two-thirds if smoking could be eliminated. If the burden of tobacco-related disease among the poor could be reduced, overall death rates in middle age would fall considerably. The policy implications of these findings are several and are dealt with in subsequent chapters.

References

Baquet, C. R., Horm, J. W., Gibbs, T., and Greenwald, P. (1991). Socio-economic factors and cancer incidence among blacks and whites. *J. Natl. Cancer. Inst.*, **83**(8), 551–7

Bobak, M., Skodova, Z., Pisa, Z., Poledne, R., and Marmot, M. (1997). Political changes and trends in cardiovascular risk factors in the Czech Republic 1985–1992. *J. Epidemiol. Comm. Hlth.*, **51**, 272–7.

Bobak, M., Hertzman, C., Skodova, Z., and Marmot, M. (1999). Socio-economic status and cardiovascular risk factors in the Czech Republic. *Int. J. Epidemiol.*, **28**, 46–52.

Caraballo, R. S., Giovino, G. A., Pechacek, T. F., Mowery, P. D., Richter, P. A., Strauss, W. J. *et al.* (1998). Racial and ethnic differences in serum cotinine levels of cigarette smokers. *JAMA*, **280**, 135–9.

Chadha, S. L., Gopinath, N., and Ramachandran, K. (1992). Epidemiological study of coronary heart disease in Gujaratis in Delhi (India). *Indian J. Med. Res.*, **96**, 115–21.

Chinese Academy of Preventive Medicine (1997). *National Prevalence Survey of Smoking Pattern*. Beijing: China Science and Technology Press.

Chung, M. H., Chung, K. K., Chung, C. S., and Raymond, J. S. (1993). Health-related behaviours in Korea: smoking, drinking, and perinatal care. *Asia-Pacific J. Publ. Health*, **6**, 10–5.

Devesa, S. S. and Diamond, E. L. (1983). Socio-economic and racial differences in lung cancer incidence. *Am. J. Epidemiol.*, **118**(6), 818–31.

Duncan, B. B., Schmidt, M. I., Achutti, A. C., Polanczyk, C. A., Benia, L. R., and Maia, A. A. (1993). Socio-economic distribution of non-communicable disease risk factors in urban Brazil: the case of Porto Alegre. *Bull. Pan American Health Organization*, **27**(4), 337–49.

English, P. B., Eskenazi, B., and Christianson, R. E. (1994). Black–white differences in serum cotinine levels among pregnant women and subsequent effects on infant birthweight. *Am. J. Public Health*, **84**(9), 1439–43.

European Commission 1996. *Tobacco consumption 1970–1994 in the member states of the European Union and in Norway and Iceland*. Stockhom: Statistics Sweden

Gajalakshmi, C. K. and Peto, R. (1997). *Studies on Tobacco in Chennai, India.* Presented at the 10th World Conference on Tobacco or Health, Chinese Medical Association, Beijing.

Garfinkel, L. (1985). Selection, follow up and analyses in the American Cancer Society prospective studies. In *Selection, Follow-up and Analyses in Prospective Studies: a Workshop* (ed. L. Garfinkel, S. Ochs and M. Mushinski), pp. 49–52. NCI Monograph 67. National Cancer Institute, NIH Publication No. 85–2713.

Gong, Y. L., Koplan, J. P., Feng, W., Chen, C. H., Zheng, P., and Harris, J. R. (1995). Cigarette smoking in China: prevalence, characteristics and attitudes in Minhang District. *JAMA*, **274**, 1232–4.

Graham, H. (1987). Women's smoking and family health. *Soc. Sci. Med.*, **25**, 47–56.

Graham, H. (1994). Gender and class as dimensions of smoking behaviour in Britain: insights from a survey of mothers. *Soc. Sci. Med.*, **38**, 691–8.

Gunther, H. K., Laguardia, A. S., Dilba, V., Piorkowski, P., and Bohm, R. (1988). Hypertension and social factors in a developing country. *J. Hypertens.*, **6** (Supplement), S608–S610.

Gupta, P. and Mehta, H. C. A cohort study of all-cause mortality among tobacco users in Mumbai, India. *Int. J. Public Health* (In press.)

Gupta, P. C. (1996). Survey of sociodemographic characteristics of tobacco use among 99,598 individuals in Bombay, India using handheld computers. *Tobacco Control*, **5**(2), 114–20.

Gupta, R., Gupta, V. P., and Ahluwalia, N. S. (1994). Educational status, coronary heart disease, and coronary risk factors prevalence in rural population of India. *BMJ*, **309**, 1332–6.

Higgins, M. (1991). Risk factors associated with chronic obstructive lung disease. *Annals of the New York Academy of Sciences*, **624**, 7–17.

Hill, D. J. and White, V. M. (1995). Australian adult smoking prevalence in 1992. *Aust. J. Public Health*, **19**(3), 305–8.

Jarvis, M. J. (1998). *Epidemiology of tobacco dependence.* Paper presented at First International Conference of the Society for Research on Nicotine and Tobacco, Copenhagen.

Jenkins, C. N., Dai, P. X., Ngoc, D. H., Kinh, H. V., Hoang, T. T., Bales, S. *et al.* Tobacco use in Vietnam: prevalence, predictors and the role of transnational tobacco corporations. JAMA. **277**: 1726–31.

Jha, P., Peto, R., Jarvis M., Lopez, A. D., Boreham, J., Zatonski, W. In press. Differences in male mortality due to smoking by education, income or social class. *British Medical Journal* (in press).

Jones, A. M. (1994). Health, addiction, social interaction and the decision to quit smoking. *J. Health Econ.*, **13**(1), 93–110.

Lund, K. E., Roenneberg, A., and Hafstad, A. (1995). The social and demographic diffusion of the tobacco epidemic in Norway. In *Tobacco and Health* (ed. K. Slama), pp. 565–71. New York: Plenum Press.

Mackenbach, J., Looman, C. W. N., and Kunst, A. E. (1989). Geographic variation in the onset of decline of male ischemic heart disease mortality in the Netherlands. *Am. J. Public Health*, **79**, 1621–7.

Marketfile. Online tobacco database. 1998. http://www.marketfile.com/market/tobacco/index.htm

Marmot, M. G. and Bobak, M. Contribution of social factors to ill health. In *Causes of Avoidable Mortality* (ed. A. Lopez). Geneva: World Health Organization. (In press.)

Marmot, M. G., Adelstein, M. M., Robinson, N., and Rose, G. A. (1978). Changing social class distribution of heart disease. *BMJ*, **2**, 1109–12.

Marmot, M. G., Davey Smith, G., Stansfeld, S., Patel, C., North, F., Head, J. *et al.* (1991). Health inequalities among British civil servants: the Whitehall II study. *Lancet*, **337**, 1387–93.

McKee, M., Bobak, M., Rose, R., Shkolnikov, V., Chenet, L., and Leon, D. (1998). Patterns of smoking in Russia. *Tobacco Control*, **7**, 22–6.

Morgenstern, H. (1980). The changing association between social status and coronary heart disease in a rural population. *Soc. Sci. Med.*, **14A**, 191–201.

Narayan, K. M., Chadha, S. L., Hanson, R. L., Tandon, R., Shekhawat, S., Fernandes, R. J. *et al.* (1996). Prevalence and patterns of smoking in Delhi: cross sectional study. *BMJ*, **312**(7046), 1576–9.

Nogueira, A., Marcopito, L., Lanas, F., Galdames, D., Jialiang, W., Jing, F. *et al.* (1994). Socio-economic status and risk factors for cardiovascular disease: a multicentre collaborative study in the International Clinical Epidemiology Network (INCLEN). *J. Clin. Epidemiol.*, **47**, 1401–9.

Novotny, T. E., Shane, P., Daynard, R., and Connolly, G. N. (1993). Tobacco use as a sociologic carcinogen: The case for a public health approach. In *Cancer Prevention.* (ed. DeVita, V.T.), pp 1–15. Philadelphia, PA: J.B. Lippencott Company.

Over, M., Ellis, R. P., Huber, J. H., and Solon, O. (1992). The consequences of adult ill-health. In *The Health of Adults in the Developing World* (ed. G. A. Feachem, T. Kjellstrom, J. L. Murray, M. Over and M. A. Phillips), pp. 161–99. New York, N.Y.: Oxford University Press.

Pamuk, E., Makuc, D., Heck, K., Reuben, C., and Lochner, K. (1988). *Socio-economic Status and Health Chart Book. Health, Unites States, 1998.* Hyattsville, Maryland: National Center for Health Statistics.

Perez-Stable, E. J., Herrera, B., Jacob, P., and Benowitz, N. L. (1998). Nicotine metabolism and intake in black and white smokers. *JAMA*, **280**, 152–6.

Peto, R., Lopez, A. D., Boreham, J., Thun, M., and Heath, C. J. (1992). Mortality from tobacco in developed countries: indirect estimation from national vital statistics. *Lancet,* **339**, 1268–78.

Peto, R., Lopez, A. D., Boreham, J., Thun, M., and Heath, C. J. (199•). *Mortality from Smoking in Developed Countries 1950–2000: Indirect Estimates from National Vital Statistics.* Oxford: Oxford University Press.

Rogers, R. G., Nam, C. B., and Hummer, R. A. (1995). Demographic and socio-economic links to cigarette smoking. *Soc. Biol.*, **42**(1–2), 1–21.

Rose, G. and Marmot, M. G. (1981). Social class and coronary heart disease. *Br. Heart J.*, **45**, 13–9.

Sarvoyatham, S. G. and Berry, J. N. (1968). Prevalence of coronary heart disease in an urban population on Northern India. *Circulation,* **37**, 939–53.

Shaper, A. G. (1973). Coronary heart disease. In *Cardiovascular Disease in the Tropics* (ed. A. G. Shaper, M. S. R. Hutt, Z. Fejfar), pp. 148–159. London: British Medical Association.

Siegrist, J., Bernhardt, R., Feng, Z. and Schettler, G. (1990). Socio-economic differences in cardiovascular risk factors in China. *Int. J. Epidemiol.*, **19**, 905–10.

Strebel, P., Kuhn, L. and Yach, D. (1989). Determinants of cigarette smoking in the black township population of Cape Town. *J. Epidemiol. Comm. Hlth.*, **43**, 209–213.

Swai, A. B., McLarty, D. G., Kitange, H. M., Kilima, P. M., Tatalla, S., Keen, N. *et al.* (1993). Low prevalence of risk factors for coronary heart disease in rural Tanzania. *Int. J. Epidemiol.*, **22**, 651–9.

Taylor, O. G., Oyediran, O. A., Bamgboye, A. E., Afolabi, B. M., and Osuntokun, B. O. (1996). Profile of some risk factors for coronary heart disease in a developing country: Nigeria. *Afr. J. Med. Sci.*, **25**, 341–6.

UK Department of Health (1998). *Smoking Kills: A White Paper on Tobacco.* London: The Stationary Office. (http://www.official-documents.co.uk/document/cm41/4177/contents.htm)

US CDC (Center for Disease Control and Prevention). (1997). Cigarette smoking among adults—United States, 1995. *MMWR Morb Mortal Wkly Rep*, **46**(51), 1217–20.

USDA (US Department of Agriculture) (1998). US Department of Agriculture Database, USDA: Washington DC, USA.

US Department of Health and Human Services (1989). *Reducing the Health Consequences of Smoking: 25 Years of Progress.* A Report of the Surgeon General, US Department of Health and Human Services, Public Health Service, Centers for Disease Control, Center for Chronic Disease Prevention and Health Promotion, Office on Smoking and Health. Rockville, Maryland. DHHS Publication No. (CDC)89–8411.

Vaughan, J. P. (1978). A review of cardiovascular diseases in developing countries. *Ann. Trop. Med. Parasitol.*, **72**, 101–9.

Wagenknecht, L. E., Cutter, G. R., Haley, N. J., Sidney, S., Manolio, T. A., Hughes, G. H. *et al.* (1990). Racial differences in serum cotinine levels among smokers in the Coronary Artery Risk Development in (Young) Adults Study. *Am. J. Public Health*, **80**(9), 1053–6.

Wardle, J., Farrell, M., Hillsdon, M., Jarvis, M. J., Sutton, S., and Thorogood, M. (1999). Smoking, drinking, physical activity and screening uptake and health inequalities. In *Inequalities in Health* (ed. Gordon, D., Shaw, M., Dorling, D., and Davey Smith, G.), pp. 213–39. Bristol: The Policy Press.

Wilkinson, R. G. (1996). *Unhealthy Societies. The Afflictions of Inequality*. London: Routledge.

World Bank (1990). *Brazil: The New Challenge of Adult Health*. Washington D.C., The World Bank.

World Bank (1997). *Sector Strategy: Health, Nutrition, and Population*. Washington DC: The World Bank Group.

World Bank. World Development Report (1993). *Investing in Health*. New York: Oxford University Press for the World Bank.

World Health Organization (1989). The MONICA project. A world-wide monitoring system for cardiovascular diseases. *Wld. Hlth. Statist. Ann.*, 27–149.

World Health Organization (1997). *Tobacco or Health: a Global Status Report*. Geneva., World Health Organization.

Yach, D., McIntyre, D., and Saloojee, Y. (1992). Smoking in South Africa: the health and economic impact. *Tobacco Control*, **1**, 272–80.

Zatonski, W. (1996). *Evolution of health in Poland since 1988*. Warsaw, Maria Sklodowska-Curie Cancer Center and Institute of Oncology.

4

Estimating the costs of tobacco use

James Lightwood, David Collins, Helen Lapsley, and Thomas E. Novotny[1]

Reliable estimates of the costs of tobacco use are valuable to policy-makers, particularly in planning health service provision and other items of public expenditure. However, such estimates are difficult to obtain because the methods used by different researchers vary and, in some respects, are controversial. Four types of cost analyses are compared here and the implications of different methods for results are explored. The literature on the healthcare costs of smoking is more extensive than for other types of cost and therefore forms the focus of this chapter. Estimates of the *gross* healthcare costs of smoking (that is, all the expenditures associated with treating diseases attributable to smoking) for high-income countries range between 0.10% and 1.1% of gross domestic product (GDP). The higher estimates occur in countries where healthcare costs account for a relatively large share of GDP. In low-income and middle-income countries, fewer studies have been performed, and often with very limited data, but the existing studies suggest that the gross costs of smoking can be as high as those in high-income countries. Studies of the *net* healthcare costs of smoking—which compare the *lifetime* healthcare costs of smokers and non-smokers and take account of the fact that smokers' lives are usually shorter than non-smokers'—reach more heterogeneous conclusions. This is because of major variations in the methods and assumptions used. However, the majority of these studies indicate that there are net costs from smoking. There is a clear need for refinement of the methods for making cost estimates, particularly for application in developing countries where the tobacco epidemic has yet to peak.

4.1 Introduction and overview

The health effects of tobacco use have been extensively documented (see Chapter 2). The costs and benefits associated with tobacco use are less well documented, and the methods used for cost estimates are complex and controversial. This chapter discusses the types of cost analysis that have been applied to tobacco consumption and reviews the existing cost estimates.

In developing countries, the relative burden of non-communicable disease is growing because of increasing life expectancies brought about by improvements in the standard of living and public health (Murray and Lopez 1996b). Also, most developing countries are at an earlier stage in the smoking epidemic than the high-income

[1] The authors gratefully acknowledge Helmut Geist and Rowena Jacobs for providing information on the environmental effects of tobacco agriculture.

countries, and the burden of tobacco-related disease is expected to treble between 1990 and 2020 (Murray and Lopez 1996a). As a result of both these trends, public health needs in developing countries will be transformed over the next 25 years. The full health consequences of smoking will not be felt until several decades after the increase in smoking prevalence, while childhood mortality and infectious diseases will be decreasing but will still be significant problems. However, because many of the consequences of smoking are not yet realized, tobacco control may not be regarded as a high priority by policy-makers. Careful analyses of the economic and financial implications of increasing tobacco use may prove valuable in planning for public health needs in the near future.

The plan of the chapter is as follows. First, three commonly used types of cost analysis will be described. The purpose, appropriate definitions of cost, and other issues will be discussed for each type of analysis. Then the application of each type of cost analysis to tobacco use will be discussed briefly. Next, existing cost estimates will be reviewed, with an emphasis on the costs of healthcare, because the literature is most extensive for this sector of the economy and because of its importance in public finance. The final section contains conclusions and suggestions for government program development, with an emphasis on important issues for developing countries.

4.2 Types of cost analysis

Confusion can arise in cost estimates because the definition of cost depends on the question that is being considered. Cost estimates using one definition will differ from those using another. Three types of analysis will be discussed and illustrated here: economic cost–benefit analysis (ECBA), GDP-based social cost analysis (GSCA), and expenditure-based cost analysis (EXBA). The approaches used in older studies may not match the prototypes presented, given changing notions of cost over time and data limitations that have forced authors to use approximations and compromises. These definitions represent broad categories that can be used to classify existing cost analyses, and for planning future research. See Leu and Schaub (1984), and Pekurinen (1992) for more detailed discussions of analyses of the costs of tobacco use. Cook (1991) is also an important discussion of the costs of substance abuse, although it is applied to alcohol.

The definition of cost employed and the type of analysis used is generally based on the policy question to be answered. For tobacco policy, key issues include optimal taxation and regulation, and the design and funding of public health campaigns (see Table 4.1). Consistency in defining costs is particularly important in avoiding double counting, aggregating costs over time, and identifying transfers of funds (as opposed to costs). The perspective from which costs are defined is also important. The perspective, for example, could be that of a government bureau, the healthcare sector of the economy, or all of society. Below, the different types of cost analysis are discussed.

4.2.1 Economic cost–benefit analysis (ECBA)

ECBA defines costs as opportunity costs. It is most often used when the policy question concerns the effect of a policy on economic welfare from the whole society's perspective. The underlying assumption is that people are rational agents who always

Table 4.1 Interpretation and use of cost estimates for tobacco policy

Type of estimate	Interpretation of results	Example of policy use
Aggregate costs	Total costs of smoking compared with alternative situation of zero smoking prevalence.	Indication of the size of the smoking problem.
Disaggregated costs	Costs of smoking disaggregated by various cost categories.	Budgetary planning for individual government units.
Avoidable costs	Potential economic benefits from harm reduction strategies.	Determination of the appropriate level of resources or best technique to be devoted to harm reduction strategies.
Cost incidence	The distribution of external costs among various community groupings.	Design of policies to correct undesirable cross-subsidies.
Cost impact	The impact of smoking on government unit's revenues and expenditures, or other group's economic welfare.	Determination of how much the tobacco industry should provide to compensate for smoking-related costs incurred by the public sector or specific groups.

Source: adapted from Table 4.1 in Collins and Lapsley (1998).

maximize their own individual welfare. In the case of tobacco, many economic costs arise from externalities in consumption or production, or from private costs due to mistaken decisions arising from imperfect information (see Chapter 7 for a detailed discussion). ECBA considers both direct and indirect, and tangible and intangible costs of tobacco use, unlike other definitions that only include monetary expenditures. However, in some ways, the ECBA definition of costs is less inclusive than others. For example, assuming utility-maximizing behavior implies that some of the medical care costs borne by the smoker of treating tobacco-related disease should not be counted. Instead, only the unexpected excess medical expenditures are included, since the tobacco user is assumed to account for the expected excess expenditures when deciding whether to consume more tobacco. This has practical significance because there is evidence that smokers do under-estimate the mortality effects of smoking (Schoenbaum 1997).

It is particularly important to avoid double counting in ECBA analyses. To do so, the analyst must identify transfer payments (which are not considered economic costs) and carefully separate primary and secondary markets in evaluating tax policy or the effects of changes in the life expectancy of tobacco users on medical and pension expenditures. Anderson (1977), Zerbe and Dively (1994), and Dinwiddy and Teal (1996) provide thorough guides to ECBA. There is no complete economic cost–benefit estimate of the aggregate cost of smoking, though some estimates of the costs that smokers impose on others (the external cost of smoking) follow the definition as closely as current data permit.

4.2.2 GDP-based social cost analysis (GSCA)

GSCA defines costs as the foregone flows of economic production, as defined by the System of National Accounts (SNA), with gross domestic product (GDP) being the most commonly used measure. The perspective for these analyses is usually that of the whole society, but it may also be that of a specific sector within an economy or government. The focus on foregone production creates differences between GDP-based costs and economic costs. For example, the economic cost of premature death is the welfare loss to the tobacco user from the unexpected increase in the annual excess probability of death from tobacco use. GDP-based costs of premature death would be based on the loss of production from the premature death of the tobacco user, whether expected or not. GDP-based cost analysis does not include intangible costs, such as non-market losses, pain and suffering from illness, other than what is reflected in market transactions.

The Canadian Centre on Substance Abuse (CCSA) has produced guidelines for adapting GDP-based costs analysis to social costs of drug use (Single *et al.* 1996a) based on the pioneering work on the cost of illness by Cooper and Rice (1976). These guidelines modify standard SNA cost definitions in two ways. First, they focus on social costs, or costs that are borne by others in society in addition to some of those borne by tobacco users. Second, they identify a threshold level of drug use that is considered addictive; use above this level is considered beyond the control of the user and, therefore, abusive. Expenditures resulting from abusive drug use are classified as costs. In the case of tobacco, almost all use is considered abusive because of the extreme potential of tobacco for addiction. The social costs of abusive consumption include the costs of morbidity and premature mortality, and the increased medical expenditures incurred by victims of environmental tobacco smoke. The CCSA guidelines also propose expanding traditional SNA-based accounts to include costs within the household and intangible costs that do not result in market transactions. These effects, such as household production lost while caring for an ill smoker, may be particularly significant in developing countries. Collins and Lapsley (1998) provide an informative discussion of this approach to estimating social costs.

4.2.3 Expenditure-based cost analysis (EXBA)

This defines costs as monetary expenditures (and revenues as benefits) that occur because of tobacco use. Intangible costs are excluded, as is the economic value of lost life. The perspective, or the definition, of the economic sector that incurs the expenditures or receives the revenues, is very important in EXBA. Many economic organizations must consider the effect of changes in revenues and expenditures on their budgets, from individual households to national health agencies. Keeping a consistent perspective is very important to avoid double counting. Transfer payments from one sector to another will be included as costs in EXBA, while transfers within a sector are not counted as costs, and neither type of transfer is an economic cost.

4.2.4 Cost-effectiveness analysis (CEA)

Smoking is associated with particular outcomes such as excess death and disability; utilization of healthcare; and costs, of the types described above. However, none of these types of analysis relates costs to particular outcomes or to changes in outcome; that is, they are not estimates of the cost of doing something so as to produce different results. That is the domain of cost-effectiveness analysis (CEA)—for example, the cost of extending smokers' lives through cessation programs. Gold *et al.* (1996) provide a comprehensive guide to CEA.

4.3 A taxonomy of costs for tobacco policy analysis

This section presents a taxonomy of costs relevant to tobacco policy. Table 4.2 provides a simple classification of aggregate costs from cigarette smoking for each of the approaches discussed in the previous section. The columns show the type of cost analysis and the rows show the various cost categories. The discussion below will compare and contrast the definition of costs used in each approach. In this section, all costs are defined in terms of the net present value arising from each individual smoker, so costs are defined as both current and expected discounted future costs. Issues concerning the treatment of future costs are discussed below.

4.3.1 Consumption

Smokers receive net benefits from that portion of consumption that can be justified by the smoker's knowledge of the health consequences, and other ill effects, of smoking, less out-of-pocket costs. In ECBA, this is usually measured by consumer surplus (see Chapter 6). There is little or no consumption benefit in GSCA since nearly all smoking is classified as abusive consumption (Collins and Lapsley 1991, 1996). In EXBA, the benefits include tax revenues and any reductions in expenditures for social insurance and medical expenditures that result from smoking.

Costs from consumption include those that fall on the smoker, arising mostly from the addictive nature of tobacco consumption and imperfect information about its consequences (see Chapter 6 for a discussion of these costs). Recently, some have described these costs as a type of externality (e.g. Stiglitz 1994b; Viscusi 1995). ECBA characterizes these costs as a welfare loss for smokers who are smoking more than they would with full information and a clear understanding of addiction. EXBA includes an analogous cost from government-funded programs for smoking cessation. Standard GSCA would exclude this type of cost as being a private cost of the smoker, rather than a social cost (Single *et al.* 1996a).

4.3.2 Health effects from smoking

These effects are overwhelmingly negative (see Chapter 2) and can be divided into direct and indirect costs. In some analyses (particularly in EXBA), premature death from adverse health effects may produce savings from reduced medical expenditures arising from the premature death of smokers. These can be divided into direct and indirect costs. For direct costs, three quantities must be measured in each of the three analyses. The first quantity is the incidence or prevalence of each disease caused by smoking. This is usually measured by the Smoking Attributable Fraction (SAF), which measures the average proportion of the occurrence of disease attributable to smoking (see Xie *et al.* 1996, section 3.3, for a good discussion of attributable fractions). Accurate estimation of

Table 4.2 Taxonomy of costs for tobacco policy

Cost category	Economic cost–benefit analysis	GDP-based social cost analysis	Expenditure based analysis
Consumption			
1. Benefit	Consumer surplus of smoker from 'informed' cigarette smoking.		Tax revenues from cigarette sales. Lower social insurance expenditures and medical expenditures from premature death due to smoking. Expenditures for smoking cessation programs and treatments.
2. Cost	Welfare loss of smokers from cigarette consumption due to unexpected addiction. Welfare loss from unexpected illness and premature death of smoker due to smoking. Welfare loss from externalities to non-smokers from illness and premature death of smokers due to smoking. Welfare loss from externalities of illness and death due to environmental tobacco smoke. Welfare loss from fires and pollution due to cigarette smoking.	Production loss of smokers from illness and premature death due to smoking. Production loss and expenses of non-smokers from illness and premature death of smokers due to smoking. Production loss and expenses from illness and death due to environmental tobacco smoke. Production and tax revenue loss from fires and pollution due to smoking.	Expenditures and tax losses from illness and premature death of smokers due to smoking. Expenditures and tax losses of non-smokers from illness and premature death of smokers due to smoking. Expenditures and tax losses from illness and premature death due to environmental tobacco smoke. Expenditures and tax losses from fires and pollution due to smoking.
Production			
3. Benefit	Producer surplus.		Producer tax revenues (that are not paid by smokers).
4. Cost	Welfare loss from unexpected illness and death of tobacco workers due to exposure to tobacco. Welfare loss from environmental pollution due to tobacco production.	Production loss from unexpected illness and death of tobacco workers due to exposure to tobacco. Production loss from environmental pollution from tobacco production.	Net expenditures and loss of tax revenue due to illness and premature death of tobacco workers due to exposure to tobacco. Net expenditures due to environmental pollution from tobacco production.

the SAF is complicated because it depends on the demographic structure, general health, and smoking habits and history of the population, as well as on the characteristics of smokers. The second quantity is the change in utilization of health and other social services as a function of the amount of smoking-related disease. This is particularly important for forecasting smoking-related costs in developing countries where current utilization rates are typically lower than in developed countries, but growing. Measured utilization depends on the health services that are included in the estimate. These services are shown in Table 4.3, and are discussed in more detail in Collins and Lapsley (1998). The third quantity is the expenditures resulting from increased utilization. In countries with good expenditure surveys, these three quantities can be estimated at once. Otherwise, they will have to be estimated separately and total costs modeled as a function of SAF, total utilization, and average cost per unit of utilization. Warner *et al.* (1999) present a detailed discussion of technical issues involved in these estimates.

In ECBA, only resources expended because of unexpected smoking-related illness

Table 4.3 Health services used in estimating direct healthcare costs of smoking

Cost center	Sources of data	Comments
Hospital services	Medical records, hospital and insurance fund bills, actual costs in public sector hospitals, DRG costs.	Usually highest share of direct costs. In developing countries, families provide significant direct unreimbursed care.
Physician/outpatient services	Fee-for-service bills, out-of-pocket expenses reported on household surveys, etiologic fraction of capitated costs.	Informal payments not accountable, but are common in many countries.
Prescription drugs	Insurance payments, sales data, out-of-pocket expenditures, and formularies.	Does not capture costs of over-the-counter drugs.
Nursing home services	Insurance payments, long-term care facility bills, actual costs in public sector facilities, and reported out-of-pocket expenses.	Many informal facilities with no diagnostic data; costs may include family transfers. Smokers in nursing homes tend to have high co-morbidity.
Home healthcare	Official home healthcare provider bills, insurance payments, and reported out-of-pocket expenses.	Many informal facilities that do not have diagnostic data, and may be part of extended family transfers. Most healthcare in developing countries is in home.
Allied healthcare (rehabilitation, respiratory therapy, nutrition care, etc.)	Insurance payments, facility bills, and reported out-of-pocket payments.	Etiologic fractions are not established in any country.

and premature death are counted as costs (see Chapter 8, for a discussion of how well informed smokers are about the risks of smoking). Economic value-of-life measures are used for evaluating this cost. In some variations of GSCA, all costs are included regardless of the smoker's expectations, and the loss of life is valued as the loss of production to society from premature death. In EXBA, costs are lost revenues from premature death, which are mostly lost tax payments and contributions to public health insurance programs.

Indirect costs include those imposed on the household from smoking-related illness or premature death. These costs cover a wide range, as shown in Table 4.4. A similar list could be constructed for indirect costs imposed on private business, or other people in society, that would include, for example, increased employee health insurance premiums. In ECBA, one example is the extra insurance premiums paid by non-smokers to cover expected smoking-related claims under policies that do not distinguish smokers from non-smokers. As with other costs in ECBA, this concerns effects on society that are unanticipated, or for which adjustment for the expected effects of smoking is not possible. In GSCA, an example of these costs is the extra insurance premiums paid by non-smokers, as well as the loss of production of family members who must care for an ill smoker, even if the probability of smoking-related illness was known by all. In EXBA, an example is the government expenditures caused by illness and premature death from smoking, and those for family members who forego employment to care for an ill smoker. Estimation of indirect economic effects in developing countries must consider the problem of incomplete insurance markets (Dinwiddy and Teal 1996).

The remaining cost categories include more familiar externalities from smoking. These are mostly from death and illness caused by exposure to environmental tobacco smoke, and property damage and injuries caused by smoking-related fires.

4.3.3 Production

On the production side, there are minor benefits. In ECBA, the benefit is producer surplus. In EXBA, the benefits might include producer tax revenues that are not passed on to smokers, although these are likely to be negligible.

The cost categories under production include externalities concerning health and environmental pollution. These costs can be particularly important for some developing countries. For example, tobacco workers may suffer nicotine poisoning known as green tobacco sickness through handling uncured tobacco leaves (Hipke 1993; Ballard *et al.* 1995).

There are three types of environmental cost associated with tobacco production. The first is soil degradation, which occurs because of the high nutrient requirement of tobacco. This high nutrient requirement can lead to pest infestation, and either 'soil mining' or environmental pollution form heavy fertilizer use (Geist 1999a). The second externality is deforestation from the intensive use of wood that is used in curing and processing tobacco leaf (Geist 1998, 1999b, 2000). Third, tobacco production requires large amounts of pesticides that may escape tobacco fields and cause ground and water pollution, and sickness among workers (Erdmann and Pinheiro 1998). Each definition of cost will lead to a different cost estimate. ECBA will define costs as

Table 4.4 Economic effects of fatal illness on the household: type and timing of impact

Type of impact	Timing of Impact			
	Before illness	During illness	Immediate effect of death	Long-term effect of death
Effect on production and earnings	Organization of economic activity Residential location	Reduced productivity of ill adult Re-allocation of labor	Lost output of deceased	Lost output of deceased Reallocation of land and labor
Effect on investment and consumption	Insurance Precautionary savings	Time and household resources use in treatment Spending savings Changes in consumption and investment	Funeral costs Legal fees	Changes in type and quantity of investment and consumption
Effect on household health and composition	Extended family Fertility	Reduced allocation of labor to health maintaining activities	Loss of deceased	Poor health of surviving household members Dissolution or reconstitution of household
Psychic costs		Disutility of ill individual	Disutility to individual Grief of loved ones	

Source: adapted from Table 4.1 in Over, M. et al. 1992 from *The Health of Adults in the Developing World*, edited by Richard Feachem et al., Copyright 1992 by International Bank for Reconstruction and Development/The World Bank. Used by permission of Oxford University Press, Inc. (1992).

welfare losses to individuals that occur because of the environmental externalities, or from unexpected effects of working in tobacco production. GSCA will count social costs, principally production losses due to production externalities. EXBA will count governmental, or other organizational, money expenditures.

4.4 Review of cost estimates of tobacco use

This section presents a critical review of estimates of the costs of cigarette smoking and other forms of tobacco use. First, several methodological issues which are used in the detailed descriptions below are discussed. Second, the individual studies and their results are reviewed. Additional reviews of estimates of the cost of smoking can be found in Markandya and Pearce (1989), and Robson and Single (1995).

4.4.1 Methodological issues

Current, future, gross, and net costs

A number of studies attempt to estimate the cost of all past and current smoking; these costs can occur in both the present and the future. Whether future expected costs should be included in the estimate depends on the question that the estimate is intended to answer. The most important element of future costs results from the decreased life expectancy of smokers. In expenditure-based estimates, the shorter life expectancies for smokers will produce cost savings through lower social insurance payments, and increase costs through reduced tax revenues. In some cases the answer to whether future costs should be included is clear: EXBA estimates to be used for budget planning should include expected future costs. However, future costs estimated for expenditure-based analyses should not be confused with economic cost–benefit estimates of economic welfare. The estimation of expected future costs differ under these two definitions. In ECBA, for example, many future costs and benefits from changes in life expectancy due to smoking will be included in the price of tobacco and other prices, to the extent that smokers and other agents in the economy understand the effects of smoking on mortality. Estimating all the costs and savings of changes in life expectancy separately and adding them to the estimate will result in double counting.

The issue of aggregation over time must be addressed whenever future costs are reported as a single summary statistic. Most estimates use the real net present value of future costs, and are therefore adjusted using a real social discount rate. The appropriate real discount rate to use is controversial. It is possible to use a zero discount rate, but if expenditure streams are aggregated over the infinite future, the sum of the costs in each period can be infinite. In developed countries, a real discount rate of between 2.5% and 5% is appropriate when changes in costs are widely dispersed throughout society, when there is a reduction in costs, or when the price of capital is not significantly affected by the proposed program change (Zerbe and Dively 1994). Where a social program uses resources that increase the price or availability of capital significantly, the real discount rate is more appropriately determined by the cost of borrowing funds for capital investment, and may be as high as 10%. Discount rates used in various studies range from 2.5% to 10%, with, 3% being the most common. The use of very low real discount rates may be interpreted as implying that all health-care is consumption and none is investment, which may not be a good assumption, particularly in developing countries (see Dinwiddy and Teal (1996) and Stiglitz (1994a) for a discussion of appropriate real discount rates).

A related issue concerns the computation of *gross* versus *net* costs. Gross costs are defined as all of the costs of treating smoking-attributable diseases and all other costs that can be attributed to smoking. They are usually an estimate of costs at any point in time, and are *not* a comparison of the lifetime costs of smokers versus those of non-smokers. Net costs, in contrast, tend to be assessed over lifetimes and are often expressed as a comparison of the lifetime costs of smokers versus those of non-smokers. Net costs take account of the fact that smokers tend to die younger than non-smokers and that they therefore avoid some healthcare costs, and forego some pension benefits, in old age. There are many approaches to calculating net costs. One approach is to estimate the net present value of smoking costs until all those people alive today who have ever smoked are dead, or until a non-smoking population is reached. Another approach is to estimate the difference between costs with the current smoking prevalence and costs in a stationary non-smoking population. A third approach deducts from gross costs the costs of dead smokers who would be alive now if they had not smoked in the past. A fourth deducts the future costs of smokers who died from tobacco-related illness in the current year. Each approach has a different interpretation, which should be considered carefully when the net cost estimate is used for policy analysis. Each approach requires strong assumptions about either the future or the past, including assumptions about smoking prevalence, patterns of healthcare utilization, relative costs, and life expectancies. Almost all studies assume that current conditions can be extrapolated over the average life span.

Life-cycle versus cross-section estimates

Two approaches have commonly been used to estimate costs: the *life-cycle approach* and the *cross-section approach*. Life-cycle studies can be considered incidence-based approaches to calculating costs. This approach estimates costs for smokers and non-smokers over their entire expected lifetimes. The estimated lifetime costs of the existing population of smokers and non-smokers is compared with those for a corresponding hypothetical non-smoking population. The life-cycle approach directly estimates the effect of the shorter life-span of smokers and the resultant change in costs. Summary estimates of current and future costs that aggregate cost flows over time are calculated using net present value analysis (Hodgson 1992). Life-cycle estimates can be used to estimate current costs by simply omitting expected future costs and savings.

Cross-section studies are based on the methodology of Cooper and Rice (Cooper and Rice 1976; Rice *et al.* 1986; Bartlett *et al.* 1994; Max and Rice 1995). The cross-section approach can be considered a prevalence-based approach: it estimates current costs as a function of the effects of all current and past smoking (Rice *et al.* 1986). Cross-section estimates are based on the costs incurred by currently living or recently deceased smokers without examining the effect of smoking on their life expectancies. They do not, therefore, capture the effects of changes in life expectancy as a function of smoking, and do not include this effect on future costs. However, cross-section estimates can be adjusted to approximate the effects of changes in life expectancy due to smoking status, and can serve as an approximation to net costs estimated with the life-cycle approach.

The quantification of future costs in life-cycle estimates can pose difficult problems. Changes in demographic structure will affect future costs, and forecasts of future demographic changes require strong assumptions because patterns of morbidity and mortality can change rapidly. It is possible, for example, that health will improve for persons in any age group, including the old and very old. This is a particularly important issue for developing countries because the percentage of the population that lives long enough to experience the chronic effects of smoking may increase rapidly (Feachem *et al.* 1995). Also, the cost of services is usually concentrated just before death. In developing countries, these costs may be less dependent on hospital care and more dependent on less-quantifiable transfers from other family members. Finally, aging populations may actually provide resources by providing care to younger ill populations and through other transfers (Normand 1998), particularly in developing countries. However, the very old may require significantly more support from the younger generation in the non-market sector of the economy (James 1994). In at least one study in a US health-maintenance organization (Scitovsky 1994), the oldest group of patients received much less resource-intensive medical care than middle-aged or younger patients, but they did receive more support from families, nursing homes, and home healthcare services. Utilization rates may also change dramatically, especially in developing countries. Similarly, it is difficult to estimate the demographic composition of hypothetical non-smoking populations for use in computing net costs in cross-section studies.

Reporting costs attributable to tobacco use

Careful attention must be paid to how costs are reported in various studies. Aggregate costs have been reported in both cross-section studies (Rice *et al.* 1986) and life-cycle studies (Leu and Schaub 1983). Hodgson (1992) reported the lifetime cost per person for tobacco use in one life-cycle study. Lippiatt (1990) reported the net change in cost per life-year gained from smoking cessation in a life-cycle study. The external cost per pack of cigarettes is often calculated for estimates of the external burden of smoking (see, for example, Manning *et al.* 1989). The cost per unit sold is a useful measure for tax planning; however, it will be difficult to estimate in countries such as Bangladesh and India where manufactured products sold in formal markets constitute a smaller part of consumption (World Health Organization 1997). Measuring costs as a fraction of GDP is a useful measure of aggregate costs, and this measure is used for comparison whenever possible in this review.

Cross-section studies that estimate only current gross costs usually report aggregate costs. Since these estimates take the population and smoking prevalence as fixed, total cost can be readily converted into the other measures. This is not true for net costs because a non-smoking population will have more life-years than one with some smoking over the expected life spans, and the size of the smoking population will usually differ from that of a non-smoking one. Therefore, the same total costs will imply different costs per person, or per life-year, for a non-smoking population than for a population in which some people smoke. This measurement issue is particularly important for developing countries where rapid demographic change is expected (for further discussion see Thompson and Forbes (1985).

Statistical issues in measuring costs attributable to tobacco use

There are two important statistical issues involved in the measurement of tobacco-related expenditures for cost analysis that need further discussion. These are the relative risks, for smokers versus non-smokers, of using healthcare services, and the possibility of confounding from other health-related characteristics of smokers that would not change if they did not smoke.

Relative risk of using healthcare services from smoking

The smoking-attributable fraction (SAF) is used to calculate the proportion of costs attributable to a given risk factor. Two components are necessary for its estimation: the relative risk of the outcome due to exposure to the risk factor, and the prevalence of the risk factor. The relative risk of healthcare utilization for smokers versus non-smokers has been estimated using two different methods. The first is called the *synthetic method*, since the estimates are built from assumptions about the relative risk and costs of smoking for individual diseases. This method selects those diseases that are known or strongly suspected to be caused by smoking and uses estimates of the relative risk of each disease and smoking prevalence to estimate a disease-specific SAF.

In high-income countries, separate disease-specific SAFs for many health care services have been estimated from survey and observational data (Rice *et al.* 1986; Miller *et al.* 1998a, 1998b). When the necessary SAF data are not available, researchers have used mortality-based or a combination of morbidity and mortality-based SAFs (Collins and Lapsley 1991). Mortality-based etiologic fractions may under-estimate the true fraction because many diseases caused by tobacco (such as chronic obstructive pulmonary disease) do not cause death until after a prolonged period of morbidity. This morbidity will cause a higher relative rate of utilization than that reflected in a mortality ratio. Alternatively, they may over-estimate it if smoking-related deaths occur after less expensive courses of treatment than non-smoking related deaths. Thus, SAFs may vary considerably across studies.

Assuming accurate disease-specific SAFs, the synthetic method produces conservative estimates of the disease burden of smoking, since it includes only conditions known to be caused by smoking. Consequently, it may significantly under-estimate smoking-related costs. The number of conditions known to be caused by smoking has increased over time (US Department of Health and Human Services (USDHHS) 1989). For example, male infertility and impotence have recently been linked to smoking. Co-morbidities (diseases where smoking is one of several contributing factors) are difficult to include using the synthetic approach, and adjustments to account for them may produce either over-estimates or under-estimates (Xie *et al.* 1996).

The second approach is the *analytic method*. This uses statistical estimates of all resources used by smokers versus non-smokers. In this approach, etiologic fractions are estimated from regression analyses employing data on healthcare utilization and expenditures, risk behavior, socio-demographic status, and health outcomes. The analytic method captures all differences in healthcare costs for smokers and non-smokers, including those from conditions and diseases that are not currently known to be caused by smoking. This approach also provides better adjustments for population characteristics, other risk behaviors, access to medical care, and co-morbidities. A disadvantage of this approach is that it may over-estimate the reduction in healthcare costs if smokers stop smoking. This is because it may be difficult to determine how much of the difference in utilization is due to smoking itself, as opposed to other unmeasured behaviors and characteristics of smokers that will not change, even if these people did not smoke. This issue is discussed further below. A disadvantage of this approach for developing countries is that the necessary data are unlikely to be available. For example, the National Medical Expenditure Survey II (NMES II), used in recent analyses in the United States, was very expensive to develop. However, methodological issues raised in studies in the high-income countries that use the analytic approach will be useful for planning and implementing future surveys in developing countries (Mackay and Crofton 1996).

Confounding from other behaviors and characteristics of smokers

Smokers differ from non-smokers in several ways that are not causally related to smoking and that may remain unchanged even if smokers become non-smokers. Smokers and non-smokers have different levels of education and income, and different rates of insurance coverage, alcohol use, physical activity, and other risk behaviors (Hodgson 1992). If smokers did not smoke but continued to engage in other risk behaviors, then their health expenditures would continue to be higher than those of non-smokers. Ignoring these differences between smokers and non-smokers could lead to an over-estimate of the costs of smoking. In order to handle this problem, investigators have modeled the so-called 'non-smoking smoker' type: that is, a person who does not smoke but has the other characteristics typical of smokers.

There have been two approaches to modeling the non-smoking smoker type. The first approach is relatively *ad hoc*, allocating a fixed proportion of the excess risk of disease to smoking itself, and the remainder to the other characteristics of smokers (Leu and Schaub 1983; Hodgson 1992). This approach has been criticized as being arbitrary (Rice *et al.* 1986; Hodgson 1992). The second approach is to adjust the data statistically for these differences. Statistical adjustment can be used with the synthetic method when estimating SAFs for particular diseases, or with the analytic method when estimating relative healthcare use and expenditures for all diseases. This approach is used when people's use of healthcare is estimated from surveys that record individual characteristics. Manning *et al.* (1989), for example, used this approach to control for drinking and other risky behaviors. That is, they estimated the non-smoking smoker types' levels of healthcare use by considering non-smokers with drinking patterns and other characteristics similar to those of smokers. This approach has the advantage of being less arbitrary than an *ad hoc* adjustment. However, it also assumes that these other factors will remain constant if smokers quit smoking. Such an assumption may be valid where education and income level are concerned, but may be less acceptable for behaviors that are affected by smoking. For example, smokers may take less exercise because of a taste for a sedentary life that is correlated with, but not caused by, smoking, but this may also be a result of the harmful respiratory effects of smoking.

4.4.2 Review of cost estimates

This section reviews cost estimates of smoking. A variety of approaches were used in these studies. Except where noted, the definitions of cost correspond most closely to expenditure-based costs from the perspective of the healthcare sector. The studies on healthcare costs are organized into groups that are reviewed in the following order: gross costs, net costs, and estimates of the external burden of healthcare costs on non-smokers. Estimates of social costs and the total social external burden of smoking are reviewed last; these estimates depend heavily on the economic organization and institutions of individual countries, so this part of the review will be selective and brief.

Estimates of gross cost

Many studies have estimated gross costs; only a few will be summarized here.[1] Whenever possible, estimates for the same region and period have been selected to increase the reliability of independent estimates and the effect of different methodologies. The studies for the United States are summarized in Table 4.5, while Table 4.6 presents the results for other high-income countries, and in Table 4.7 the results for developing countries. The US Centers for Disease Control and Prevention has distributed several versions of a computer program (SAMMEC: Smoking-Attributable Mortality, Morbidity, and Economic Costs) for use in cross-section estimates of smoking costs (Shultz 1985; Shultz *et al.* 1991). Many estimates for single regions or states in the United States using this software have appeared in the public health literature (Robson and Single 1995), and they are too numerous to review here. The SAMMEC methodology is based on the attributable-risk methodology developed for the United States (Cooper and Rice 1976; Hodgson and Meiners 1982; and Rice *et al.* 1986). Therefore it is appropriate only for use in economies with relatively well-developed healthcare systems and relatively mature smoking epidemics.

The United States

Luce and Schweitzer (1978) were among the first to estimate current gross costs for the United States. They used a synthetic cross-section approach with disease specific SAFs for malignant neoplasms, circulatory and respiratory diseases, and injuries from fires. These SAFs were applied to the average cost of each of these illnesses. No adjustment was made for smoking related characteristics. Their estimated direct costs of smoking for 1976 were US$8.2 billion, or 0.46% of GDP. This early study provides the basic methodology used by many synthetic studies based on aggregate data. A strength

---

[1] One influential cost estimate from the US Office of Technology Assessment (Merdman *et al.* 1993), and a subsequent controversial and poorly documented revision, is not discussed here because of space limitations (for a detailed discussion of these estimates see: Warner *et al.* 1999).

Table 4.5 Estimates of gross healthcare costs, United States

Study	Year of estimate	Services included[a]	Diseases included[b]	Tobacco attributable medical care costs (US$ billion)	% of GDP	Method: analytic vs. synthetic	Method: cross-section vs. life-cycle
Luce and Schweitzer (1978)	1976	F H L M O P[c]	C M R F	8.2	0.46	Synthetic	Cross-section
Rice *et al.* (1986)	1984	F H L M O P	C M R	23.3	0.62	Synthetic	Cross-section
Bartlett *et al.* (1994)	1993	F H L M P	C M R[d]	50.0	0.79	Synthetic	Cross-section
Miller *et al.* (1998b)	1993	F H L M O P	[e]	72.7	1.15	Both	Cross-section
Miller *et al.* (1999)	1993	F H L M O P	[f]	53.4	0.84	Analytic	Cross-section

[a] Services are: F, other professional medical fees; H, hospital; L, long-term care; M, medicine; O, outpatient visits; P, physician fees.
[b] Diseases are: C, cardiovascular and circulatory diseases; M, malignant neoplasms; R, non-malignant respiratory disease; F, health costs from fires.
[c] All costs included in Cooper and Rice (1976).
[d] Emphysema only included in non-malignant respiratory illness (R).
[e] Diseases included in Bartlett (1994), plus all diseases associated with poor health states due to smoking.
[f] All diseases reported in survey.

of their estimate was the use of cost-of-illness estimates from Cooper and Rice (1976), which covered many health services. The study's principal weakness is the use of relatively informal judgmental estimates for SAFs developed by an expert consensus panel.

Similarly, Rice *et al.* (1986) estimated gross costs for 1984 using a synthetic cross-section approach. This study reports aggregate costs to the healthcare system for three broad disease categories: cardiovascular disease, respiratory disease, and malignant neoplasms. The SAFs were estimated using the US National Health Interview Survey (USNHIS). Both current and former smokers were defined as smokers. These SAFs were applied to average national expenditures for various services. This study included a relatively complete list of healthcare services: hospital services, services from a physician or other professionals, nursing-home care, home healthcare, and medications. Due to a lack of data, SAFs for hospital care were applied to several other healthcare services. No adjustment was made for the non-smoking smoker type. They estimated that US$23.3 billion in healthcare costs, or 0.62% of GDP, were attributable to smoking in 1984. The use of SAFs estimated from survey data on utililization, rather than the more subjective estimates used by Luce and Schweitzer (1978) was a significant advance. The principal shortcoming of the study was that no adjustments were attempted for the non-smoker smoking type.

Bartlett *et al.* (1994) estimated gross costs for 1993 using more detailed survey data on health expenditures and characteristics of smokers versus non-smokers. SAFs were estimated for cardiovascular and cerebrovascular disease, cancer, and emphysema. The SAFs were estimated in three stages: the first stage estimated the effect of smoking on the presence of a smoking-related disease; the second estimated the probability of expenditure in each disease type; and the third estimated conditional smoking-related expenditures. Data on expenditures were taken from the 1987 NMES-II. NMES-II included all medical expenditures reported by the respondents along with extensive demographic, socioeconomic and behavioral information. NMES-II also included a survey of medical service providers reporting healthcare expenditures that respondents might not be able to report, thereby increasing the accuracy of the expenditure estimates. The study also addressed the issue of the non-smoking smoker, as well as other possible sources of bias, by extensive statistical adjustment after categorizing respondents into four categories: current smokers, those who never smoked, and two categories of ex-smokers. Health services considered included: hospital services, ambulatory care, physician services, prescription medications, and home healthcare. They estimated total costs for 1987 and extrapolated them to 1993 using expenditure data from the Health Care Financing Agency (HCFA). Their estimated cost attributable to smoking in 1993 was US$50 billion, or 0.79% of GDP. This study contained the most sophisticated adjustments for other characteristics that might differ among smokers and non-smokers and that might influence expenditures, and used the most complete survey data on individual health expenditures available. However, it limited the analysis to only a few smoking-related disease categories, and omitted other conditions known to be related to smoking (e.g. chronic bronchitis, low birthweight from maternal smoking, and ulcers). Also, SAFs for hospitals had to be used for long-term care costs given the lack of appropriate data on SAFs for long-term care.

Leonard Miller *et al.* (1998a, 1998b) developed and used a more complicated methodology. Their approach combined the synthetic and analytic methods to estimate SAFs. In the synthetic portion of the estimate, expenditures associated with known smoking-related disease categories were estimated in the same way to those of Bartlett *et al.* (1994). These estimates were adjusted based on data on demographic and socioeconomic characteristics, and risk attitudes. In addition, all other health expenditures associated with smoking were estimated, controlling for health status and health insurance status. This was intended to cover health effects associated with smoking that are not included in the major disease categories known to be caused by smoking. The analytic portion of the estimate was obtained in two steps: first, the probability of any expenditure was estimated; second, conditional health expenditures were estimated. Data from the 1987 NMES-II, the Behavioral Risk Factor Surveillance System (BRFSS) and the Current Population Survey (CPS) were used. The problem of the non-smoking smoker type was addressed by statistical adjustment in the synthetic portion of the estimate. Healthcare expenditures were estimated by applying state-specific SAFs to state healthcare expenditures supplied by HCFA. Leonard Miller *et al.* estimated the gross costs of smoking for the United States in 1993 to be US$72.7 billion or 1.15% of GDP.

This estimate was considerably higher than earlier estimates (although the 95% confidence interval for their estimates included some of the earlier estimates). One reason for this may be the use of both the synthetic and analytic approach to estimating SAFs.

The analytic portion of the estimate is supposed to account for health status. However, to the extent that self-reported health status is related to smoking, there may be some double counting of expenditures. In addition, since the study used the same expenditure data as Bartlett *et al.* (1994), the problems associated with estimating long-term care costs remain.

Vincent Miller *et al.* (1999) provides the most recent estimate of gross costs for the United States. These researchers used an analytic approach and estimated costs directly from the 1987 NMES-II. SAFs were calculated from expenditures predicted for the current population and a hypothetical non-smoking population. State-specific SAFs were calculated and applied to 1993 expenditure data to estimate state costs, then summed for the national total. The estimation approach employed is simpler than of Leonard Miller *et al.* (1998b). Two equations are estimated for each of four expenditure categories: ambulatory care, hospital care, prescription medications, and other expenses. One equation predicts the probability of a positive expenditure in each cost category; the second estimates the size of the expenditure, conditional on a positive expenditure. Expenditures attributable to smoking are adjusted for smokers' other characteristics that may influence health expenditures. These include demographic, socio-economic, and life-style characteristics, as well as health insurance status. Their estimate of costs for 1993 was US$53.4 billion, or 0.84% of GDP.

The estimate by Vincent Miller *et al.* (1999). was much lower than that of Leonard Miller *et al.* (1998b), even though the two studies used similar data and methods. Part of the difference results from the simpler statistical specification of the more recent study that they describe as a set of reduced-form equations in which all explanatory variables are exogenous. However, the authors neither justify the chosen reduced-form specifications, nor do they perform any exogeneity tests. Examination of the regression specification reveals some variables that may well not be exogenous. For example, both self-reported taste for risk, as well as specific risk behaviors, such as seat-belt use were included in the specification, which cannot occur in a true reduced form. Also, self-reported physical activity is used as an explanatory variable; however, the level of physical activity is probably affected by smoking as well as being an indicator of smokers' tastes. Failing to account for endogeneity can easily result in biased estimates.

High-income countries other than the United States

Australia   Collins and Lapsley (1991, 1996) provide cross-section estimates using the synthetic approach, closely following a GDP-based definition of social costs. Both gross and net costs are estimated; the gross cost estimates are discussed here, and net costs are discussed below. SAFs for current and ex-smokers are estimated from meta-analyses of the relative risks for smoking-related conditions (although some of the SAFs used in the 1991 study were based on relative risks of mortality). No adjustment is made for the non-smoking smoker type. Medical care included hospital care, the services of physicians and other professionals, medications, nursing homes, home and community health services, and allied healthcare services. The costs of healthcare were estimated from the average costs of professional encounters or institutional bed-days. Their original (1991) gross cost estimate for 1988 was Aust$759.5 million, or 0.24% of

Table 4.6 Estimates of gross health care costs, other high-income countries

Authors	Year of estimate	Services included[a]	Diseases included[b]	Tobacco attributable medical care costs	% of GDP	Method: analytic vs. synthetic	Method: cross section vs. life cycle
Australia				Aust$ million			
Collins and Lapsley (1991)	1988	F H L M O P	C G M O R	759.5	0.24	Synthetic	Cross-section
Collins and Lapsley (1996)	1988	F H L M O P	C G M O R	910.9	0.29	Synthetic	Cross-section
Collins and Lapsley (1996)	1992	F H L M O P	C G M O R	1597.5	0.41	Synthetic	Cross-section
Canada				Can$ million			
Collishaw and Myers (1984)	1979	H P	[c]	1118.0	0.40	Analytic	Cross-section
Choi and Nethercott (1988) (Ontario)	1979	H P	[c]	261.0	0.25	Analytic	Cross-section
Raynauld and Vidal (1992)	1986	H[d]	Is MR[e]	615.0	0.12	Synthetic	Cross-section
Choi and Pak (1996) (Ontario)	1988	H P	[c]	765.0	0.30	Analytic	Cross-section
Xie et al. (1996) (Ontario)	1992	F H L M O P	C G M O R	1073.0	0.38	Synthetic	Cross-section
Kaiserman (1997)	1991	H L M O P	[c]	3798.0	0.56	Analytic	Life-cycle
Finland				FIM million			
Pekurinen (1992)	1987	H M O P	C M R	524–594	0.14–0.15	Both	Cross-section
Pekurinen (1999)	1995	H M O P	C M R	924.0	0.17	Both	Cross-section
New Zealand				NZ$ million			
Gray et al. (1988)	1984	H	C M R O[f]	61	0.16	Synthetic	Cross-section
Phillips et al. (1992)	1989	H M O P	C M R O[f]	185.4	0.29	Synthetic	Cross-section
United Kingdom				£ million			
Maynard et al. (1987)	1985–86	[g]	C G M R	290–497	0.08–0.13	Synthetic	Cross-section

[a] Services are: F, other professional medical fees; H, hospital; L, long-term care; M, medicine; O, outpatient visits; P, physician fees.

[b] Diseases are: C, cardiovascular and circulatory disease; G, gastrointestinal diseases; Is, ischemic heart disease; M, malignant neoplasms; R, non-malignant respiratory disease; O, other. (C includes Is.)

[c] Estimates of attributable risk for hospitalization for all causes due to tobacco use from survey data. Includes medical costs from fires.

[d] Includes other unspecified health service expenditures. See text for discussion.

[e] Non-malignant respiratory disease (R) includes COPD only.

[f] Other diseases (O) includes fire injuries and perinatal complications.

[g] Estimated inpatient, outpatient, and general practice expenditures to National Health Service.

GDP. Their revised (1996) estimate for 1988 increased to Aust$910.9 million, or 0.29% of GDP. The estimate in the 1996 report for 1992 was Aust$1.6 billion, or 0.41% of that year's GDP. They attributed the increase in costs to an increase in the number of diseases that are known to be caused by smoking, increases in SAFs, and the use of disease-specific averages for hospital costs. A strength of these synthetic estimates is the use of a comprehensive list of smoking related diseases.

Canada   Collishaw and Myers (1984) estimated gross costs for 1979 using the analytic method. The costs of hospitalization and physicians' services were estimated with SAFs for utilization calculated from the Canada Health Survey. These SAFs were applied to total days of hospital care and physician visits and the average cost per hospital separation or visit. No adjustments were made for the non-smoking smoker type. They concluded that smoking increased healthcare costs in Canada by Can$1.12 billion in 1979, or 0.4% of GDP.

Choi and Nethercott (1988) and Choi and Pak (1996) adapted the approach of Collishaw and Myers to Ontario Province, Canada for 1979 and 1988, respectively, using local estimates of the costs of using hospitals' and physicians' services. Estimated costs for 1979 and 1988 were 0.25% and 0.30% of Ontario's GDP, much lower than the national estimates of Collishaw and Myers.

Raynauld and Vidal (1992) conducted a synthetic study that included ischemic heart disease, cancer and chronic obstructive pulmonary disease. SAFs were calculated using data from the United States. Hospitalization costs are included. Other healthcare services are included but these are not clearly specified and apparently do not include long-term care for the elderly. These other costs are estimated by extrapolating costs for Saskatchewan to all of Canada and applying the SAFs to that estimate. No adjustments are made for the non-smoking smoker type. The estimate of gross costs for 1986 is Can$ 615 million, or 0.12% of Canadian GDP. This low estimate may be due to the restricted number of diseases included. However, it is difficult to evaluate the estimate because of the incomplete specification of the medical services included.

Xie *et al.* (1996, also reported in Xie *et al.* 1999) provide a more recent estimate for Ontario, based on the CCSA guidelines and using the synthetic approach. They used relative risks for smoking-related disease taken from the literature, and used separate SAFs for morbidity and mortality. Separate age-specific and gender-specific SAFs were calculated for current and former smokers and those who had never smoked, using relative risks from the literature, and prevalence rates for Ontario. An unusual feature of the estimates is an attempt to include the costs of co-morbidity due to tobacco. All major health services were included in the estimate. Total utilization levels were from Ontario health reports, or estimated from Canadian data. The cost data were average costs per episode of care, or average per capita costs. The SAFs were applied to total levels of utilization, and costs were estimated from average cost data. No adjustments were made for the non-smoking smoker type. Xie *et al.* estimated that the gross costs for 1992 were Can$1.1 billion or 0.38% of Ontario GDP. Two strengths of this study are the careful use of relative risks for morbidity in estimating the SAFs, and the comprehensive list of diseases used.

The same team of authors also produced an estimate for all of Canada (Single *et al.*

1996b) that also very closely follows the CCSA guidelines for cost estimates. The results are quite close to the estimates of Xie *et al.* (1996): the gross medical costs for Canada were Can$2 676 million in 1992, or 0.39% of that year's GDP.

Kaiserman (1997) estimated both gross and net costs for 1986 using the approach of Rice *et al.* (1986). The gross cost estimates are reported here. Costs were estimated using the analytic method by comparing smokers' and non-smokers' use of health services. Relative risks for hospital admissions, outpatient visits, and prescription drugs were calculated from Canadian national survey data. SAFs were calculated from these relative risks and Canadian smoking prevalence. Average hospital costs were estimated from published reports from Canadian survey data. The Canadian Medical Association estimated average outpatient costs, and the average prescription cost was estimated from Ontario data. No adjustment was made for the non-smoking smoker type. Kaiserman estimated that direct medical costs in 1991 were Can$3.8 billion, or 0.56% of GDP, much higher than the other Canadian estimates. The differences result, in part, from Kaiserman's exclusion of observations that implied lower costs for smokers, which likely biased the estimates upward.

Finland Pekurinen (1992) conducted a cross-section study for Finland that reported both gross and net costs. The gross costs are discussed here. Hospital care, prescription medicine, outpatient visits, and physician services are included in the analysis. The study used both analytic and synthetic approaches. Hospitalization costs were estimated using the synthetic method; the diseases included were smoking-related cancers, cardiovascular disease, and respiratory disease (bronchitis and chronic obstructive pulmonary disease). Low and high estimates of SAFs were chosen from previous studies, and generally limited to those diseases with long-established evidence of a causal association with smoking. Average daily hospital costs and total utilization were estimated from Finnish survey data. The costs of visits to physicians and outpatient care were estimated using the analytic method from Finnish survey data that included information on smoking status, combined with average costs per visit estimated from separate data sources. Prescription medicine costs were estimated using Finnish survey data using the same methods as for physician costs. There was no adjustment for the non-smoking smoker type. Pekurinen's estimated gross costs for 1987 ranged from FIM524 to FIM594 million, or between 0.14% and 0.15% of GDP, respectively.

Pekurinen (1999) recently updated these estimates, using more recent relative risk estimates for smoking-related disease and new national data. The estimated costs for 1995 were FIM924 million, or 0.17% of GDP. The estimated total cost thus remained approximately the same as a percentage of GDP. However, the apparent similarity of the earlier and later estimates hid several significant changes that had taken place in Finland over the period: decreased smoking prevalence, increased hospital utilization and increased average costs.

New Zealand Gray *et al.* (1988) used a synthetic approach to estimating gross costs from cardiovascular and cerebrovascular disease, smoking related cancers, chronic obstructive pulmonary disease, low birthweight, and fire injuries. The only healthcare service included was hospitalization for acute care. Age- and gender-specific SAFs for hospitalization were calculated from relative risks for mortality attributable to smoking, using prevalence data from the New Zealand census. Costs were estimated by applying the SAFs to total utilization and average cost per hospital day from national survey data. No adjustment was made for the non-smoking smoker type. Direct hospital costs were estimated to be NZ$61 million for 1984, or 0.16% of GDP. This early study provides conservative estimates because it is limited to hospital costs and includes only the major smoking-related diseases.

Phillips *et al.* (1992) used a synthetic approach to update and refine the estimates of Gray *et al.* (1988). They included the same diseases but also took account of outpatient visits, professional services and prescription drugs, as well as hospitalization for acute care. Their SAFs for hospitalization were taken from previous studies for Australia and New Zealand. Their SAF for prescription drugs were estimated from a random sample within a private practice, while that for outpatient care was based on data from a regional survey. Average costs of hospitalization were disease-specific estimates taken from hospital cost-reporting systems. The costs of an average outpatient visit and prescription drugs were calculated from published fee schedules. No adjustment was made for the non-smoking smoker type. Their estimated direct medical costs of smoking for 1989 were NZ$185.4 million, or 0.29% of GDP.

United Kingdom   Maynard *et al.* (1987) estimated the 1985–86 budgetary cost of smoking for the National Health Service (NHS) in the United Kingdom. This study used the synthetic method applied to cardiovascular, malignant and benign respiratory disease, other cancers, and gastrointestinal disease. The SAFs were taken from studies by the Royal College of Physicians, and cost data for hospitalization, outpatient services, and visits to general practitioners were obtained from the NHS. No adjustment was made for the non-smoking smoker type. The researchers estimated that smoking cost between £290 million and £497 million in 1985–86, or between 0.08% and 0.13% of GDP. Their estimate is surprisingly low, given that the prevalence of smoking in the United Kingdom is comparable to that in other developed countries, even after considering the relatively low rate of national health expenditure in the United Kingdom as a percentage of GDP. Few details are provided, however, making it difficult to assess the quality of the estimates.

Middle-income and low-income countries

South Africa   Yach (1982) estimated gross costs using the synthetic approach, and included costs from ischemic heart disease, cancer, and bronchitis. SAFs specific to South Africa's different racial and ethnic groups were calculated from relative risk statistics in the literature. Estimates of smoking prevalence in South Africa were also made separately for each racial and ethnic group. Of healthcare services, only hospital costs were included, and these were estimated from the average length of stay and average cost per day in South African hospitals. There was no adjustment for the non-smoking smoker type. The total estimated smoking-attributable costs were 17.6 million Rand, or 0.03% of GDP. This is a very early study based on limited data; hence, it is likely to have under-estimated smoking-related costs.

McIntyre and Taylor (1989) provide a synthetic estimate for South Africa that includes the costs of circulatory and benign respiratory diseases, chronic obstructive

Table 4.7 Estimates of gross healthcare costs for developing countries

Study	Year of estimate[a]	Services included[a]	Diseases included[b]	Tobacco attributable medical care costs	% of GDP	Method: analytic vs. synthetic	Method: cross section vs. life cycle
South Africa				Rand million			
Yach (1982)	1980–81	H	Is M R[c]	17.6	0.03	Synthetic	Cross-section
McIntyre and Taylor (1989)	1985	H O P	C M R[d]	128.5	0.10	Synthetic	Cross-section
Puerto Rico				US$ million			
Dietz et al. (1991)	1983	F H L M O P	C G M R O[e]	55.9	0.43	Synthetic	Cross-section
India				Rupees million			
Rath and Chaudry (1995)	1990–91	H P	M[f]	833.0	0.02	Synthetic	Cross-section
Peoples Republic of China				Yuan billion			
Jin et al. (1995)	1989	H O	C G M R	6.94	0.43	Synthetic	Cross-section
Venezuela				Bolivares billion			
Pan American Sanitary Bureau (1998)	1997	H[g]	C M R O	129.0	0.30	Synthetic	Cross-section

[a] Services are: F, other professional medical fees; H, hospital; L, long-term care; M, medicine; O, outpatient visits; P, physician fees.
[b] Diseases are: C, cardiovascular and circulatory diseases; G, gastrointestinal diseases; Is, ischemic heart disease; M, malignant neoplasms; R, non-malignant respiratory disease; O, other. (C includes Is.)
[c] Non-malignant respiratory disease (R) includes bronchitis only.
[d] Non-malignant respiratory disease (R) includes COPD only.
[e] Other disease (O) includes tuberculosis and pediatric conditions.
[f] Costs for first 3 years of treatment only for cancers of oral cavity, pharynx, larynx, and lungs.
[g] Includes basic hospital room and board services only; omits tests, examinations, intensive care and other services.

pulmonary disease, and cancer. The SAFs for hospitalizations and outpatient visits were assumed to be equal to the SAF for mortality. The cost of a hospital day and an outpatient visit were estimated from costs in the Cape Province. The researchers' estimated gross costs for 1985 were 128.5 million Rand, or 0.10% of GDP. Although this figure is higher than that of Yach (1982) it is also based on very limited data and is likely to have under-estimated gross costs.

Puerto Rico   Dietz *et al.* (1991) estimated costs for 1983 using the synthetic approach. The diseases considered were cancer, diseases of the circulatory, respiratory and digestive organs, tuberculosis, and pediatric and infant conditions. SAFs were calculated from US mortality data and Puerto Rican rates of smoking. Healthcare utilization rates were taken from US data. Average cost data were from the HCFA and the Puerto Rican Department of Health. There was no adjustment for the non-smoking smoker type. The health services considered were the same as in Rice *et al.* (1986). The estimated cost for 1983 was US$ 55.9 million, or 0.43% of GDP. This study is one of the most complete for a developing country, but the use of US data for relative risk and healthcare utilization is an important limitation.

India   Rath and Chaudry (1995) estimated the cost of treatment for the first three years of care for cancers that have a high SAF. These include cancers of the oral cavity, larynx, pharynx, and lungs. The data are from a sequential sample of 342 patients in a New Delhi cancer center who were followed until death or 3 years from their initial hospital visit. All expenditures for diagnosis, hospital treatment, and physician consultation were recorded. Estimates for India were derived from the costs per patient in the sample, from the total number of the sample members' hospital admissions for the cancers, and the SAF of the cancers. The total estimated cost of cancer care due to tobacco use for these cancers in India was 833 million Rupees, or 0.02% of GDP.

People's Republic of China   Jin *et al.* (1995) estimated the gross costs of smoking using the synthetic method. They included smoking-related cancers, coronary heart disease, stroke, hypertension, respiratory diseases, and ulcers. SAFs were calculated from age-specific and gender-specific smoking rates and relative risks for death and morbidity from previous research in China. Estimates of the level of healthcare use were made for each disease, using a 1985–86 survey on health services that included both urban and rural areas. Costs for outpatient visits and hospitalization were taken from national data on fees, categorized by disease and type of institution. No adjustment was made for the non-smoking smoker type. Estimated costs were 6.94 billion Yuan in 1989, or 0.43% of GDP. Rural areas accounted for 62% and urban areas 38% of the total. Men accounted for most of the costs because of the higher prevalence and longer history of smoking in men (see Chapter 2).

The breakdown of direct costs by each disease is interesting. Respiratory illness (other than cancer) accounted for 58.8% of the total direct cost. Circulatory disease accounted for 14.5% and all cancers accounted for only 6.1%. The relatively high proportion of costs due to non-malignant respiratory illness may be related to the joint effects of smoking and air pollution (both indoor and outdoor) in China. This study is one of the most complete for developing countries. Its greatest strength is the use of data from national surveys and health censuses to estimate SAFs, utilization rates and costs.

Venezuela The Pan American Sanitary Bureau (1998), part of the Pan-American Health Organization, provided a recent estimate of costs for 1967–97 and part of 1998 using the synthetic method. The conditions included are smoking-related cancers, cardiovascular disease, other benign respiratory disease, and childhood diseases resulting from active and passive smoking. The services included are: hospital inpatient care, medications, and selected outpatient treatments (such as radiation therapy and cardiac rehabilitation). The non-smoking smoker type is not discussed. The estimated costs for basic services in 1997 are 129 billion Bolivares, or 0.30% of GDP. Other hospital-based expenditures for tests, prescriptions, intensive care, and other services are not broken down by year. The total costs for all hospital services for 1967–97 implies a ratio of 1.55 of these other cost categories for every Bolivare spent in basic service costs. Applying this ratio produces a total hospital cost of 200 billion Bolivares, or 0.47% of GDP in 1997.

Estimates of net costs

We turn now to a review of the existing estimates of net costs, which, as we have seen, take account of the impact of smokers' tendency to die earlier than non-smokers. These are summarized in Table 4.8. Several are quite controversial, because they include cost savings resulting from premature tobacco-related death. Several techniques have been used to calculate net costs, making comparison between studies difficult. This review reports the cost estimates contained in the studies, along with, where possible, estimates that could be calculated without using additional assumptions not stated in the study. For cross-section studies, the net estimates reported in the study will be given. The results of life-cycle studies that report the costs of stationary populations depend heavily on current smoking prevalence. Therefore, the ratio of the lifetime costs of a smoker versus a non-smoker will be reported whenever available. Otherwise the net present value of the costs of the current cohort of smokers will be reported. Adjusted cross-section studies will be discussed first, followed by a review of the life-cycle studies.

Cross-section estimates

Australia Collins and Lapsley (1991, 1996) estimated net costs for 1988 by estimating the healthcare costs of people who would have been alive in 1988 had they not smoked. They note that these calculations are speculative because there are no relative risk estimates for tobacco-related mortality for older individuals. In their 1991 study, they used SAFs from Holman and Armstrong (1990). The resulting net costs for 1988 were Aust$610 million or 0.19 of GDP, about four-fifths of gross costs. The method employed in their 1996 study was the same, except that it used revised SAF estimates from English *et al.* (1995). The resulting estimate of net cost for 1988 is Aust$484 million, just over half of their gross costs estimate. The estimate for 1992 is Aust$833 million, or 0.21% of GDP for that year. The increase in estimated smoking-related mortality rates accounts for the difference in their estimates.

Table 4.8 Estimates of net healthcare costs for high-income countries

Study	Year of estimate	Services included[a]	Diseases included[b]	Discount rate (%)	Annual tobacco-attributable medical care costs[c]	% of GDP	Smoker/non-smoker costs	Method: analytic vs. synthetic
Adjusted cross-section								
Australia					Aust$ million			
Collins and Lapsley (1991)	1988	F H L M O P	C G M O R	—	609.6	0.19	—	Synthetic
Collins and Lapsley (1996)	1988	F H L M O P	C G M O R	—	484.1	0.15	—	Synthetic
Collins and Lapsley (1996)	1992	F H L M O P	C G M O R	—	832.5	0.21	—	Synthetic
Canada					Can$ billon			
Forbes and Thompson (1983)	1980	H L P	[d]	—	1.16	0.37	Men: 1.25 Women: 1.15	Both
Kaiserman (1997)	1991	H L M P	[e]	4	2.3	0.34	—	Analytic
Finland					FIM million			
Pekurinen (1992)	1987	H M O P	C M R	4	(16) to 93	<0.024	—	Both
Life-cycle								
Switzerland					Swiss Franc million			
Leu and Schaub (1983)	1976	H P	Is M R	0	0	0	0.93–1.00[g]	Synthetic
Leu and Schaub (1985)	1976	H P	[e]	0–10	—	—	0.83–0.97[g]	Analytic
United States					US$ billion			
Lippiatt (1990)	1986	F H L M O P	Is M R	3–5	(49.5)–(22.3)[h]	—	—	Synthetic
Manning et al. (1991)	1986	F H L M O P[f]	[e]	5	9.2	0.22	—	Analytic
Hodgson (1992)	1985	F H L O P	[e]	3–5 3 for ratio	501–473[h]	—	Men: 1.32 Women: 1.24	Analytic
Netherlands					Guilders billion			
Barendregt et al. (1997)	1988	F H L M O P	C M R[j]	0	—	—	Men: 0.87 Women: 0.85	Synthetic

[a] Services are: F, other professional medical fees; H, hospital; L, long-term care; M, medicine; O, outpatient visits; P, physician fees.

[b] Diseases are: C, cardiovascular and circulatory diseases; G, gastrointestinal diseases; Is, ischemic heart disease; M, malignant neoplasms; R, non-malignant respiratory disease; O, other. (C includes Is.)

[c] See text for explanation of these columns (parentheses indicates negative cost, or net savings from smoking).

[d] Excess expenditures for all diseases inferred from excess mortality rates of smokers. Smoking-related illnesses used for children.

[e] Includes all excess expenditures of smokers estimated from survey data or health census data.

[f] Only lung cancer included in malignant neoplasm (M), only COPD included in respiratory illness (R).

[g] Range includes ratio of smokers to non-smoker and smoker to non-smoking smoking type.

[h] Present value of costs incurred by current cohort of smokers.

[j] R includes COPD Only.

Canada   Forbes and Thompson (1983) also estimated net costs using a cross-section approach. Cost is expressed as the difference in per capita healthcare costs in the current population and per capita costs in a hypothetical stationary population with no smoking. This approach has been criticized as difficult to interpret (Leu and Schaub 1985; Pekurinen 1992). Both the synthetic and analytic approaches have been used to estimate levels of use of healthcare services that result from smoking. The synthetic approach is used, and the researchers include some effects of parents' smoking on children, including some children's diseases, medical care for newborns, and complications of pregnancy. Relative risks for various smoking-related conditions of newborns and children are taken from the literature and used to calculate SAFs. These SAFs are applied to disease-specific average hospital costs per diagnosis. For adults, the SAF for hospitalization was calculated from the relative risk for hospitalization due to smoking, and the latter was assumed to be equal to the relative risks of smoking-related death in the United States. The long-term care costs of the elderly were estimated by calculating the relative proportion of elderly institutionalized smokers to the elderly proportion of the population in general, and then attributing the costs pro rata accordingly. The services included are hospitalization and long-term care for adults, and physicians' visits for children. Forbes and Thompson estimated that smoking increased the 1980 per capita medical care costs of Canadian men by 16%, and of women by 10%. This implies a net cost of Can$1.16 billion, or 0.37% of GDP. The fact that less than 30% of Canadians smoke, together with the reported average costs for the current and the hypothetical population, implies that the ratio of lifetime costs for smokers versus non-smokers is rather high: 1.25 for men and 1.15 for women.

Kaiserman (1997) estimated net costs from gross cross-section estimates by calculating the net present value of future savings from people who had died from smoking during the year, using a 4% discount rate. The SAFs for mortality were taken from a US study. The net cost for Canada is 2.3 Can$ billion, or 0.34% of GDP. Kaiserman's net cost estimate is 60% of that for gross costs. A major drawback is that this approach does not seem to account for the shorter life expectancies of smokers who survived the year.

Finland   Pekurinen (1992) estimated the net present value of savings from smoking-related deaths in 1987. As in the case of Kaiserman, this does not represent a complete analysis of net costs, and in fact Pekurinen only reports gross costs in his final results. The number of deaths from smoking was calculated using SAFs derived from the literature for selected diseases and applied to Finnish cause-of-death statistics. Net present value was calculated using a 4% discount rate. The estimated discounted future healthcare cost savings from smoking-related deaths in 1987 is between FIM430 million and FIM 610 million. Subtracting this from the gross costs results in somewhere between a net savings of FIM16 million and a net cost of FIM93 million (less than 0.024% of GDP).

Life-cycle approach

Switzerland   Leu and Schaub (1983) provide an early and well-known life-cycle cost estimate using the synthetic method. Their study used two approaches to estimating net costs. The first was a comparison between the total healthcare costs that would have been incurred for the male Swiss population in 1976, if no one who had been born after 1876 had ever smoked, with actual male healthcare costs for the same year. The second analyzed the lifetime costs of a smoker versus those of a person who had never smoked. Both of these approaches used the life-cycle approach to net costs. The SAFs were calculated from the relative risks of smoking-related mortality for various specific diseases, and were applied to the utilization rates of hospital services and physicians' services for Swiss males. The issue of the non-smoking smoker is addressed by assuming that 65% of smokers' additional use of healthcare is due to smoking. Only hospital costs and physicians' fees were included in the estimate. Net cost was estimated using two methods: the expected value of the life-cycle costs of a smoker versus a non-smoking smoker type; and simulation of a hypothetical non-smoking population. Excess mortality due to smoking was estimated using US mortality ratios stratified by age and amount smoked per day. The researchers concluded that lifetime healthcare costs are between 6% and 7% higher for non-smokers than for smokers, and that past smoking did not increase costs in 1976.

Leu and Schaub's results were controversial. The researchers have been criticized for using mortality data to estimate the SAFs, for their use of fixed, multiplicative, factors to adjust SAFs, and for the inclusion of only two major healthcare services. An additional criticism of their methods is as follows. Leu and Schaub relied on only a few smoking-related diseases to calculate the excess costs of living smokers, but used all-cause differences in mortality rates for smokers versus non-smokers. The result is that they under-estimate the lifetime costs of smoking. There are two reasons for this. First, some costs of smoking-related disease among living smokers will be missed, but will implicitly be counted as cost savings when smokers die early. Second, conditions that are considered associated with, but not caused by, smoking will be omitted from the costs of living smokers, but will be counted as costs savings after smokers die. The implication of this is that the mortality data used for life-cycle estimates must undergo the same statistical adjustments as the data for healthcare utilization and costs. Finally, the estimated health care expenditure patterns in Switzerland were very different than those in the United States, so critics have questioned the extent to which the results can be generalized to elsewhere (Hodgson 1992).

Leu and Schaub (1985) addressed most of these issues in further research. Details were not provided, but the revised estimates are based on a multi-equation econometric model for healthcare expenditures developed by Leu and Doppmann (1984) using data from the first comprehensive Swiss healthcare survey. Visits to physicians and hospitalization remained the only services included in this study, which uses the analytic approach. The lifetime costs of 35-year-old males are calculated by smoking status using discount rates from 0 to 10%. The ratio of lifetime costs of 35-year-old male smokers to non-smoking smoker types was 0.91 to 0.97 (for discount rates of 0 to 10%, respectively). The cost ratios of smokers to non-smokers ranged from 0.83 to 0.94. The non-smoking smokers had higher lifetime costs than non-smokers. These estimates answered most of the previous criticisms. However, only two major health services were still included, and it is unclear whether comparable statistical adjustments were done for estimated health utilization and mortality rates by smoking status.

United States Lippiatt (1990) conducted a life-cycle study that estimated the change in the net present value of healthcare costs for the US population aged between 25 and 79 years as a function of changes in cigarette consumption. Effects of both changes in smoking prevalence and in the average amount smoked were modeled. The synthetic approach was used to calculate excess use of healthcare services for three disease categories: lung cancer, coronary heart disease, and chronic obstructive pulmonary disease. There was no adjustment for the non-smoking smoker type. Healthcare costs included were: hospital costs, physicians' fees, and insurance fees. Changes in life-span from smoking were estimated with the life-table approach, using data from Oster *et al.* (1984a, 1984b). Average medical costs were estimated from several sources, including Leu and Schaub (1983). Lippiatt's estimates indicated that the net present value of increased healthcare costs of longer-lived ex-smokers was greater than the cost savings from reduced smoking and smoking cessation. A decrease in cigarette sales of 1% would increase the net present value of healthcare costs by between approximately US$191 million and $ 405 million (with discount rates of 5% and 3%, respectively). These estimates implied a healthcare cost of smoking cessation of between $280 and $132 per life-year gained. These estimates implied a net present value of medical care savings of between $22.3 and $49.5 billion from smoking in 1986. A strength of Lippiatt's approach is the detailed modeling of the effects of smoking based on Oster *et al.* (1984a, 1984b), particularly the estimation of the change in life expectancy of ex-smokers. The important weaknesses of the study are the very limited number of diseases included, and the use of Leu and Schaub's (1983) estimates of average medical costs.

Manning *et al.* (1989, 1991) reported a life-cycle study that estimated the net present value of the external healthcare burden in terms of cost per pack of cigarettes sold, as well as aggregate net healthcare costs. Their studies used the analytic approach to estimate excess utilization by smokers using data from the RAND Health Insurance Experiment (HIE) and the US NHIS. Statistical adjustment was used to model the cost savings for the non-smoking smoker type using socio-demographic, life-style and clinical information. A unique feature of this approach is the researchers' adjustment for two other major risk behaviors for ill health in the United States: heavy alcohol consumption and physical inactivity. The life-table method was used to model changes in population age structure from changes in smoking prevalence. Excess mortality risk was estimated from a 1984 health risk appraisal program developed by the Centers for Disease Control and Prevention. This allowed the same types of adjustments to be made for mortality rates as for healthcare use, another unique feature of this study. Data on the utilization and cost of healthcare came from the RAND HIE, and included all costs except those for maternity care, infant care, and dental care. Utilization rates for the elderly (who were omitted from the HIE) were obtained from the NHIS. Manning *et al.*'s estimates were used for an analysis of the tax rate needed to cover the net annual social costs of cigarette smoking. Therefore the costs are expressed in cents per pack. They estimated that aggregate net healthcare costs, including the costs of infant morbidity from maternal smoking, were 32 cents per pack in 1986, at a discount rate of 5%, implying total costs of US$9.2 billion, or 0.22% of GDP. The main strength of these estimates was the consistent analysis of smoking-related mortality and morbidity. The inclusion of measures of alcohol intake and physical activity may or may not be a strength in the base-case estimate. As noted in the discussion on Vincent Miller *et al.* (1999), there are unresolved issues in adjustment for these potentially endogenous variables. Manning *et al.* (1989, 1991) were aware of this problem and performed a sensitivity analysis for smoking-related characteristics in their estimates of external burden, which is discussed below.

Hodgson (1992) estimated the expected lifetime medical expenditures of smokers (defined as current and former smokers) versus those who had never smoked, and the total net present value of costs for the current cohort of smokers. Relative risks of healthcare utilization were estimated using the analytic approach. A unique aspect of Hodgson's approach was the separate estimation of costs for survivors and decedents. Hodgson described this as important because only survivors are represented in most healthcare utilization surveys, a factor that may introduce a bias in the estimates. Hospitalization and use of physicians' and outpatient services for survivors were based on data from the NHIS. Hospital utilization for decedents was estimated using the US National Medical Care Utilization and Expenditure Survey (NMCUES). Age-specific and sex-specific average hospital costs were estimated using NMCUES. Long-term care utilization by the elderly was estimated using the National Nursing Home Survey, and several other health and demographic surveys. There is no adjustment for the non-smoking smoker in the main analysis. The effects of smoking on mortality are modeled using the life-table approach, using data from the American Cancer Society's Cancer Prevention Study II. The results of this study are that the excess health care costs of smokers outweigh the increased cost of medical care over the longer lives of non-smokers.

Hodgson estimated that the smoking population over 25 years of age increased the net present value of lifetime health expenditures by US$473 to 501 million (with discount rates of 3% and 5%, respectively). Hodgson used Manning *et al.*'s (1989) estimate that adjustment for the non-smoking smoker would reduce excess costs by about 13%, producing a lower bound estimate of between $412 million and $436 million. At a 3% discount rate, he estimated that the ratio of lifetime costs of smokers to non-smokers was 1.32 for men and 1.24 for women. Hodgson did not provide an estimate of gross costs, but an approximation of annual gross costs can be derived from some of the estimates in the paper. For the period of the study, gross costs were approximately $40 billion per year from 1985 to 1989 (see Warner *et al.* 1999), or between 0.7% and 1.0% of GDP (0.6–0.9% with the adjustment for the non-smoking smoker). This tends towards the higher end of the range of gross cost estimates for the United States, especially since the estimates omit some of the total US healthcare expenditure because of the omission of other services (such as dentistry) and medicines. The main drawback of the study is the use of a fixed adjustment factor for the non-smoking smoker type.

Netherlands Barendregt *et al.* (1997) estimated costs over time from 1988 onwards for the Dutch population compared to a hypothetical population of non-smokers, using the synthetic approach. The diseases included were heart disease, stroke, smoking-related cancer, and COPD. The life-table method was used to model the Dutch population in the absence of smoking. Details of the population modeling were not reported, but adjustments for the non-smoking smoker type appear to have been made in both. This study did not estimate a net present value of future costs, but rather reports the length of time it takes for the cost savings from smoking cessation to be just balanced by the increased costs from the longer life expectancies of non-smokers, using discount rates of 0–10%. With no discounting, savings are balanced by costs for males in 26 years, and after 50 years the healthcare costs are about 7% higher. The results for women are similar, with costs ultimately 4% higher. Using discount rates of 3% and 5% produces similar results. These results imply that smoking reduces net healthcare costs with a discount rate of up to 5%. At 10%, the break-even point becomes very large, and smoking begins to increase net costs. The ratio of undiscounted costs of smokers to non-smokers is 0.87 for men and 0.85 for women. The small number of tobacco-related diseases included in this study, however, may result in a substantial under-estimate of costs.

Estimates of external burden

Estimates of the external burden of cigarette smoking (shown in Table 4.9) do not address the total cost of smoking, but rather the costs borne by the non-smoking population. These estimates attempt to follow the economic cost–benefit approach as much as possible. Under the usual economic definition, costs incurred to anyone within the same household are not considered external costs, possibly leading to an under-estimate of the external burden under other definitions of cost. In this review, costs incurred within the household are also reported whenever available. The results reported below do not include the effect of tobacco tax revenues.

Canada

Stoddart *et al.* (1986) presents a cross-section estimate of gross costs for Ontario, Canada in 1978. Their study used the synthetic approach to estimate excess healthcare utilization. The diseases considered were lung cancer, coronary heart disease, bronchitis, and emphysema. A sensitivity analysis also considered non-respiratory smoking-related cancers (cancers of the oral cavity, esophagus, larynx, pharynx, bladder, and pancreas); stroke; aortic aneurysm; pneumonia and influenza; pulmonary tuberculosis; digestive ulcers; and pulmonary disease. There was no adjustment for the non-smoking smoker type. The conclusion of the study is that smoking imposes an external burden of between Can$39.1 and $81.1 million. A sensitivity analysis that increased the costs of hospital care per day, included more healthcare services, and increased the SAFs of disease to the highest plausible values resulted in an estimate of Can$145.0 million. These estimates imply external gross costs of between 0.04% and 0.16% of GDP. The main weakness of the base case of this study is its very conservative selection of diseases.

Raynauld and Vidal (1992) calculate an estimate of external burden for Canada in 1986 from their gross cost estimate discussed above. The external burden is calculated by estimating the current and future medical care costs, and savings due to premature death from smoking between 1986 and 2071, using 3% for the discount rate. The estimated external burden is Can$153 million or 0.03% of Canadian GDP. Their method may be inconsistent because they appear to assume that current smoking does

Table 4.9 Estimates of external healthcare cost burden for high-income countries

Study	Year of estimate	Services included[a]	Diseases included[b]	Discount rate (%)	Tobacco-attributable costs	% of GDP	Method: analytic vs. synthetic
Gross costs cross-section							
Canada (Ontario)					Can$ million		
Stoddart et al. (1986)	1978	H O P	C G M R	—	39.1–145.0	0.04–0.16	Synthetic
Raynauld and Vidal (1992)	1986	H[c]	Is M R[d]	3	153	0.03	Synthetic
Finland					FIM million		
Perkurinen (1992)	1987	HOM	C M R	—	255–294	0.07–0.08	Synthetic
Net costs life-cycle					US$ billion		
United States							
Manning et al. (1991)	1986	F H L M O P	[e]	0	3.5 (in home costs excluded)	0.08	Analytic
				5	3.5–8.1	0.08–0.19	
				10	4.6	0.11	
				5	4.0 (low birthweight included)	0.09	
Viscusi (1995)	1993	F H L M O P	[e]	0–5	1.9–9.2 (from Manning)	0.03–0.15	Analytic
				0–5	2.8–10.4 (tar adjusted)	0.04–0.16	
				0–5	1.9–8.5 (lag tar adjusted)	0.03–0.13	

[a] Services are: F, other professional medical fees; H, hospital; L, long-term care; M, medicine; O, outpatient visits; P, physician fees.
[b] Diseases are: C, cardiovascular and circulatory diseases; G, gastrointestinal diseases; Is, ischemic heart disease; M, malignant neoplasms; R, non-malignant respiratory disease; O, other. (C includes Is.)
[c] Includes other unspecified health service expenditures. See text for discussion.
[d] Non-malignant respiratory (R) disease includes COPD only.
[e] Includes all expenditures for all conditions attributable to smokers.

not cause any increase in the use of long-term care among the living, yet they include reduced use of long-term care due to premature death in the savings.

Finland

Pekurinen (1992) reported the gross external burden of smoking from the cross-section estimates for 1987 reported above. The estimated external costs (after adjustments for cross-subsidization in healthcare) are between FIM255 million and FIM294 million, or 0.07–0.08% of GDP.

United States

Manning *et al.* (1989, 1991) reported net external costs from the life-cycle estimates discussed above. The external costs are calculated in the same way as aggregate net costs. These researchers' base-case cost, discounted at 5%, was US$6.6 billion, or 0.15% of GDP. A sensitivity analysis that varied discount rates and included the different assumptions for non-smoking characteristics of smokers, among other things, produced a range of between US$3.5 and $8.1 billion, or 0.08–0.19% of GDP.

Viscusi (1995) performed a life-cycle study of the excess smoking-attributable social burden per pack of cigarettes. His base case consisted of updated estimates based on Manning *et al.* (1989, 1991). The new analysis consists of two adjustments. One is for changes in the tar levels of cigarettes over time, on the theory that tar levels have dropped dramatically and that cigarettes should therefore have less severe health effects than indicated by SAFs that were estimated for a population that smoked higher-tar cigarettes. The second adjustment was the use of lags in health effects to account for the fact that the effects of cumulative exposure to smoke represented in estimated SAFs often take place decades after consumption. Viscusi estimated the cost, in cents per pack, in order to calculate the tax needed to cover annual net costs from smoking. His base-case estimate of external costs ranged between US$1.9 and $9.2 billion, or 0.03–0.15% of GDP. With the tar adjustment, costs are from $2.8 to $10.4 billion. With the tar adjustment and lagged health effects, the costs range from $1.9 to $8.5 billion, or 0.03–0.13% of GDP. Viscusi's estimates are largely the same as those of Manning *et al.* except that the lower-bound external cost is smaller.

Viscusi's adjustments to the standard analysis, however, are controversial. The problem with his adjustment for lower tar levels is that nicotine and tar levels dropped together, and there is substantial new evidence that smokers compensate for lower nicotine levels by smoking cigarettes more intensely. Therefore any tar adjustment may be inappropriate (Parish *et al.* 1995). The use of lags is also disputable in the case of some smoking-related diseases such as heart attack and stroke, which are likely to be the result of current as well as past smoking.

Review of existing studies on the social costs of smoking

Several of the studies discussed here also report estimates of the total social costs of smoking: that is, all the indirect costs of morbidity and premature mortality, as well as direct medical costs. The review will be selective and brief because the definition of social cost can vary greatly. The reader should consult the original studies for more detailed discussions. There are several analyses of the costs of tobacco use on old-age pensions and medical plans, which will not be reviewed here since the results depend on the details of the specific programs (Wright 1986; Shoven *et al.* 1987; Herdman *et al.* 1993).

Cross-section estimates of gross social costs in Canada and the United States follow a conceptual framework that is broadly similar to that of the 'cost of illness' concept as described by Hodgson and Meiners (1982). This preceded the GDP-based social definition of cost. Luce and Schweitzer (1978), for example, estimated the total social cost of annual consumption for the United States to be 1.6% of GDP, while Rice *et al.* (1986) estimated it to be 1.4%. The Canadian social cost estimates range from 1.3% of Ontario GDP (Choi and Pak 1996; Xie *et al.* 1996) to 2.2% for all Canada (Kaiserman 1997). The lowest estimates are from Pekurinen (1992, 1999) for Finland, where costs were 1.2–1.3% of GDP in 1987, but fell to 0.8% in 1995. Pekurinen attributed this decline to a large drop in smoking prevalence during the intervening years. This seems to place a very large emphasis on current (as opposed to past) smoking in the cost estimate, but it is a direct result of using SAFs calculated using current smoking prevalence to estimate costs. The only comprehensive estimate based on local data for a developing country is Jin *et al.*'s (1995) estimate of 1.7% of GDP for China. The estimates of net social cost by Collins and Lapsley (1991, 1996) for Australia, range between 2.1% and 3.4% of GDP. These estimates follow the CCSA definitions closely and are not directly comparable with the estimates for Canada and the United States. They are more comprehensive than other estimates in that they attempt to estimate the social cost of unwanted nicotine addiction.

Estimates of external burden are lower. Pekurinen's (1992, 1999) estimates of gross external costs for Finland ranged from 0.3% to 0.5% of GDP. The net cost estimates of Manning *et al.* (1989, 1991) ranged from a saving of 0.6% to a cost of 0.2% of GDP, with a base-case estimate of a cost of 0.1%. Savings occur in the base case when the discount rate is less than 3.5%. If internal costs that occur within the family, such as the effects of parental smoking on children's health, were included, the break-even discount rate would be higher. If the costs of morbidity and mortality to others within the family are included, but the mortality costs to the smoker are excluded, the base-case estimate rises from 0.1% of GDP to 0.3%. Viscusi (1995) includes a sensitivity analysis on the effect of including costs of mortality from environmental tobacco smoke (ETS) on non-family members, which results in a wide range of estimates: from a saving of 0.11% of GDP to a cost of 0.36% of GDP. Viscusi considers the upper-bound estimates of the costs due to environmental tobacco smoke to be extremely unlikely, and concludes that the median estimate of approximately no net external costs is a realistic upper bound.

Some estimates indicate that any external social costs of smoking are recovered from tax revenue from tobacco users. This question, however, is beyond the scope of this chapter. The estimates of net extenal burden on non-smokers that include the effects of taxes paid by smokers are not discussed here. See the individual studies for these estimates. It is very difficult to compare studies across different countries since the results depend heavily on the characteristics of the individual tax systems and social insurance programs, and studies do not analyse tax incidence consistently. Also, the results for high-income countries assume a tobacco tax system which can be administered with high compliance; this may not be characteristic of developing countries where formal tobacco markets are still relatively small.

4.5 Conclusion

Estimates of the gross healthcare costs of smoking for high-income countries range from around 0.10–1.1% of GDP, with relatively higher estimates in countries where healthcare costs account for a greater share of GDP. The relatively small number of studies from developing countries suggests that the gross cost of smoking can be as high in these countries as in developed countries. However, these studies are of uneven quality and are often based on very limited data, making it impossible to draw overall conclusions at this time.

As far as studies of the net costs of smoking are concerned, it is difficult to reach conclusions for any group of countries. This is because of differences in the methodologies used. The majority of the cross-section studies indicate that the net costs of smoking are positive, with only the low estimates for Finland implying healthcare cost savings from smoking. The life-cycle cost studies show little agreement and are very sensitive to the details of the study. We consider that the most methodologically sound of these studies are Hodgson (1992) and Manning *et al.* (1991). The main strength of Hodgson's study is the separate estimation of survivors' and decedents' costs. The main strength of the study by Manning *et al.* is the careful modeling of, and sensitivity analysis for, the non-smoking smoker type, both for disease incidence and mortality. Both Hodgson and Manning (for the base cose) conclude that there are net costs from smoking. The results of the studies of the external costs of smoking indicate that there are external burdens for gross and net healthcare costs due to tobacco use.

The estimates of both gross and net total social costs are fairly high because of the large costs of deaths caused by smoking, and they indicate that productive assets (i.e. smokers' lives) equal to 1% or more of GDP are lost each year due to smoking. In contrast, the estimates of the external burden of social costs have a very wide range, and there is no clear consensus. As with net cost estimates, these estimates are sensitive to the assumptions used. Overall, however, the cost estimates agree that smoking increases the current medical and social costs of living individuals. There is less consistency concerning how much these costs are reduced by savings from the shorter life-spans of smokers.

There are several methodological considerations that are important for developing countries. The first is that the definition of costs used in the study will have an important influence on the result. The first task in any estimation of the costs associated with tobacco use is to carefully state the policy question that the estimate is intended to answer, so that the most appropriate definition of costs and perspective can be chosen.

Second is the issue of gross versus net costs. The estimates of gross costs are much more consistent than the estimates of net and external costs, and should therefore be reported separately with a carefully documented sensitivity analysis of all estimates. This permits policy-makers to evaluate the tradeoffs between the almost certain short-run costs of smoking and the more uncertain longer-run effects that occur with longer life expectancies in a population with less smoking.

Third is the calculation of net costs. There are several methods for estimating net costs, which range from estimates of the future net present value of costs from current smokers, to the comparison of healthcare costs in populations with and without smoking. These different approaches have different interpretations, though some may turn out to be equivalent in special cases. Interpretations of the concept of net cost used in some estimates for high-income countries are shown in Table 4.10. The choice of the type of net cost analysis should be carefully justified and its connection to the policy question being answered should be explained. If the life-cycle approach is chosen then the very large uncertainties involved in forecasting healthcare utilization

Table 4.10 Net health cost interpretations from research studies in developed countries

Author	Country	Conclusion
Leu and Schaub (1983)	Switzerland	Male smokers' lifetime healthcare expenditures are slightly lower than if they had never smoked. In 1976, aggregate male medical care expenditure was the same as it would have been if nobody born after 1876 had ever smoked
Leu and Schaub (1985)	Switzerland	The ratio of lifetime medical care costs of male Swiss smokers to comparable non-smokers is between 0.91 and 0.97, for discount rates of 0 to 10%.
Manning *et al.* (1991)	United States	Each pack of cigarettes consumed increases the net present value of current and future health costs by about 30 cents, discounted at 5%.
Pekurinen (1992)	Finland	The total cost of health expenditures in 1987 attributed to smoking was in the range FIM524–594 million. The net present value of health care expenditure avoided due to deaths attributed to smoking in that year was in the range FIM431–610 million.
Hodgson (1992)	United States	The current population of smokers will increase the cost of health care by about 500 US$ billion (discounted at 3%) spread out over their remaining lifetimes.
Collins and Lapsley (1996)	Australia	In 1992 the healthcare benefits resulting from past and current premature deaths of smokers accounted for about 48% of the gross healthcare costs attributable to smoking (Aust$1600 million).
Barendregt *et al.* (1997)	Netherlands	The ratio of undiscounted medical costs of smokers to non-smokers is 0.87 for men and 0.85 for women. The discounted lifetime medical cost of smokers is less than non-smokers until the discount rate is about 10%.

and costs should be kept in mind when designing the sensitivity analysis. This is a particularly important consideration for developing countries.

The fourth issue concerns the use of the synthetic and analytic approaches. The analytic approach depends on availability of national survey data, and is difficult even in countries with extensive survey databases, such as the United States and Canada. For countries with limited survey data, the synthetic approach may be most practical. However, the diseases selected should be the result of careful epidemiological analysis in order to identify all conditions that are causally related to tobacco use. The estimates should be identified as lower bounds, since this review suggests that including only the most obvious tobacco-related diseases produces a downward bias in the estimated costs. The services included also have an important effect on costs, and this issue should also be considered in evaluating whether the estimate is a lower bound. The treatment of healthcare services is especially important for developing countries where many healthcare services are likely to move from the household to the formal market sector within the lifetimes of current smokers.

Adjusting for the non-smoking characteristics of smokers (that is, accounting for the non-smoking smoker type) is a difficult and still-unresolved issue that requires careful analysis of smoking patterns and their interaction with other behaviors and life-style. Kato *et al.* (1989) and Thornton *et al.* (1994) report that ex-smokers do change important non-smoking behaviors, such as diet, as time since smoking cessation increases. Therefore, some non-smoking characteristics of current smokers are not completely exogenous. This issue needs further research because it has had a significant impact on existing cost estimates.

While this review recommends that the synthetic approach be taken in countries with limited resources for national health surveys, the goal should be to use all available information regarding healthcare utilization and smoking status. The strengths and weaknesses of existing cost estimates should be critically examined in order to improve future efforts. In countries where surveys are being developed, there is an opportunity for researchers to contribute to their design in order to collect the information needed for better estimates at a reasonable cost. New developments in the epidemiology of tobacco-related disease will suggest modifications. For example, the duration of smoking and the age at which smoking was started may be important determinants of the development of lung cancer (Peto 1986; Wiencke *et al.* 1999). Therefore, information on individuals' history of smoking and changes in their risk behaviors as a function of smoking status may be as important as estimates of current prevalence, and modification of future surveys to collect this information should be seriously considered.

References

Anderson, L. (1977). *Benefit-Cost Analysis: a Practical Guide.* Lexington, MA, Lexington Books.

Ballard, T., Ehlers, J., Freund, E. *et al.* (1995). Green tobacco sickness: occupational nicotine poisoning in tobacco workers. *Archives of Environmental Health*, **50**(5), 384–9.

Barendregt, J. J., Bonneux, L., and Van der Maas, P. J. (1997). The health care costs of smoking. *New England Journal of Medicine*, **337**(15), 1052–7.

Bartlett, J. C., Miller, L. S., Rice, D. P. (1994). Medical care expenditures attributable to cigarette smoking–United States, 1993. *Morbidity and Mortality Weekly Report*, **43**(26), 469–72.

Choi, B. C. K. and Nethercott, J. R. (1988). The economic impact of smoking in Canada. *International Journal of Health Planning and Management*, **3**, 197–205.

Choi, B. and Pak, A. W. (1996). Health and social costs of tobacco use in Ontario, Canada, 1979 and 1988. *Journal of Epidemiology and Community Health*, **50**(1), 81–5.

Collins, D. and Lapsley, H. (1998). Estimating and disaggregating the social costs of tobacco. In *The Economics of Tobacco Control: Towards an Optimal Policy Mix* (ed. I. Abedian, R. van der Merwe, N. Wilkins, and P. Jha.), pp. 155–78. Cape Town, Applied Fiscal Research Centre: University of Cape Town.

Collins, D. J. and Lapsley, H. M. (1991). *Estimating the Economic Costs of Drug Abuse in Australia*. Monograph Series no. 15. Sydney, Australia, Commonwealth Department of Human Services and Health.

Collins, D. J. and Lapsley, H. M. (1996). *The Social Costs of Drug Abuse in Australia in 1988 and 1992*. Monograph Series no. 30. Sydney, Australia, Commonwealth Department of Human Services and Health.

Collishaw, N. E. and Myers, G. (1984). Dollar estimates of the consequences of tobacco use in Canada, 1979. *Canadian Journal of Public Health*, **75**, 192–9.

Cook, P. J. (1991). The Social Costs of Drinking. In *Tne Negative Social Consequences of Alcohol Use*. Oslo, Norway, Norwegian Ministry of Health and Social Affairs.

Cooper, B. S. and Rice, D. P. (1976). The economic cost of illness revisited. *Social Security Bulletin*, **39**(2), 21–36.

Dietz, V. J., Novotny, T. E., Rigau-Perez, J. G. *et al.* (1991). Smoking-attributable mortality, years of potential life lost, and direct health care costs for Puerto Rico, 1983. *Bulletin of PAHO*, **25**(1), 77–86.

Dinwiddy, C. and Teal, F. (1996). *Principles of Cost Benefit Analysis for Developing Countries*. Cambridge, Cambridge University Press.

English, D., Holman, C. D. J., Milne, E. *et al.* (1995). *The quantification of drug caused morbidity and mortality in Australia*, 1995 edition. Canberra, Australia, Commonwealth Department of Human Services and Health.

Erdmann, C. and Pinheiro, S. (1998). *Special Communication: Pesticides used on tobacco crops in southern Brazil*. Berkeley, California, Division of Public Health Biology and Epidemiology, School of Public Public Health, University of California.

Feachem, R., Kjellstrom, T., Murray, C. *et al.* (ed.) (1995). *The Health of Adults in Developing Countries*. Oxford, The World Bank and Oxford University Press.

Forbes, W. F. and Thompson, M. E. (1983). Estimating the health care costs of smokers. *Canadian Journal of Public Health*, **74**(3), 183–90.

Geist, H. (1998). How tobacco farming contributes to tropical deforestation. In *The Economics of Tobacco Control: Towards an Optimal Policy Mix* (ed. I. Abedian, R. van der Merwe, N. Wilkins, and P. Jha), pp. 232–44. Cape Town, Applied Fiscal Research Centre: University of Cape Town.

Geist, H. (1999a). Soil mining and societal responses: The case of tobacco in Eastern Miombo Highlands. In *Coping with changing environments: Social dimensions of endangered ecosystems in the developing world* (ed. B. Lohnert and H. Geist), pp. 119–148. Ashgate, Aldershot.

Geist, H. (1999b). Global assessment of deforestation related to tobacco farming. *Tobacco Control*, **8**(1), 18–28.

Geist, H. (2000). Transforming the fringe: Tobacco-related wood usage and its environmental implications. In *Marginality, landscape, and environment* (ed. R. Majoral, F. Delgado-Cravidão, H. Jussila). Ashgate, Aldershot (in press).

Gold, M., Siegal, J. E., Russell, L. B. *et al.* (ed.) (1996). *Cost-Effectiveness in Health and Medicine*. New York, Oxford University Press.

Gray, A. J., Reinken, J. A., and Laugesen, M. (1988). The cost of cigarette smoking in New Zealand. *New Zealand Medical Journal*, **101**(846), 270–3.

Herdman, R., Hewitt, M., and Laschober, M. (1993). *Smoking-related Deaths and Financial Costs: Office of Technology Assessment Estimates for 1990*. Washington, DC, Office of Technology Assessment.

Hipke, M. (1993). Green tobacco sickness. *Southern Medical Journal*, **86**(9), 989–92.

Hodgson, T. A. (1992). Cigarette smoking and lifetime medical expenditures. *Milbank Quarterly*, **70**(1), 81–125.

Hodgson, T. and Meiners, M. (1982). Cost-of-illness methodology: a guide to current practices and procedures. *Milbank Memorial Fund Quarterly*, **60**(3), 429–62.

Holman, C. and Armstrong, B. K. (1990). *The Quantification of Drug-Caused Morbidity and Mortality in Australia, 1989*. Canberra, Australia, Commonwealth Department of Human Services and Health.

James, E. (1994). *Averting the Old Age Crisis*. World Bank, Washington, D.C., World Bank: Investing in Health, World Development Report 1993, Washington DC).

Jin, S., Lu, B. Y., Yan, D. Y. *et al.* (1995). An Evaluation on Smoking-induced Health Costs in China (1988–1989). *Biomedical And Environmental Sciences*, **8**, 342–9.

Kaiserman, M. J. (1997). The cost of smoking in Canada, 1991. *Chronic Diseases in Canada*, **18**(1), 13–9.

Kato, I., Tominga, S., and Suzuki, T. (1989). Characteristics of past smokers. *International Journal of Epidemiology*, **18**(2), 345–54.

Leu, R. E. and Doppmann, R. J. (1984). The demand for health care in Switzerland—a latent variable approach. In *System Science in Health Care* (ed. W. von Eimeren, R. Engelbrecht, and C. D. Flagle), pp. 932–5, Heidelberg, Springer.

Leu, R. E. and Schaub, T. (1983). Does smoking increase medical care expenditure? *Social Science and Medicine*, **17**(23), 1907–14.

Leu, R. E. and Schaub, T. (1984). Ecopnomic aspects of smoking. *Effective Health Care*, **2**(3), 111–23.

Leu, R. E. and Schaub, T. (1985). More on the impact of smoking on medical expenditure. *Social Science and Medicine*, **21**(7), 825–7.

Lippiatt, B. C. (1990). Measuring medical cost and life expectancy impacts of changes in cigarette sales. *Preventive Medicine*, **19**, 515–32.

Luce, B. R. and Schweitzer, S. O. (1978). Smoking and alcohol abuse: a comparison of their economic consequences. *New England Journal of Medicine*, **298**(10), 569–71.

Mackay, J. and Crofton, J. (1996). Tobacco and health: tobacco and the developing world. *British Medical Bulletin*, **52**(1), 206–21.

Manning, W., Keeler, E. B., Newhouse, J. P. *et al.* (1989). The taxes of sin: do smokers pay their way? *JAMA*, **261**(11), 1604–9.

Manning, W., Keeler, E. B., Newhouse, J. P. *et al.* (1991). *The Costs of Poor Health Habits*. Cambridge, MA, Harvard University Press.

Markandya, A. and Pearce, D. (1989). The social costs of tobacco smoking. *British Journal of Addiction*, **84**, 1139–50.

Max, W. and Rice, D. P. (1995). The cost of smoking in California. *Tobacco Control*, **4**(supplement 1), S39–S46.

Maynard, A., Hardman, G., and Whelan, A. (1987). Measuring the social costs of addictive substances. *British Journal of Addiction*, **82**, 701–6.

McIntyre, D. E. and Taylor, S. P. (1989). Economic aspects of smoking in South Africa. *South African Medical Journal*, **75**(9), 432–5.

Miller, L., Zhang, X., Novotny, T. *et al.* (1998a). State estimates of Medicaid expenditure attributable to cigarette smoking, Fiscal year 1993. *Public Health Reports*, **113**(2), 140–51.

Miller, L., Zhang, X., Rice, D. P. *et al.* (1998b). State estimates of total medical expenditures attributable to cigarette smoking, 1993. *Public Health Reports*, **113**(5), 447–58.

Miller, V. P., Ernst, C., and Collin, F. (1999). Smoking-attributable medical care costs in the USA. *Social Science and Medicine*, **48**(3), 375–91.

Murray, C. J. L. and Lopez, A. D. (ed.) (1996a). *The Global Burden of Disease: a Comprehensive*

Assessment of Mortality and Disability from Diseases, Injuries, and Risk Factors in 1990 and Projected to 2020. Global Burden of Disease; 1. Cambridge MA, Harvard University Press.

Murray, C. J. L. and Lopez, A. D. (ed.) (1996b). *Global Health Statistics: a Compendium of Incidence, Prevalence and Mortality for Over 200 Conditions.* Global Burden of Disease; 2. Cambridge MA, Harvard University Press.

Normand, C. (1998). Ten popular health economic fallacies. *Journal of Public Health Medicine*, **20**(2), 129–32.

Oster, G., Colditz, G. A., and Kelly, N. L. (1984a). *The Economic Costs of Smoking and Benefits of Quitting.* Lexington, MA, D. C. Health.

Oster, G., Colditz, G. A., and Kelly, N. L. (1984b). The economic costs of smoking and the benefits of quitting for individual smokers. *Preventive Medicine*, **13**, 377–89.

Over, M., Ellis, R., Huber, J. H. *et al.* (1992). The Consequences of Adult Ill-Health. In *The Health of Adults in the Developing World.* (ed. R. Feachem, T. Kjellstrom, C. Murray, M. Over and M. Phillips), pp. 161–207, New York, Oxford University Press.

Pan American Sanitary Bureau (1998). *Cost–benefit Analysis of Smoking. Caracas, Venezuela.* Pan American Health Organization.

Parish, S., Collins, R., Peto, R., *et al.* (1995). Cigarette smoking, tar yields, and non-fatal myocardial infarction:14,000 cases and 32,000 controls in the United Kingdom. The International Studies of Infarct Survival (ISIS) Collaborators. *BMJ*, **311**(7003), 471–7.

Pekurinen (1992). *Economic Aspects of Smoking. Is There a Case for Government Intervention in Finland?* Helsinki, VAPK Publishing.

Pekurinen, M. (1999). *The Economic Consequences of Smoking in Finland 1987–1995.* Helsinki, Health Services Research, Ltd.

Peto, R. (1986) Influence of dose and duration of smoking on lung cancer rates. In *Tobacco: a major international health hazard* (ed. R. Peto and D. Zaridze), pp. 23–33. Lyon, International Agency for Research on Cancer, 1986. IARC Scientific Publications, no. 74.

Phillips, D., Kawachi, I., and Tilyard, M. (1992). The costs of smoking revisited. *New Zealand Medical Journal*, **105**, 240–2.

Rath, G. K. and Chaudry, K. (1995). Cost of management of tobacco-related cancers in India. In *Tobacco and Health* (ed. K. Slama), pp. 559–564. New York, Plenum.

Raynauld, A. and Vidal, J.-P. (1992). Smokers burden on society: myth and reality in Canada. *Canadian Public Policy*, **18**(3), 300–17.

Rice, D. P., Hodgson, T. A., Sinsheimer, P. *et al.* (1986). The economic costs of the health effects of smoking, 1984. *Milbank Quarterly*, **64**(4), 489–547.

Robson, L. and Single, E. (1995). *Literature Review of Studies on the Economic Costs of Substance Abuse.* Toronto, Canadian Centre on Substance Abuse.

Schoenbaum, M. (1997). Do smokers understand the mortality effects of smoking? Evidence from the health and retirement survey. *American Journal of Public Health*, **87**(5), 755–9.

Scitovsky, A. A. (1994). The high cost of dying revisited. *Milbank Quarterly*, **72**(4), 561–91.

Shoven, J. B., Sundberg, J. O. *et al.* (1987). *The Social Security Cost of Smoking.* NBER Working Paper Series, no. 2234. Cambridge, MA, National Bureau of Economic Research.

Shultz, J. M. (1985). *SAMMEC: Smoking-Attributable Mortality, Morbidity, and Economic Costs.* (Computer software and documentation.) Minneapolis, MN, Minnesota Center for Nonsmoking and Health, Minnesota Department of Health.

Shultz, J. M., Novotny, T. E., and Rice, D. P. (1991). Quantifying the disease impact of cigarette smoking with SMMEC II software. *Public Health Reports*, **106**(3), 326–33.

Single, E., Collins, D., Easton, B. *et al.* (1996a). *International Guidelines for Estimating the Costs of Substance Abuse.* At <http://www.ccsa.ca/intguide.htm>. Ottawa, Canada, Canadian Centre on Substance Abuse: accessed January, 1999.

Single, E., Robson, L., Xie, X. *et al.* (1996b). *The Costs of Substance Abuse in Canada. A Cost Estimation Study.* Ottawa, Canada, Canadian Centre on Substance Abuse.

Stiglitz, J. E. (1994a). Discount rates: the rate of discount and the theory of the second best. In *Cost–benefit Analysis* (ed. R. Layard and S. Glaister), pp. 116–59, Cambridge, Cambridge University Press.

Stiglitz, J. E. (1994b). *Whither Socialism?* Cambridge, MA, MIT Press.

Stoddart, G. L., Labelle, R. J., Barer, M. L. *et al.* (1986). Tobacco taxes and health care costs: do Canadian smokers pay their way? *Journal of Health Care Economics*, **5**, 63–80.

Thompson, M. E. and Forbes, W. F. (1985). Reasons for the disagreements on the impact of smoking on medical care expenditures: a proposal for a uniform approach. *Social Science and Medicine*, **21**(7), 771–3.

Thornton, A., Lee, P., and Fry, J. *et al.* (1994). Differences between smokers, ex-smokers, passive smokers and non-smokers. *Journal of Clinical Epidemiology*, **47**(10), 1143–62.

US Department of Health and Human Services (1989). *Reducing the Health Consequences of Smoking: 25 Years of Progress.* A report of the Surgeon General, DHHS publication no (CDC) 90–8416, US Department of Health and Human Services, Public Health Service, Centers for Disease Control and Prevention, Center for Chronic Disease Prevention and Control, Office of Smoking and Health.

Viscusi, W. K. (1995). Cigarette taxation and the social consequences of smoking. *Tax Policy and the Economy* (ed. J. M. Poterba), Cambridge, MA, MIT Press. **9**: 51–101.

Warner, K. E., Hodgson, T. A., and Carroll, C. E. (1999). The medical costs of smoking in the United States: estimates, their validity, and their implications. *Tobacco Control*, **8**(3), 290–300.

Wiencke, J. K., Thurston, S. W., Kelsey, K. T. *et al.* (1999). Early age at smoking initiation and tobacco carcinogen DNA damage in the lung. *Journal of the National Cancer Institute.* **91**(7), 614–9.

World Health Organization (1997). *Tobacco or Health: A Global Status Report.* Geneva, World Health Organization.

Wright, V. B. (1986). Will quitting smoking help Medicare solve its financial problems? *Inquiry*, **23**, 76–82.

Xie, X., Rehm, J., Single, E. *et al.* (1996). *The Economic Costs of Alcohol, Tobacco, and Illicit Drug Abuse in Ontario: 1992.* Toronto, Canada, Addiction Research Foundation.

Xie, X., Robson, J., Single, E. *et al.* (1999). The economic consequences of smoking in Ontario. *Pharmacological Research*, **39**(3), 185–91.

Yach, D. (1982). Economic aspects of smoking in South Africa. *South African Medical Journal*, **62**, 167–70.

Zerbe, R. O. and D. D. Dively (1994). *Benefit-Cost Analysis.* New York, Harper Collins.

Section II
Analytics of tobacco use

5

The economics of addiction

Frank J. Chaloupka, John A. Tauras, and Michael Grossman

Non-technical summary

This chapter reviews economic models of addiction and their empirical applications to cigarette smoking and other tobacco use. These models can help in understanding the impact of prices and tobacco-control policies on individuals' smoking behavior, including their decisions to start, continue, reduce, quit, or re-start smoking. The discussion of economic models is technical and assumes some knowledge of economics. Here we provide a summary for the reader interested in the key implications from the various models.

Introduction. Economic theory assumes that individuals demand goods or services to maximize their happiness (or 'utility' in economic terms), taking into account prices, income, and other factors. For most products, consumption decisions at a given point in time are independent of past choices. Cigarettes and other tobacco products, unlike nearly all other consumer goods, are highly addictive, implying that decisions regarding their consumption at any moment depend on previous choices. In other words, a consumer who is addicted to a particular product, such as cigarettes, must by definition have bought the product before and will require the same or larger quantities as before to maintain the addiction. Likewise, the consumer will suffer significant adjustment costs if consumption is stopped or reduced.

Different models of addiction. Economic models in the past either ignored addiction or treated it as an irrational behavior not subject to basic laws of economics. Thus, for example, many assumed that higher prices for an addictive product would not, in fact, reduce its consumption.

Over the past few decades, economists have increasingly examined addictive behaviors, including smoking, in theoretical and empirical models. These models differ largely in the assumptions made about the extent of rationality among consumers of addictive products. Three groups of these models are discussed in this chapter.

The first approach models addiction as an imperfectly rational behavior. In these models, individuals' preferences are not consistent over their life-cycle. Some, for example, assume that people have two competing sets of preferences: one for good health and long life; and the other for the pleasure of smoking. This leads people to choose different actions at different ages. For example, people may prefer to smoke at one age with the intention of quitting later, but then change their mind later in life. These models have not been applied empirically to smoking or other addictions.

The second approach models addicts as myopic. These models generally assume that people know that their current smoking is based on their past smoking (i.e. that smoking is addictive), but do not take account of the future consequences of their addiction when making current choices. Empirical applications of this model in several high-income countries have confirmed that cigarettes are addictive in an 'economic' sense; that is, current cigarette smoking is increased by past consumption. These studies also confirm that higher prices reduce smoking.

The third approach models addiction as a fully rational behavior. That is, addicts are both aware of the dependence of current choices on past behavior (as in the myopic-addiction models) and consider the future implications of their addictions when making current choices. This model has generated considerable debate both within and outside of economics. Several empirical applications of the rational-addiction model confirm that smoking is an addictive behavior and that increases in cigarette prices lead to reductions in cigarette smoking. The evidence is mixed, however, when it comes to the 'rationality' of cigarette smoking.

These models, particularly the rational-addiction model, have been criticized for not fully taking into account some aspects of addictive behavior. One frequently criticized feature of the rational-addiction model is that it assumes perfect foresight, implying that people fully understand the future implications of decisions concerning the consumption of addictive products. The reality, however, is that most addictions begin in adolescence, and young people have, at best, a limited understanding of addiction. Recent extensions of the rational-addiction model attempt to account for this, concluding that this lack of information for some individuals will lead many to regret becoming addicted. Other extensions of the economic models of addiction attempt to explain cessation behavior, such as the use of nicotine-replacement therapies, and focus on the 'adjustment costs' associated with overcoming withdrawal. This approach suggests that aging, by raising the immediacy of the health consequences of smoking, will result in some people quitting, and suggests that, in economic terms, it may be easier for the heaviest smokers to quit 'cold-turkey'. Finally, other recent models have examined the impact of differing approaches to modeling time-preferences, and suggest that youth onset is heavily influenced by a desire for immediate gratification and lack of self-control. These models, however, have only begun to be empirically tested.

Policy implications. These models have important implications for policy. Most importantly, because of the dependence of current consumption on past consumption, they indicate that the effect of a permanent change in price will be greater in the long-run than in the short-run, suggesting that permanent real price increases and strong tobacco-control efforts, which raise the actual and perceived costs of smoking, can be effective in significantly reducing smoking. By nature, the economic models of addiction will tend to simplify what are, in reality, very complex decisions about starting to smoke, continuing, quitting, or re-starting. Moreover, this research is at a relatively early stage and interesting theoretical developments remain to be tested empirically. Further research is likely to yield even more policy-relevant answers on smoking and addiction.

5.1 Introduction

Whether a commodity conforms to the law of diminishing or increasing return, the increase in consumption arising from a fall in price is gradual; and, further, habits which have once grown up around the use of a commodity while its price is low are not so quickly abandoned when its price rises again (Marshall 1920, appendix H, section 3, p. 807).

Standard economic theory implies that the demand for any product will depend on its price, the prices of other products, incomes, tastes, and other factors. For years, however, the conventional wisdom was that the basic principles of economics did not apply to addictive products, such as cigarettes and other tobacco products (which, because of the nicotine contained in them, are highly addictive; see Chapter 2 and Chapter 12). As the quotation from Marshall above indicates, the impact of addiction on demand is something that economists have considered for many years. However, they have largely either ignored the addictive nature of goods such as cigarettes when estimating demand or have assumed that behaviors such as smoking were irrational and could not be analyzed in the rational, constrained utility maximizing framework of economics.

Many theoretical and empirical studies from the past three decades, however, explicitly address the unique dimensions of the consumption of addictive goods. In economic analyses of addiction, the consumption of a good is considered addictive if an increase in the past consumption of that good leads to an increase in current consumption. Most analyses of addictive consumption have focused on the use of harmful substances, including tobacco products, alcohol, and illicit drugs. However, applications of the economic models of addiction are not limited to harmful consumption, but can also include more 'positive' addictions, including those to jogging, classical music, religion, and more that do not impose harm on others and that may yield future benefits (Becker and Murphy 1988; Grossman *et al.* 1998). These models clearly indicate that addiction has important implications for the impact of price and other control efforts on the demands for tobacco, alcohol, drugs, and other addictive substances.

This chapter provides an overview of economic models of addiction, their empirical applications to tobacco use, and recent innovations in the economic modeling of addiction. The chapter begins with a brief discussion of the physiological and psychological aspects of nicotine addiction, followed by a review of the most widely used economic models of addiction. Economic models of addiction can be divided into three basic groups: imperfectly rational models of addictive behavior; models of myopic addictive behavior; and models of rational addictive behavior. Each of these is discussed, along with a selected review of their empirical applications to cigarette smoking. This is followed by a discussion of several recent theoretical developments in the economic modeling of addictive behavior that focus on the initiation of addiction, the role of adjustment costs, and the time inconsistency of addictive behavior. Finally, several conclusions are provided.

5.2 Physiological and psychological dimensions of nicotine addiction

Over the past several decades, extensive biomedical, pharmacological, psychological, and other research have clearly demonstrated that cigarettes and other tobacco products are addictive, primarily because of the nicotine contained in them (US

Department of Health and Human Services/USDHHS 1988; Food and Drug Administration/USFDA 1996). The presence of three key factors—tolerance, reinforcement, and withdrawal—are often used to distinguish addictive consumption from the consumption of other goods and services (for more detailed reviews see: Ashton and Stepney 1982; Chaloupka 1988; USDHHS 1988). Other definitions are also employed that emphasize compulsive consumption, intoxication, and impairment of control (Hughes and Bickel 1999).

Tolerance reflects the body's adaptation to taking a drug. In the case of most drugs, tolerance implies that a given level of consumption yields less satisfaction as cumulative past consumption is higher. In other words, more of the drug must be consumed to achieve the same level of satisfaction from drug taking. Tolerance is exhibited somewhat differently in the case of cigarettes and other tobacco products. In part, tolerance reflects the overcoming of the initially unpleasant physical reactions to early consumption experiences. Moreover, in the case of tobacco use, tolerance does not result in a continuing escalation of use, but rather in the maintenance of a plateau.

Reinforcement reflects the learned responses to consumption and the rewards associated with it. In the case of cigarette smoking, reinforcement may be positive or negative (Ashton and Stepney 1982). Positive reinforcement comes from the pleasure or satisfaction that results from consuming cigarettes, including the pharmacological effects produced by nicotine and the psychological benefits associated with the act of smoking. Negative reinforcement is reflected by cigarette smoking to avoid a negative stimulus, such as smoking to avoid stress, weight gain, or nicotine withdrawal.

Finally, withdrawal reflects the negative physical reactions to the cessation, interruption, or reduction of consumption. In the case of cigarette smoking, these include increased irritability, inability to concentrate, increased anxiety, elevated blood pressure and heart rate, and much more, with a craving for tobacco the most common. As Ashton and Stepney (1982, p.61) describe it, the presence of withdrawal leads to the evolution from 'taking the drug in order to feel better to taking it in order to avoid feeling worse'.

The risk that the consumption of tobacco products can lead to nicotine addiction is exacerbated by the fact that most tobacco use begins at an early age (see Chapter 2) and that most young users are likely to underestimate their potential for addiction (see Chapter 7 and Chapter 8). In the United States, for example, surveys of youth indicate that most young smokers do not expect to be smoking regularly in the future; in follow-up surveys 5 years later, however, fewer than two out of five who expected to quit have actually done so (USDHHS 1994).

Over the past several decades, significant advances have been made in understanding the neuropsychological, pharmacological, and genetic mechanisms underlying nicotine addiction (see, for example, the proceedings from the National Institute on Drug Abuse's 1998 conference *Addicted to Nicotine* (Swan and Balfour 1999) for an excellent collection of multidisciplinary reviews of the state of the science on nicotine addiction). In contrast, economic models of addiction are at a relatively earlier stage of their development and are the subject of much debate among economists and others.

5.3 Economic models of addiction

For years, most economists treated the consumption of addictive goods no differently from other consumption even though the factors discussed above that are unique to addictive consumption were well known. These aspects of consumption were ignored, in part, because addiction was considered an irrational behavior not subject to standard economic analysis. As a result, many thought that the consumption of addictive substances, including tobacco products, was not subject to the same laws of economics that guided the consumption of other goods and services. That is, many thought that increases in prices and changes in other costs associated with the consumption of addictive goods would have little or no impact on their use. This is in contrast to the use of a typical consumer good that falls as prices and other costs associated with use rise.

However, over the past three decades, economists have begun to apply the standard framework of rational, constrained utility maximization to the study of the consumption of addictive substances. The economists who have studied addictions have made differing assumptions concerning the rationality of addictive behavior, where rationality in the context of these models largely reflects the degree to which the addict considers the future implications of current addictive consumption decisions. This chapter groups these studies into three basic categories depending on their assumptions about rationality: imperfectly rational addiction models, myopic-addiction models, and rational-addiction models. Other approaches that rely on more unusual approaches to modeling utility or the technology associated with addictive production are not discussed here (e.g. Barthold and Hochman 1988; Michaels 1988).

5.3.1 Imperfectly rational addiction models

Elster (1979), McKenzie (1979), Winston (1980), and Schelling (1978, 1980, 1984a, 1984b) best exemplify the economic models of imperfectly rational addictive behavior. These models generally assume stable but inconsistent short-run and long-run preferences. This is seen, for example, in Schelling's (1978, p. 290) description of a smoker trying to 'kick the habit':

Everybody behaves like two people, one who wants clean lungs and long life and another who adores tobacco. . . . The two are in a continual contest for control; the 'straight' one often in command most of the time, but the wayward one needing only to get occasional control to spoil the other's best laid plan.

Thus, the farsighted personality may enroll in a smoking-cessation program, only to be undone by the short-sighted personality's relapse in a weak moment. Winston (1980) formally modeled this behavior and described how this contest between personalities leads to the evolution of what he called 'anti-markets', which he defined as firms or institutions that individuals will pay to help them stop consuming (e.g. smoking cessation programs or pharmaceutical companies producing nicotine-replacement products).

Strotz (1956) was the first to develop a formal model of such behavior, describing the constrained utility-maximization process as one in which an individual chooses a future consumption path that maximizes current utility, but later in life changes this plan 'even though his original expectations of future desires and means of consumption are verified' (p. 165). This inconsistency between current and future preferences arises when a non-exponential discount function is used (this is discussed further below). Strotz went on to suggest that rational persons will recognize this inconsistency and plan accordingly, by pre-committing their future behavior or by modifying consumption plans to be consistent with future preferences when unable to pre-commit.

Pollak (1968) went one step further, arguing that an individual may behave naively even when using an exponential discount function. Thaler and Shefrin (1981) described the problem similarly, referring to an individual at any point in time as both a 'far-sighted planner and a myopic doer' (p. 392), with the two in continual conflict. While these models present interesting discussions of some aspects of addictive behavior, they have not yet been applied empirically to cigarette smoking or other addictions.

5.3.2 Myopic-addiction models

The naive behavior described in some of the imperfectly rational models of addiction is the basis for many of the myopic models of addictive behavior. As Pollak (1975) observed, behavior is naive in the sense that an individual recognizes the dependence of current addictive consumption decisions on past consumption, but then ignores the impact of current and past choices on future consumption decisions when making current choices. Many of these models treat preferences as endogenous, allowing tastes to change over time in response to past consumption (Gorman 1967; Pollak 1970, 1976, 1978; von Weizsacker 1971; El-Safty 1976a, 1976b; Hammond 1976a, 1976b). These models are similar in spirit to those in which tastes change in response to factors other than past consumption, including advertising (Galbraith 1958, 1972; Dixit and Norman 1978) and prices (Pollak 1977).

In some implementations of these models, past consumption affects current consumption through an accumulated stock of past consumption (e.g. Houthakker and Taylor 1966, 1970). These models are comparable to those of the demand for durable consumer goods that use a stock adjustment process (e.g. Chow's (1960) model of the demand for automobiles, and Garcia dos Santos' (1972) analysis of the demands for household durables). As Phlips (1983) noted, however, the distinction between models with endogenous tastes and those with stable preferences within a household production framework is purely semantic, since the underlying mathematics of the two are the same.

The earliest theoretical models of demand in the context of myopic addiction can be traced to the irreversible demand models (Haavelmo 1944; Duesenberry 1949; Modigliani 1949; Farrell 1952). Farrell, for example, described an irreversible demand function as one in which current demand depends on all past price and income combinations. As a result, price and income elasticities are constant, but may differ for increases and decreases in price and income. Farrell tested this model empirically, using data from the United Kingdom on the demands for tobacco and beer from 1870 through 1938, in a model that included not only current price and income, but also price, income, and consumption in the prior year. In general, his estimates were inconclusive, although he did find limited evidence of habit formation for tobacco use.

The notion of asymmetric responses to price and income reappeared in Scitovsky (1976) and was applied to cigarette demand by Young (1983), using US data from 1929–73. The basic notion was that the response to a price increase or drop in income will be smaller in absolute value than the response to a comparable price reduction or increase in income. Young asserted that this was due to the addictive nature of cigarette smoking. Young's empirical model included separate variables for price increases, price reductions, income increases, and income reductions, as well as a variety of other factors affecting demand. Using Ridge regression methods, Young obtained estimates consistent with his hypotheses. His estimated price elasticity of demand for price increases (–0.33) was slightly more than half of his estimate for price decreases (–0.61), with a comparable relationship for income (income elasticity of 0.30 for increases and 0.15 for reductions). Pekurinen (1989) took the same approach to estimating cigarette demand in Finland, concluding that Finnish smoking was almost twice as responsive to price reductions (elasticity of –0.94) as it was to price increases (elasticity of –0.49).

In the Young and Pekurinen models, myopic behavior is captured by the asymmetric responses to changes in price and income. In contrast to the earlier work by Farrell (1952), these models are essentially atheoretical and ignore the effect of past consumption on current consumption that is emphasized in most theoretical models of addiction. As Godfrey (1989) noted, this mis-specification of demand is likely to produce biased estimates of the effect of price on cigarette demand.

Most empirical applications of myopic models of addiction are based on the pioneering work by Houthakker and Taylor (1966, 1970). They formally introduced the dependence of current consumption of an addictive good on its past consumption by modeling current demand as a function of a 'stock of habits':

$$C(t) = a + \beta S(t) + \mathbf{X}(t)\Gamma, \tag{5.1}$$

where $C(t)$ is consumption of the addictive good at time t, $\mathbf{X}(t)$ is a vector of factors influencing demand, and $S(t)$ is the stock of habits at time t, defined as:

$$S(t) = C(t-1) + (1-\delta)S(t-1), \tag{5.2}$$

where δ is the rate of depreciation. This stock of habits, or 'addictive stock,' represents the depreciated sum of all past consumption of the addictive good and explicitly captures the dependence of current consumption on past consumption. Making appropriate substitutions, Houthakker and Taylor derived the following demand equation:

$$C(t) = \pi + \tau C(t-1) + [\mathbf{X}(t) - \mathbf{X}(t-1)]\varphi + \mathbf{X}(t)\theta. \tag{5.3}$$

Thus, after simplification, the addictive nature of demand is captured by making current consumption dependent on past consumption. Houthakker and Taylor predicted that τ will be positive for addictive or habit forming goods like tobacco products. Houthakker and Taylor estimated alternative versions of eqn 5.3 for a number of goods, including cigarettes, using annual aggregates for the US and several Western

European countries. Their estimates provided considerable support for their hypothesis of habit formation in demand, with positive estimates of the structural stock coefficient (β) for almost all of the non-durable consumer goods, including cigarettes, they examined.

Mullahy (1985) took a similar approach in his empirical examination of cigarette demand using US survey data. In his model, the stock of past cigarette consumption has a negative impact on the production of commodities such as health and the satisfaction received from current smoking. Mullahy used a two-part model to estimate cigarette demand, as well as instrumental variables methods to account for the unobserved individual heterogeneity likely to be correlated with the stock of past consumption. Mullahy found strong support for the hypothesis that cigarette smoking is an addictive behavior, as shown by the positive and significant estimates he obtained for the addictive stock in both the smoking participation and conditional demand equations. His estimates for price are quite similar to those obtained by Lewit and Coate (1982), with the overall price elasticity of demand centered on –0.47. In addition, Mullahy estimated that men were more price-responsive than women (total price elasticities of –0.56 and –0.39, respectively). Finally, using an interaction between the addictive stock and price, Mullahy concluded that more-addicted smokers (defined as those with a larger addictive stock) were less responsive to price than their less-addicted counterparts.

Using an approach that combined aspects of the Houthakker and Taylor model with Deaton and Muellbauer's (1980) Almost Ideal Demand System, Jones (1989) explicitly modeled the acquired tolerance characteristic of addictive consumption. Tolerance, in his model, is captured by replacing the money prices of addictive goods, including cigarettes, with their shadow prices, which include a variety of other costs associated with addictive consumption, including future health consequences and reduced productivity. Jones used quarterly data from the UK to estimate this model for cigarettes and various other goods, as well as an alternative model that ignores the addictive or habitual nature of cigarette demand. He found that the more conventional model, with an own-price elasticity of cigarette demand of –0.29, provided a better statistical fit than the habit model, with an own-price elasticity of –0.60. Nonetheless, Jones concluded that addiction was an important factor in cigarette smoking, speculating that the effects of withdrawal are more important than those of tolerance.

In a model reminiscent of the partial adjustment process described by Marshall (1920), Baltagi and Levin (1986) estimated cigarette demand using a time-series of annual state-cross-sections for the period 1964–80. In their model, changes in cigarette consumption over time depend on the divergence between 'desired' cigarette consumption and actual consumption, where desired consumption depends on prices, income, current and lagged advertising, and other factors. They estimated a coefficient on lagged cigarette consumption of 0.9, which they interpret as evidence of addiction, while estimating an own-price elasticity of cigarette demand of –0.22.

5.3.3 Rational-addiction models

Several researchers have modeled addiction as a rational behavior. In this context, rationality simply implies that individuals incorporate the interdependence between past, current, and future consumption into their utility-maximization process. This is in contrast to the assumption, implicit in myopic models of addictive behavior, that future implications are ignored when making current decisions. In other words, myopic behavior implies an infinite discounting of the future, while rational behavior implies that future implications are considered, while not ruling out a relatively high discount rate. Several of the rational-addiction models, including those of Lluch (1974), Spinnewyn (1981), and Boyer (1983), assume that tastes are endogenous. These models build on the significant contributions of Ryder and Heal (1973), Boyer (1978), and others in the optimal growth literature who have developed endogenous taste models with rational behavior.

Spinnewyn (1981) and Phlips and Spinnewyn (1982) argued that incorporating rational decision-making into models of habit formation results in models that are 'formally equivalent to models without habit formation' (Spinnewyn 1981, p. 92). This observational equivalence is obtained by redefining wealth and the cost of current consumption, so as to account for the additional costs associated with the addictive stock. The demand equations that result are equivalent to those obtained from myopic models of addictive behavior. Thus, they argue, assuming rationality only leads to unnecessary complications.

This assertion was challenged by Pashardes (1986) in his empirical test of the myopic versus rational models in the context of the Almost Ideal Demand System. In his model, myopic and rational demand equations are the limiting cases of a more general model. In the context of his general model, Pashardes derived demand equations for a rational consumer in which current consumption is determined by past consumption and current preferences with full knowledge about the impact of current decisions on the future costs of consumption. He then tested for rational and myopic behavior using British data for nine groups of commodities, including tobacco products, alcohol, food, and others, for the period 1947–80. Pashardes found considerable evidence to support the hypothesis of rational behavior in general, as well as evidence that cigarette smoking is an addictive behavior. Finally, he noted that expectations concerning the future price and other costs of consumption played an important role in consumer behavior.

Becker and Murphy (1988) similarly rejected the notion that myopic behavior is empirically indistinguishable from rational behavior in their theory of rational addiction. They assumed that individuals consistently maximize utility over their life-cycle, taking into account the future consequences of their choices. At any point in time t, an individual's utility, $U(t)$, depends on current addictive consumption, $C(t)$, current consumption of a composite of non-addictive consumption, $Y(t)$, and the stock of past consumption, $S(t)$:

$$U(t) = U[C(t), Y(t), S(t)].$$ (5.4)

They assumed that $U(t)$ is a strongly concave function of C, Y, and S, and that the lifetime utility function is separable over time in C, Y, and S, but not in C and Y alone. Tolerance is incorporated by assuming that the marginal utility of the addictive stock is negative. Reinforcement is modeled by assuming that an increase in the addictive stock raises the marginal utility of current addictive consumption. Finally, eqn 5.4 captures withdrawal, since total utility falls with the cessation of addictive consumption.

Becker and Murphy define the stock accumulation process as:

$$\partial S(t)/\partial t = C(t) - \delta S(t) - h[D(t)]. \tag{5.5}$$

This is comparable to the stock accumulation process described in other models of addiction, with the exception of the D(t) term representing endogenous attempts to reduce the addictive stock.

Maximizing lifetime utility subject to an appropriate budget constraint and the stock accumulation process described by eqn 5.5 yields the following first order condition for the addictive good:

$$U_C(t) = \mu \pi_C(t), \tag{5.6}$$

where μ is the marginal utility of wealth and $\pi_C(t)$ is the full price of the addictive good, which depends on the money price of the good and the future utility costs (or shadow price) of the addictive stock. For harmful addictions, the full price of addictive consumption exceeds its money price due to the effects of tolerance and the health consequences of consumption, for example. Moreover, the full price is lower as depreciation on the addictive stock is faster or as the rate of time-preference is higher.

Becker and Murphy (1988) and Becker *et al.* (1991) developed several hypotheses from this basic model. First, addictive consumption displays 'adjacent complementarity'; that is, due to reinforcement, the quantities of the addictive good consumed in different time periods are complements. As a result, current consumption of the addictive good will be inversely related not only to the current price of the good but also to all past and future prices. Consequently, the long-run effect of a permanent change in price will exceed the short-run effect. In addition, price responsiveness varies with time-preference: addicts with higher discount rates will be relatively more responsive to changes in money price than those with lower discount rates. The opposite will be true with respect to the effects of information concerning the future consequences of addictive consumption. Thus, the model suggests that younger, less educated persons and those on lower incomes will be relatively more responsive to changes in the money price of cigarettes, while older, more educated persons and those on higher incomes will be relatively more responsive to new information on the health consequences of cigarette smoking.

Strong adjacent complementarity, reflecting strong addiction, can lead to unstable steady states in the Becker and Murphy model. This is a key feature of their rational addiction theory, helping to explain the binge behavior and 'cold turkey' quit behavior observed among addicts. Furthermore, these unstable steady states imply that there will be a bimodal distribution of consumption, again something that is observed for many addictive goods. In addition, Becker and Murphy's model implies that temporary events, including price reductions, peer pressure, or stressful events, can lead to permanent addictions.

Given a quadratic utility function (which has the useful property that the first order conditions for each of the arguments are linear), and the individual's rate of time-preference, σ, being equal to the market interest rate, a structural demand function for the consumption of the addictive good is derived as:

$$C(t) = \alpha_0 + \alpha_1 P_C(t) + \alpha_2 P_C(t-1) + \beta\alpha_2 P_C(t+1) + \alpha_3 C(t-1) + \beta\alpha_3 C(t+1), \quad (5.7)$$

where β is a discount factor that depends on the rate of time-preference ($\beta = 1/(1 + \sigma)$). Equation 5.7 is the basis for most of the empirical applications of the rational-addiction model. In this equation, current consumption of the addictive substance is inversely related to its current price, but positively related to past and future prices. As Becker *et al.* (1994) noted, the positive past and future price effects seem contra-dictory, given the discussion of adjacent complementarity. However, eqn 5.7 holds past and future consumption constant, eliminating the mechanism through which past and future prices affect current consumption. If past consumption did not change as past prices rose, then some other factor must have led to an increase in past consumption, offsetting the decrease caused by the price increase. This increase in past consumption is what causes current consumption to be positively related to past price when past and future consumption are held constant.

For addictive goods, eqn 5.7 implies that current consumption is positively related to past consumption, with the degree of addiction reflected by α_3. Similarly, given the assumption of rational behavior and the symmetry present in the model, future consumption has a positive impact on current consumption. Finally, the effects of future consumption and future price on current consumption are expected to be smaller than those of past consumption and price by a factor that depends on the rate of time-preference.

The demand equation given by eqn 5.7 allows for direct tests of addiction and ratio-nality. If a good is not addictive, in the sense that its past consumption has no impact on current consumption, then α_2 and α_3 will be equal to zero. Similarly, if a good is addictive, but individuals behave myopically ($\sigma \to \infty$), then past consumption and price will have a positive impact on current consumption, but future consumption and price should have no effect, and the resulting demand equations would be comparable to those estimated by Mullahy (1985) and others described above. Clearly, the demand equations obtained when rationality is assumed are not observationally equivalent to those resulting from the alternative assumption of myopic behavior.

Given the endogeneity of past and future consumption in eqn 5.7, ordinary least squares estimation would lead to biased estimates of the key parameters. Fortunately, the theoretical model provides a solution to this problem. In the full reduced form, addictive consumption at any point in time is a function of all past, current, and future prices, while in the structural demand equation, it is a function of the current, once lagged, and once led price. Thus, further leads and lags of price are appropriate instru-ments for past and future consumption. In addition, many empirical applications of the Becker and Murphy rational-addiction model impose the additional assumption that the depreciation rate on the addictive stock is equal to one. When this assumption is imposed, $\alpha_2 = 0$, and current consumption is a function of the current price only, as well as past and future consumption.

The Becker and Murphy rational-addiction model has several interesting implica-tions with respect to the effects of price on demand for an addictive good that can be obtained from the solution to the second-order difference equation given in eqn 5.7. For one, the effect of an anticipated price change is expected to exceed that of an unanticipated change in price, while the effect of a permanent price change will exceed that of a temporary change. Perhaps most interestingly, the Becker and Murphy model predicts that the long-run effect of a permanent change in price will exceed its short-run effect. Moreover, the ratio of the long-run to short-run price effects rises as the degree of addiction rises (Becker *et al.* 1991, 1994).

Chaloupka (1988, 1990, 1991, 1992) was the first to use individual level data to estimate cigarette demand equations derived from the Becker and Murphy rational-addiction model. His data were taken from the Second National Health and Nutrition Examination Survey for the United States conducted in the late 1970s. Although a cross-sectional survey, information on past cigarette consumption was collected retrospectively, which enabled Chaloupka to construct measures of past, current, and future cigarette consumption for all survey respondents ages 18 years and older. In addition to estimating a version of eqn 5.7, Chaloupka estimated an alternative version that replaced the past consumption and price variable with the stock of past cigarette consumption. In all of the estimated models, past cigarette consumption had a significant positive impact on current consumption, consistent with the notion that cigarette smoking is an addictive behavior. Similarly, consistent with the hypothesis of rational behavior, future cigarette consumption had a significant positive effect on current consumption. The relatively low rates of time-preference implied by these estimates are also consistent with the hypothesis of non-myopic or rational behavior.

Chaloupka's (1991) estimates of the long-run price elasticity of demand fell in the range from –0.27 to –0.48, larger than the elasticities obtained from conventional demand equations using the same data. In addition to estimating the rational addiction demand equations for the full sample, Chaloupka also explored the implications of the Becker and Murphy model with respect to the rate of time-preference by estimating comparable demand equations for subsamples based on age and educational attainment. Chaloupka's (1991) estimates were generally consistent with the hypothesis that less educated or younger persons behave more myopically than their more educated or older counterparts. In addition, less educated persons were more price responsive, with long-run price elasticities ranging from –0.57 to –0.62, than were more educated persons, who were generally unresponsive to price. Chaloupka (1990) also estimated separate demand equations for subsamples based on gender, concluding that men behaved more myopically and were relatively more responsive to price (long-run price elasticity centered on –0.60) than women (statistically insignificant effect of price on demand).

Becker *et al.* (1994) estimated a version of eqn 5.7 that assumed a depreciation rate of 1 on the stock of past cigarette consumption, as well as a comparable myopic demand equation, using a pooled time-series of annual US state cross-sections for the period 1955–85. They also found clear evidence that cigarette smoking is addictive as well as evidence of non-myopic behavior. However, estimates from unrestricted models containing past and future cigarette prices and taxes as instruments for past consumption produced relatively high estimates of the discount factor, implying less than fully rational behavior. Becker *et al.* presented a variety of other estimates to address this issue, including those from models that exclude future variables from the set of instruments and others that impose more reasonable discount rates. The authors concluded that there was insufficient information in the data to accurately estimate the discount rate, and that their estimates were clearly inconsistent with myopic behavior. The authors' estimates of the short-run price elasticity of demand, ranging from −0.36 to −0.44, are generally consistent with the estimates from conventional demand models. However, they found that, due to the addictive nature of smoking, the demand for cigarettes was nearly twice as responsive in the long-run (long-run elasticity estimates ranging from −0.73 to −0.79).

Sung *et al.* (1994) used similar data for 11 Western United States states for the years 1967–90 in an interesting application of the Becker and Murphy model that simultaneously estimated cigarette demand and supply. Their estimates for demand were generally consistent with those of Becker *et al.* (1994) and hence with the hypothesis of rational addiction. In addition, they found that when cigarette taxes increased, because of the oligopolistic nature of the cigarette industry and the addictive nature of cigarette demand, cigarette prices rose by more than the amount of the tax increase. This is consistent with Becker *et al.*'s (1994) theoretical model of a monopolist producing cigarettes.

Several other applications of the Becker and Murphy model have employed aggregate time-series data for various countries or other jurisdictions. Keeler *et al.* (1993), using data from California, Pekurinen (1991), using data for Finland, and Bardsley and Olekalns (1998), with data for Australia, produced estimates consistent with the hypothesis of rational addiction. Duffy (1996), Cameron (1997), and Conniffe (1995), using annual time-series data for the United Kingdom, Greece, and Ireland, respectively, found little support for the rational-addiction model. However, the latter two studies were limited by the relatively small number of observations available for their analyses, while all three have problems resulting from the use of several highly correlated regressors.

Finally, Douglas (1998) used hazard models to examine the determinants of smoking initiation and cessation in the context of the Becker and Murphy (1988) rational-addiction model. In contrast to his finding that price does not significantly affect the hazard of smoking initiation, Douglas concluded that increases in price significantly increase the likelihood (hazard) of smoking cessation. He estimated a price elasticity for the duration of the smoking habit of 1.07 with respect to future price, consistent with the hypothesis of rational addiction; paradoxically, past and current prices were not found to have a statistically significant effect on cessation. Similarly, his parametric and non-parametric results imply that the hazard of smoking cessation has a positive duration dependence, a finding Douglas suggested is consistent with rational addiction in that the rational smoker will discount future health costs less as they become more imminent.

5.4 Recent developments in the economic modeling of addiction

While the rational-addiction model has been more widely used in empirical examinations of addiction than any of the other models, many object to several of the assumptions that provide the foundation for these studies. Perhaps the most criticized aspect of the model is the assumption of perfect foresight. As Winston (1980, p.302) explained, in the context of the Stigler and Becker (1977) model:

[T]he addict looks strange because he sits down at period j = 0, surveys future income, production technologies, investment/addiction functions, and consumption preferences over his lifetime to period T, maximizes the discounted value of his expected utility, and decides to be an alcoholic. That's the way he will get the greatest satisfaction out of life. Alcoholics are alcoholics because they want to be alcoholics, *ex ante*, with full knowledge of its consequences.

Similarly, Akerlof (1991) noted that, in the rational-addiction models, individuals who become addicted do not regret their past decisions, given that they are assumed to have been fully aware of the consequences of their consumption of a potentially addictive good when making these decisions. A few recent theoretical papers have addressed both the concerns about the 'decision' to become addicted and the apparent lack of regret among addicts that arise from the rational-addiction model.

5.4.1 The initiation of addiction

As discussed by Jha *et al.* (see Chapter 7), young people generally have a poor understanding of the addictiveness of tobacco use. This, coupled with the fact that most smokers begin before the age of 20, suggests that the rational-addiction model is ill-suited to describing smoking initiation. A recent theoretical paper by Orphanides and Zervos (1995) addressed this and other perceived inconsistencies of the rational-addiction model that arise largely from the assumption of perfect foresight. In particular, the authors introduced uncertainty into the model by assuming that inexperienced users are not fully aware of the potential harm associated with consuming an addictive substance. In their model, an individual's knowledge comes from the observed effects of the addictive good on others as well as through his or her own experimentation with that good. More specifically, they assume that the harmful effects (including addiction) of consuming a potentially addictive good are not the same for all individuals, that each individual possesses a subjective understanding of his or her potential to become addicted, and that this subjective belief is updated via a Bayesian learning process as the individual consumes the addictive good. Thus, an individual who underestimates his or her potential for addiction and experiments with an addictive substance can end up becoming addicted. Rather than the 'happy addicts' implied by the rational-addiction model (Winston 1980), these addicts will regret becoming addicted. As Orphanides and Zervos describe it (1995, p.750), individuals 'simply *risk* the possibility of addiction because the good is perhaps not harmful to them individually, and they enjoy the immediate rewards of its consumption. Since individuals who become addicts regret having taken that risk, they are naturally unhappy *ex post*'.

As Orphanides and Zervos noted, the incorporation of subjective beliefs into the rational-addiction model helps explain youthful experimentation, the importance of peer influences, and other commonly observed facets of addiction. They go on to note that their model provides important implications for public policy, notably with respect to the control of advertising, the importance of information dissemination programs, and public support of 'rehabilitation programs' aimed at helping addicts break their addiction. However, they note that their model does not go far enough to address other observed behavior of addicts that is inconsistent with the rational-addiction model (specifically decisions to quit and reinitiate addictive consumption).

5.4.2 Adjustment costs

More recent efforts attempt to deal explicitly with cessation decisions in the context of models that focus on the role of adjustment costs (Jones 1999; Suranovic *et al.* 1999). Suranovic and his colleagues, for example, reconsidered the adjacent complementarity of the Becker and Murphy (1988) model, noting that one implication of adjacent complementarity is that efforts to reduce current consumption will lead to reductions in utility. These 'quitting costs' are an important feature of their model and help explain the seeming inconsistency between smokers' stated wishes to quit smoking and their continued cigarette consumption. For example, they help explain why smokers engage in various behavior modification treatments, such as the use of the nicotine patch, which help make quitting easier.

A second point of departure from the Becker and Murphy model concerns the timing of the consequences of smoking, which Suranovic *et al.* assume are concentrated at the end of a smoker's life. In addition, rather than assuming that individuals choose a lifetime consumption path that maximizes the present value of their lifetime utility, Suranovic *et al.* assume 'boundedly rational' behavior, implying that individuals choose current consumption only rather than their lifetime consumption path. As a result, their model suggests that aging is enough to induce cessation among some smokers. That is, as the health consequences of smoking become more immediate, raising the perceived benefits of cessation, smokers will be more likely to quit, an hypothesis that is confirmed by Douglas' (1998) finding of positive duration dependence (described above). As in the Becker and Murphy model, their model implies that quitting 'cold-turkey' is likely in the case of a strong addiction (one where quitting costs rise rapidly for small reductions in consumption). However, in contrast to Becker and Murphy, Suranovic *et al.* predicted gradual reductions in consumption progressing to quitting in the case of relatively weak addictions.

Jones and his colleagues have conducted empirical analyses implementing the notion of adjustment costs as an important determinant of smoking cessation (Jones 1994; Yen and Jones 1996; Contoyannis and Jones 1999). Yen and Jones (1996), for example, estimate a double-hurdle model for smokers that considers separately their decisions concerning how much to smoke and whether or not to quit, where both decisions are based, in part, on past consumption. In this model, the net benefits of quitting are a key determinant of whether or not a smoker will quit. Net benefits are determined by comparing the health and other benefits associated with quitting to the withdrawal costs associated with cessation. Their estimates provide some empirical support that greater adjustment costs and/or lower benefits from quitting significantly reduce the likelihood of cessation. Interestingly, and contrary to general perceptions, they find that the heaviest smokers have the greatest incentive to quit once the adjustment costs are accounted for. Contoyannis and Jones (1999) extend this analysis to examine the Suranovic *et al.* hypotheses concerning the impact of age and the perceived bene-fits of quitting on smoking cessation. Their analysis of UK data provides support for the hypothesis that the probability of cessation rises with age. In addition, they find that the probability of quitting is higher for both the lightest smokers and heaviest smokers than it is for more moderate smokers. They do not, however, find that increases in the perceived benefits of quitting—as measured by the perceived improve-ment in life expectancy resulting from cessation—significantly raise the probability of quitting.

Most recently, Goldbaum (in press) builds on the Becker and Murphy (1988) and Suranovic *et al.* (1999) approaches in a model that allows for fully rational behavior by a consumer whose lifetime is finite. The key difference between his model and the others is the introduction of a second stock variable that captures the delayed health consequences that result from addictive cigarette consumption. In Goldbaum's model, a young person may rationally decide to become addicted, trading off the immediate gratification associated with current cigarette consumption against the future conse-quences associated with addiction and the distant health consequences of smoking. The optimal consumption path that results from this model can include quitting at some future point in response to the accumulating stock of smoking-attributable health consequences. While this model does address some of the limitations of the earlier eco-nomic models of addiction, it appears to be based on a relatively naïve description of the initiation process.

5.4.3 Addiction and time-preference

A separate but related stream of recent research has focused on the role of time-preference in modeling addictive behavior. As noted above, the early work by Strotz (1956) considered the 'time-inconsistency' of preferences in helping to explain the regret associated with addiction. In his model, this time-inconsistency resulted from the use of a non-exponential discount function. Repeating from above, time-inconsis-tency in Strotz's model is reflected by an individual changing his consumption path at some point in time 'even though his original expectations of future desires and means of consumption are verified' (p. 165). Put differently, even with full information, perfect foresight, stable preferences, and rational behavior at initiation that results in a plan that would have the person smoking in all future periods, a smoker may eventually decide to quit.

Much empirical evidence, generally from disciplines other than economics, indicates that preferences are often time-inconsistent. Vuchinich and Simpson (1999), for exam-ple, show that a hyperbolic discount function (that results in time-inconsistencies), rather than the more commonly used exponential function (which is always time-consistent), better describes the nature of discounting among drinkers. In addition, they find that heavy social and problem drinkers have higher discount rates (a stronger preference for the present) than lighter drinkers; Bretteville-Jensen (1999) finds similar differences among current and former heroin and amphetamine users and non-users. However, the direction of causality accounting for the differences in rates of time-preference is unclear. Recent work by Becker and Mulligan (1997) on the endogeneity of time-preference, for example, suggests that addiction itself can lead to heavier discounting, while at the same time a greater preference for the present can make addiction more likely (Becker *et al.* 1991). As Grossman *et al.* (1998) describe, these interactions between time-preference and addiction, coupled with imperfect information, youthful initiation, and the importance of peer influences, provide strong justifications for government interventions to reduce youth tobacco use.

O'Donoghue and Rabin (1999a, b, c), building on earlier work by Phelps and Pollak (1968) and Laibson (1994), as well as the imperfectly rational addiction models described above, present an interesting discussion of time-inconsistency and self-control that has implications for the economic modeling of addiction. In a model incorporating the two key elements of most economic models of addiction—the dependence of current consumption decisions on past consumption and the presence of what they call 'negative internalities' or the negative impact of the addictive stock on current utility—they allow for time-inconsistent preferences (O'Donoghue and Rabin, 1999b). As they describe it (p. 2):

These preferences give rise to a self-control problem because at any moment the person pursues immediate gratification more than she would have preferred if asked at any previous moment.

In addition, they allow for two extreme types of persons—the 'sophisticated' person, who understands her self-control problems and, as a result, knows how she will behave in the future, and the 'naïve' person, who is completely unaware of his self-control problems and does not fully understand how he will behave in the future—in addition to persons with time-consistent preferences. In their model, the naïve person may end up consuming more than they otherwise would if they had no self-control problem, while some sophisticated persons may end up consuming less because they understand their self-control problem and fear becoming addicted. Finally, as the authors note, the introduction of self-control problems into the economic models of addiction is of particular importance because this leads to a much different implication for welfare than that resulting from the rational addiction type models. Specifically, for both sophisticated and naïve persons, self-control problems lead to behavior that causes severe harm (something that would not happen in the rational-addiction models with time-consistent preferences).

Laux (1999) also examines the welfare implications of nicotine addiction using the estimates obtained in various empirical applications of the rational-addiction model. His approach emphasizes three basic arguments: that youths do not adequately understand the costs that youthful smoking decisions will impose on their adult selves, in large part because of their relatively myopic behavior; that adult smoking reflects myopic, or at least less than fully rational behavior, given the rates of time-preference implied from empirical applications of the rational-addiction model; and that the importance of peer effects exacerbate the welfare problems resulting from youth smoking. This leads Laux to treat the internal costs associated with youthful decisions to start smoking and subsequent addiction as a type of externality (the magnitude of which swamps the more conventional externalities from smoking). It should be noted that his approach depends heavily on the assumptions that societies should not treat youth as sovereign and that the impact of decisions made by minors on their smoking as adults can be quantified using the estimates from the rational-addiction model described above. Following this approach, Laux concludes that there are significant social costs arising from cigarette smoking and that government intervention to reduce these costs is warranted (see Chapter 6 for a welfare analysis of tobacco use that is similar in spirit to Laux's analysis).

5.5 Policy implications

While addiction was once considered a problem not conducive to standard economic analysis, this is clearly no longer the case. After sporadic past efforts to theoretically and empirically model addiction, the last decade has seen a growing number of economists devote substantial effort to more fully understanding the impact of addiction on the consumption of tobacco products, alcoholic beverages, illicit drugs, and other addictive commodities. While these models have generated much debate, both within and outside of economics, this debate has stimulated new research that has made and promises further important theoretical and empirical contributions. One thing, however, is clear from both the theoretical models and their empirical applications: the basic laws of economics do apply to addictive goods, including tobacco products.

By necessity, the economic models of addiction are highly stylized and include many simplifying assumptions. These assumptions have led many to object to these models (e.g. the assumptions of perfect foresight, full information, and rational behavior in the rational-addiction model). In some cases, however, these objections have led to new theoretical developments, with different models emphasizing particular aspects of addictive behavior. For example, the recent work by Suranovic and his colleagues (1999) emphasizing the role of adjustment costs seems better suited to examining decisions to continue smoking or to quit (as in the empirical application by Contoyannis and Jones 1999) than it does to examining smoking-initiation decisions. In contrast, the theoretical model employed by Orphanides and Zervos (1995) provides interesting insights into youthful decisions to initiate addictive behaviors, including smoking, and the subsequent regretting of these decisions, but does little to explain cessation efforts. Many of the most promising of these theoretical advances have yet to be tested empirically, in part because the necessary data to test them are not available.

Despite its limitations, the economic analysis of addiction has contributed to a better understanding of the impact of prices and control policies on addictive behaviors, including tobacco use. All of the theoretical models emphasize the role of price and the importance of past consumption as determinants of current smoking decisions. Empirical applications of these models clearly show that higher prices will lead to reductions in cigarette smoking and other tobacco use, while increases in past cigarette consumption (that may have resulted, for example, from lower past prices) will raise current smoking. Price, in the context of these models, includes many dimensions that reflect the costs associated with smoking, including those that result from restrictions on smoking in public and private places, limits on the availability of tobacco products, and new information that raises perceptions of the long-term health and other consequences of smoking. While this is true for non-addictive goods as well, the key implication of the addiction models is that the long-run impact of permanent price changes will be larger than would be expected based on estimates that ignore the role of addiction. Thus, significant permanent real increases in tobacco taxes, strong restrictions on smoking in public places and other control efforts can lead to significant reductions in smoking in the short-run, with even larger reductions in the long-run. In addition, these models generally provide theoretical support for the hypothesis that the dissemination of information on the consequences of tobacco use and/or limits on the provision of misleading information can lead to significant reductions in tobacco use. Moreover, many of the more recent theoretical developments in the economic modeling of addiction contain interesting insights concerning the welfare effects of addictive consumption that provide strong support for government intervention to reduce tobacco use, particularly among youth.

The empirical application of recent theoretical developments, and the continued refinement and expansion of the economic modeling of addiction, promises to further improve our understanding of the role of prices and control policies in affecting smoking initiation, cessation, cigarette consumption, and other aspects of tobacco use. This further research is likely to produce additional, policy-relevant findings on the determinants of cigarette smoking and other tobacco use.

References

Akerlof, G. A. (1991). Procrastination and obedience. *American Economic Review*, **81**, 1–19.

Ashton, H. and Stepney, R. (1982). *Smoking: Psychology and Pharmacology*. London: Tavistock Press.

Baltagi, B. H. and Levin, D. (1986). Estimating dynamic demand for cigarettes using panel data: the effects of bootlegging, taxation, and advertising reconsidered. *Review of Economics and Statistics*, **68**(1), 148–55.

Bardsley, P. and Olekalns, N. (1998). *Cigarette and Tobacco Consumption: Have Anti-smoking Policies Made a Difference?* Working Paper. Department of Economics, The University of Melbourne.

Barthold, T. and Hochman, H. (1988). Addiction as extreme seeking. *Economic Inquiry*, **26**(1), 89–106.

Becker, G. S. and Mulligan, C. B. (1997). The endogeous determination of time-preference. *Quarterly Journal of Economics*, **112**(3), 729–58.

Becker, G. S. and Murphy, K. M. (1988). A theory of rational addiction. *Journal of Political Economy*, **96**(4), 675–700.

Becker, G. S., Grossman, M., and Murphy, K. M. (1991). Rational addiction and the effect of price on consumption. *American Economic Review*, **81**, 237–41.

Becker, G. S., Grossman, M., and Murphy, K. M. (1994). An empirical analysis of cigarette addiction. *American Economic Review*, **84**(3), 396–418.

Boyer, M. (1978). A habit forming optimal growth model. *International Economic Review*, **19**, 585–609.

Boyer, M. (1983). Rational demand and expenditures patterns under habit formation. *Journal of Economic Theory*, **31**, 27–53.

Bretteville-Jensen, A. L. (1999). Addiction and discounting. *Journal of Health Economics*, **18**(4), 393–408.

Cameron, S. (1997). Are Greek smokers rational addicts? *Applied Economics Letters*, **4**(7), 401–2.

Chaloupka, F. J. (1988). *An Economic Analysis of Addictive Behavior: The Case of Cigarette Smoking* [dissertation]. New York: City University of New York Graduate School.

Chaloupka, F. J. (1990). *Men, Women, and Addiction: The Case of Cigarette Smoking*. Working paper no. 3267. Cambridge (MA): National Bureau of Economic Research.

Chaloupka, F. J. (1991). Rational addictive behavior and cigarette smoking. *Journal of Political Economy*, **99**(4), 722–42.

Chaloupka, F. J. (1992). Clean indoor air laws, addiction, and cigarette smoking. *Applied Economics*, **24**(2), 193–205.

Chow, G. (1960). Statistical demand functions for automobiles and their use for forecasting. In *The Demand for Durable Goods* (ed. A. C. Harberger), pp. 149–178. Chicago: University of Chicago Press.

Conniffe, D. (1995). Models of Irish tobacco consumption. *Economic and Social Review*, **26**(4), 331–47.

Contoyannis, P. and Jones, A. M. (1999). *Rationality, Addiction, and Adjustment costs*. Manuscript presented at the International Workshop on Nicotine Dependence, Lausanne, Switzerland, May 27.

Deaton, A. S. and Muellbauer, J. (1980). An almost ideal demand system. *American Economic Review*, **70**, 312–26.

Dixit, A. and Norman, V. (1978). Advertising and welfare. *Bell Journal of Economics*, **9**, 1–17.

Douglas, S. (1998). The duration of the smoking habit. *Economic Inquiry*, **36**(1), 49–64.

Duesenberry, J. S. (1949). *Income, Saving, and the Theory of Consumer Behavior*. Cambridge (MA): Harvard University Press.

Duffy, M. (1996). An econometric study of advertising and cigarette demand in the United Kingdom. *International Journal of Advertising*, **15**, 1–23.

El-Safty, A. E. (1976a). Adaptive behavior, demand, and preferences. *Journal of Economic Theory*, **13**, 298–318.

El-Safty, A. E. (1976b). Adaptive behavior and the existence of Weizsäcker's Long-Run Indifference Curves. *Journal of Economic Theory*, **13**, 319–28.

Elster, J. (1979). *Ulysses and the Sirens: Studies in Rationality and Irrationality*. Cambridge: Cambridge University Press.

Farrell, M. J. (1952). Irreversible demand functions. *Econometrica*, **20**, 171–86.

Galbraith, J. K. (1958). *The Affluent Society*. Cambridge (MA): Houghton Mifflin Company.

Galbraith, J. K. (1972). *The New Industrial State*. 2nd edition. New York: Pelican Books.

Garcia dos Santos, J. (1972). Estimating the durability of consumers' durable goods. *Review of Economics and Statistics*, **54**, 475–9.

Godfrey, C. (1989). Factors influencing the consumption of alcohol and tobacco: the use and abuse of economic models. *British Journal of Addiction*, **84**, 1123–38.

Goldbaum, D. Life cycle consumption of a harmful and addictive good. *Economic Inquiry*. (In press.)

Gorman, W. M. (1967). Tastes, habits, and choices. *International Economic Review*, **8**, 218–22.

Grossman, M., Chaloupka, F. J., and Anderson, R. (1998). A survey of economic models of addictive behavior. *Journal of Drug Issues*, **28**(3), 631–644.

Haavelmo, T. (1944). The probability approach in econometrics. *Econometrica*, **12**, 96–124.

Hammond, P. J. (1976a). Changing tastes and coherent dynamic choice. *Review of Economic Studies*, **43**, 159–73.

Hammond, P. J. (1976b). Endogenous tastes and stable long-run choice. *Journal of Economic Theory*, **13**, 329–40.

Houthakker, H. S. and Taylor, L. D. (1966). *Consumer Demand in the United States, 1929–1970: Analyses and Projections.* Cambridge (MA): Harvard University Press.

Houthakker, H, S. and Taylor, L. D. (1970). *Consumer Demand in the United States, 1929–1970: Analyses and Projections.* 2nd ed. Cambridge (MA): Harvard University Press.

Hughes, J. and Bickel, W. K. (1999). *Medical Models of Dependence.* Manuscript presented at the International Workshop on Nicotine Dependence, Lausanne, Switzerland, May 27.

Jones, A. M. (1989). A systems approach to the demand for alcohol and tobacco. *Bulletin of Economic Research*, **41**, 85–105.

Jones, A. M. (1994). Health, addiction, social interaction and the decision to quit smoking. *Journal of Health Economics*, **13**, 93–110.

Jones, A. M. (1999). Adjustment costs, withdrawal effects, and cigarette addiction. *Journal of Health Economics*, **18**(1), 125–37.

Keeler, T. E., Hu, T.-W., Barnett, P. G., and Manning, W. G. (1993). Taxation, regulation and addiction: a demand function for cigarettes based on time-series evidence. *Journal of Health Economics*, **12**(1), 1–18.

Laibson, D. (1994). *Essays in Hyperbolic Discounting* [dissertation]. Cambridge (MA): MIT.

Laux, F. L. (1999). *Addiction as a Market Failure: Using Rational Addiction Results to Justify Tobacco Regulation.* Manuscript, School of Business, Instituto Tecnologico Autonomo de Mexico.

Lewit, E. M. and Coate, D. (1982). The potential for using excise taxes to reduce smoking. *Journal of Health Economics*, **1**(2), 121–45.

Lluch, C. (1974). Expenditure, savings, and habit formation. *International Economic Review*, **15**, 786–97.

Marshall, A. (1920). *Principles of Economics.* 8th ed. London: Macmillan and Co.

McKenzie, R. B. (1979). The non-rational domain and the limits of economic analysis. *Southern Economic Journal*, **46**(1), 145–57.

Michaels, R. (1988). Addiction, compulsion, and the technology of consumption. *Economic Inquiry*, **26**(1), 74–88.

Modigliani, F. (1949). Fluctuations in the savings-income ratio: a problem in economic forecasting. In *Studies in Income and Wealth*, vol. 11, pp. 371–443. New York: National Bureau of Economic Research.

Mullahy, J. (1985). *Cigarette Smoking: Habits, Health Concerns, and Heterogeneous Unobservables in a Micro-econometric Analysis of Consumer Demand* [dissertation]. Charlottesville (VA): University of Virginia.

O'Donoghue, T. and Rabin, M. (1999a). Doing it now or later. *American Economic Review*, **89**(1), 103–24.

O'Donoghue, T. and Rabin, M. (1999b). *Addiction and Self-control.* Manuscript, Department of Economics, Cornell University.

O'Donoghue, T. and Rabin, M. (1999c). *The Economics of Immediate Gratification.* Manuscript, Department of Economics, Cornell University.

Orphanides, A. and Zervos, D. (1995). Rational addiction with learning and regret. *Journal of Political Economy*, **103**, 739–58.

Pashardes, P. (1986). Myopic and forward looking behavior in a dynamic demand system. *International Economic Review*, **27**, 387–97.

Pekurinen, M. (1989). The demand for tobacco products in Finland. *British Journal of Addiction*, **84**, 1183–92.

Pekurinen, M. (1991). *Economic Aspects of Smoking: Is There a Case for Government Intervention in Finland?* Helsinki: Vapk-Publishing.

Phelps, E. S. and Pollak, R. A. (1968). On second-best national saving and game-equilibrium growth. *Review of Economic Studies*, **35**(2), 185–99.

Phlips, L. (1983). *Applied Consumption Analysis.* Advanced Textbooks in Economics. Amsterdam: North-Holland Publishing Company.

Phlips, L. and Spinnewyn, F. (1982). Rationality versus myopia in dynamic demand systems. In *Advances in Econometrics*, vol. 1 (ed. R. L. Basman and G. F. Rhodes Jr.), pp. 3–33. Greenwich (CT): JAI Press.

Pollak, R. A. (1968). Consistent planning. *Review of Economic Studies*, **35**, 201–8.

Pollak, R. A. (1970). Habit formation and dynamic demand functions. *Journal of Political Economy*, **78**, 745–63.

Pollak, R. A. (1975). The intertemporal cost of living index. *Annals of Economic and Social Measurement*, **4**, 179–95.

Pollak, R. A. (1976). Habit formation and long-run utility functions. *Journal of Economic Theory*, **13**, 272–97.

Pollak, R. A. (1977). Price dependent preferences. *American Economic Review*, **67**, 64–75.

Pollak, R. A. (1978). Endogenous tastes in demand and welfare analysis. *American Economic Review*, **68**, 374–9.

Ryder, H. E. and Heal, G. M. (1973). Optimal growth with intertemporally dependent preferences. *Review of Economic Studies*, **40**, 1–31.

Schelling, T. C. (1978). Egonomics, or the art of self-management. *American Economic Review*, **68**, 290–4.

Schelling, T. C. (1980). The intimate contest for self-command. *The Public Interest*, **60**, 94–113.

Schelling, T. C. (1984a). *Choice and Consequence*. Cambridge (MA): Harvard University Press.

Schelling, T. C. (1984b). Self-command in practice, in policy, and in a theory of rational choice. *American Economic Review*, **74**, 1–11.

Scitovsky, T. (1976). *The Joyless Economy: An Inquiry into Consumer Satisfaction and Human Dissatisfaction*. Oxford: Oxford University Press.

Spinnewyn, F. (1981). Rational habit formation. *European Economic Review*, **15**, 91–109.

Stigler, G. and Becker, G. S. (1977). De gustibus non est disputandum. *American Economic Review*, **67**, 76–90.

Strotz, R. H. (1956). Myopia and inconsistency in dynamic utility maximization. *Review of Economic Studies*, **23**, 165–80.

Sung, H.-Y., Hu, T.-W., and Keeler, T. E. (1994). Cigarette taxation and demand: an empirical model. *Contemporary Economic Policy*, **12**(3), 91–100.

Suranovic, S. M., Goldfarb, R. S., and Leonard, T. C. (1999). An economic theory of cigarette addiction. *Journal of Health Economics*, **18**(1), 1–29.

Swan, G. E. and Balfour, D. J. K. (ed.) (1999). *Nicotine and tobacco research: Proceedings from "Addicted to Nicotine: A National Research Forum"*, Bethesda, MD, July 27–28, 1998.

Thaler, R. and Shefrin, H. M. (1981). An economic theory of self-control. *Journal of Policial Economy*, **89**, 392–406.

US Department of Health and Human Services (1988). *The Health Consequences of Smoking: Nicotine Addiction. A Report of the Surgeon General*. Rockville (MD): US Department of Health and Human Services, Public Health Service, Centers for Disease Control, Center for Health Promotion and Education, Office on Smoking and Health.

US Department of Health Human Services (1994). *Preventing tobacco use among young people: a report of the Surgeon General*. Atlanta (GA): US Department of Health and Human Services, Public Health Service, Centers for Discase Control and Prevention, and Health Promotion, Office on Smoking and Health.

US Food and Drug Administration (1996). *Regulations Restricting the Sale and Distribution of Cigarettes and Smokeless Tobacco to Protect Children and Adolescents; Final Rule*. Washington, DC: US Department of Health and Human Services, Food and Drug Administration.

von Weizsäcker, C. C. (1971). Notes on endogenous change of tastes. *Journal of Economic Theory*, **3**, 345–72.

Vuchinich, R. E. and Simpson, C. A. (1999). Delayed-reward discounting in alcohol abuse. In *The Economic Analysis of Substance Use and Abuse: an Integration of Econometric and Behavioral Economic Research* (ed. F. J. Chaloupka, M. Grossman, W. K. Bickel, and H. Saffer H), pp. 103–22. Chicago: University of Chicago Press for the National Bureau of Economic Research.

Winston, G. C. (1980). Addiction and backsliding: a theory of compulsive consumption. *Journal of Economic Behavior and Organization*, **1**(4), 295–324.

Yen, S. and Jones, A. M. (1996). Individual cigarette consumption and addiction: a flexible limited dependent variable approach. *Health Economics*, **5**(1), 105–17.

Young, T. (1983). The demand for cigarettes: alternative specifications of Fujii's model. *Applied Economics*, **15**, 203–11.

6

A welfare analysis of tobacco use

*Richard Peck, Frank J. Chaloupka, Prabhat Jha,
and James Lightwood*

Non-technical summary

This chapter examines the costs and benefits of smoking with the aim of asking whether, in economic terms, tobacco on net makes the world better or worse off. Given that the analysis is relatively complex and technical, we provide a summary for the reader interested in the key findings and an outline of the methods used.

Introduction. Like most consumer goods, cigarettes have both costs and benefits. The chief benefits are the satisfaction and enjoyment that smokers receive from smoking. There are also profits to producers. The chief costs are death and disability among smokers themselves. Other costs, which are much smaller, include health damage to non-smokers from passive smoking.

In conventional economics, consumers are assumed to weigh the personal costs and benefits of any purchase. It is assumed that, in buying something, a consumer has judged the personal benefits to outweigh the personal costs. Therefore, conventional cost–benefit analyses exclude consumers' own costs and analyze only the costs that their consumption choices impose on others. In the case of smoking, the costs to smokers themselves— including the premature loss of life and health—should thus theoretically be excluded, because they are assumed to have been taken into account. However, it is argued here that smokers cannot be assumed to have taken all their personal costs into account, given the nature of tobacco as a consumer good. Most smokers start young, become addicted, and then face significant adjustment costs when trying to stop their addiction. In high-income countries, most adult smokers say they regret starting. The aim of this paper is to analyze the costs and benefits of smoking in a way that goes beyond the traditional approach and accounts for these factors.

Benefits. By examining the relationship between the price of a good and the demand for it (demand-elasticity), economists can approximate, but not precisely measure, the benefits people assign to that good. This is called consumer surplus, defined as the amount that people are prepared to pay for a product over and above its price. (The more benefits people assign to the product, the less willing they are to give it up at higher prices.) Cigarettes are addictive, so, in this analysis, we take addiction into account by assessing the demand-elasticity for tobacco over a long period rather than a short one, because consumers of addictive products will take longer than consumers of non-addictive products to adjust their demand for the product in response to price changes.

For producers, economists can approximate the benefits by examining the relationship between the price of a good and the amount of it supplied (supply-elasticity). This is called producer surplus, and is calculated by estimating how much money could be taken from producers without reducing the amount that they would supply. Using empirical data on price, expenditures on cigarettes, and demand- and supply-elasticities, we can calculate estimates of consumers' and producers' surpluses in dollar terms.

Costs. While it is relatively easy to estimate the benefits of cigarettes, estimating costs is much more difficult. We use the following approach. First and most importantly, we assume that people are willing to pay to avoid death and disability. Thus, a smoker who fully understands the risks of smoking would be considered to have taken the loss of life and health into account. But an uninformed smoker would be considered not to have taken the loss of life into account, and would be willing to pay something to buy it back. Second, we assign a monetary value to what each year of healthy life would be worth to smokers. We use a standard measure, the disability-adjusted life-year, or DALY. This unit expresses the sum of years lost due to premature mortality and years lived with disability adjusted for severity. One DALY is thus one lost year of healthy life. We use a base value of $7750 per DALY, which is average global per capita gross domestic product (GDP) weighted for tobacco consumption. This, according to various studies, is a very conservative value of what people are actually willing to pay to live an extra year. Third, using projections of the number of DALYs that will be attributed worldwide due to tobacco, if current smoking patterns continue between 1990 and 2020, we can estimate the monetary value of the future costs of smoking-attributable DALYs. Fourth, we determine what proportion of today's smokers would need to be uninformed about their health risks for the total smoking-attributable DALY burden to have the same dollar value as the sum of the consumer and producer surpluses. In other words, we ask what proportion of smokers would have to be uninformed about their risks for the costs of smoking to rise as high as the benefits—the point at which smoking would be considered to have no social benefits. It should be noted that other smoking-attributable costs, including external costs, are not considered in this analysis. Finally, we subject these values to various sensitivity analyses.

Key results. Depending on different assumptions, the proportion of smokers worldwide who would have to be uninformed for there to be no social benefits from smoking ranges from 3% to 23%. This may also be considered in terms of individual smokers' risk perceptions. If a typical or average smoker under-estimates his or her own health costs of smoking by 3 to 23%, then the net benefits are zero. We also use this framework to examine the impact of higher taxes on cigarettes. The resulting higher prices lead to loss of satisfaction, as some smokers give up or reduce smoking in response to the higher prices. This loss of satisfaction has a dollar value. However, if only 3% of smokers are uninformed about the risks of smoking, then the avoided costs of ill health exceed the costs of lost satisfaction that would be associated with a price rise of 10% due to tax. This suggests that modest tax increases are likely to enhance global welfare.

Discussion. The framework presented here is illustrative. The actual numeric results depend on several assumptions and limited data. The analyses do suggest that any discussion of benefits of smoking to smokers or producers must take into account that people are willing to pay to avoid death and disability and that there are substantial information problems in using tobacco. Given the evidence that many smokers do underestimate their future health costs, our analyses raise questions as to the validity of traditional assessments of the benefits of smoking.

6.1 Introduction

For determining policy toward tobacco, an estimate of the net social benefit of tobacco consumption—that is, an estimate of both costs and benefits—is very useful. Such an estimate provides an answer to the question: Does the presence of tobacco, on net, make the world better off or worse off? With the data currently available, this question is difficult to answer directly, but this paper develops an alternative approach that indirectly addresses this question. Conventional economic analysis defines total benefits as the sum of the consumers' total willingness to pay for tobacco products, net of expenditures, and all economic profits generated by tobacco production. Net benefits are determined by subtracting the relevant social costs from total benefits. Usually, the relevant social costs are so-called external costs (the value of resources utilized in the production or consumption of tobacco that are not taken into account by consumers or producers because they are borne by others). For example, smokers may not take into account the impact of environmental tobacco smoke (ETS) on the health of non-smokers who are present when they smoke. However, there are other costs that smokers may fail to take into account because they are uninformed or only partially informed about them. These costs have been omitted from previous studies, but we argue that they should be considered. The costs arise from consumers' lack of information about the health risks of tobacco. Most smokers start young, become addicted, and then face significant adjustment costs when trying to stop their addiction. Rather than determining the size of costs arising from uninformed tobacco use directly, which would be difficult given available data, we determine instead the fraction of the smoking population that would need to be uninformed for the total net benefits of tobacco use to be zero. To illustrate our approach we calculate this threshold percentage of uninformed smokers using World Bank data. Depending on various assumptions, this threshold percentage of uninformed smokers ranges from 3% to about 23%. These initial estimates mean that if more than one-quarter of the world's smokers are uninformed about smoking risks, then the net benefits of smoking are negative. An alternative interpretation is that if the typical or average smoker under-estimates the cost of smoking by between 3% and 23%, then there are net social costs. The approach parallels the classical cost–benefit technique of determining an internal rate of return, that is, finding an interest rate that equates net benefits with zero.

The analysis also underscores an important direction for future research. To assess and understand the impact of tobacco consumption, we need to have a better understanding of how well-informed individuals are about the addiction and the health consequences of tobacco consumption. There is already significant evidence indicating that many smokers initially under-estimate the addictive potential and health consequences of tobacco (see Chapter 8).

We also examine the incremental benefits and costs associated with a 10% increase in the retail price of cigarettes. The social cost of raising cigarette prices is the net reduction in consumer welfare and producer profits, the so-called deadweight loss. The social benefits of higher cigarette price arise from reductions in either external or uninformed costs. We find that the deadweight loss is an order of magnitude smaller than the decline in tobacco-related death and disability. Accordingly, a price rise of 10% will generate net positive benefits if more than 3% of smokers are uninformed.

The paper is organized as follows. First, the theoretical underpinnings of measuring consumer benefits are briefly reviewed. We then present our estimates of net consumer benefits, i.e. consumer surplus. We then turn to producer benefits, i.e. producer surplus. Next we discuss costs and, in particular, explain the distinction between external and internal costs. We then present our estimates of the threshold percentage of smokers who would need to be uninformed about the health risks of smoking for the social benefits to be zero. Following this is a discussion of the incremental benefits and costs of a 10% increase in the price of tobacco. The paper closes with discussion of some implications and suggestions for further research.

6.2 The benefits of tobacco consumption

6.2.1 Introduction

The benefits of tobacco consumption flow from two sources. First, there are the profits earned by producers. While these are non-trivial amounts, of the order of US$40 billion to $50 billion per year, they are dwarfed by the primary source of benefits: the satisfaction derived by the consumers of tobacco products. Our results are sensitive to elasticity of demand, a concept discussed below, but our best guess is that annual consumer surplus (also considered below) is about $236 billion (measured in 1990 prices). In this section, consumer surplus is discussed first, followed by a discussion of producer surplus.

6.2.2 Consumer surplus

For any standard economic commodity, there are two distinct, equally legitimate ways to measure the benefits to consumers. The first approach considers willingness to accept payment. One can ask, what is the total amount of compensation required by consumers so that they are just willing to give up tobacco products? Here, we are considering the cash amount that makes a consumer indifferent between consuming the product and not consuming the product. This benefit measure is referred to as compensating variation. In the case of tobacco products, this is equivalent to determining the size of the bribe or payment required to induce smokers to quit.

The second approach is based on willingness to pay. In particular, one measures benefits by determining the maximum amount consumers are willing to pay to prevent the loss of tobacco products. In this approach, we are asking how much a consumer would be willing to pay to continue smoking. This measure of consumer benefit is called equivalent variation. Both approaches are equally sound, but give different answers. In particular, willingness to accept payment is always larger than the willingness to pay.[1] For reasonable preferences, these two measures tend to move together: a large compensating variation implies a large equivalent variation. For cigarettes, however, the gap between equivalent variation and compensating variation may be

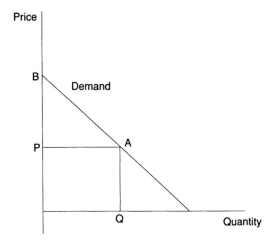

Fig. **6.1** Demand curve with consumer surplus PBA.

quite large; an addicted smoker may require infinite compensation to quit, yet his willingness to pay, since it is bounded by the smoker's income, may be finite. The two measures do assume different entitlements. In measuring compensating variation, one is implicitly assuming that individuals have the right to smoke and that one must pay people not to smoke. In contrast, equivalent variation, it has been argued, implicitly assumes that smokers do not possess the right to smoke and therefore must purchase this right.

When there is insufficient data available, it is standard to approximate benefits by considering consumer surplus.[2] The justification for such an approximation in the case of a non-addictive good is provided by Willig (1976), though the applicability of the Willig results for addictive goods remains an open research area. The standard interpretation of consumer surplus is that it gives net willingness to pay for a given amount of the commodity, that is, total willingness to pay minus what is actually spent. For a given price, consumer surplus is geometrically the area under the demand curve up to the amount consumed at the specified price minus the total amount paid for tobacco; this is shown as area of the triangle PBA in Fig. 6.1.

Consumer surplus is estimated as follows. The long-run demand curve is assumed to be linear, that is:

$$P = a - bQ. \tag{6.1}$$

[1] A statement and proof of this well-known result can be found in Hausman (1981).
[2] The framework we have outlined for determining consumer benefits is very general and can be applied to a variety of consumer goods. Many have argued, however, that the demand for tobacco is distinctive and special because tobacco is an addictive substance. A natural question to ask is what willingness to pay and willingness to accept payment mean for a good that is addictive. For economists, the analytical definition of an addictive good is that it is a good for which current consumption depends on past consumption, as well as on current price and other factors. Since past consumption depends on past prices, this implies that for

With a linear demand curve, if the current price is P and current consumption is Q and the price elasticity in absolute value at P and Q is e, then annual consumer surplus, CS, is:

$$CS = PQ/2e. \tag{6.2}$$

Price elasticity, e, measures the sensitivity of quantity demanded to changes in price; formally it is the percentage change in quantity demanded for a 1% increase in price. This consumer surplus formula indicates that consumer surplus varies inversely with the price elasticity.[3] When the price elasticity is infinite, consumer surplus is zero and when the price elasticity is less than 0.5 in absolute value, consumer surplus exceeds total expenditures. This formula is very useful when data are limited, since consumer surplus can be calculated with only two variables: expenditures and price elasticity. Put differently, by assuming linear demand curves, there is sufficient structure to estimate consumer surplus with very limited data.

The principle shortcoming of linear demand curves is that they may not accurately portray behavior when tobacco prices are very high. Of course, we have no direct observations about the behavior of demand when prices are extremely high. However, for a linear demand curve, the price intercept is given by:

$$a = P(1+1/e), \tag{6.3}$$

where a is the price at which the demand for tobacco products is zero. This formula implies that if the price of cigarettes is $2.00 and the observed elasticity at $2.00 is –0.8, then at a price of $4.50, the long-run demand for tobacco products would be zero. The fact that this is not a very plausible conclusion can be taken as evidence that the assumption of linear demand curves may, for this reason, lead to an under-estimation of total consumer surplus. However, as outlined below, there are also reasons to believe that linear demand curves over-estimate total consumer surplus.

In implementing this formula, we take into account the fact that the retail price of cigarettes and the quantity of cigarettes consumed vary across regions. It also likely that the price elasticity will vary from region to region, since per capita incomes vary considerably across regions. To compute total world annual consumer benefits over n regions, we have:

$$CS_{world} = 1/2[p_1 q_1/e_1 + p_2 q_2/e_2 + ... + p_n q_n/e_n]. \tag{6.4}$$

an addictive good, current consumption levels are determined by past and current prices. For 'rational' addicts, future prices are also an important determinant of current consumption (see Chapter 5). In our analysis, we compare long-run steady-states so that prices and the long-run use of tobacco remain constant over time. Thus, when we talk about willingness to pay, we mean how much an individual is willing to pay to maintain smoking with the long-run price of tobacco at its current level. The compensating variation measure of benefits, when the long-run price is fixed at p, is the amount required to ensure that utility remains constant if the long-run price is raised arbitrarily high.

[3] With a linear demand curve, the elasticity increases as the price rises, i.e the elasticity varies along the demand curve. If the consumer surplus is computed at a different P and Q, then the elasticity has to be re-computed for that particular price and quantity combination.

This approach to consumer surplus takes into account the addictive nature of tobacco products in the following way. Economic theories of addiction indicate that for an addictive good, the elasticity of demand is greater in the long-run than in the short-run. Hence, for an addictive good, the long-run consumer surplus is smaller than the short-run consumer surplus. In determining the elasticity of demand, we distinguish two regions: the high-income countries, known as the established market economies (EME); and the rest of the world (Non-EME). For the established market economies, based on a large literature from high-income countries, we use a long-run price elasticity of –0.8 (see Chapter 10). For the rest of the world, we use a long-run price elasticity of –1.2, based on the higher short-run elasticities in these countries and the finding from high-income countries that long-run demand is more elastic than short-run demand (see Chapter 10).[4] The price of a pack of cigarettes in 1990 employed for EME countries is $1.80. For India and China, the prices employed are $0.40 and $0.20, respectively. Finally, for the rest of the world, price is set at $0.60 per pack. These estimated prices are based on data from the World Bank's tobacco database.

The level of expenditures for each World Bank region is given in Table 6.1. The annual consumer surplus for each region is given in column three of Table 6.2. The average annual per capita consumer surplus implied by our parameter values is $108. One can think of this amount as approximately the average amount that would have to be paid to induce each smoker to quit for one year; this amount is bounded above by approximately $3600.[5] This is, of course, a global average and will vary from region to region, as well as varying from one individual to the next.

To convert this annual stream of consumer surplus into a discounted present value, annual consumer surplus is divided by the social discount rate, that is:

$$\text{Discounted Present Value of Consumer Surplus} = CS/r. \qquad (6.5)$$

Here we are assuming that the annual stream of consumer surplus, denoted by CS, extends indefinitely; that is, the implicit time period over which we are discounting is infinite. Using a value of 0.03 for the social discount rate, the discounted sum of future consumer surplus is $4.2 trillion.[6] Table 6.2 presents the annual and discounted present value of consumer surplus for a range of price elasticities. The table indicates that our results are sensitive to assumptions about the price elasticity of demand. For example, if the demand elasticities in EME and non-EME countries are –0.2 and –0.4, respectively, our estimates rise by a factor of 3.7. Geometrically this arises because, as demand becomes more inelastic, the demand curve becomes steeper and the area under the demand curve increases. The underlying economics is straightforward: more inelastic demand indicates that consumers are willing to continue purchasing the product at higher prices, indicating a greater willingness to pay. Because expenditures are high in the EME, the price elasticity assumed for this region is of particular importance.

---

[4] This estimate for price elasticity is also consistent with estimates for US teenagers, who can be regarded as a lower income group relative to the remainder of the US population.

[5] Here we assume that an individual is paid in one lump sum an amount equal to the present discounted value of an annual flow $108 in perpetuity with an interest rate of 3%. If the interest rate is 5%, this is equal to $2160.

[6] Trillion is here defined as 1000 billion.

Table 6.1 Expenditures on tobacco

1990 Expenditures (Billions of 1990 US$)	
Established market economies	148.2
Formally socialist economies	11.6
India	14.9
China	15.8
Other Asia and islands	15.3
Sub-Saharan Africa	3.7
Latin America and Caribbean	10.2
Middle Eastern Crescent	8.7

Table 6.2 The consumer surplus of tobacco use

EME price elasticity	Non-EME price elasticity	Annual consumer surplus (Billions$)	Discounted consumer surplus (Billions$)
0.2	0.4	471	15 692
0.4	0.8	236	7 846
0.6	1.0	156	5 453
0.8	1.2	119	4 201
1.0	1.4	97	3 425
1.2	1.6	82	2 894

All prices are in 1990 US$.

The choice of a discount rate also affects our estimates of total discounted consumer benefits. The traditional range for the social rate of discount is between 3% and 6%. The fact that discounted benefits become arbitrarily large when the discount rate falls close to zero is an artifact of assuming an infinite horizon. With an infinite horizon, as the discount rate drops toward zero, the discounted value of benefits becomes unbounded. If we used a fixed horizon, say 30 years, then benefits have a finite upper bound, even as the discount rate approaches zero. The problem with using such a fixed horizon is, however, that this implicitly assumes that the flow of benefits beyond the horizon is zero, which is a problematic assumption.[7]

---

[7] A shortcoming of the approach, as outlined, is that it does not account for economic growth or population growth, which will shift out the demand curve and lead to higher estimates of consumer surplus. It is straightforward to amend our framework, however, to account for growth. A simple way to account for economic growth is to assume that real expenditures are growing at fixed annual rate, say g. This means that the discounted consumer surplus will be given by approximately:

Discounted Present Value of Consumer Surplus = CS/(r-g).

For example, if real expenditures are growing at 2% annually, the discount rate is 3%, and the annual consumer surplus in 1990 equal to $119 billion, then the discounted present value of consumer surplus will be $11.9 trillion. This calculation assumes that the elasticities remain constant; if they fall over time then discounted consumer surplus will be higher.

Table 6.3 Per capita consumer surplus

	Per capita annual consumer surplus (1990 US$)
Established market economies	173
Formerly socialist economies	22
India	12
China	9
Other Asia and islands	17
Sub-Saharan Africa	7
Latin America and Caribbean	17
Middle Eastern Crescent	15

Table 6.3 shows per capita annual consumer surplus by region (the total population, non-smokers and smokers, is included here). The most striking aspect of this table is the large disparity between per capita consumer surplus in established market economies (so-called EME countries) and per capita consumer surplus in the other regions: annual per capita consumer surpluses for the EME and non-EME regions differ by more than a factor of 10. The per capita annual consumer surplus in the EME countries is $173, while for the other regions the average annual per capita consumer surplus is $16.50. This reflects the higher expenditures for smokers in the EME; expenditures for EME countries are roughly 10 times as great as those of non-EME countries. This implies that, on a per capita basis, consumers in the EME currently receive a disproportionate share of the benefits from the consumption of tobacco products. After the established market economies, the formerly socialist economies have, at $22 per person per year, the second highest per capita annual consumer surplus. This reflects the high per capita consumption of cigarettes in these countries (including the Czech Republic and Poland, which have the highest per capita consumption levels in the world). Sub-Saharan Africa, China, and India have relatively lower per capita annual consumer surplus, primarily reflecting lower cigarette prices.

The measurement and interpretation of consumer surplus is complicated by two confounding factors.[8] The first is the addictive nature of cigarettes. Suppose that initially a consumer is not addicted and is deciding whether or not to try cigarettes. An individual may be uncertain about how she or he will respond to cigarettes. In particular, before trying cigarettes, the individual may not know his or her own addictive potential and how much he or she will like smoking. Depending on what type of person an individual is, there are a number of possible outcomes that arise when the individual experiments with cigarettes. For instance, one possible outcome is that cigarettes will be highly addictive for the individual but the individual may not, on net, like smoking. Here, experimentation would lead to addiction but the individual will regret his or

---

[8] While we do not present a complete model of addiction, we discuss some relevant issues employing the framework of Orphanides and Zervos (1995) closely; see Chapter 5 for a more extensive discussion of economic models of addiction.

her decision to experiment with cigarettes. A second possibility is that an individual becomes addicted, but likes cigarettes, so that the individual becomes a 'happy addict' and does not regret the decision to try cigarettes. There is also a possibility that the individual will not like cigarettes and will not become addicted and will stop smoking. Thus consumers must make a decision about whether to try cigarettes under uncertainty, since they do not know which of these outcomes is most likely to apply to them personally. The individual has a subjective probability distribution over types and on the basis of this distribution, makes a consumption decision that maximizes expected utility subject to a budget constraint. For example, some individuals may believe that the probability of regretting the decision to try cigarettes is very high; that is, they believe that it is very likely that they will become addicted and not like cigarettes. Such individuals will accordingly decide not to experiment.

There is evidence that many individuals who try cigarettes consistently under-estimate the addictive potential of cigarettes and over-estimate the benefits from cigarette smoking. On the assumption that the evidence is correct, the smoking population consists in part of individuals who are addicted but regret their decision to start smoking. A recent survey indicates that from 75% to 85% of current smokers in the United States would quit if they could, and regret their decision to start smoking. The 1994 Surgeon General's Report indicates that only 15% of teenagers smoking less than a pack a day think that they will be still smoking in 5 years. In fact, 5 years later, 42% of such teenagers are smoking at least one cigarette per day. Thus there is ample evidence that individuals under-estimate their propensity for addiction and over-estimate the utility that they will receive from smoking, leading to a high percentage of individuals expressing regret over the decision to begin smoking. For these individuals, the willingness to pay for cigarettes arises from the need to avoid the cost of ending their addiction to cigarettes, that is, the physical and psychological costs of withdrawing from cigarette use. Accordingly, addicted individuals who regret their decision to try cigarettes may have a positive willingness to pay for painless tobacco cessation. This suggests that one can argue that, for these individuals, the willingness to pay for cigarettes should be regarded as part of the cost of smoking and not a net economic benefit. Attempting to systematically take this into account in estimating consumer surplus would involve novel and somewhat speculative adjustments, and so is not pursued further. Nonetheless, this discussion strongly indicates that the consumer surplus estimates provided below should be regarded as upper bounds on the true consumer surplus.

The second caveat to keep in mind is that consumers may not be fully informed about all the adverse effects of tobacco consumption. In particular, to the extent that consumers lack complete information about the adverse health effects of tobacco consumption, consumer surplus is overstated.[9] This can be seen as follows by noting that the individual demand curve takes into account perceived health costs in the following way. Associated with varying levels of consumption are the consumer's perceived

---

[9] Of course, some individuals may overestimate the dangers of smoking (see Viscusi 1992); to the extent that these individuals do not smoke, they will receive no benefit from cigarette consumption and consumer surplus will be unaffected.

marginal benefits; the marginal benefit is measured as the incremental willingness to pay for an additional unit of consumption, given the current amount consumed. The consumer's consumption level is determined by comparing marginal benefits with marginal costs. Marginal costs consist of two components: market and non-market costs. The market marginal cost is just the market price of an additional unit of the product. The second component of marginal cost is the expected non-market marginal costs of tobacco consumption. These include the expected adverse health consequences of smoking, the increased probability of fire, as well as the cost of time involved in consumption. The consumer's consumption level is determined by comparing marginal benefits and marginal costs from tobacco consumption to those for consumption of other goods and services. Note that if marginal costs are sufficiently high or marginal benefits sufficiently low, the consumption level will be zero.

The demand curve in Fig. 6.1 is equal to the marginal benefits minus the perceived non-market marginal costs; that is, the marginal costs associated with adverse health consequences. The consumer's consumption level is determined by equating this net marginal benefit curve with the price of the commodity. The area shown as consumer surplus is the area under the net marginal benefit curve minus expenditures, and measures the net benefits to cigarette consumption. These are defined as the total benefits minus total health costs and total expenditures. If the perceived marginal costs due to adverse health effects rise, the net demand curve shown in Fig. 6.1 shifts in toward the origin. This inward shift means that consumer surplus is smaller. If the perceived marginal costs are lower than the 'true' marginal costs—that is, the consumer is under-informed about the true health consequences of smoking—then the demand curve will be shifted out and consumer surplus will be overstated. Thus, misinformed consumers will result in consumer surplus estimates that are too high. For the United States, Ippolito *et al.* (1979) estimate that the release of the Surgeon General's 1964 report on the health consequences of smoking led, over time, to a decline in annual tobacco consumption of around 30%, suggesting that the lack of consumer information would have led to excessive estimates of consumer surplus in the 1950s. This is another reason why the estimates of consumer surplus reported above should be regarded as upper bounds on true consumer surplus.

6.2.3 Producer surplus

Net economic benefits to tobacco producers and cigarette manufacturers depend on the alternative products that can be grown or manufactured with the assets currently used for tobacco products. Producer surplus is the payment that producers receive in excess of their opportunity cost. Producer surplus is also equivalent to economic rent, which is the amount that a payment exceeds the minimum amount necessary to ensure that the goods are supplied at the specified quantity. Thus, if a star basketball player receives a salary of $1 million but would be willing to play for only $50 000, then $950 000 of his $1-million-dollar salary is said to be economic rent. This connection between economic rent and producer surplus is made clear in the following alternative definition of producer surplus: producer surplus is the amount that can be taken from producers without diminishing the amount supplied.

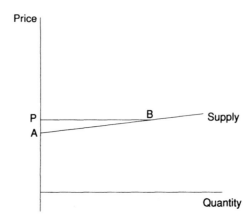

Fig. 6.2 Elastic supply curve with producer surplus PAB.

As a measure of economic profits, producer surplus is simply revenue minus opportunity costs.[10] Geometrically, producer surplus is the area between price P and the supply curve; that is, the area above the supply curve and below the price line. Producer surplus arises from the production of tobacco leaf and from the manufacture of cigarettes. As a first approximation we assume that production of tobacco leaf occurs under competitive conditions. For the manufacture of cigarettes, this assumption is less tenable and we modify our approach to take into account the market power of cigarette manufacturers.

With a standard supply curve diagram, the connection between producer surplus and ease with which assets can be redeployed in the production of alternative products is easy to see. For example, if it is easy for tobacco growers to produce a lucrative alternative product, then small changes in price will lead to big changes in output. As the price for the product declines, producers will quickly shift assets into the production of the lucrative alternative product. In this case, the supply of tobacco will be relatively elastic as indicated in the Fig. 6.2. Total producer surplus will, all else being equal, be relatively small (shown in Fig. 6.2 as PAB). On the other hand, if there are no alternative products, producers will not be able to readily redeploy assets in the event of price decline. The supply curve, in this case, will be relatively inelastic. Here, producer surplus will be relatively large.

In general, producer surplus is given by the area between price and the supply curve; accordingly, given a supply curve, generating producer surplus is a matter of computing the appropriate integral. Modeling leaf production of tobacco as a competitive industry is, of course, only a first approximation to a much more complicated reality. We assume that supply curves are iso-elastic (this is the same assumption as Barnum (1993)), that is:

---

[10] In general, the area underneath the supply curve is total variable cost. If firms are infinitesimal, i.e efficient scale is small relative to total market demand, then one can show that the area under the supply curve is exactly total costs. For monopolies and oligopolies, supply curves may not be well-defined; for these cases the best approach is to compute profits directly.

Table 6.4 The producer surplus of tobacco

Supply elasticity	Annual producer surplus	Discounted producer surplus (1990 US$ (millions))
0.1	51.2	1570
0.2	49.2	1503
0.3	47.5	1448
0.4	46.1	1400
0.5	44.8	1358
0.6	43.7	1321
0.7	42.8	1289
0.8	41.9	1260
0.9	41.1	1234
1.0	40.5	1212

$$Q_s = Ap^\eta, \tag{6.6}$$

where η is the supply-elasticity. For this supply curve, producer surplus, PS, is given by:

$$PS = PQ/(1+\eta). \tag{6.7}$$

In this particular case, we only need the supply-elasticity, output, and the market price to determine producer surplus. This is the annual producer surplus. To convert this flow into a stock, we compute the present discounted value of the flow of producer surplus as follows:

$$\text{Discounted Present Value of Producer Surplus} = PS/r, \tag{6.8}$$

where r is the social discount rate.

We estimated agricultural supply functions from the World Bank data using country and year fixed-effects models. Our estimated supply elasticities were relatively low (0.2); the literature gives estimates that range from 0.4 to 0.8. We attribute these low-elasticity estimates to two factors. First, we are estimating short-run elasticities and, second, there is some measurement error in the price data. Measurement error tends to bias estimates downwards. Our base case assumes that the supply-elasticity is 0.6, which is consistent with estimates of supply elasticities for agricultural goods.[11] Accordingly, we find the annual producer surplus associated with the agricultural production of tobacco leaf to be about $16 billion in 1990 (Table 6.4). To account for cigarette manufacturer profits, we assume that profits average $0.10 per pack; this implies profits of about $27 billion per year.[12] Accordingly, total producer benefits are $43 billion per year. With a social discount rate of 3%, the discounted value of future producer surplus

[11] Estimates used in World Bank commodity price projections (World Bank 1991) suggest a supply-elasticity of 0.6; Dean (1966) estimates a supply-elasticity of 0.5 for tobacco farmers in Malawi. Johnson (1984) finds a supply-elasticity of 1.0 for US farmers.

[12] In the late 1990s, the estimated profit on a $3.50 package of Marlboro cigarettes was $0.28, a profit rate of 8% (Newman 1999). If we apply this rate to world production, total world profits are about $16.9 billion, lower than our $27 billion estimate.

Table 6.5 Per capita producer surplus

	Per capita producer surplus (1990 US$)
Established market economies	197.7
Formerly socialist economies	7.6
India	2.7
China	17.5
Other Asia and islands	12.7
Sub-Saharan Africa	25.6
Latin America and Caribbean	11.3
Middle Eastern Crescent	8.4

Supply elasticity = 0.6.

is about \$1321 billion. The per capita producer surplus is shown for each region in Table 6.5.

One way to interpret this figure is that it is the minimum lump payment necessary to induce tobacco growers and manufacturers to voluntarily quit their activities and use their assets in other, non-tobacco activities. Sensitivity analysis indicates that when the supply-elasticity is 0.1, annual agricultural producer surplus is \$26 billion, and when the elasticity is twice our base-case value, i.e. 1.2, it is about \$12 billion. The discounted sum of producer surplus ranges from \$1570 billion, when the elasticity is 0.1, to \$1172 billion, when the elasticity is 1.2. While not particularly sensitive to assumptions about the supply-elasticity, the total discounted producer surplus does vary significantly with the social discount rate.

6.3 Cost of tobacco consumption

6.3.1 Internal and external costs

The central issue in calculating the social costs of tobacco consumption is determining which costs are already accounted for in consumer and producer decisions and which costs are not taken into account. Costs that are already accounted for should not be explicitly subtracted in the analysis, since this would lead to double counting. Costs that are not counted in consumer or supplier decisions, however, need to be explicitly taken into account by the analysis. In determining what costs should be taken into account, the following taxonomy is useful. Internal costs are costs that are taken into account and are typically borne by the smoker. The reason why these costs are not subtracted from measured benefits in determining the net social benefit or loss from smoking has been explained in our discussion of consumer surplus. External costs are costs that are not taken into account by the decision-maker because they do not affect the decision-maker; as such, they must be imposed on others in order to be external costs. External costs need to be counted explicitly as part of the social costs. Finally, if individuals choose to smoke but are not fully informed about the consequences of their decision, some costs may not be fully reflected in demand and supply curves. If individuals are completely uninformed about the adverse consequences of tobacco consumption, then the costs associated with premature death and higher morbidity may be explicitly subtracted as an additional uncounted cost. We refer to this category of uncounted costs as uninformed costs.

The following simple matrix summarizes the discussion. The rows indicate whether the decision-maker is uninformed or informed, while the columns are labeled internal and external costs. 'Uninformed' implies that the decision-maker is not aware of the relevant cost and does not take the cost into account in his decision-making. 'Informed' means that the individual is aware of the cost, and takes the cost into account in making a decision. If a cost is uncounted, then that cost needs to be explicitly accounted for in our analysis; if the cost is counted, it has already been taken into account by the decision-maker and is accordingly reflected in consumer or producer surplus. Informed, internal costs are taken into account by consumers and are already measured by standard consumer surplus. As the matrix indicates, there are three other possible configurations that give rise to costs that are uncounted in conventional measures of consumer and producer surplus.[13] These costs should be subtracted from consumer and producer surplus to determine the net social costs of tobacco consumption. In our analysis, we assume away all external costs and focus on uncounted internal costs.

	Internal cost	External cost
Informed decision-maker	Counted cost	Uncounted cost
Uninformed decision-maker	Uncounted cost	Uncounted cost

6.4 The social cost of smoking

If the total discounted stream of benefits from tobacco consumption is B and the total discounted stream of uncounted costs of tobacco consumption, external and uninformed cost, is C, then B–C is the net discounted flow of social benefits from tobacco consumption. This represents the net amount that society would be better off, from the initial point of time measured into the indefinite future when tobacco products are present. If this sum is negative, then society is on net worse off with tobacco products than without them. It is, of course, conceptually and empirically difficult to measure all uncounted costs. To address the difficulties of distinguishing counted and uncounted costs directly, we propose the following alternative procedure that focuses on the uncounted costs arising from a lack of consumer information. It is standard to measure the aggregate health impact of tobacco use in units called DALYs. DALY is an acronym for disability-adjusted life-year; DALYs capture in a

---

[13] External costs generated by an informed individual may become internalized if his utility function is interdependent, i.e. the individual cares about his impact on others.

single time-based unit, years lost due to premature mortality and years lived with
disability, adjusted for severity. One DALY is thus one lost year of healthy life.
Estimates for DALYs attributable to smoking were provided by WHO (1996, 1999).
DALYS caused by smoking refer only to disease among smokers and exclude the
effects of smoking on non-smokers. They are derived from the smoking-impact ratio
model (SIR) (Peto *et al.* 1994; see Chapter 2, for a more detailed discussion). DALY
projections from 1990 to 2030 are also provided by WHO (1996; Lopez, personal
communication).

Uncounted costs result when consumers make uninformed or under-informed decisions to consume tobacco products. Here, we regard uninformed consumers as assuming that the expected DALY cost of smoking is zero, when in fact such costs are positive. We compute the percentage of the population that must be uninformed so that
the net social benefits are zero. Thus if a fraction α of the smoking population is uninformed and the value of one DALY(D) is L, then there is a total uninformed cost of:

$$\sum_{t=0}^{\infty} \alpha LD_t \bigg/ (1+r)^t, \tag{6.9}$$

that needs to be subtracted from total benefits to determine net benefits. We then
consider:

$$B - \sum_{t=0}^{\infty} \alpha LD_t \bigg/ (1+r)^t = 0. \tag{6.10}$$

This equation gives the level of uninformed costs resulting in a net social benefit of
zero.[14] Note that this calculation assumes all other uncounted costs are zero. The solution of this equation, α^*, is given by:

$$\alpha^* = B \bigg/ \left(\sum_{t=0}^{\infty} LD_t \bigg/ (1+r)^t \right). \tag{6.11}$$

This fraction can be interpreted as the percentage of the smoking population that must
be uninformed so that net benefits are zero. If the fraction uninformed exceeds α^*,
then the total uncounted cost will be larger than the above sum, and the net social
benefit will be negative.

6.5 Empirical findings

Our base case is as follows. We assume a supply-elasticity of 0.6 and demand-
elasticity for EME countries of –0.8, and a demand-elasticity of –1.2 for non-EME
countries. The discount rate is set at 3%. We compute the threshold level of uninformed
individuals for our base case and find that it is 23%. Thus, if more than a quarter of
the population is consuming tobacco products without fully realizing the addiction and

---

[14] Note that though the interpretation is different, this is algebraically equivalent to assuming that the
uncounted costs associated with each DALY, L*, are equal to α^*L, so that net benefits of smoking equal
zero. To see this, merely substitute $\alpha^*L = L^*$ into the summation given in eqn 6.10.

Table 6.6 The percentage of smokers who would need to be uninformed of the health risks for social benefits of smoking to be zero

Discount rate	EME price elasticity	Non-EME price elasticity	Fraction of the population uninformed (DALY= US$7750)	Fraction of the population uninformed (DALY = US$15 500)
0.01	0.2	0.4	0.59	0.25
0.01	0.4	0.8	0.32	0.16
0.01	0.8	1.2	0.20	0.10
0.01	1.0	1.6	0.17	0.09
0.03	0.2	0.4	0.70	0.35
0.03	0.4	0.8	0.38	0.19
0.03	0.8	1.2	0.23	0.12
0.03	1.0	1.6	0.19	0.10
0.05	0.2	0.4	0.79	0.39
0.05	0.4	0.8	0.43	0.21
0.05	0.8	1.2	0.26	0.13
0.05	1.0	1.6	0.22	0.11
0.07	0.2	0.4	0.86	0.43
0.07	0.4	0.8	0.47	0.23
0.07	0.8	1.2	0.29	0.14
0.07	1.0	1.6	0.24	0.12

health consequences (i.e. is not cognizant of the full DALY cost of tobacco use), then we conclude that there are net social costs. In reaching these estimates, we assume that the value of one DALY is US$7750, which is the global average per capita gross domestic product (GDP) weighted for tobacco consumption. This assumption is extremely conservative,[15] for instance, if the value of one DALY is doubled, the threshold level of uninformed individuals falls to 13%. Sensitivity analyses indicate that our results depend fairly heavily on our assumption regarding price elasticity, particularly our choice of the price elasticity for the EME countries (see Table 6.6). This arises because tobacco consumption in the EME countries is high, relative to the rest of the world, which means that consumer surplus in the EME countries dominates the expression for benefits, B. On the other hand, our conclusions are not very sensitive to the choice of the social discount rate; this is because the social discount rate enters both the numerator and the denominator of the expression that determines α.

[15] This is an extremely conservative choice in the following sense. In a survey of 23 studies using US data (Viscusi 1993) the average value of a life is $5.8 million (typically derived from labor-market data), while the average income in these studies is $22 600. Assuming that one life translates into 40 healthy life-years (allowing for age weighting and discounting), this implies that the value of a DALY is about $320 000. Accordingly, the ratio of a DALY to income for the United States is about 14.3. If we assume that the value of a DALY is 14.3 times per capita GNP, the threshold percentage who would have to be uninformed for the net benefits of tobacco to be zero is 3%.

6.6 Incremental analysis

We also consider the welfare effects of a 10% increase in the price of cigarettes arising from a tax increase. This exercise is relevant for two reasons. First, tobacco tax increases are a widely discussed policy option, so it is useful to measure its welfare effects in the context of our framework. Second, an incremental analysis of this type does not involve extrapolation into situations that have not been observed. In particular, the global analysis of the previous section may make untenable assumptions about the behavior of demand when prices are extremely high. An incremental analysis of the type proposed here makes much more modest extrapolations about the behavior of demand.

We suppose that the 10% increase in the price of tobacco arises because of the imposition of a tax. This means that there is a reduction in the quantity of tobacco products produced and consumed. There are also significant money transfers from tobacco consumers and producers to governments. Transfers are not included in the assessment of costs and benefits because, while they represent a cost to consumers, they also generate an equal sized benefit to taxpayers and the beneficiaries of government programs financed by the tax revenues. Accordingly, transfers net out to zero. Losses to consumers and producers, however, exceed the amount collected in tax revenue and this extra burden is referred to as a deadweight loss. Deadweight losses are the net social costs generated by the taxation of tobacco products. We first calculate the deadweight loss that arises from the reduction in consumer demand, denoted as DWL_c. DWL_c can be expressed as a function of the elasticity parameter e as follows:

$$DWL_C = 1/2\,PQe(\Delta P/P)^2. \tag{6.12}$$

The most salient feature of this formula is that the percentage change in price is squared. This implies that the deadweight loss will be an order of magnitude smaller than the drop in DALYs that is roughly proportional to the percentage change of price.

The next step is the computation of the deadweight loss of producer surplus for tobacco producers, denoted as DWLP. This is the net reduction in producer profits; that is, the decline in producer profits minus transfers to the government sector. The formula for this computation is:

$$DWL_P = PQ/(1+\eta) - P_1 Q_1/(1+\eta) - Q_1(P - P_1), \tag{6.13}$$

where P and Q are the original price and quantity, and P_1 and Q_1 are the new price and quantity that arise after the 10% increase in cigarette prices is put into place. P_1 and Q_1 are computed as follows. A 10% increase in the price of cigarettes leads to a lower quantity of cigarettes sold, based on the shape of the demand curve for cigarettes. We assume that the reduction in tobacco leaf is proportional to the reduction in cigarettes, so that if cigarette consumption falls by $\Delta Q/Q\%$, then tobacco leaf production also falls by $\Delta Q/Q\%$. Given the equation for the supply curve $Q = AP^\eta$, the market price that corresponds to reduced level of production can be computed.

The final set of calculations concerns DALYs. We estimated the relationship between consumption and mortality at the country level based on cigarette smoking in 1970 and lung cancer in 1990 (see Chapter 2, Figure 2.4) as follows:

$$Y = 0.0248X + 5.5, \qquad (6.14)$$

where Y equals lung cancer deaths per 100 000 at ages 35–69, and X is total cigarette consumption. For every lung cancer death there are approximately 36 DALYs (Murray and Lopez 1996). Based on these figures, we estimated the percentage decline in DALYs that results from a 10% increase in cigarette prices, using the above estimates of price elasticity. In particular, we took original DALYs in the year 2020, and assumed that they would fall by the percentage amount predicted by eqn 6.14. When properly discounted, this produces an 8% decline in discounted DALYs.

The results are summarized in Table 6.7. For our base case of a demand-elasticity of –0.8 for the EME countries and –1.2 for the non-EME countries, and a supply-elasticity of 0.6, the discounted deadweight loss is US$44 billion. We compute a break-even percentage of uninformed smokers for a range of demand and supply elasticities. For our base case, the break-even percentage of uninformed smokers is 2.2%. The most striking feature of Table 6.7 is that the numbers are an order of magnitude lower than the numbers for the global analysis, i.e. the figures presented in Table 6.6. This is basically because the deadweight losses are, as pointed out earlier, an order of magnitude smaller than the change in producer and consumer surplus. (Most of the change in producer and consumer surplus results from the transfer of funds from the private to public sector, assuming that the 10% increase is the result of a tax increase.) On the other hand, the reduction in DALYs is on the same order of magnitude as the change in price and hence much bigger.

Table 6.7 Incremental cost–benefit analysis

Supply elasticity	EME price elasticity	Non-EME price elasticity	Deadweight loss (Billions $)	Breakeven % uninformed (DALY = US$7750)
0.3	0.2	0.4	26.1	1.3
0.3	0.4	0.8	36.4	1.8
0.3	0.8	1.2	51.6	2.5
0.3	1.0	1.6	61.9	3.0
0.6	0.2	0.4	18.6	0.9
0.6	0.4	0.8	28.9	1.4
0.6	0.8	1.2	44.1	2.2
0.6	1.0	1.6	54.4	2.7
1.2	0.2	0.4	14.6	0.7
1.2	0.4	0.8	24.9	1.2
1.2	0.8	1.2	40.1	2.0
1.2	1.0	1.6	50.4	2.5

Discount rate = 0.03.

6.7 Comparison with earlier analyses

Barnum (1993, 1994) estimated the costs and benefits of smoking, using a different methodology, and reached somewhat different conclusions. His approach is designed to answer the question: What are the net benefits of additional investments in tobacco production capability? Accordingly, Barnum takes an incremental approach; also his treatment of the costs of cigarette consumption is very different than the approach we have taken. Barnum assumes that there is a one-time increase in tobacco production of 1000 metric tonnes that results in a one-time net increase in output of 500 metric tonnes. The incremental producer and consumer surplus occurs for just the initial year; Barnum does not consider a discounted stream of consumer and producer surplus. Barnum then assumes that this increase in production is consumed in the initial year. As a result of this one-time increase in consumption, there are subsequent rises in the death and morbidity rates. The incremental cost of additional deaths, in the Barnum analysis, is $3.1 million. The incremental cost due to disability and morbidity is $3.4 million. Barnum also considers the direct cost of added morbidity, at $2.3 million. The net change in consumer and producer surplus is 1.7 million. Adding the Barnum figures together, we reach a total of $7.2 million costs per 1000 metric tonnes. Assuming that this marginal rate is also the average rate, this implies a total annual cost of $46.8 billion per year (6500 × $7.2 million). If we assume that this cost occurs each year, i.e. costs are constant over time, the total discounted costs are $1.6 trillion. The Barnum estimate is for a one-time increase in tobacco production of 1000 metric tonnes. If this were sustained indefinitely, then the marginal increase in present discounted value of net benefits would be −7.2/0.03 or −$240 million. In contrast, we determine total consumer and producer surplus, rather than marginal quantities. We also highlight the proportion of the smoking population that must be uninformed for net benefits to equal zero and thereby stress the uncounted costs that arise from smokers' lack of information about the health risks. Thus our analysis takes into account explicitly the distinction between internal and uncounted social costs. In determining these quantities we use total DALYs attributable to tobacco consumption, rather than the marginal DALYs utilized by Barnum in his work.

6.8 Conclusion

The approach we have outlined here provides a framework for assessing the economic impact of tobacco consumption. It also suggests important areas for future work. This study suggests that better estimates of demand and supply functions, along with estimates of regional demand and supply elasticities, are needed. We would also like to have a better understanding of how various government interventions affect demand and supply. Finally we need to have better measures of the degree to which consumers are informed about the health consequences of tobacco consumption. Our approach is different from Barnum's and has some novel features. Instead of considering an incremental change in tobacco production and then determining the marginal consumer and producer surplus and the incremental costs, we consider total consumer surplus and total producer surplus. We then consider the percentage of the smoking population that needs to be completely uninformed so that net social benefits to tobacco consumption are equal to zero. To illustrate our approach we provide calculations and find that, for our base case, this number is 23%. Thus we conclude that if individual smokers underestimate the cost of smoking by more than 23%, the net social benefit will also be negative. Given what we know about the levels of consumer information on the health risks of tobacco, these figures are consistent with the notion that, on net, consumption of tobacco products leads to a net decline in economic welfare.

We also consider the effect on social welfare of an incremental increase of 10% in the retail price of cigarettes. Here the results are very striking: if only a very small percentage of the population is uninformed, 2.2%, then increasing tobacco prices by relatively modest amounts raises economic welfare. Again, given what we know about levels of consumer information on tobacco health risks, this result is consistent with arguments in favor of moderate increases in tobacco taxes.

References

Barnum, H. (1993). *The Economic Costs and Benefits of Investing in Tobacco.* Unpublished manuscript, Human Development Department, The World Bank.

Barnum, H. (1994). The economic burden of the global trade in tobacco. *Tobacco Control,* 3(4), 358–61.

Dean, E. (1966). *The Supply Responses of African Farmers: Theory and Measurement in Malawi,* Amsterdam, North Holland.

Hausman, J. (1981). Exact consumer surplus and deadweight loss. *American Economic Review,* **71**, 662–76.

Ippolito, R. A., Murphy, R. D., and Sant, D. (1979). *Staff Report on Consumer Responses to Cigarette Health Information.* Washington DC: Federal Trade Commission.

Johnson, P. R. (1984). *The Economics of the Tobacco Industry,* New York, Praeger.

Murray, C. J. L. and Lopez A. D. (ed) (1996). *The Global Burden of Disease.* Cambridge, MA: Harvard University Press, 1996.

Newman, A. (1999). The economics of cigarettes: smoke on for the tax man. *New York Times,* February 28.

Orphanides, A. and Zervos, D. Rational Addiction with Learning and Regret, *Journal of Political Economy,* **103**, 739–58.

Peto, R., Lopez, A. D., Boreham, J., Thun, M., and Heath, C. Jr. (1994). *Mortality from smoking in developed countries,* 1950–2000. Oxford, Oxford University Press.

Viscusi, W. K. (1992). *Smoking: Making the Risky Decision,* New York, Oxford University Press.

Viscusi, W. K. (1993). The value of risks to life and health. *Journal of Economic Literature,* **31**, 1912–46.

Willig, R. (1976). Consumer surplus without apology. *American Economic Review,* 66(4), 589–97.

World Bank (1991). *Price Prospects for Major Primary Commodities, 1990–2005,* Washington, D.C., World Bank.

World Health Organization (1996). Investing in Health Research and Development, report of the Ad Hoc Committee on Health Research Relating to Future Intervention Options (Document TDR/Gen/96.1). Geneva, World Health Organization.

World Health Organization (1999). *World Health Report: Making a Difference.* Geneva, World Health Organization.

7

The economic rationale for intervention in the tobacco market

Prabhat Jha, Philip Musgrove, Frank J. Chaloupka, and Ayda Yurekli

Economic theory starts with the assumption that a consumer usually knows what is best for him or herself—the notion of 'consumer sovereignty'. The theory also assumes that privately-determined consumption choices, including the decision whether to consume a particular product at all within a free competitive market, will most efficiently allocate society's scarce resources. Within this framework, economic theory holds that if smokers consume tobacco with full information about its health consequences and addictive potential, and bear all costs and benefits of their choice themselves, there is no justification, on the grounds of inefficiency, for governments to interfere. However, in practice, the market for tobacco is characterized by three specific 'market failures'—that is, features that result in economic inefficiencies and that may therefore justify public intervention. First, there is an 'information failure' about the health risks of smoking: some consumers do not know the risks, and, even where consumers are informed, they may not appreciate the scale of those risks or apply the knowledge to themselves. Second, there is an information failure about the addictive potential of tobacco. Many smokers, and especially adolescents, under-estimate the risk of becoming addicted and, once addicted, face very high costs in trying to quit. These two information failures result in high private costs of death and disability for smokers. The third market failure is the external costs of smoking—that is, the costs imposed by smokers on others. External costs are most clearly apparent as the health effects of passive smoking. There are several ways that governments may intervene. In economic theory, 'first-best' interventions, which specifically address the identified inefficiency, should ideally be pursued. In the tobacco market, the first-best interventions would probably be to educate young people about the risks of addiction and disease from smoking, or to restrict their access to tobacco. However, evidence suggests that these measures are largely ineffective. In contrast, taxation, albeit a blunt instrument and thus a 'second-best intervention', is highly effective at protecting children from taking up smoking. Taxation is also an effective means of correcting external health costs, and, possibly, also external financial costs. However, taxation and various other interventions impose costs on a wide range of smokers. The policy options available to governments are discussed.

7.1 Introduction

There is no doubt that prolonged smoking is an important cause of premature mortality and disability worldwide (see Chapter 2). Strictly on health terms, then, there is a strong reason to intervene to reduce this damage.

However, smoking is voluntary and is not illegal for adults, so the existence of an enormous health problem is not, *prima facie*, sufficient to justify interference with people's choice to smoke. An *economic* rationale for such intervention requires that failures in tobacco markets are sufficiently large to justify the costs of such interference. Despite the strong consensus that smoking harms health, there is much debate about proper government roles, if any, in reducing smoking (see, for example, *The Economist* 1997).

In this chapter, we explore the economic rationale for government intervention in tobacco markets. We first discuss the two key market failures that justify government intervention on efficiency grounds: first, consumers' incomplete information about the risks of addiction and disease; and, second, external costs. We do not deal with supply-side market failures, such as the monopoly power of the tobacco industry. Next, we discuss which interventions are available to governments to correct these market failures, noting their specificity and effectiveness and their economic costs. We focus in this section on interventions that would protect children and adult non-smokers, and that would inform adult smokers. Third, we discuss whether government intervention in tobacco markets is appropriate to reduce inequity between rich and poor.

This exploration will take account of particular epidemiological features of the tobacco epidemic that are relevant to the economic arguments. The first of these is the early age at which people typically start smoking, which, in high-income countries at least, is during the teen years. The risk of lung cancer is far higher in individuals who start smoking at age 15 and smoke one pack a day for 40 years than among those who start at age 35 and smoke two packs a day for 20 years (Peto 1986). Therefore, the early age of onset has a direct bearing on individuals' health risks. From the standpoint of economics, the early typical age of onset is also relevant because the standard economic concept of consumer sovereignty, which holds that the consumer knows what is best for him or her, may not apply so forcefully to adolescents as to adults. The second key epidemiological feature of the tobacco epidemic is that fully half of smoking-related deaths occur in productive middle age (defined as 35–69 years) (Peto *et al.* 1994). This is relevant to the economic debate about smoking, since it dispels the notion that smoking kills people mostly in old age, when the economic losses (as well as the health losses) are small.

7.2 Inefficiences in the tobacco market

Smokers clearly receive benefits from smoking; otherwise they would not pay to do it. The perceived benefits include pleasure and satisfaction, stress relief (presumably derived in part from the nicotine content of the smoke), peer acceptance, and a sense of maturity and sophistication (most important for adolescent smokers, and derived from the act of smoking as such). An additional important benefit for the addicted smoker is the avoidance of nicotine withdrawal. There is little that economics can say about the preferences that determine smoking, except to try to understand how the addictive nature of cigarettes influences subsequent consumption (see Chapter 5). As with other addictive behaviors, the decision to start and the 'decision' to continue are quite different, and different economic arguments may be relevant to each. The private costs to be weighed against those benefits include money spent on tobacco products, damage to health, and nicotine addiction. Defined this way, the *perceived* benefits evidently outweigh the *perceived* costs for at least 1.1 billion people who smoke today.

Economic theory assumes that the consumer knows best and that privately-determined consumption will most efficiently allocate society's scarce resources. Thus, *if* smokers know their risks and internalize all their costs and benefits, there is no justification, on the grounds of inefficiency, for governments to interfere (Pekurinen 1991).

However, these assumptions may not hold for several reasons, leading to market failures. (Note that even efficient markets do not necessarily achieve equity, and that inequity is not normally classified as market failure. We discuss equity issues later in the chapter.) Below, we analyze three failures in the tobacco market. The first is incomplete information about health risks. The second is incomplete information about addiction, specifically the complex issue of children's tendency to under-estimate the addictive potential of smoking (and therefore the costs of quitting). The third failure consists of costs imposed on others.

7.2.1 Incomplete information about health consequences

Incomplete information about the risks of smoking leads to behavior that smokers would not otherwise choose for themselves. Poorly-informed smokers often under-estimate the risks of their action (Weinstein 1998). Since people usually react to known risks by reducing the risky consumption, incomplete information means more smoking than would otherwise occur. There are two principal reasons why smokers tend to be inadequately informed. The first is that the market, far from providing information, has actually hidden or distorted it. The second is the long delay between starting to smoke and the onset of obvious disease, which has obscured the link between the two. Each of these are discussed in turn.

The tobacco industry, like other industries, has no financial incentive to provide health information that would reduce consumption of its products. On the contrary, the industry has consistently hidden product information on the ill effects of smoking or actively misinformed smokers about risks (Sweda and Daynard 1996). Notably, the industry has used advertising and promotion to promote its products as 'safe' despite internal evidence that all types of smoking are harmful. For example, the industry has tried to advertise filter cigarettes as 'healthier' (USDHHS 1989). The industry has also used advertising to reach young smokers (Institute of Medicine 1994). Other tactics of the industry to leave smokers uninformed or misinformed include dissuading lay journals from reporting on smoking's health effects Warner *et al.* 1992, and sponsoring biased scientific research (Bero *et al.* 1994). Internal industry documents uncovered in recent lawsuits in the United States confirm such practices (Glantz *et al.* 1995).

Second, consumers derive information on the costs and benefits of smoking primarily from their own experience and what happens to their peers, as well as from studies largely financed by the public sector. However, the obvious health damage from smoking usually emerges at least 20–30 years after exposure. This differs from most other risky behaviors, such as fast driving, where the costs and benefits are more readily and immediately appreciated.

The long delay between exposure and effect has also impeded the growth of scientific knowledge. In the United States, the 1960s evidence suggested that only one in four smokers died from smoking. When risks were re-assessed decades later, when the epidemic had matured, the evidence showed that the risks were actually much higher: one in two long-term smokers die from smoking (see Chapter 2; Doll *et al.* 1994; Peto *et al.* 1999). Anyone who considered starting or continuing smoking 20 or 30 years ago in high-income countries would, therefore, have under-estimated the risks, even if he or she had based the decision on the best available information. Moreover, as the list of diseases and conditions associated with smoking expands, smokers continue to under-estimate the risks. Most developing countries still do not have estimates of the health hazards of smoking for their own populations. It is, therefore, not surprising that even respectable journals, such as *The Economist* (1997), reveal their confusion about the scale of the true risks or the high proportion of smokers who die in middle age:

... most smokers (two-thirds or more) do not die of smoking-related disease. They gamble and win. Moreover, the years lost to smoking come from the end of life, when people are most likely to die of something else anyway.

As Kenkel and Chen discuss in Chapter 8, there are two key features of consumers' incomplete information: first, in low-income and middle-income countries, absolute awareness of the health risks is still comparatively low. For example, in China, about two-thirds of adult smokers surveyed in 1996 believed that cigarettes did them 'little or no harm' (Chinese Academy of Preventive Medicine 1997). Second, consumers in all countries may not clearly internalize the risks, even when they have been informed about them, nor may they accurately judge the risks of smoking relative to other environmental exposures, such as 'stress' or radiation.

Children and teenagers generally know less about the health effects of smoking than adults. A recent survey of 15- and 16-year-olds in Moscow found that more than half either knew of no smoking-related diseases or could name only one, lung cancer (Levshin and Droggachih 1999). Even in the United States, where young people might be expected to have received more information, almost half of 13-year-olds today think that smoking a pack of cigarettes a day will not cause them great harm (National Cancer Policy Board 1998).

In addition, teenagers–even those with good understanding of the risks of smoking–may have a limited capacity to use information wisely. Teenagers behave myopically, or short-sightedly. It is difficult for most teenagers to imagine being 25, let alone 55, and warnings about the damage that smoking will inflict on their health at some distant date are unlikely to reduce their desire to smoke.

In developing countries, there is less awareness of the hazards of smoking at all ages, including among adults, for several reasons. Education levels are lower, and, since education leads to more rapid and thorough absorption of information, it is reasonable to conclude that less-educated populations will be less receptive to health information.

There are fewer local data on the hazards of smoking and less dissemination of existing data on health risks. Governments less often regulate industry information practices, such as advertising and promotion. For all these reasons, it is unlikely that current smokers and potential smokers in low-income and middle-income countries have adequate knowledge from which to make informed decisions.

7.2.2 Inadequate information about addiction

The second major information failure in the tobacco market involves inadequate information about nicotine addiction. Smokers acquire *psychological addiction* to the act of smoking itself, and *physical addiction* to nicotine (Kessler *et al.* 1997). Psychological addiction to cigarettes is hardly different from habit formation with respect to other products or practices. Nicotine addiction, however, is not simply a matter of choice or taste reinforced by repetition, such as choosing to listen to certain music or keeping company with dangerous friends. Of course, as with all biologically addictive goods, many people can change their behavior and quit using nicotine, as the decline in smoking among adults in high-income countries demonstrates (see Chapter 2 and Chapter 12). However, the costs of quitting are significant, so much so that some people find quitting virtually impossible. Most smokers who quit have to make several attempts before they succeed, and former smokers remain vulnerable to resuming smoking at times of stress (USDHHS 1990).

The addictive properties of nicotine and the fact that most smoking starts early in life have important implications for tobacco markets. Chaloupka *et al.* discuss the economics of addiction in more detail in Chapter 5. Here we elaborate on nicotine's influence on demand and its impact on young people, particularly as concerns their tendency to under-estimate the costs of quitting.

Is addiction alone reason enough for governments to intervene against smoking? If children had full information about the likelihood of becoming addicted and understood the long-run implications of their addiction, they might conceivably become 'happy addicts' who are maximizing their own welfare by smoking. For example, the teenager might argue that it would be 'better to suffer lung cancer at age 60 than to suffer Alzheimer's disease at age 80'. Models of so-called 'rational addiction' (Becker and Murphy 1988) assume that individuals maximize utility over their lifetime, taking into account the future consequences of their choices. However, the key assumptions of the model are that people are fully rational, that they are far-sighted about their choices, and that they have full information on the costs and benefits of their choices. These assumptions are not satisfied in the case of smoking. Children are more myopic, or 'short-sighted', than adults, and they typically have less information. Recent extensions to the rational addiction model by Orphanides and Zervos (1995) take some of this into account when looking at youthful 'decisions' to become addicted. In their model, imperfect information about addiction early in life can result in seemingly rational decisions that are later viewed with regret.

Other recent theoretical work emphasizes the role of 'adjustment costs' for addictive goods (Suranovic *et al.* 1999). The presence of these adjustment costs, in the context of less than fully rational behavior, implies that smokers may continue to smoke while regretting this decision, given that the costs of stopping are greater than the costs of continuing. In this context, rather than providing benefits, continued smoking for an addicted smoker is the lesser of two evils. Some might interpret the differences between the short- and long-run price elasticities of demand for an addictive good as reflecting the magnitude of these adjustment costs. That is, much of the difference between the long-run and short-run consumer surplus may be thought to reflect the adjustment costs. Assuming a linear demand curve, and given the evidence that the long-run elasticity for cigarette demand is about double the short-run elasticity, this suggests that as much as half of perceived consumer surplus (based on short-run demand) reflects the adjustment costs associated with addiction (see Chapter 6).

Perhaps most importantly, there is clear evidence that young people under-estimate the risk of becoming addicted to nicotine, and, therefore, grossly under-estimate their future costs from smoking. Among high-school seniors in the United States who smoke but believe that they will quit within five years, fewer than two out of five actually do quit. The rest are still smoking five years later (Institute of Medicine 1994). In high-income countries, about seven out of ten adult smokers say they regret their choice to start smoking and two-thirds make serious attempts to quit during their life (USDHHS 1989). In sum, it is the combination of imperfect information about addiction and myopia that results in significant under-estimation of the risks of future health damage. In the absence of addiction, teenagers could more easily quit later, when they become aware of the health risks, as they tend to do where other risky behaviors are concerned. We discuss this further below.The risk that young people will make unwise decisions is recognized by most societies and is not unique to choices about smoking, although in the case of smoking it is compounded by addiction and inadequate information. Therefore, most societies restrict young people's power to make certain decisions. For example, most democracies prevent their young people from voting before a certain age; some societies make education compulsory up to a certain age; and many prevent marriage before a certain age. The consensus across most societies is that some decisions are best left until adulthood. Likewise, many societies consider that the freedom of young people to choose to become addicted should be restricted.

It might be argued that young people are attracted to many risky behaviors, such as fast driving or alcohol binge-drinking, and that there is nothing special about smoking. However, few other risky behaviors carry the high risk of addiction that is seen with smoking, and most others are easier to abandon or modify, and are abandoned or modified in maturity (O'Malley *et al.* 1998; Bachman *et al.* 1997). For example, teenagers often binge drink, but most grow to be responsible moderate drinkers later in life. Driving motor vehicles is risky, but most young drivers survive long enough to learn to drive more responsibly. With smoking, there is no comparable way to behave more prudently, except to quit; even cutting back somewhat on consumption does not reduce the risks proportionally. Also, compared with other risky behaviors, such as alcohol use, new recruits to smoking face a very high probability of premature death. These factors combined create a probability of addiction and premature death that is higher than for other risk behaviors. Using estimates from Murray and Lopez (1996) and WHO (1999), and studies in high-income countries, we estimate that of 1000 15-year-old males currently living in middle-income and low-income countries, 125 will be killed by smoking before age 70 if they continue to smoke regularly. By comparison, before age 70, 10 will die because of road accidents, 10 will die because of violence, and about 30 will die of alcohol-related causes, including some road accidents and violent deaths.

The tobacco industry has a clear incentive to subsidize or to give away free cigarettes to potential smokers, especially young people, in order to induce them to smoke and become addicted to nicotine (Becker *et al.* 1994; Ensor 1992). The same incentive applies to creating addiction among adults in low-income and middle-income countries by manipulating price.

Thus, at best, nicotine addiction greatly weakens the argument that smokers should exercise consumer sovereignty. Given the myopia of young consumers and the likelihood of information failure for all smokers, it is inappropriate to regard an addiction-induced demand as representing genuine welfare gains to the smoker.

7.2.3 External costs

Consumers and producers in any transaction may impose costs or benefits on others, which are known as externalities. The costs—or benefits—imposed by smokers on others are of three types. First are the direct physical costs for non-smokers who are exposed to others' smoke. Second are the financial externalities that cause monetary loss (or gain) for non-smokers, whether or not they are exposed to smoke. Last (and most difficult to assess) are the so-called 'caring externalities' or 'existence value' effects of smoking, whereby non-smokers suffer emotionally from the illness and death of smokers unrelated to them personally.

Physical externalities

Physical externalities from smokers involve both health effects for non-smokers, such as a higher risk of disease or death, and other effects, such as the nuisance of unpleasant smells, physical irritation, and smoke residues on clothes, and the greater risks of fire and property damage. The health effects are briefly summarized. They include, for children born to smoking mothers, low birthweight and an increased risk of various diseases (USDHHS 1986; Charlton 1996), and an increased risk of various diseases in children and adults chronically exposed to environmental tobacco smoke either at home or in the workplace (Environmental Protection Agency 1992; Wald and Hackshaw 1996). Importantly, the list of diseases and conditions associated with environmental tobacco smoke is expanding (California Environmental Protection Agency 1997).

Financial externalities

Financial externalities are costs that are imposed by smokers but at least partly financed by non-smokers. In countries where there is an element of publicly financed healthcare, these include medical costs, among them the costs of treating the newborns of mothers who smoke during pregnancy. Non-smokers also help to pay for the damage from fires and the higher maintenance costs of workplaces and homes where smokers are present. Here we briefly summarize the key arguments related to healthcare costs and to pensions.

In high-income countries, the overall annual cost of healthcare that may be attributed to smoking has been estimated to be between 6% and 15% of total health-care costs. In most low-income and middle-income countries today, the annual costs of healthcare attributable to smoking are lower than this, partly because the epidemic of tobacco-related diseases is at an earlier stage, and partly because of other factors, such as the kinds of tobacco-related diseases that are most prevalent and the treatments that they require. However, these countries are likely to see their annual smoking-related healthcare costs rise in the future as the tobacco epidemic matures (World Bank 1992).

For those concerned with public spending budgets, it is vital to know these annual healthcare costs and the fraction borne by the public sector, because they represent real resources that cannot be used for other goods and services. For individual con-sumers, on the other hand, the key issue is the extent to which the costs will be borne by themselves or by others. As the following discussion shows, the assessment of these costs is complex, and therefore it is not possible yet to draw definitive conclusions about whether or how they may influence smokers' consumption choices.

In any given year, on average, a smoker's healthcare is likely to cost more than that of a non-smoker of the same age and sex. However, because smokers tend to die earlier than non-smokers, the *lifetime* healthcare costs of smokers and non-smokers in high-income countries may be fairly similar. Studies that measure the lifetime healthcare costs of smokers and non-smokers in high-income countries have reached conflicting conclusions (see Chapter 4 for more details). In the Netherlands (Barendregdt *et al.* 1997) and Switzerland (Leu and Schwab 1983), for example, smokers and non-smokers have been found to have similar costs, while in the United Kingdom (Atkinson and Townsend 1977) and the United States (Hodgson 1992), some studies have concluded that smokers' lifetime costs are, in fact, higher. Part of this confusion stems from the fact that it is relatively easy to make actuarial estimates of the potential for smokers' earlier deaths to bring savings in public health or pension expenditures. In contrast, the external financial costs of smoking are more difficult to measure reliably, and may be considerably under-estimated (Chaloupka and Warner, in press). Recent reviews that take account of the growing number of tobacco-attributable diseases and other factors conclude that, overall, smokers' lifetime costs in high-income countries are somewhat greater than those of non-smokers, despite their earlier deaths (Chapter 4; Chaloupka and Warner, in press). There are no such reliable studies on lifetime health-care costs in low-income and middle-income countries.

Clearly, for all regions of the world, smokers who assume the full costs of their medical services will not impose costs on others, however much greater those costs may be than non-smokers'. In developing countries, higher proportions of healthcare costs are borne by private individuals, rather than by the public system (Bos *et al.* 1999). Nonetheless, even in low-income countries, a significant percentage of medical care, especially that associated with hospital treatment, is financed either through govern-ment budgets or through private insurance. To the extent that taxes, co-payments, or social insurance premiums are not differentially higher for smokers, the higher medical costs attributable to smokers will be at least partly borne by non-smokers. To the extent that private business healthcare costs are passed on to consumers in the form of higher prices, or to workers in the form of lower wages, any costs incurred by workers who smoke will similarly be partly passed on to non-smokers. However, such costs are small in low-income and middle-income countries (Collins and Lapsley 1998). Out-of-pocket payments and risk-adjusted insurance schemes do not burden non-smokers with some of the costs of smokers. For private insurance, where premiums for non-smokers are lower than for smokers, there may be little economic justification for public intervention. In reality, however, most health insurance plans are increasingly group-based and contain no risk-adjustment for smoking.

In low-income and middle-income countries, intra-household transfers of income or welfare may be as important a source of externalities as formal, extra-household transfers (James 1994). Manning *et al.* (1991) and others argue that intra-household transfers are irrelevant, since adults' decisions to smoke are made on behalf of a whole household, and reflect the preferences of all family members. This is implausible, since adults are likely to become smokers before marrying or having children. They are likely to find it difficult to quit later—even if spouses or children urge them to. Furthermore, very young children, who may be the most severely affected by exposure to others' smoke, have no voice in such decisions. Spouses may, in deciding to marry, have taken into account the addiction of their partner, and may, therefore, be said to acquiesce in the decision; but that is not the same thing as helping to make the decision or approving of it.

In high-income countries, public expenditure on health accounts for about 65% of all health expenditures, or about 6% of GDP (Bos *et al.* 1999). If smokers have higher net lifetime healthcare costs, then non-smokers will subsidize the healthcare costs of smokers. The exact contribution is complex and variable, depending on the type of coverage, and the source of taxation that is used to pay for public expenditures. If, for example, only the healthcare costs of those over 65 are publicly funded, then the net use of public revenues by smokers may be small, to the extent that many require smoking-related medical care and die *before* they reach this age. Equally, if public expenditure is financed out of consumption taxes, including cigarette taxes, or if third-party private insurance adjusts smokers' premiums because of their higher health risks, then their costs may not be imposed on others. Once again, the situation differs in low-income and middle-income countries, where the public component of total healthcare expenditure is on average lower than in high-income countries, at around 44% of the total, or 2% of GDP (Bos *et al.* 1999). However, as countries spend more on health, the share of total expenditure that is met by public finance tends to rise too (World Bank 1993).

While it is difficult to assess the relative healthcare costs of smokers and non-smokers, the issue of pensions has proved at least as contentious, and has attracted some popular debate. For example, an editorial in *The Economist* (1995) expressed the view that smokers 'pay their way'. It continued:

... what they cost in medical bills, fires and so on, they more than repay in pensions they do not live to collect.

This assertion is based on analyses from high-income countries that suggest that smokers contribute more than non-smokers to pension schemes, because many pay contributions until around retirement age and then die before they can claim a substantial proportion of their benefits (Manning 1989; Viscusi 1995). There are several problems with this assertion. First, there is an ongoing academic debate over definitions of the social costs of smoking, and particularly the extent to which 'savings' from not collecting pensions should be included. Depending on differing assumptions, other studies (see, for example, Atkinson and Townsend 1977) have not found net costs for smokers to be lower. Second, the issue is not currently relevant to many of the low-income and middle-income countries where most of the world's smokers live. In low-income countries, only about one in ten adults has a public pension, and in middle-income countries the proportion is between a quarter and half of the population, depending on the income level of the country; private pension plans are less common (James 1994). Finally, and perhaps most importantly, most of these studies have followed traditional notions of economic externalities, and have not placed any value on life *per se*. Even if smokers do reduce the net costs imposed on others by dying young, it would be misleading to suggest that society is better off because of these premature deaths. To do so would be to accept a logic that says society is better off without its older adults (Harris 1994).

Caring externalities

The third group of externalities that we consider are those that are the most difficult to assess: they are known as 'existence value' or 'caring' externalities (Krutilla 1967). There is evidence that people are willing to pay for another's well being, even if they do not know the person and even if they do not benefit directly themselves. Public spending on health partly reflects such externalities. Existence value is most readily applied to children, whom society typically protects more than adults. In contrast, caring externalities for adults almost directly contradict the notion of consumer sovereignty. Clearly, caring externalities differ across cultures and countries, depending among other things on the importance society assigns to individual sovereignty. Non-smokers may be willing to subsidize efforts to prevent people taking up smoking or efforts to help smokers quit. They may also be prepared to contribute towards the care of sick smokers, even when these represent a financial burden. However, their attitudes may change over time as knowledge about the health effects of smoking becomes more widespread and non-smokers' tolerance for smokers may decline (Gorovitz *et al.* 1998). In any case, there is little solid information of such willingness, so it is difficult to use it to formulate public policies.

In sum, there are clearly direct costs imposed by smokers on non-smokers, such as health damage. There are probably also financial costs, although it is more difficult to identify or quantify these.

7.3 Government responses to market failure: what, for whom and at what price?

Given that, as we have argued, the markets for tobacco products suffer efficiency failures that result in premature death and illness, and costs imposed on others, it is appropriate to ask if government intervention can correct them. Here we ask whether governments have interventions available to correct these failures, and discuss the costs and effectiveness of these interventions.

Below we describe briefly those interventions that respond to, or deal with, each of the types of inefficiency in the tobacco market that we have described above. Governments can use information, regulation, taxation, or subsidies to address these market failures.

Government responses to *incomplete or erroneous information* include, specifically, mass information campaigns, warning labels, and publicly-financed research to create more, or better, or more easily assimilated, information. All are public goods, which the market is unlikely to provide adequately. Public responses to existing addiction in adults include, specifically, incentives to quit, such as cessation programs (with or without pharmacological therapies) offered free or at subsidized prices, and education campaigns that raise awareness of the risks of smoking and the benefits of cessation. In addition, governments can encourage deregulation of the market for nicotine replacement therapy (see Chapter 12). Public responses to preventing new addiction in children (discussed in more detail below) include education campaigns about the danger of addiction, restricting children's access to tobacco products, bans on the advertising and promotion of tobacco products, and taxation. Increased taxation will also increase cessation rates among adults.

Government responses to *direct physical externalities* include education campaigns emphasizing the right of non-smokers to a smoke-free environment, restrictions on smoking in public places and workplaces, and taxes. Government responses to *financial externalities* may include risk-adjusted health or pension premiums, or anything that restricts tobacco consumption, whether or not in the presence of non-smokers. These may include taxation, information campaigns, and restrictions on where people can smoke.

Government responses to '*existence value*' externalities also include any intervention that restricts consumption and thereby reduces the health damage from smoking. Concern for smokers at highest risk—those already addicted who have smoked for many years—would lead to specific subsidies for cessation programs, the deregulation of nicotine replacement markets, and information campaigns emphasizing the dangers of long-term smoking. However, in reality, governments do not always aim interventions directly at the sources of market failures themselves, but to particular constituencies or population groups affected by those market failures. In the case of the tobacco market, government intervention is often designed to protect children.

We turn now to a discussion of the appropriateness of the various available interventions.

7.4.1 Choosing 'first-best' and 'second-best' interventions

Government intervention in the tobacco market is most easily justified to deter children and adolescents from smoking and to protect non-smokers. But it is also justified for the purposes of giving adults all the information they need to make an informed choice. Ideally, government interventions should address each identified problem with a specific intervention tailored to solve that particular problem and none other. These may be thought of as first-best interventions. However, a neat one-to-one correspondence between problems and solutions is not always possible, and some interventions may have broader effects. We discuss first-best interventions, their effectiveness, and their limitations, first for protecting children, then for correcting the physical and financial costs imposed by smokers on others, and lastly for informing adult smokers. A common theme emerges: the use of taxes, though a second-best and more blunt instrument, is more effective.

Protecting children

Several economists have suggested that protection of children is the most compelling economic argument for higher taxes (Warner *et al.* 1995). Governments can choose to protect children for several reasons. First, childhood is when nicotine addiction is likely to begin. Second, children are not yet sovereign adults making informed choices, so the principal argument for *not* intervening does not apply to them as strongly as to adults. Third, there is evidence that the tobacco industry targets children with glamorous advertisements and promotion. Fourth, compared with many consumer goods that may appear desirable to children, such as automobiles, cigarettes are generally affordable and accessible: thus the market does not spontaneously protect children from them. Finally, children have no way to become better or safer smokers as they mature, except by quitting.

A priori, parents would ideally always be willing and able to protect children from tobacco themselves. If this happened, there would be little need for governments to duplicate such efforts (Musgrove 1999). Perfect parents, however, are rare. Adults may smoke themselves, thereby modeling this behavior for their children, and, even though few would actually encourage their children to start smoking, they may also fail to educate them about the risks. Parents' responsibilities on the question of smoking are not comparable to, say, their responsibilities to ensure their children are immunized. In the latter case, the parent or caregiver has a defined responsibility to protect the child through a fairly simple action, and where the child's lack of information is irrelevant.

The next best public or non-parental interventions would be to try to educate children, restrict advertising and promotion targeted to children, and to restrict their access to tobacco products. As discussed above and in more detail by Kenkel and Chen (Chapter 8), information campaigns have had an important impact on overall declines in smoking in high-income countries. But information campaigns targeted at children are likely to be less effective than those targeted at adults, because children discount the future more, and have difficulty considering consequences of today's behavior that may not take effect for three or four decades. Individual youth-centered programs, including school health programs, have often been found ineffective (Reid 1996).

For a specific campaign aimed at children, governments would need to ban advertising and promotion of tobacco products in the media that children are most often exposed to, such as television or radio. Empirical evidence cited by Saffer (Chapter 9), suggests that partial bans cause the tobacco industry to shift to other media, including promotional goods (such as free samples), and sponsorship of sports events, which do influence children (Charlton *et al.* 1997). Finally, efforts to restrict young people's access to tobacco products in shops, restaurants, and bars appear to have had mixed success to date, given that the enforcement of bans is difficult. Moreover, youth restrictions have relatively high administrative costs (Chapter 11; Reid 1996).

In contrast to these measures, there is ample evidence that tax increases are the single most effective policy measure for reducing children's consumption of tobacco products (see Chapter 10). Young people are more sensitive to price changes than older people. Estimates suggest that a tax increase of $2 per pack in the United States would reduce overall youth smoking by about two-thirds (National Cancer Policy Board 1998). To the extent that low-income and middle-income countries have younger populations than high-income countries, tax increases would be expected to be effective in these countries too (see Chapter 18).

In theory, if cigarette taxes are to be used mainly to deter children and adolescents from smoking, then the tax on children should be higher than any tax on adults. Such differential tax treatment would, however, be virtually impossible to implement. Yet a uniform rate for children and adults, the practical option, would impose a burden on adults. Societies may nevertheless consider that it is justifiable to impose this burden on adults in order to protect children. Moreover, if adults reduce their cigarette consumption, children may smoke less, given evidence that children's propensity to smoke is influenced by whether their parents, and other adult role-models, smoke (Murray *et al.* 1983).

Physical costs imposed on non-smokers

Governments can choose to protect non-smokers from the health effects of exposure to environmental tobacco smoke, including the effects on children and babies born to smoking parents. The externalities of maternal smoking for infants are less clear than for other non-smokers exposed to others' smoke, at least where mothers are assumed to have rights over fetuses, including the right to submit them to risks. However, the literature on the attitudes of pregnant women to their own health and that of their fetuses suggests that those who are informed about healthy behaviors are more likely to act to protect their fetuses' health (Charlton 1996).

Costs to non-smokers' health would appear, a priori, to be easily reduced through bans on public and workplace smoking. These 'clean-air' restrictions have the advantage that they limit the conditions under which people can smoke, without directly addressing the choice of whether to smoke. It should be noted that direct physical externalities do not by themselves justify widespread government interventions, such as advertising and promotion bans, and tax increases, since what matters is not how much people smoke, but whether others are exposed to tobacco smoke. As discussed by Woollery and others (Chapter 11), restrictions in high-income countries on smoking in public places and private workplaces reduce both smoking prevalence and average daily cigarette consumption. Data from developing countries are much less complete, but experience from South Africa suggests that restrictions do reduce smoking (Van der Merwe 1998). Such restrictions are clearly weakened where there is a lack of enforcement, or a reliance on self enforcement. However, a more significant problem with this approach is that the vast majority of exposure to environmental tobacco smoke is in homes, and this is where children are also more likely to be exposed. (Mannino *et al.* 1996; NCI 1999). In contrast to clean-air restrictions, tax increases, by significantly reducing smoking in all settings, could lower this cost to children.

Financial costs borne by non-smokers would, a priori, be best reduced through adjusted risk premiums on health services or pension services. Financial costs could be calculated over short intervals, but lifetime medical costs for today's young smokers are more unpredictable. Private insurance markets sometimes include such price differentials, without requiring regulation; publicly-financed insurance seldom or never does. As the administrative costs for adjusting risk premiums are high, a less precise but more efficient method would be to simply tax cigarettes at the source. Note that in contrast to physical externalities, financial externalities would justify such general consumption-reducing measures, since what matters is how much people smoke rather than where they do it.

Giving adult smokers information

Governments can use a number of measures to protect adult smokers' health by inducing them to quit or to smoke less, but this most directly conflicts with the assumption of consumer sovereignty, except in the case of smokers who want to quit but find it difficult because they are already addicted. Public policy responses include information about the health risks, subsidization of cessation programs and tax increases. Only the last of these conflicts with permitting individuals to take risky decisions (such as . playing dangerous sports, or associating with dangerous friends) on the assumption that individuals know their risks and bear the costs of their choices. Providing information, and helping individual smokers who want to quit, are not in conflict with the principal of consumer sovereignty.

Publicly financed information campaigns and research on the health risks of smoking for adults are justified as a 'first-best' intervention. As Kenkel and Chen elaborate (Chapter 8), such information has had a powerful impact on smoking in high-income countries, although the effects take time to appear. Statutory warnings on tobacco products and regulations on tar and nicotine content are also common throughout the world, but few countries use strong and varied warning labels that convey meaningful information on the hazards of smoking (WHO 1997). An extension of information measures are bans on advertising and promotion. Such bans can help smokers to quit or to avoid starting again (USDHHS 1990). As discussed above, historically the tobacco industry has used advertising to make misleading claims about the health risks. Thus, bans on advertising and promotion are justified as a more intrusive but effective intervention.

Governments may also deregulate nicotine replacement, finance, or provide cessation advice, or even subsidize cessation treatment. As discussed by Novotny *et al.* (Chapter 12) and Gajalakshmi *et al.* (Chapter 2), an individual's risk of premature mortality drops sharply on quitting, especially at younger ages (Doll *et al.* 1994). Note that nicotine replacement products are not public goods, and are in fact provided by the private market: smokers wanting to quit can buy private cessation-help programs and nicotine-delivering patches to ease withdrawal. The argument for public intervention is only that the private market's response may be sub-optimal, partly due to regulation that restricts the public's access to cessation aids.

Taxation is also an effective intervention. Cigarettes are taxed in nearly all countries, sometimes heavily, but mainly because of the administrative ease of collecting tobacco taxes and the relatively inelastic demand. Adults are less price-responsive than children to increases in tobacco tax.

7.3.2 The economic costs of intervening

Given that the effective interventions do not neatly correspond to the market failures they were designed to correct, an important consideration is whether they also generate further economic costs that may be worse than the original market failure. This specifically applies to taxes, given that they are the most blunt, and also most effective, measure to protect children. Below we discuss the key economic costs of intervening, including the costs of foregone pleasure from smoking. Unfortunately, there are few empirical studies of the economic costs of intervening (Warner 1997). We focus on the conceptual framework of costs from various interventions, emphasizing the costs to individuals. We do not discuss costs to producers. Estimates by Peck *et al.* (Chapter 6) suggest that consumer satisfaction is the lion's share of any plausible estimate of benefits from smoking, with producers' benefits being much smaller. Ranson *et al.* (Chapter 18) provide estimates of cost-effectiveness from the perspective of the public sector.

Control measures would cause regular smokers to forego the pleasure of smoking, or incur the costs of quitting, or both. A priori, this loss of consumer surplus would appear to be the same as it would be for bread or any other consumer good. However, tobacco is not a typical consumer good with typical benefits. For the addicted smoker who regrets smoking and expresses a desire to quit, the benefits of smoking are largely the avoidance of the costs of withdrawal. If tobacco control measures reduce individual smokers' consumption, those smokers will face significant withdrawal costs. Furthermore, the costs would differ between current smokers and potential smokers who have not yet begun.

Clean-air restrictions impose costs on smokers by reducing their opportunities to consume cigarettes, or by forcing them outdoors to smoke, raising the time and discomfort associated with smoking, or by imposing fines for smoking in restricted areas. Such restrictions raise the individual's costs relative to his or her benefits, and prompt some smokers to quit or cut back their consumption. For non-smokers, however, restrictions on smoking in public places will bring welfare gains. Given that most regular smokers express a desire to quit but few are successful on their own, it seems likely that the perceived costs of quitting are greater than the perceived costs of continuing to smoke, such as damage to health. By making the costs of continued smoking greater than the costs of withdrawal, higher taxes can induce some smokers to quit. However, smokers who quit or cut back would face withdrawal costs from higher taxes. The extent of the loss depends on levels of tax already paid, price responsiveness, and other factors (see Chaloupka and Warner, in press, for a related discussion on the distributional impacts of taxes).

The provision of information about the health consequences of smoking would increase the perceived costs of continuing to smoke, and alert smokers to the benefits of quitting. Widened access to nicotine replacement therapy and other cessation interventions would help also to reduce the costs of quitting.

In considering economic costs to smokers, it is important to distinguish between regular smokers and others. For children and adolescents who are either beginners or merely potential smokers, the costs of avoiding tobacco are likely to be less severe, since addiction may not yet have taken hold and, therefore, withdrawal costs are likely to be lower. Other costs may include, for example, reduced acceptance by peers, less satisfaction from the thwarted desire to rebel against parents, and the curtailment of other pleasures of smoking.

Bans on advertising and promotion might be expected to increase the costs for smokers of obtaining information about their preferred products. However, to the extent that tobacco advertising focuses more on establishing brand loyalty among the new smokers it attracts rather than on providing information of value to current smokers, even established adult smokers would suffer little information loss or search costs if advertising and promotion were banned (Chapman 1996).

In sum, interventions in the smoking market vary by specificity to the market failure and groups most affected. It is obvious that some interventions are fairly specific to particular problems. This is notably the case for bans on smoking in public places, which are intended to control physical externalities. It is also the case for measures to make smokers pay any additional medical costs due to their behavior, which are intended to control financial externalities. But measures that are aimed at reducing cigarette consumption, rather than controlling where it occurs or who pays the associated costs, are much more general. Taxation and information campaigns are both measures of this type. When it comes to protecting or affecting particular population groups, there is similarly a mixture of more specific and more general connections between an intervention and the group(s) it is meant to affect.

7.4 Government interventions to protect the poor

Aside from government interventions to correct for market failures, intervention to protect the poor is a well-recognized government role (Musgrove 1999). Investing in health is one method but another is to reduce poverty or alleviate its consequences (World Bank 1993). We examine next the issues of how smoking burdens are distributed and the equity implications of some of the interventions analysed above.

In most countries of the world, tobacco consumption is highest among poorer socio-economic groups, and, accordingly, so is the incidence of tobacco-related disease (Chapter 3). Comparison between countries reveals that the poor have higher death rates from smoking-related diseases. Moreover, the poor spend a considerable amount on tobacco as a percentage of their household income, which adversely affects household consumption of items beneficial to children's health (Cohen 1981; World Bank 1993). To some extent, the market failure of incomplete information is more pronounced among the poor (Townsend *et al.* 1994).

Government interventions to reduce the impact of smoking among the poor include taxation, information, and subsidizing access to cessation advice or nicotine replacement therapies (NRT). Differences in the relative importance of different problems imply that the optimal combination of interventions should probably be different for poor and non-poor populations. Several studies suggest that information is less effective in reducing smoking among poor groups than among richer groups (see, for example, USDHHS 1989; Townsend 1998). Smoking prevalence has declined much faster among higher socio-economic groups than among lower groups (Chapter 3). The provision of information (such as mass information campaigns and warning labels), and bans on advertising and promotion are justified on efficiency grounds. There is little doubt, however, that the poor would use such information less, or less quickly, than would the rich. Another strategy would be to finance or provide cessation advice and cessation aids to help the poor quit smoking if they could not afford to pay for them (Musgrove 1999), provided the effects justify the costs. Delivering these services may be costly or difficult, however, since the poor tend to have less access to basic health services than the rich, and the costs of expanding these services to reach the poor might be considerable.

In contrast to information, tax increases on tobacco reduce consumption more among the poor and less educated than among the rich and more educated. Evidence from the United Kingdom and the United States (CDC 1998; Townsend 1998; Chaloupka 1991) suggests that price elasticities in the lowest income groups are significantly higher than in the highest income groups. Tobacco taxation would thus narrow the difference in consumption between rich and poor (Warner *et al.* 1995). In high-income countries, the poor usually spend a larger share of their incomes on tobacco than do the rich. Thus, a tax on tobacco is necessarily regressive *among those who continue to smoke*. Whether the overall effect of tax increases is regressive, depends on what share of each group, poor and non-poor, would react to the higher price by quitting. If more of the poor quit, then the tax effect could even be progressive. Tobacco taxes, like any other single tax, need to work within the goal of ensuring that the entire system or tax and expenditure is proportional or progressive. (Townsend 1998; Chaloupka and Warner, in press). Studies of tobacco taxation in the United States and the United Kingdom suggest that tax increases are less regressive than presumed, and may even be progressive (see Chapter 10). In contrast to the taxation of other goods, when the poor reduce their consumption of tobacco they gain a health benefit in return for the tax burden they continue to pay. Finally, the poor may benefit in another way from increased tobacco taxes, if health and social services are targeted to the poor and financed by those taxes (Saxenian and McGreevey 1996; WHO 1999).

It might be argued that taxes and other tobacco control measures would impose bigger costs on poor individuals. But if this is true for tobacco, it is not unique in public health. Compliance with many health interventions, such as child immunization or family planning, is often more costly for poor households. For example, poor families may have to walk longer distances to clinics than rich families and may lose income in the process. Yet health officials do not hesitate to argue that the health benefits of most interventions, such as immunization, are worth the cost, provided the costs do not rise so high that poor individuals are deterred from using services.

In summary, the fact that the poor devote relatively more of their income to tobacco does not provide any strong equity-based argument against the tobacco control measures analyzed here.

7.5 Conclusion

We have described specific failures in the tobacco market: first, inadequate information about the health risks of smoking; second, inadequate information about the risks of addiction (and particularly the youthful onset of use of an addictive product); and, third, the external costs of smoking. We argue that because of these market failures, government intervention is justified on economic grounds. However, the interventions themselves are often non-precise and impose costs on even informed adult smokers. What then do these findings imply for public policy?

First, the public health arguments and the economic arguments for tobacco control differ on goals. Public health goals would, rationally, be to eradicate smoking if possible, given that tobacco hazards increase with increasing exposure and overwhelm any possible beneficial effects on health. In contrast, the economic arguments suggest that the socially-optimal level of consumption of tobacco would not be zero. Ideally in economic terms, children would not smoke, but adults who knew their risks and bore their costs entirely themselves could smoke (Warner 1998).

Such a situation would involve considerably less smoking than at present, but would stop well short of eradication. Preventing children from smoking could, in theory, eventually lead to the epidemic disappearing. In reality, slightly older cohorts may take up smoking, and it is unlikely that the recruitment of new smokers would cease. Several of the interventions discussed here, particularly those designed to prevent smoking in youth, protect non-smokers from externalities, and leave smokers better informed.

However, a major problem for the 'economically optimal' view of smoking is the fact that nicotine is addictive. This undermines the consumer-sovereignty argument against intervention, because all evidence suggests that the conditions for a rational choice to become addicted are not met, and the addicted smoker is to some degree a different person from the one who decided to start smoking. If addiction is taken into account, a 'middle-ground' rationale that is justifiable by both economic and public-health arguments becomes feasible. It still falls short of eradication, but is more realistic and justifiable than a purely economics-led view that defines adult consumers as rational and informed. The economic rationale for intervention described here largely involves information and regulation, and not direct public finance or the provision of private goods, except perhaps to the poor. As such, it leaves much room for private choice.

As with other areas of public policy, governments have to make choices, drawing here on economics, epidemiology, and public health. Even limited reductions in the prevalence of smoking, achieved as the result of interventions to correct market failures, would, by any measure, constitute an enormous public health victory, avoiding millions of deaths per year.

References

Atkinson, A. B. and Townsend, J. L. (1977). Economic aspects of reduced smoking. *Lancet*, **2**(8036), 492–5.

Bachman, J. G., Wadsworth, K. N., O'Malley, P. M., Johnston, L. D., and Schulenberg, J. (1997). *Smoking, drinking, and drug use in young adulthood: The impacts of new freedoms and new responsibilities*. Mahwah, NJ: Lawrence Erlbaum Associates.

Barendregt, J. J., Bonneux, L., and van der Maas, P. J. (1997). The health care costs of smoking. *New England Journal of Medicine*, **337**(15), 1052–7.

Becker, G. S. and Murphy, K. M. (1988). A theory of rational addiction. *Journal of Political Economy*, **96**(4), 675–700.

Becker, G. S., Grossman, M., and Murphy, K. M. (1994). An empirical analysis of cigarette addiction. *American Economic Review*, **84**(3), 396–418.

Bero, L. A., Glantz, S. A., and Rennie, D. (1994). Publication bias and public health policy on environmental tobacco smoke. *JAMA*, **13**, 133–6.

Bos, E. R., Hon, V., Maeda, A., Chellaraj, G., and Preker, A. (1999). *Health, Nutrition, and Population Indicators: a Statistical Handbook*. Washington, DC : World Bank.

California Environmental Protection Agency (1997). *Health Effects of Exposure to Environmental Tobacco Smoke: Final Report*. Office of Environmental Health Hazard Assessment (OEHHA). http://www.oehha.org/scientific/ets/finalets.htm

Centers for Disease Control and Prevention (CDC) (1998). Response to increases in cigarette prices by race/ethnicity, income, and age groups – United States, 1976–1993. *Morbidity and Mortality Weekly Report*, **47**(29), 405–9.

Chaloupka, F. J. (1991). Rational addictive behavior and cigarette smoking. *Journal of Political Economy*, **99**(4), 722–42.

Chaloupka, F. J. and K. E. Warner. The economics of smoking. In *The Handbook of Health Economics* (ed. J. Newhouse and A. Culyer). Amsterdam: North Holland. (In press.)

Chapman, S. (1996). The ethics of tobacco advertising and advertising bans. *Br. Med. Bull.*, **52**(1), 121–31.

Charlton, A. (1996). Children and smoking: the family circle. *Br. Med. Bull.*, **52**(1), 90–107.

Charlton, A., While, D., and Kelly, S. (1997). Boys smoking and cigarette-brand-sponsored motor racing. *Lancet*, **350**(9089), 1474.

Chinese Academy of Preventive Medicine (1997). *Smoking in China: 1996 National Prevalence Survey of Smoking Pattern*. Beijing: China Science and Technology Press.

Cohen, N. (1981). Smoking, health, and survival: prospects in Bangladesh. *Lancet*, **1**(8229), 1090–3.

Collins, D. and Lapsley, H. (1998). estimating and disaggregating the social costs of tobacco. In *The Economics of Tobacco Control: Towards an Optimal Policy Mix* (ed. I. Abedian, R. van der Merwe, N. Wilkins and P. Jha), pp. 155–78. Cape Town, Applied Fiscal Research Centre: University of Cape Town.

Doll, R., Peto, R., Wheatley, K., Gray, R., and Sutherland, I. (1994). Mortality in relation to smoking: 40 years observations on male british doctors. *British Medical Journal*, **309**(6959), 901–11.

The Economist (1995). An anti-smoking wheeze: Washington needs a sensible all-drugs policy, not a 'war on teenage smoking'. 19 August, pp. 14–15.

The Economist (1997). Tobacco and tolerance. 20 December, pp. 59–61.

Ensor, T. (1992). Regulating tobacco consumption in developing countries. *Health Policy and Planning*, **7**, 375–81.

Environmental Protection Agency (1992). *Respiratory Health Effects of Passive Smoking: Lung Cancer and Other Disorders*. EPA, Office of Research and Development, Office of Air and Radiation. EPA/600/6–90/006F.

Glantz, S. A., Barnes, D. E., Bero, L., Hanauer, P., and Slade, J. (1995). Looking through a keyhole at the tobacco industry. The Brown and Williamson documents. *JAMA*, **274**(3), 219–24.

Gorovitz, E., Mosher, J., and Pertschuk, M. (1998). Pre-emption or prevention?: lessons from efforts to control firearms, alcohol, and tobacco. *Journal of Public Health Policy*, **19**(1), 36–50.

Harris, J. E. (1994). *A Working Model for Predicting the Consumption and Revenue Impacts of Large Increases in the U.S. Federal Cigarette Excise Tax*. Working paper no. 4803. Cambridge (MA): National Bureau of Economic Research.

Hodgson, T. A. (1992). Cigarette smoking and lifetime medical expenditures. *Milbank Quarterly*, **70**(1), 81–125.

Institute of Medicine (1994). *Growing Up Tobacco Free*. National Academy Press: Washington DC.

James, E. (1994). *Averting the Old Age Crisis: Policies to Protect the Old and Promote Growth*. Oxford and New York: World Bank and Oxford University Press.

Kessler, D. A., Barnett, P. S., Witt, A., Zeller, M. R., Mande, J. R., and Schultz, W. B. (1997). The legal and scientific basis of FDA's assertion of jurisdiction over cigarettes and smokeless tobacco. *JAMA*, **277**, 405–9.

Krutilla, J. V. (1967). Conservations reconsidered. *American Economic Review*, **57**, 776–86.

Leu, R. E. and Schaub, T. (1983). Does smoking increase medical care expenditure? *Social Science and Medicine*, **17**(23), 1907–14.

Levshin, V. and Droggachih, V. (1999). *Knowledge and Education Regarding Smoking Among Moscow Teenagers*. Paper presented at the workshop on Tobacco Control in Central and Eastern Europe. Las Palmas de Gran Canaria. February 26.

Manning, W. G. (1989). The taxes of sin: do smokers and drinkers pay their way? *Journal of the American Medical Association*, **261**(11), 1604–09.

Manning, W. G., Keeler, E. B., Newhouse, J. P., Sloss, E. M., and Wasserman, J. (1991). *The Costs of Poor Health Habits*. Cambridge, Mass.: Harvard University Press.

Mannino, D. M., Siegel, M., Husten, C., Rose, D., and Etzel, R. (1996). Environmental tobacco smoke exposure and health effects in children: results from the 1991 National Health Interview Survey. *Tob. Control*, **5**(1), 13–18.

Murray, C. J. and Lopez, A. D. (ed.) (1996). *The Global Burden of Disease: a Comprehensive Assessment of Mortality and Disability from Diseases, Injuries, and Risk Factors in 1990 and Projected to 2020*. Cambridge, Mass.: Harvard School of Public Health.

Murray, M., Swan, A. V., Johnson, M. R., and Bewley, B. R. (1983). Some factors associated with increased risk of smoking by children. *Journal of Child Psychology and Psychiatry*, **24**(2), 223–32.

Musgrove P. Public spending on health care: how are different criteria related? *Health Policy* 1999 Jun. 47(3):207–23.

National Cancer Institute (NCI) (1999). *Health Effects of Exposure to Environmental Tobacco Smok*. The Report of the California Environmental Protection Agency. Smoking and Tobacco Control Monograph no. 10. Bethesda, MD. US Department of Health and Human Services, National Institutes of Health, National Cancer Institute, NIH Pub. No. 99–4645.

National Cancer Policy Board (1998). *Taking Action to Reduce Tobacco Use*. Washington, DC: National Academy Press.

O'Malley, P.M., Bachman, J.G., and Johnston, L.D. (1988). Period, age and cohort effects on substance use among young Americans: a decade of change, 1976–86. *American Journal of Public Health*, **78**(10), 1315–21.

Orphanides, A., and Zervos, D. (1995). Rational addiction with learning and regret. *Journal of Political Economy*, **103**(4), 739–58.

Pekurinen, M. (1991). *Economic Aspects of Smoking: Is There a Case for Government Intervention in Finland?* Helsinki: Vapk-Publishing.

Peto, R. (1986). Influence of dose and duration of smoking on lung cancer rates. In *Tobacco: a Major International Health Hazard*. (ed. R. Peto, and D. Zaridze), pp. 23–34. International Agency for Research on Cancer, 1986 (IARC Scientific Publications, no. 74).

Peto, R., Lopez, A. D., Boreham, J., Thun, M., and Heath, C. Jr. (1994). *Mortality from Smoking in Developed Countries 1950–2000*. Oxford: Oxford University Press.

Peto, R., Chen, Z. M., and Boreham, J. (1999). Tobacco: the growing epidemic. *Nature Medicine*, **5**(1), 15–7.

Reid, D. (1996). Tobacco control: overview. *British Medical Bulletin*, **52**(1), 108–20.

Saxenian, H. and McGreevey, B. (1996). *China: Issues and Options in Health Financing.* World Bank Report No. 15278-CHA, Washington, DC.

Suranovic, S. M., Goldfarb, R. S., and Leonard, T. C. (1999). An economic theory of cigarette addiction. *Journal of Health Economics*, **18,** 1–29.

Sweda, E. L. Jr. and Daynard, R. A. (1996). Tobacco industry tactics. *Br. Med. Bull.*, **52**(1), 183–92.

Townsend, J., Roderick, P., and Cooper, J. (1994). Cigarette smoking by socioeconomic group, sex, and age: effects of price, income, and health publicity. *British Medical Journal*, **309**(6959), 923–27.

Townsend (1998). The role of taxation policy in tobacco control. In *The Economics of Tobacco Control* (ed. I. Abedian, R. van der Merwe, N. Wilkins, and P. Jha), pp. 85–101. Cape Town, South Africa: Applied Fiscal Research Centre, University of Cape Town.

US Department of Health and Human Services (1986). *The Health Consequences of Smoking For Women.* US Department of Health and Human Services, Public Health Service, Office of the Assistant Secretary for Health, Office on smoking and Health. Rockville, Maryland

US Department of Health and Human Services (1989). *Reducing the Health Consequences of Smoking: 25 Years of Progress. A Report of the Surgeon General.* Rockville, Maryland: US Department of Health and Human Services, Public Health Service, Centers for Disease Control, Center for Chronic Disease Prevention and Health Promotion, Office on Smoking and Health. DHHS Publication No. (CDC)89–8411.

US Department of Health and Human Services (1990). *The Health Benefits of Smoking Cessation: A Report of the Surgeon General.* Rockville, Maryland: US Department of Health and Human Services, Public Health Service, Centers for Disease Control, Center for Chronic Disease Prevention and Health Promotion, Office on Smoking and Health. DHHS Publication No. (CDC) 90–8416.

Van der Merwe, R. (1998). The economics of tobacco control in South Africa. In *The Economics of Tobacco Control* (ed. I. Abedian, R. van der Merwe, N. Wilkins, and P. Jha), pp. 251–71. Cape Town, South Africa: Applied Fiscal Research Centre, University of Cape Town.

Viscusi, W. K. (1995). Cigarette taxation and the social consequences of smoking. In *Tax Policy and the Economy.* (ed. J. M. Poterba). Cambridge, MA, MIT Press. **9**, 51–101.

Wald, N. J. and Hackshaw, A. K. (1996). Cigarette smoking: an epidemiological overview. *British Medical Bulletin*, **52**(1), 3–11.

Warner, K. E., Goldenhar, L. M., and McLaughlin, C. G. (1992). Cigarette advertising and magazine coverage of the hazards of smoking. A statistical analysis. *N. Engl. J. Med.*, **326**, 305–9.

Warner, K. E. (1997). Cost-effectiveness of smoking cessation therapies: interpretation of the evidence and implications for coverage. *PharmacoEconomics*, **11**, 538–49.

Warner, K. E. (1998). The economics of tobacco and health: an overview. In *The Economics of Tobacco Control* (ed. I. Abedian, R. van der Merwe, N. Wilkins and P. Jha), pp. 55–75. Cape Town, South Africa: Applied Fiscal Research Centre, University of Cape Town.

Warner, K. E., Chaloupka, F. J., Cook, P. J., Manning W. G., Newhouse, J. P., Novotny, T. E. *et al.* (1995). Criteria for determining an optimal cigarette tax: the economist's perspective. *Tobacco Control*, **4**, 80–6.

Weinstein, N. D. (1998). Accuracy of smokers risk perceptions. *Annals of Behavioral Medicine*, **20**(2), 135–40.

World Bank (1992). *China: Long-term Issues and Options in the Health Transition.* Washington, DC.

World Bank (1993). *The World Development Report 1993: Investing in Health.* New York: Oxford University Press.

World Health Organization (1997). *Tobacco or Health: a Global Status Report.* Geneva, Switzerland.

World Health Organization (1999). *The World Health Report 1999: Making a difference.* Geneva, Switzerland.

Zatonski, W. (1996). *Evolution of Health in Poland Since 1988.* Warsaw: Marie Skeodowska-Curie Cancer Center and Institute of Oncology, Department of Epidemiology and Cancer Prevention.

Section III
Demand for tobacco

8

Consumer information and tobacco use

Donald Kenkel and Likwang Chen

This chapter addresses two related questions: first, are consumers well-informed about the consequences of tobacco use?; and, second, can public policies to improve consumer information reduce tobacco use? Although in many countries people are generally aware of the health risks of smoking, there are gaps in their perceptions of those risks. Individuals tend to under-estimate the risk of smoking relative to other causes of death. In addition, many smokers appear not to apply their knowledge of the health risks to themselves personally. Finally, evidence suggests that young people under-estimate the addictive properties of tobacco. In some countries significant improvements in consumer information about the links between tobacco use and disease are still possible; while in other countries consumers are probably as fully informed as is realistically possible. In many countries, so-called 'information shocks'—such as the publication of new reports on the health effects of smoking—have reduced tobacco consumption. If the experience of these countries can be applied elsewhere, consumer information policies appear to be effective instruments for tobacco control. This conclusion is buttressed by the success of specific interventions including mass-media campaigns and warning labels on cigarette packs.

8.1 Overview

This chapter asks whether and how information about the risks of smoking can influence consumers' use of tobacco and how the answers may affect tobacco-control policy. Smokers are like other consumers in that they face problems in learning about the price and quality of their prospective purchases. However, they are unlike most other consumers in that their purchased goods, tobacco products, are addictive and have serious health consequences. Smokers who are unaware of either the addictive properties or the health consequences of tobacco are not buying the products they think they are. In essence, each purchase of a tobacco product involves two components: the good to be consumed in the present, and the flow of future consequences from that consumption. Poorly informed consumers do not place enough weight on the flow of future consequences. As a result, they make purchases of tobacco products that they later regret or would judge not to be in their best interests if they had had more information (see Chapter 5).

The plan of the chapter is as follows. Sections 8.2 and 8.3 address the first of the chapter's two questions, on how well-informed consumers are. Section 8.2 discusses how scientific information on the effects of tobacco is discovered and disseminated to consumers. Section 8.3 reviews the evidence on what consumers know and understand about the risks. Sections 8.4 and 8.5 turn to the second question of whether improving consumer information can reduce tobacco use in countries where important information gaps remain. Section 8.4 reviews econometric studies on the impacts of 'information shocks' on tobacco markets over time, and on the extent to which differences in consumer information at a point in time are related to tobacco use. Section 8.5 summarizes the evidence on the effectiveness of specific health information interventions. In general, the message of both Sections 8.4 and 8.5 is positive: the provision of consumer information appears to be an effective tobacco control measure. Section 8.6 concludes the chapter and raises some of the remaining questions for research.

8.2 The process of information discovery and dissemination

8.2.1 Information discovery

This section describes how information about the health consequences of tobacco use has been discovered and disseminated. A simplified view of the process is as follows: scientists discover new facts about tobacco and announce their research findings to the scientific community through conferences and publications in academic journals. Important research findings are then disseminated more broadly to the public, often with the help of various government programs and initiatives.

This description of the process is somewhat misleading in several respects. First, it assumes a naïve view of the scientific process, where facts are simply discovered. Instead, starting from around the 1950s, research on the health consequences of tobacco use has steadily accumulated, leading to a scientific consensus about what the 'facts' about tobacco and health probably are. The nature of the consensus changed over time. For example, by the late 1950s there might have been a consensus that smoking is probably dangerous. Currently, there is a consensus that smoking is definitely dangerous. The consensus about the magnitude of the risks involved continues to change over time (see Chapter 1 for a detailed discussion). Whether a process of 'fact discovery' or 'consensus formation', from the 1950s onwards research established solid evidence linking tobacco use to heart disease, lung cancer, emphysema, and other cancers. More recent research has established additional health effects from smoking during pregnancy and from second-hand smoke. Smokers also appear to face a greater risk of death from tuberculosis than non-smokers.

Another complication is the influence of the tobacco industry on the process of information discovery. The industry has obvious incentives to try to block the formation of a scientific consensus that its products are harmful. In 1954, US tobacco companies formed the Tobacco Industry Research Committee, later re-named the Council for Tobacco Research. The tobacco industry has used several vehicles for publishing the findings of their sponsored research, including symposia proceedings, books, journal articles, and letters-to-the-editor in medical journals. Bero *et al.* (1994) have studied tobacco-industry sponsored symposia on passive smoking in detail. Compared to a random sample of articles on passive smoking from the scientific literature, Bero and colleagues find that symposia articles on passive smoking were more likely to agree with the tobacco industry's position that passive smoking is not harmful. Recently, however, tobacco companies are moving in the direction of accepting the consensus that smoking is dangerous to health, partly in response to litigation in the United States. For example, Philip Morris's web site states the overwhelming medical and scientific consensus that cigarette smoking causes lung cancer, heart disease, emphysema, and other serious diseases in smokers. It also states that cigarette smoking is addictive, and acknowledges that official government reports have concluded that second-hand smoke is harmful, although it continues to dispute many of their conclusions. So while the tobacco industry tried to influence research on tobacco and health in the past, recent trends suggest it may play less of a role in the future.

8.2.2 Information dissemination

Governments in many countries have played active roles in disseminating information about the health consequences of tobacco use. Information policies range from the publication of official reports, to a requirement for warning labels on packages and advertisements, to school health education and mass-media campaigns.[1] Although there are exceptions, the trend has been from inexpensive interventions, such as the publication of official reports, to more direct and expensive efforts to inform the public, such as mass-media campaigns. As the philosopher Robert Goodin (1989) points out, the strategy of providing information about health consequences is usually seen as less intrusive and less paternalistic than many other tobacco control policies.

Publication of official reports by the Royal College of Physicians in Britain in 1962 and by the United States Surgeon General in 1964 (USDHEW 1964) are milestones in tobacco control in high-income countries, and mark the beginning of serious efforts to improve consumer information about smoking and health. Many of the subsequent official Surgeon General reports mainly confirm the main message that smoking is unhealthy, but certain reports have new information. For example, the 1986 report was the first to identify a health risk from second-hand smoke (USDHHS 1986). The 1988 report concluded that tobacco use is an addiction rather than a habit (USDHHS 1988). The function of official government reports is not so much to disseminate the newest research findings, as to have an official statement of current consensus judgements.

Following the official reports of the health consequences of tobacco use, many countries required warning labels on tobacco-product packaging and advertising. The United States required warning labels on all cigarette packages beginning January 1, 1966, with somewhat stronger wording introduced in 1970. In 1972 all print advertisements were required to carry the warnings as well. In 1985, instead of a general warning about health consequences, packages and print advertisements were required to contain one of four rotating texts with statements about specific health hazards. As of 1991, 77 countries required health warnings on tobacco-product packages (Roemer

---

[1] Saffer (Chapter 9) discusses advertising bans. While banning advertisements can have implications for information, the dissemination of health information to consumers is not the primary goal of this type of tobacco control policy.

1993; WHO 1997). In most of these countries (48), the warnings are relatively incon-spicuous and contain little information, such as a general statement that smoking is hazardous. But a growing number of countries (27 in 1991, the most recent date for which figures are available) require rotating or strong warnings, and a few (such as Iceland and Norway) include pictures to enhance the likely effectiveness of warning labels. Many governments have also launched school health education and mass-media public information campaigns about the health consequences of tobacco use. These efforts are difficult to summarize because they have varied considerably over time and continue to vary from country to country.

In describing how research findings on tobacco and health have been disseminated to the public, it is important to recognize that people as consumers are not passive recipients of information. In everyday life people continually learn about the health consequences of consumption choices by evaluating their own experiences and the experiences of their families and friends. Even without hard scientific evidence, tobacco use has long been considered unhealthy (Corti 1931). To explore the media's role in information dissemination, Viscusi (1992) tallies the number of articles on smoking hazards that appeared in *Reader's Digest* from 1950 to 1989. By decade, the number of articles increased over the period: 12 from 1950 to1959; 17 from 1960 to 1969; 19 from 1970 to 1979; and 23 from 1980 to 1989. Counted differently, out of 71 articles on smoking hazards from 1950 to 1989, 18 appeared before the 1964 Surgeon General's report.

The tally of magazine articles on smoking hazard supports the more general point that in the US the media provided a great deal of information on tobacco and health to the public before the government began its information campaign. Clearly, the media, including the world wide web, continue to be important sources of health infor-mation. More generally, it should be stressed that consumers are not passive and the public sector is not the only source of health information. In its history of anti-smoking efforts, the United States Department of Health and Human Services (1989, p. 413) notes that the three major voluntary health organizations, American Cancer Society (ACS), American Lung Association (ALA), and American Heart Association (AHA), have played an important role over the last 25 years in disseminating information about the hazards of smoking. Their role was particularly prominent in the late 1960s after the Federal Communications Commission ruled that under the Fairness Doctrine broadcasters must present anti-smoking public service messages to balance cigarette advertising. Ironically, the frequency of anti-smoking messages fell dramatically in 1971 when broadcast advertising for cigarettes was banned.

To improve profitability, firms in many industries promote their products, so it is not surprising that the tobacco industry has a history of efforts to influence consumer infor-mation about the consequences of tobacco use.[2] For much of the past 50 years there has also been a history of public policy efforts in response. Until at least the 1950s, many cigarette advertisements fairly explicitly promoted the advertised brand as healthy, or at least healthier than other brands. The United States Federal Trade Com-mission (FTC) began to respond to these claims long before the 1964 report of the Surgeon General on smoking and health. At first the public-sector response was in the

---

[2] The discussion that follows draws heavily on USDHHS (1989).

form of cease-and-desist orders against false and misleading health claims made in advertising. Industry-wide cigarette advertising guidelines were enacted in 1955; additional regulations followed the 1964 Surgeon General's report; and eventually a ban on broadcast-media advertising became effective in 1971. However, many observers see the shift towards low-tar and low-nicotine cigarettes during the 1970s as an example of how tobacco-industry efforts continued to mislead consumers (USDHHS 1989). Although advertisements for these products contained only implicit health claims, surveys in the 1970s found that large proportions of smokers believed low-tar and low-nicotine products posed little or no health risk (FTC 1988). In many countries the tobacco industry's ability to influence consumer information about the health consequences of tobacco use has become more limited by regulations and bans on advertising, although the ability to spread misinformation remains considerable (see Chapter 9 for a discussion on the ineffectiveness of partial advertising bans).

8.3 Are consumers informed about the consequences of tobacco use?

This section provides an overview of the evidence on whether consumers are well-informed about the consequences of tobacco use. To begin, it is useful to define what a potential consumer would have to understand to make well-informed decisions about tobacco use. To be well-informed, the consumer would need to know which diseases are linked to the use of different tobacco products and to second-hand smoke, the morbidity and mortality associated with each disease, and the extent to which tobacco use increases their risks of each disease. In addition, when making the decision to start tobacco use, the well-informed consumer would need to understand addiction and how difficult it will be to quit if he or she decides to attempt this at a future date. Some of these pieces of information may not matter to some consumers. For example, simply knowing that smoking is linked to lung cancer without knowing much about the disease or the magnitude of the risks may itself discourage many from smoking. But to other consumers, the gaps in their information may be critical. For example, they may decide to smoke knowing that the practice carries an increased risk of lung cancer, because they under-estimate the increase in that risk or because they over-estimate the chances of surviving the disease.

This section first addresses whether consumers are informed at the most basic level about the major health consequences of tobacco use. The discussion then turns to other aspects of consumer information that may help explain how people actually respond to the risks. A difficult question is whether consumers accurately assess the quantitative risks of tobacco use, both in general and for themselves personally. A related question is whether consumers accurately judge the risks of tobacco use relative to other risks. If smokers believe their personal risks are low, or believe that the risks of tobacco use are low relative to other threats to health, they may place little importance on changing their own behavior, despite their awareness of the health consequences. The last part of the section discusses consumer information about addiction and the information available to young people—the age group in which the decision to start smoking is most common.

8.3.1 Consumer information about the links between tobacco use and disease

Recent research conducted in a number of countries provides a fairly broad international perspective on what consumers know about the health consequences of tobacco use. Most of the studies used similar measures of whether consumers were aware of the health consequences of smoking. However, the specific measures of consumer information vary. As a result, there is considerable heterogeneity in the proportions of the survey respondents who are 'well-informed' depending in large part on what questions are posed.

The 1996 National Prevalence Survey on Smoking, a representative national survey of over 122 000 Chinese, included four questions about their knowledge of the health consequences of tobacco use. At the most general level, 55% of Chinese non-smokers and 69% of Chinese smokers surveyed believed that cigarettes did them 'little or no harm' (Chinese Academy of Preventive Medicine 1997). About the same percentages believed that passive smoking does little or no harm to their health. The specific disease linked to tobacco use most often was bronchitis, with about 70% of both Chinese non-smokers and smokers aware of the link. But only about 40% of both groups said that smoking causes lung cancer and only 4% said that smoking causes heart disease. However, Gong *et al.* (1995) report very different patterns for consumer awareness in one district of China. The results are from a survey of 3423 males and 3593 females in the Minhang District, near Shanghai. In this sample, consumer awareness of the health risks of smoking seems to be widespread, with almost 90% of respondents reporting that they believe that smoking is harmful for both the smoker and those exposed passively to smoke. Current smokers are only somewhat less likely to agree that smoking is a health hazard, with 82% of male smokers so responding. Presumably, the differences between the results reported by the Chinese Academy of Preventive Medicine (1997) and Gong *et al.* (1995) reflect different sampling frames, and the fact that education and income levels are higher in Shanghai than in the rest of China. Gong *et al.* report several additional interesting results. Despite the apparently widespread awareness of the health hazards, smoking is very common among men (67%), but very rare among women (2%). Even more puzzling is that only 14% of current smokers report wanting to quit, and even fewer had ever tried.

Osler and Kirchhoff (1995) report the results of two independent cross-sectional surveys of Danish adults conducted in 1982 (N = 4807) and 1992 (N = 2226). Knowledge is measured by the number of times the respondent agreed with a series of statements about the health consequences of smoking. In 1982, about a quarter of both men and women scored five or more (out of a possible 11) on this knowledge scale. In 1992, the proportions had increased so that about one-third of both men and women scored five or more. More than 90% of the respondents agreed that smoking increases the risks of lung cancer. But knowledge of other consequences of smoking was much less widespread: for example, in 1982, slightly fewer than half of the respondents agreed that smoking increased the risk of cancer of the mouth and throat, although this increased to 57% of the sample by 1992.

According to a 1996 survey of 500 adults from Szekesfehervar, Hungary, about three-quarters of the respondents think that smoking damages health to a large extent. Another 19% think that it damages health, but only to a small extent. Only 2% think that smoking is absolutely harmless. For current smokers, reported awareness is lower: only 56% responded that smoking damages health to a large extent, while 36% responded that it damages health to a small extent and 6% responded that it does not damage health at all. About 80% of respondents had already heard of passive smoking, and awareness of the health hazards of passive smoking was relatively widespread. Three-quarters of respondents said that breathing others' smoke could certainly or probably increase the risks of asthma; 81% responded that breathing others' smoke could certainly or probably increase the risks of heart disease; and 91% responded that breathing others' smoke could certainly or probably increase the risks of pulmonary cancer.

Two recent studies measuring consumer information about tobacco in South African populations demonstrate the incomplete nature of knowledge about smoking risks. Reddy *et al.* (1996) report the results of a 1995 survey that provides a nationally representative sample of 2238 adults. The vast majority of respondents, 87%, agreed with the general statement that the health effects of smoking are serious. Jones and Kirigia (1999) report a very similar finding from a sample of about 3500 female respondents in South Africa: 86% of the sample knew that smoking has negative health consequences. Reddy *et al.* (1996) find that knowledge of many specific health consequences of smoking was much less widespread in South Africa than was general awareness, however. While 67% and 58% of respondents knew that smoking was associated with lung disease and cancer, respectively, only 31% knew that smoking was associated with heart disease. Knowledge about passive smoking was more widespread but far from complete, with 82% agreeing that babies' health is affected by mothers' smoking and 71% agreeing that the health of non-smokers is affected by smokers in the household.

A study of smoking practices and attitudes in Vietnam finds that consumer awareness about the hazards of smoking is fairly widespread (Jenkins *et al.* 1997). The survey was conducted in 1995, with random samples totaling 2004 adults from Hanoi, Ho Chi Minh City, and two rural communes in Vietnam. Of the respondents, 87% agreed that smoking harms health, and 81% agreed that smokers die at a younger age than non-smokers. Almost 80% agreed that environmental tobacco smoke harms health. With this apparently high level of consumer information, it seems puzzling that 73% of men (but only 4% of women) smoke. Their awareness of the health consequences could be reflected in the fact that 61% of current smokers reported wanting to quit, although only 44% report that they had ever tried to quit.

In the United States, the evidence suggests that consumer information about the health consequences of tobacco use has improved dramatically from the 1950s and 1960s onwards. The improvements parallel the government information campaigns described in Section 8.2.2 and suggest the overall effectiveness of these campaigns. However, the trend analysis below does not attempt to determine the impacts of specific interventions on consumer information.

Figure 8.1 shows estimates from national surveys conducted between 1954 and 1990 on public knowledge about the link between cigarette smoking and lung cancer. Although the surveys are not all identical, they are fairly comparable over

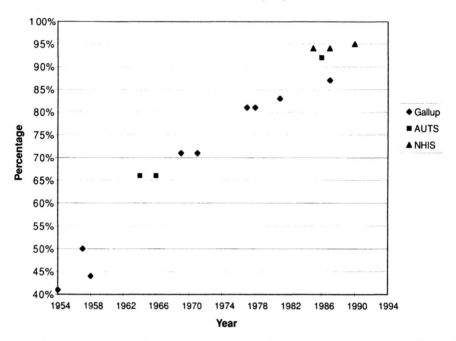

Fig. 8.1 Trends in public knowledge about smoking and lung cancer—all adults (% believing in a health risk).

Data sources: US Department of Health and Human Services (1989); authors' calculations using National Health Interview Surveys (NIHS).

Note: Actual questions:

1954, 1957, 1958, 1969, 1971, 1977, 1978, and 1981 Gallup surveys: Do you think that cigarette smoking is or is not one of the causes of lung cancer? (Yes, is a cause; no, is not a cause; no opinion.)

1964 and 1966 AUTSs: Would you say that cigarette smoking is definitely, probably, probably not, or definitely not a major cause of lung cancer, or that you have no opinion either way? (Percentages include those who say smoking is 'definitely' or 'probably' a major cause of lung cancer.)

1985 NHIS: Tell me if you think cigarette smoking definitely increases, probably increases, probably does not increase, or definitely does not increase a person's chances of getting lung cancer? (Percentages include those who say smoking 'definitely' or 'probably' increases the risk.)

1986 AUTS: Do you think a person who smokes in any more likely to get lung cancer than a person who doesn't smoke? (Much more likely, somewhat more likely, no, don't know.) (Percentages include those who say smokers are 'much more likely' or 'somewhat more likely' to get lung cancer.)

1987 Gallup survey: Do you think smoking is a cause of lung cancer? (Yes, no, don't know.)

1987 NHIS: People have different beliefs about the relationship between smoking and health. Do you believe cigarette smoking is related to lung cancer? (Yes, no, maybe, unknown.) (Percentages include those who say yes or maybe.)

1990 NHIS: Cigarette smoking definitely increases, probably increases, probably does not increase, or definitely does not increase chance of developing lung cancer? (Percentages include those who say smoking 'definitely' or 'probably' increases the risk.)

time.[3] Gallup surveys conducted in the 1950s found that between 40% and 50% of respondents agreed that smoking is one of the causes of lung cancer. In a 1969 Gallup poll this percentage had increased to above 70%. Other surveys conducted over the period show similar trends, so that by 1990, between 90% and 95% of respondents stated that they are aware of the link between smoking and lung cancer. The trend in public knowledge about smoking and heart disease (Fig. 8.2) is similar. In the early- to mid- 1960s, between 40% and 55% of respondents agreed that the chances of heart disease are higher for cigarette smokers. In the 1985 and 1990 National Health Interview Surveys, about 90% of respondents indicated that smoking either definitely or probably increases the risks of heart disease. Similarly, the percentage of respondents indicating that smoking increases the risk of emphysema/chronic bronchitis increased from 50% to 60% during the 1960s, and reached about 90% by 1990.

There are somewhat fewer data available on trends in consumer information about the other health consequences of tobacco use. By the late 1980s or early 1990s, about 80% of respondents to various surveys indicated awareness that smoking causes cancer of the mouth/throat/larynx/esophagus; by 1992 almost 90% indicated that smoking during pregnancy is hazardous.

A detailed chronology of research findings establishing the links between smoking and each of these health consequences is beyond the scope of this chapter. In broad terms, however, it is clear that the public awareness of the risks follows the publication of research findings.

Public knowledge about passive smoking and health is of special interest, because of the efforts of tobacco industry on this topic. Despite a growing consensus that passive smoking is harmful, a study of newspaper and magazine articles published between 1981 and 1995 found that most of the articles left the impression that there is still a controversy on the issue (Kennedy and Bero 1996). However, as shown in Fig. 8.3, the trend in public knowledge of the link between passive smoke and ill health generally parallels trends in the public understanding of other health consequences of tobacco. In surveys conducted in the 1970s only about half of the respondents agreed that passive smoking was harmful. By the late 1980s the proportion who were aware of the risks had reached more than 80%, and by 1992 it had reached 87%.

Comparing Fig. 8.3 with Figs 8.1 and 8.2 reveals that awareness of the risks of passive smoking is not quite as widespread as is awareness of the risks of active smoking. Although this may be in part due to the tobacco industry's efforts, it is also not unexpected because the scientific evidence about passive smoke accumulated only after the other risks of smoking had already been well established. For example, the 1972 report of the Surgeon General (USDHEW 1972) contained only cautious statements about possible health effects of passive smoke, and the 1986 report (USDHHS 1986) was the first to focus on involuntary or passive smoking. Of course, the formation of the consensus in the scientific community may also have been slowed by the tobacco industry's efforts. But once that consensus was formed and signaled by official publications, the evidence suggests that public awareness of the risks of passive smoking became very widespread.

---

[3] Details on the survey organizations, texts of the questions, and survey dates are provided in footnotes to the Figure.

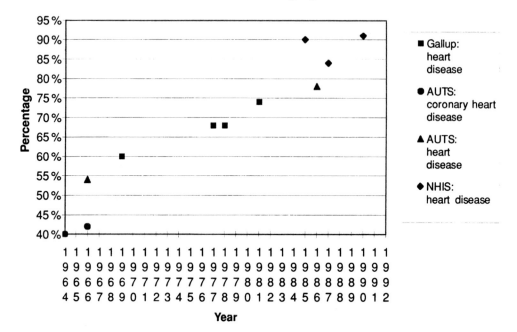

Fig. 8.2 Trends in public knowledge about smoking and heart disease—all adults (% believing in a health risk).

Data sources: US Department of Health and Human Services (1989); authors' calculations using National Health Interview Surveys (NHIS).

Note: Actual questions:

1964 and 1966 AUTSs: Do you think the chances of getting coronary heart disease are the same for people who don't smoke cigarettes as they are for people who do smoke cigarettes? Who would be more likely to get it, people who don't smoke cigarettes or people who do smoke cigarettes?

1966 AUTS: Cigarette smokers are more likely to die from heart disease than people who don't smoke cigarettes. (Strongly agree, mildly agree, no opinion, mildly disagree, strongly disagree.) (Percentages include those who 'strongly agree' or 'mildly agree'.)

1969, 1977, 1978, and 1981 Gallup surveys: Do you think that cigarette smoking is or is not one of the causes of heart disease?

1985 NHIS: Do you think cigarette smoking definitely increases, probably increases, probably does not increase, or definitely does not increase a person's chances of getting heart disease? (Percentages include those who say smoking 'definitely' or 'probably' increases the risk.)

1986 AUTS: Do you think a person who smokes is any more likely to get heart disease than a person who doesn't smoke? (Much more likely, somewhat more likely, no, don't know.) (Percentages include those who say smokers are 'much more likely' or 'somewhat more likely' to get heart disease.)

1987 NHIS: People have different beliefs about the relationship between smoking and health. Do you believe cigarette smoking is related to heart disease? (Yes, no, maybe, unknown.) (Percentages include those who say yes or maybe.)

1990 NHIS: Cigarette smoking definitely increases, probably increases, probably does not increase, or definitely does not increase chance of developing heart disease? (Percentages include those who say smoking 'definitely' or 'probably' increases the risk.)

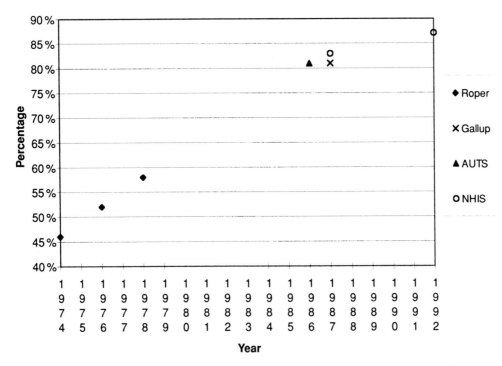

Fig. 8.3 Trends in public knowledge about the health risks of passive smoking—all adults
(% believing in a health risk).

Data sources: US Department of Health and Human Services (1989); authors' calculations using
National Health Interview Surveys.
Note: Actual questions:
1974, 1976, and 1978 Roper surveys: Is smoking hazardous to nonsmokers' health? (Probably is hazardous, probably doesn't have any real effect, don't know.)
1986 AUTS: Think now for a moment about a nonsmoker who lives or works with smokers ... do
you think that exposure to tobacco smoke is harmful or not harmful to the nonsmoker's health?
1987 NHIS: The smoke from someone else's cigarette is harmful to you. (Strongly agree, agree, disagree, strongly disagree.) (Percentages include those who 'strongly agree' or 'agree.')
1987 Gallup survey: If people smoke, do you think that it is harmful or is not harmful to people who
are near them? (Yes, harmful; no, not harmful; can't say/no opinion.)
1992 NHIS: Other people's smoke is harmful. (Agree/yes, disagree/no, not ascertained or no
opinion/don't know.)

8.3.2 Consumer information about the magnitude of health risks from tobacco

An additional concern is whether consumers who are aware of the health effects of
tobacco use have accurate perceptions of the magnitudes of the risks. This is a difficult
research question, but available evidence suggests that some consumers over-estimate
the health risks of smoking, while others under-estimate these risks. In a series of
studies, Viscusi presents evidence that most people, including most smokers, over-estimate the health risks of cigarette smoking. He reports (1990, 1991, 1992) analyses of

national US survey data collected in 1985, where perceived lung cancer risk is measured based on answers to the question: 'Among 100 cigarette smokers, how many of them do you think will get lung cancer *because* they smoke?'. Viscusi (1998) reports additional analyses of survey data on people's perceptions of the total mortality risk of smoking, based on answers to the question: 'Out of every 100 cigarette smokers, how many of them do you think will die from lung cancer, heart disease, throat cancer, or any other illness *because* they smoke cigarettes?'. Dividing the answers by 100 yields the perceived lung cancer and total mortality risk.

In the 1985 sample, the average perceived lung cancer risk was 0.426, and when the sample was restricted to current smokers the average was 0.368. In the 1997 sample the average perceived total mortality risk was 0.501 for the full sample, and 0.424 for the sample restricted to current smokers. Viscusi (1992) also reports the results of a series of smaller-scale surveys conducted in 1990 and 1991 that explored the sensitivity of the risk responses to several variations in question formulation. For example, he presents evidence that the risk of death from lung cancer due to smoking was perceived to be similar to the perceived risk of the incidence of lung cancer due to smoking. Viscusi (1992, p. 83) concludes that 'the similarity of the responses for [six] different question formulations suggests that the empirical findings are not an artifact tied to some specific question phrasing'.

Part of the difficulty in determining the accuracy of consumers' perceptions of the risks of smoking is that the true risk level is unknown, and the state of scientific knowledge of the risks changes over time. Based on the state of scientific knowledge at the time of the surveys, Viscusi (1992, 1998) argues that reasonable scientific reference ranges are from 0.05 to 0.10 for the lifetime risk of dying of lung cancer, and 0.18 to 0.36 for the lifetime risk of dying from any tobacco-related disease. However, the current consensus is that the risks of smoking are higher, with a consensus estimate of the total mortality risk being around 0.5. Hanson and Logue (1998, pp. 1355–56) criticize Viscusi's reference point as 'probably too low'; in which case fewer people over-estimate the risks of smoking than Viscusi reports. The appropriate reference point depends, of course, on the question being asked. Viscusi uses a different reference point from Hanson and Logue because he is addressing a different question. By focusing on the consensus at the time of the survey, Viscusi's comparisons address whether consumers understood the available scientific information about smoking. Hanson and Logue argue that, in order to address whether those smokers were well-informed by current standards, their perceptions of the risks should be compared with the current range of risks agreed by scientific consensus.

If the distribution of perceived risks in these samples is compared with Viscusi's reference points it may be concluded that most people and most smokers over-estimate the mortality risks of smoking. Moreover, Viscusi's evidence suggests that over-estimation of risks remains an important empirical phenomenon using any plausible estimate of the true risk of death from smoking. For example, a little over 5% of both the full sample and current smokers perceive a smoking mortality risk of 1, and 20.5% of the full sample and 12.8% of smokers perceive a risk of 0.8 or above.

Liu and Hsieh (1995) use Viscusi's approach to measure the risk perceptions of smokers and non-smokers in Taiwan. A survey of a random sample of adults in the metropolitan area of Taipei was undertaken in 1993. Perceptions of the risk of lung cancer were measured using the same question wording as Viscusi (1990). The average perceived risk of lung cancer in the full sample is 0.363, while the average perceived risk of lung cancer in the sample restricted to current smokers is 0.288. The researchers compare these estimates to one for the 'true risk', which, based on evidence from Taiwan, is judged to be 0.025. Using this scientific reference point, they conclude that only 10.8% of the full sample and 19.2% of the smokers under-estimate risks, while the rest over-estimate risks. The percentages of the Taiwanese sample that perceived extremely high risks are smaller than in Viscusi's US samples; for example, only 1.5% of the full sample reported a risk perception of 1.

A limitation to Viscusi's approach is that the measures he uses are based on asking individuals to assess the risk in a hypothetical population of smokers. People may feel that the risks they face personally are lower. Weinstein (1998) reports an attempt to locate and review all studies that investigated smokers' risk perceptions. Most of the reviewed studies appear to have been conducted in the United States and the United Kingdom. A number of conclusions emerge from Weinstein's review. The review 'shows unequivocally that smokers acknowledge that smokers' risks of various health problems are higher than non-smokers' risks'. At the same time, however, the reviewed studies indicate that non-smokers rate smoking as riskier than do smokers. The evidence on the accuracy of smokers' quantitative risk assessments is decidedly mixed, with two of the reviewed studies finding that smokers over-estimate the risks of smoking, two finding that smokers either over-estimate or under-estimate the risks depending on how the question is asked, one finding that smokers' risks perceptions are accurate or under-estimates, and one finding that smokers under-estimate the risk of smoking. In contrast, the evidence is very consistent that smokers minimize their personal risks. For example, various studies find that, on average, smokers report that their personal risks are lower than the average smoker, and only slightly above the risks of non-smokers.

Given the importance of survey design, it should be noted that Hanson and Logue (1998, appendix) offer a set of specific criticisms of such surveys. The criticisms were made in the specific context of Viscusi's surveys on people's perceptions of the risks of smoking, but are relevant to all such studies. Their overarching concern seems to be that (p. 1361):

... respondents did not operate with precise quantitative risk assessments. Instead, they had only foggy qualitative assessments ... [so] the numeric responses do not mean what they appear to mean.

This implies that this line of research is not likely to yield valid conclusions one way or the other on whether smokers under-estimate or over-estimate the risks of smoking.

More recently, Ayanian and Cleary (1999) find that most current smokers do not believe that their personal risks of heart disease and cancer are higher than the risks faced by other people of the same age and sex. For example, only 29% of current smokers believed they have a higher-than-average risk of myocardial infarction, and this increases to only about 50% among smokers with identified risk factors of hypertension and angina. These findings are consistent with other evidence of unrealistic optimism in survey responses. Weinstein (1980) surveyed college students on how their estimated chances of experiencing 42 events differed from the chances of their class-mates. On average, the surveyed college students estimated that they were more likely than average to live past the age of 80 and to experience other positive events. Con-versely, on average, the college students estimated that they were less likely than average to have a heart attack or experience other negative events.

The Health and Retirement Survey (HRS) has been analyzed to provide more evi-dence on the magnitude of the poor information (or unrealistic optimism) in older smokers' expectations of reaching age 75 (Schoenbaum 1997; Sloan et al. 1999). The HRS is a data set used by many health and labor economists, and is based on a national sample of adults aged 50–62. Respondents were asked the following question: 'Using any number from zero to ten, what do you think are the chances that you will live to be 75 or more?', where zero was labeled 'no chance at all'and 10 was labeled 'absolutely certain'. Dividing by ten provides an estimate of the subjective probability of survival to age 75. Although respondents could view this question as an ordinal ranking rather than a probability assessment, Hurd and McGarry (1995) present additional evidence that responses to this question behave like probabilities. Schoenbaum (1997) and Sloan et al. (1999) compare the subjective estimates to estimates of the 'true' survival prob-abilities from life-tables. Using life-table values, the mean probability of survival to age 75 for men who are current heavy smokers is 0.263, while the mean subjective value is 0.501. Similarly, the life-table mean survival probability for women who are current heavy smokers to age 75 is 0.308, while the mean subjective value is 0.601. Among men who were never smokers, former smokers, and current light smokers, subjective sur-vival probabilities correspond quite closely to the relevant life-table values, but for women in these categories, subjective survival probabilities are below the life-table values. The pattern of results suggests that heavy smokers over-estimate their survival probability and hence must under-estimate the risks of smoking; other groups either appear to have accurate perceptions or to over-estimate all risks, including the risks of death unrelated to smoking.

The fact that Viscusi reached opposing conclusions to those of the researchers ana-lyzing the HRS data illustrates the inherent difficulty of research into whether con-sumer-risk perceptions are accurate. However, it is also important not to overstate the degree of difference between these studies. Some of the difference is to be expected, given differences in the composition of the samples studied. Evidence from the HRS data suggests that older (aged 50–62) heavy smokers under-estimate the risks of smoking. The smokers in Viscusi's studies are much younger, as they are representative of the population aged over 16. If smokers with higher risk perceptions are more likely to quit, it is to be expected that people who remain smokers at older ages will have lower-than-average risk perceptions. In addition, Viscusi (1991) finds evidence that younger people are particularly likely to overestimate the risks of smoking, and sug-gests that it may result from their greater exposure to the public anti-smoking campaign. However, it has been suggested that young people act as if they feel invulnerable to many risks (see Chapter 7 for a detailed discusion). Young people may, therefore, have a greater divergence than older people between their perceptions of hypothetical risks (measured by Viscusi) and their estimates of personal risks (mea-sured by Schoenbaum). This question could be explored by collecting data on the per-sonal risk perceptions of people of a variety of ages, similar to the data used in the HRS.

It should also be pointed out that in the HRS data, Schoenbaum finds that light smokers on average appear to have accurate risk perceptions, and, by the definition used, light smokers make up the majority of smokers in the sample (59% of male smokers and 77% of female smokers). Given the distribution around the average subjective survival probabilities, there are many light smokers who under-estimate their survival probability in Schoenbaum's sample. Unfortunately, Schoenbaum (1997) does not present much information on the distribution of responses. Because there are also many non-smokers who under-estimate their survival probabilities, it is difficult to determine whether light smokers who under-estimate their survival probability over-estimate the risks of smoking or over-estimate other risks. Of course, they could have private information, in which case their personal estimates may be more accurate than the life-table values. Viscusi's method has some advantages in interpretation over this approach, but its weakness is that it does not take into account the individual's internalization of the risks.

In sum, both Viscusi and Schoenbaum present evidence that some smokers over-estimate the risks of smoking, while others under-estimate them. There is more disagreement about the extent of the information problem and the relative frequencies of the types of mistakes that consumers make.

8.3.3 Consumer information about the relative risks from tobacco and other hazards

Another approach to measuring risk perceptions focuses on relative risks rather than absolute magnitudes. Well-known systematic biases in individual risk perceptions suggest that perceptions of the relative risks of smoking are likely to be inaccurate. As Hanson and Logue (1998, pp. 1190–2) point out, consumer information about the relative risks of smoking compared to other threats to their health is an essential part of well-informed consumer decision-making:

> If in fact, consumers tend to over-estimate some or all of the other risks to which they are exposed, they may well behave *as if* they under-estimate the risks of smoking.

Evidence shows that people tend to under-estimate the risks of common causes of death, while they tend to over-estimate the risks of rare causes of death (Lichtenstein *et al.* 1978; Slovic *et al.* 1979, 1985; Slovic 1987). In one experiment reported by Lichtenstein *et al.* (1978), participants were told the frequency of deaths in the United States due to motor vehicle accidents, and with this standard were asked to estimate the frequency of 40 other lethal events. On average, the risks of high-frequency lethal events, such as cancer and heart disease, were substantially under-estimated, often by a factor of 10 or more, depending upon the cause of death. The risks of low-frequency lethal events, such as botulism and tornadoes, were over-estimated, again often substantially. In another study, lay people's perceptions of relative risks were compared to the perceptions of a group of experts chosen for their professional involvement with risk assessment (Slovic *et al.* 1979). As an example of how much lay and expert risk assessments diverged, members of the League of Women Voters and a group of college students ranked nuclear power as the most risky activity or technology, but the experts' ranking placed nuclear power as the twentieth most risky activity or technology. For the cases where technical estimates of the frequency of death were available, the experts' perceived risks were closely related to annual fatalities, but the risk perceptions of lay people showed only a moderate relationship.

As a relatively common cause of death, there is some evidence that people tend to under-estimate the risks of smoking. For example, Lichtenstein *et al.* (1979) found that in two groups of subjects, the geometric mean of their estimated frequencies of death from lung cancer responses implied about 10 000 annual deaths, compared to a true frequency of about 76 000 annual deaths at that time. In the study by Slovic *et al.* (1979), the experts ranked smoking as the second riskiest activity or technology, but the groups of lay people put smoking in third or fourth place. With the widespread publicity given to smoking, these results about people's risk perceptions in the 1970s may no longer be relevant. But a more recent 1993 Harris poll in the United States had similar findings. When asked to rank activities that 'help people in general to live a long and healthy life', avoidance of smoking was ranked tenth, far behind good air quality, good water quality, domestic fire detectors, and other factors with statistically marginal effects on survival. A 1996 survey of 500 adults from Szekesfehervar, Hungary, measured respondents' perceptions of the relative risks of various factors, based on a scale measuring the extent of the perceived broad influence on health of each of those factors.[4] On average, smoking ranked fourth, slightly behind daily stress, alcohol consumption, and environmental damages. Only 33% of respondents ranked smoking first, compared to 50% who ranked stress first.

Benjamin and Dougan (1997) point out a limitation of many of the studies that find systematic biases in individual risk perceptions: the aggregate annual numbers of deaths due to various causes are not very relevant to peoples' decisions about their own health and safety. Benjamin and Dougan argue that people can be well-informed about the risks they face but relatively uninformed about aggregate, population-wide fatality rates. Benjamin and Dougan build a a model where people have good information on their age-specific mortality rates. The model further assumes that people use this information on their age-specific mortality rates to estimate population-wide rates. Calculating optimal estimates this way, Benjamin and Dougan re-analyze the data that Lichtenstein used. They find no important differences between actual responses and the optimal estimates, given the assumed information set of the respondents. Hakes and Viscusi (1997) argue that risk perceptions fit a Bayesian learning model. These studies suggest that inaccurate risk perceptions may result more from the inherent difficulties of learning about risks than from systematic departures from rationality. This interpretation, in turn, suggests that appropriate information policies have potential to influence smoking behavior.

8.3.4 Information about addiction

The preceding discussion has shown that people may not fully realize the health consequences of tobacco consumption. Here we turn to discuss the possibility that people

---

[4] Other results from this survey on Hungarians' general awareness of the risks of smoking are discussed above.

may also be poorly informed about addiction. In 1964, tobacco use was considered habituating. Perhaps surprisingly, it was not until 1988 that the US Surgeon General established nicotine as 'a highly addictive substance, comparable in its physiological and psychological properties to other addictive substances of abuse'. In terms of consumer information, the 1992 National Health Interview Survey Cancer Control Supplement asked respondents if they thought smoking is a habit or an addiction. The most common response was that smoking is both a habit and an addiction, given by 54.4% of the sample. Another 22.4% of the sample identified smoking as an addiction. Only 17.8% of the sample thought smoking was just a habit, and a fairly trivial number (1.2%) responded that it was neither.

Interestingly, the patterns of responses to the 1992 National Health Interview Survey about the addictiveness of smoking are very similar when the sample is broken down by smoking status (current smokers, those who never smoked ('never-smokers'), and former smokers). About 55% of current smokers, never smokers, and former smokers identify smoking as both a habit and an addiction. About 21% of current smokers respond that smoking is a habit, slightly more than the percentages of former smokers, and never-smokers who gave that response (19% and 16%, respectively). In sum, most adults in the United States, and most smokers, identify smoking as an addiction or as an addiction and a habit. However, it should be noted that it is unclear how the distinctions that the lay population makes—between an addiction, a habit, or both—correspond to the concept of addiction used by medical professionals.

Whether teenagers are well-informed about the addictiveness of tobacco when they decide to start smoking is obviously of crucial importance because virtually all smokers in high-income countries, and many smokers in low-income and middle-income countries (see Chapter 2), start their addictions before the age of 20. There are several pieces of evidence suggesting that a lack of information about addiction is a common problem among youth smokers. One comes from the 1989 Teenage Attitudes and Practices Survey in the United States. In this survey of 12–18-year-olds, 39% of smokers—but only 11% of never-smokers—believed that they would be able to quit at any time they wanted (USDHHS 1994, p. 81). Using data from Tobacco Use Supplements to the Consumer Population Survey in 1992 and 1993, Hersch (1998) found that young people aged 15–20, who believe smoking is not an addiction, are much more likely to smoke than those who believe it is an addiction, or both an addiction and a habit. For example, among white males in this age group who believe smoking is an addiction, only 12.3% smoke, while the proportion among those who believe it is neither an addiction or a habit is 39%.

Additional important evidence on youth information about addiction comes from analysis of data from the Monitoring the Future Project surveys (USDHHS 1994, pp. 84–7). Teen smokers are optimistic about their personal chances of quitting smoking: 55% of past-month smokers and 45% of daily smokers predicted that they probably would not, or definitely would not, be smoking in 5 years. Data from longitudinal follow-up surveys of these same students provides direct evidence on whether their predictions were accurate. The typical pattern was for the teen smokers to maintain or increase the amount they smoked. In particular, the expectations about quitting showed very little connection to actual smoking behavior 5 or 6 years later. These patterns are again suggestive that teens under-estimate the addictiveness of smoking.

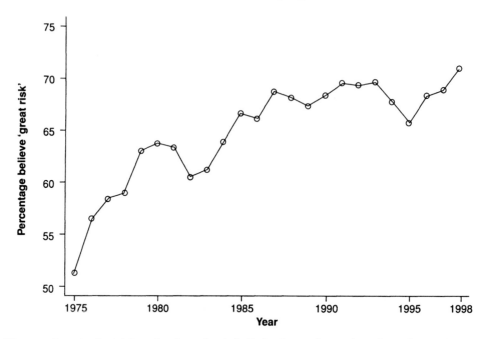

Fig. 8.4 Trends in high school seniors' beliefs about the risks of smoking. Source: Moniting the Future Project, USDHHS (1994).

A study of 191 adolescent girls in the United Kingdom found that 71% of daily smokers and 72% of occasional smokers made at least one attempt to quit, but failed (McNeil *et al.* 1986). Similar British data are reported by Townsend and colleagues (1991).

8.3.5 Adolescents' awareness of the health risks of tobacco

While it is clear that young people may consistently under-estimate the risk of becoming addicted to smoking, it is also worthwhile to note that their understanding of the health risks may also be somewhat different from that of older adults. Data from the Monitoring the Future Project (MTFP), a national survey, (USDHHS 1994) show that in 1975 just over 50% of high-school seniors indicated that they believed people are putting themselves at 'great risk' by smoking one or more packs of cigarettes a day. Although progress has not always been steady, the general trend shows higher percentages responding this way over time (Fig. 8. 4). By 1991, almost 70% of high-school seniors in the MTFP data indicated that smokers put themselves at great risk. However, during the 1990s this trend did not continue, and for much of the decade slightly lower percentages of high-school seniors reported believing that smokers put themselves at great risk. In 1995 the percentage perceiving a great risk had dipped to a low of 65.6%. The percentage began to increase again after 1995, so that by 1998, 70.8% of high-school seniors perceived a great risk from smoking.

8.3.6 Summary

In sum, then, an optimist would note that high rates of knowledge about the general health risks of smoking have been found in surveys of populations as diverse as those of Denmark, Hungary, South Africa, Vietnam, and Taiwan. Trends in high-income countries, such as the United States, show consumer information increasing steadily over time, in parallel with scientific discoveries of the health consequences of smoking and policy efforts to disseminate this information. By the 1990s, the evidence suggests that over 90% of the US population is aware that smoking increases the risks of lung cancer, heart disease, and emphysema/bronchitis. Nearly 90% agree that passive smoke is harmful, and almost 80% believe that smoking is addictive.

However, a pessimist would point out many remaining gaps in consumer information about tobacco. In some countries, such as China, many people are unaware of many of its health consequences. In the United States, young people seem to under-estimate the addictiveness of tobacco. In many countries, even though consumers are aware of general health hazards from smoking, knowledge about many specific health consequences is inadequate. Psychological research finds systematic biases in individual risk perceptions, where people tend to under-estimate the riskiness of the most common causes of death, of which prolonged tobacco use is one. Some evidence also suggests that people who appear to be well-informed fail to apply the information to themselves.

It is difficult to compare the extent of consumer information between different countries because of the lack of comparable survey data. Nevertheless, some preliminary comparisons can be suggested. Broadly speaking, where surveys have been done, low-income and middle-income countries do not have the consistently high levels of awareness seen in the United States. However, the pattern is not consistent, and some countries, such as Vietnam, report high awareness of risk, whereas others, notably China, report very low levels of awareness in the general population. Moreover, even if there are apparently similar levels of awareness, smoking behavior is very different in the United States, where smokers are more likely to report intentions to quit, more likely to attempt to quit, and more likely to do so. Much of this could be related to gaps between awareness of risks and the degree to which it is internalized and translated into action. Studying the determinants of quitting behavior in different countries is a promising direction for future research.

When thinking about the future potential for consumer information policies to reduce tobacco use, it is necessary to consider why information gaps remain. In this regard, it seems appropriate to sound a note of cautious optimism. Psychologists and economists are gaining a better understanding of the formation of risk perceptions and how policy interventions can help. Slovic *et al.* (1985, p. 259) argue that while some of the broad results of psychological research on the difficulties people have in comprehending and estimating risks seem pessimistic, the details give some cause for optimism: people understand some things quite well, although their path to knowledge may be quite different from that of the technical experts. In situations where misunderstanding appears to be rampant, errors can often be traced to inadequate information and biased experiences, which education may be able to counter. Taking an economic approach, Taylor *et al.* (1999) provide evidence that survey respondents' expectations of survival to a given age are strongly related to the actual observed mortality subsequent to the survey. This result suggests that respondents were rational in anticipating their own deaths, and that the relationships are consistent with Bayesian updating models of risk perceptions. In a related study, Smith *et al.* (1999) use new information from their own health experiences to update their expectations of survival to a particular age. These results are consistent with the argument by Slovic and his colleagues that people do learn about risks, and give cause for more optimism about the potential of information campaigns.

8.4 Econometric studies of the link between consumer information and tobacco use

This section begins by reviewing the common conceptual framework underlying economic analyses of consumer information and tobacco use, then reviews two strands of econometric research on the empirical relationships between these variables. The first approach estimates the impact of so-called 'information shocks', such as the 1964 report of the US Surgeon General, on tobacco markets over time. The second approach examines the relationship between consumer information and smoking behavior in a cross-section of the population at a point in time.

8.4.1 Conceptual framework

The effects of health information on tobacco use can be analyzed in an extended version of the standard economic model of consumer behavior. Each consumer is assumed to compare the monetary price of tobacco products to the utility (pleasure or satisfaction) received in the present, taking into account the effects of addiction and smoking-related health problems on future utility. The individual demand curve summarizes consumer behavior by showing that, holding other factors constant, the quantity demanded declines as the price of tobacco products increases. The impact of changes in consumer information about the addiction and health consequences of tobacco use are examples of what happens when other factors are not held constant. Each individual consumer demand curve will shift down and to the left, meaning that because of the new information for any given price, the quantity demanded is lower. Market demand is the aggregate of individual demand and shifts in the same way in response to new information.

The use of this framework of consumer demand to analyze tobacco use raises some special practical and conceptual issues. On the practical side, it is important to note that the quantity of tobacco products sold depends on the number of users and the quantity demanded by each user. Considering the addictive properties of tobacco, the number of users can be thought of as being determined by consumer decisions to start and to quit. So health information can decrease aggregate tobacco demand in four ways:

(1) it discourages non-users from starting;
(2) it encourages current users to cut down;
(3) it encourages current users to quit; and
(4) it discourages relapse (re-starting) among former smokers.

The different types of consumer response to information influence aggregate tobacco sales with different time lags. The short-run response is dominated by the reactions of currents smokers who either cut down or stop their use of tobacco products in response to new health information. The extent to which new information discourages non-users from starting is less of a factor in the short-run because the flow of potential new smokers is small compared to the stock of existing smokers. For example, the Congressional Budget Office (1998) estimates that in the United States, established adult smokers (defined as those age 18 and over) account for 98% of cigarette sales. However, the degree to which starting behavior is responsive to health information determines the long-run market demand. For example, information will have less of an impact on tobacco markets if young people continue to start smoking at rates that can replace the lost demand from older users who cut down, quit, or die. The empirical studies reviewed below mainly provide evidence on the broad impact of information on total tobacco use.

It is important to note that consumer information is only one of many influences on tobacco use. Tobacco use is also influenced by policy-manipulable factors, such as price and regulations on public smoking, other economic factors, such as income and labor-market conditions, and demographic factors, such as schooling and age. The challenge for the empirical studies reviewed below is to disentangle these effects. It is difficult to make estimates of the extent to which tobacco use would fall if health information changed but all other factors were held constant. In reality other factors are not held constant.

The difficulty is compounded because information about the health consequences of tobacco use may actually cause other important factors to change. Warner (1977, 1981, 1989) argues that scientific evidence establishing tobacco as a major public health problem helped change the context of the political debate about tobacco control in the United States. In this way, the anti-smoking information campaign induced other policy changes. For example, Warner (1977, p. 648) points out that in 1965, just after the 1964 Surgeon General's report, there were 23 state and local cigarette tax increases, compared to no more than a dozen in any of the preceding 14 years. Although there was a period of tax inactivity during the 1970s in the United States, for the past two decades tax increases and other tobacco control measures have continued to be associated with increased anti-smoking sentiment in many state and federal legislatures (Warner 1989). The full impact of information campaigns on tobacco use reflects the direct effect of health information on consumer demand, plus any indirect effects when information changes public anti-smoking sentiment and thus facilitates tobacco control policies. An important topic for research in political science or political economy will be to estimate the extent to which tobacco control measures have resulted from campaigns in this way: the conclusions will be important considerations for policy-makers. The discussion here, however, is more narrow and reviews studies that use the economic framework of consumer demand to estimate the direct effect of health information on tobacco use.

A further complication is that the impact of new health information can depend on, and interact with, other factors that determine tobacco use. For example, the effectiveness of mass-media information campaigns may depend on the general levels of literacy and schooling in the population. Factors such as prices and income may place less obvious but also important roles in interaction with consumer information. Section 8.6 of this chapter discusses these issues in more depth to help judge what developing countries can learn from other countries about health information as tobacco control policy.

A final conceptual issue to be noted concerns the relevance of the economic approach to understanding tobacco use. In Becker's (1976) famous definition, rational maximizing behavior is one of the assumptions that, when 'used relentlessly and unflinchingly, form the heart of the economic approach . . .'. In contrast, the economic approach does *not* assume that individuals are perfectly informed. Analysis of tobacco use by poorly-informed consumers fits into a rich tradition of theoretical and empirical economics research into markets with information problems.. Becker and Murphy (1988) develop a model of so-called 'rational addiction' that demonstrates how many of the phenomena of addiction can be analysed in an economic model (see Chapter 5 for a detailed discussion).

The correct policy response depends on whether tobacco use results from a lack of information or from a lack of rationality. Orphanides and Zervos (1995) show how policies to improve information, such as prohibitions of misleading advertisements by the tobacco industry, can improve social welfare in the Paretian sense. If information about addiction were not an issue, advertising bans would increase the information search costs for smokers and decrease their welfare. However, in the framework developed by Orphanides and Zervos, advertisements can lead more people to mistakenly begin addictive behaviors. In this situation, advertising bans are desirable policies whenever the potential of advertising 'to mislead produces more harm than its potential to inform' (Orphanides and Zervos 1995, p. 753). The economic approach and the rational model do not imply that tobacco control policies necessarily make consumers worse off.

In a world with imperfect information and scarce resources, the role of economic policy analysis is to help evaluate whether the benefits of additional information are worth the costs of providing it. But as a final note on the economic approach, it also should be recognized that economic models allow for the possibility that some rational, well-informed people may decide to begin and continue an addiction to a substance with serious health consequences. As mentioned elsewhere in Chapter 7, it appears that most countries do not have in place policies that would address the specific market failures from smoking, but which would still leave such room for optimal consumption by informed smokers.

8.4.2 The impact of 'information shocks'

Studies to explore the impact of anti-smoking publicity started in the early 1970s. Table 8.1 summarizes the results of selected studies from a number of countries. Because it is hard to quantify the volume of tobacco-related health information, the studies generally explore whether events such as the publication of the 1964 US Surgeon General's report shifted cigarette consumption away from its time-trend. Many of the studies also explore and control for the role of cigarette advertising, discussed in more detail by Saffer (Chapter 9).

In an influential study, Hamilton (1972) studied the impact of what he terms the 'health scare' on the per capita demand for cigarettes of the US population aged 14 and older, from 1926 to 1970. He estimates several specifications for the periods

Table 8.1 The effect of anti-smoking publicity and health information on demand for cigarettes

Country	Time	Event regarding anti-smoking publicity and health information	Effect
The United States	1954–55	The release of the Hammond and Horn Study in 1954, and a book by Koskowski in 1955.	A decrease in per capita consumption by 6.9% to 8.8% cigarettes in each of the two years, fading away.
	1964	The publication of the 1964 Surgeon General's Report about Smoking.	Reducing per capita consumption by 1% to 1.3% cigarettes in that year.
	1971	Ban on television and radio advertising of cigarettes.	Reducing per capita consumption by 2.2% to 2.9% cigarettes in that year.
The United Kingdom	1962	The first report of the Royal College of Physicians.	A sudden 4.6% reduction, recovering 1% a year.
	1965	Ban on television advertising of cigarettes, and considerable public discussion of the issue.	A sudden 4.9% reduction, recovering 1% a year.
	1971	The second report of the Royal College of Physicians.	A sudden 4.9% reduction, returning back later.
Switzerland	1964	The publication of the US Surgeon General's Report.	An immediate 15% reduction, 4% of which had faded away by 1972.
	1966	Anti-smoking publicity in the mass media and various anti-smoking activities following the largest single increase in the tobacco tax in January 1966.	An immediate but temporary 11% reduction.
	1978–79	The mass debates regarding a public vote on a complete advertising ban for tobacco products before this vote, which took place in 1979.	An immediate but temporary 9% reduction.
Finland	1964	The publication of a short report on the health risks of smoking by the National Board of Health, and the publication of the Terry report.	An immediate but temporary 6% reduction.
	1971	Ban on television tobacco advertising.	No effect.
	1976–77	The *1976 Tobacco Act*, the total advertising ban in 1977, and an	A permanant 7% reduction.

Table 8.1 (*cont.*)

Country	Time	Event regarding anti-smoking publicity and health information	Effect
		extensive public debate about the health risks of smoking in 1977.	
Greece	1979	A systematic anti-smoking campaign including health education, non-smoking in public offices, and non-advertising of cigarettes on television.	A 7.3% reduction in the short-run.
Turkey	1982	Starting to put health warnings on cigarette packages.	A reduction of about 8% in the short-run.
	1986	An anti-smoking campaign by a national newspaper.	Additional reduction.
	1988	An anti-smoking campaign by the government.	Additional reduction.
South Africa	1991	Starting to have anti-smoking advertising and health warnings on cigarette packages.	Some effect on reducing demand for cigarettes.

Sources: For the United Kingdom, Atkinson and Skegg (1973); for Switzerland, Leu (1984); for Greece, Stavrinos (1987); for Finland, Pekurinen (1989); for Turkey, Tansel (1993); for the United States, Blaine and Reed (1994); for South Africa, Abedian (1996).

1926–70 and 1953–70. He assumes that once a message regarding the health consequences of smoking had been sent to the public, its impact on cigarette consumption stayed stable from year to year in his observation period. His results show that the 1964 Surgeon General's report decreased per capita cigarette consumption by between 146 and 253 cigarettes per year on average during 1964–70. Expressed differently, these decreases are from 3.7% to 6.5% of the average per capita consumption from 1968 to 1970. He also estimates a significant impact due to the advent of large-volume broadcast anti-smoking messages required by the Federal Communication Commission's Fairness Doctrine (to counterbalance cigarette broadcast advertising) from 1968 to 1970. His results indicate that this publicity reduced per capita cigarette consumption by between 9.9% and 13.7% per year on average over the period 1968–70. In addition, he estimates that the Fairness Doctrine anti-smoking messages had a larger impact on cigarette consumption than broadcast advertising by the tobacco industry. When the United States banned the industry's broadcast advertisements, an unintended consequence was that the Fairness Doctrine no longer required broadcast media to air anti-smoking messages. Based on his results, Hamilton (1972) predicted that the ban on broadcast advertising would therefore not reduce cigarette consumption.

In additional analysis of US time-series data from 1930 to 1978, Schneider *et al.* (1981) estimate that consumers responded to three information shocks: a 1953 publication by the American Cancer Society; the 1964 Surgeon General's report; and the anti-smoking messages broadcast during the Fairness Doctrine era (1968–70). They estimate that the cumulative effect of these shocks was a 30% relative decrease in cigarette consumption.

Blaine and Reed (1994) have updated earlier studies to estimate the impacts of health-related information about smoking in the United States after World War II by using data on cigarette consumption per US adult aged 18 or over, from 1946 to 1992. They have estimated the effects of health publicity 'events' in three periods:

(1) the release of the Hammond and Horn paper in 1954, and a book by Koskowski in 1955, which reported the relationship between smoking and mortality;
(2) the publication of the 1964 Surgeon General's Report about the health consequences of smoking and subsequent efforts by the government to reduce tobacco consumption from 1965 to 1970; and
(3) a ban on television and radio advertising of cigarettes in 1971 and anti-smoking activities since 1971 to the end of the study period (i.e. 1992).

The researchers imposed some assumptions in their specifications. First, they allowed the 'information shock' effect related to the 1954–55 health publicity event to decay gradually after these two years. Second, they allowed the health-scare effect related to the 1964 event and subsequent warnings to increase from year to year during 1964–70 and then fade away. Third, they allowed the health-scare effect related to the 1971 event, and those that followed, to increase from year to year until the end of the observation period. They found that repeated health warnings about smoking have considerably reduced consumption. The 1954–55 health scare reduced per capita consumption by between 6.9% and 8.8% in each of the two years, and the effect gradually faded away. The 1964 publicity decreased per capita consumption by between 1% and 1.3% in that year, and the annual effect from this publicity and anti-smoking efforts during 1965–70 increased from year to year until 1970 and then died away. The 1971 event reduced per capita consumption by between 2.2% and 2.9% in that year, and the annual effect from this event and following anti-smoking activities increased until the end of the study period.

Chen (1998) takes a somewhat different approach and extends this earlier line of research to explore a new information shock that is expected to have a disproportionate impact on smoking in a particular segment of the population: parents with children at home. To the extent that parents understand the consequences of second-hand smoke for their children's health, they can invest in their children's health by cutting down or quitting. Chen uses several approaches to explore whether the dissemination of information on the health consequences of second-hand smoke in the United States changed parents' demand for cigarettes. Her first approach is to calculate ratios of expenditures on tobacco per adult in households consisting of husband, wife, and children to expenditures on tobacco in households with single adults. This ratio falls fairly steadily over time, from 1.45 in 1960 to 0.83 in 1994, suggesting that parents' demand for cigarettes is falling much faster than that of single persons. Additional analysis of repeated cross-sections of the American population from several years of the National Health Interview Survey provides further support for this interpretation (Kenkel and Chen 1999). For example, over time, the impact of having young children

in the household further reduces the prevalence of smoking in parents. This is important evidence that information released after the early findings reported in the 1964
Surgeon General's report continued to influence smoking patterns in the United States
for some years.

In the United Kingdom, Atkinson and Skegg (1973) use aggregate data on tobacco
consumption from 1951 to 1972 to examine the effects of anti-smoking publicity. They
investigate three events related to anti-smoking publicity:

(1) the publication of the first report of the Royal College of Physicians in 1962;
(2) the ban on television advertising of cigarettes and considerable public discussion
     of the issue in 1965; and
(3) the publication of the second report of the Royal College of Physicians in 1971.

Based on their results from models using data on the numbers of cigarettes consumed,
they maintain that the 1962 event caused a sudden reduction of 4.6% in consumption,
which recovered at a rate of about 1% a year; the 1965 event caused a sudden
reduction of 4.9% in consumption, which also died away at a rate of about 1% a
year; and the 1971 event again resulted in a fall of 4.9% in consumption in that year
and the effect again faded away. These effects appeared to be for men rather than
women.

Leu (1984) analyzes the impact of anti-smoking publicity in the mass media in
Switzerland by using data of annual per capita cigarette consumption of adults aged
over 15, between 1954 and 1981. He examines the effects of three events:

(1) the publication of the US Surgeon General's Report, which had an important
     impact in Switzerland;
(2) anti-smoking publicity in the mass media and various anti-smoking activities fol-
     lowing the largest single increase in the tobacco tax in January 1966; and
(3) mass debates that took place in the run-up to a public vote on a complete adver-
     tising ban for tobacco products in 1979.

Leu argues that anti-smoking publicity in the mass media had an important effect on
decreasing cigarette consumption and had permanently reduced consumption by 11%
in 1984.

Stavrinos (1987) employs aggregate data of the number of cigarettes consumed per
adult in Greece from 1960 to 1982 to examine the effect of a systematic anti-smoking
campaign in 1979, including health education, non-smoking in public offices, and non-
advertising of cigarettes on television. The empirical model adopts a partial adjustment
specification, which considers the habit-forming nature of cigarettes and time-lags in
reaching the desired consumption level. The results suggest that the anti-smoking campaign reduced consumption of cigarettes by 7.3% initially and by 13.5% in the long run.

Pekurinen (1989) applies Finnish aggregate data of the number of cigarettes consumed per capita for the population aged over 15 from 1960 to 1987 to estimate the
effect of anti-smoking publicity. He considers four publicity events:

(1) the Terry report and the report about the health consequences of smoking by the
     National Board of Health in 1964;
(2) the ban on television tobacco advertising in 1971;

(3) the *1976 Tobacco Act*; and
(4) the total advertising ban in 1977.

He concludes that the 1964 publicity event decreased consumption immediately, but temporarily, by 6%; that the 1971 ban on television tobacco advertising did not have any significant effect; and that the events in 1976 and 1977 permanently reduced consumption by 7%.

Tansel (1993) uses Turkish annual time-series data of the weight of cigarettes consumed per person aged over 15, between 1960 and 1988, to estimate the effects of three events:

(1) health warnings after 1981;
(2) a 1986 anti-smoking campaign by a national newspaper; and
(3) a short-lived anti-smoking campaign mounted by the government in 1988.

The results suggest that the health warnings, on average, decreased cigarette consumption by about 8% for the period 1982–88. The 1986 and the 1988 publicity events appeared to induce additional reduction in consumption in the 1986–88 period. In addition, the author argues that health warnings can produce an effect larger than the opposing effect of advertising, and maintains that public education about the health consequences of smoking may be a more effective way to reduce cigarette consumption than increasing the price of cigarettes.

Abedian (1996) explores the effect of anti-smoking advertising in South Africa by using data on the real per capita numbers of cigarettes consumed domestically from 1970 to 1993. He examines the decline in per capita consumption and assesses whether the decline can be explained by changes in price, income, advertising, and anti-smoking campaigns. Because the decline can not be explained by the first three factors alone, he argues that anti-smoking publicity has contributed to the decline.

8.4.3 Studies of the link between consumer information and smoking in cross-section

Instead of focusing on information shocks and tobacco use over time, another approach examines the relationship between consumer information and smoking behavior in a cross-section of the population at a point in time. Given different costs in acquiring information, it is reasonable to expect variation in the degree to which different members of society are informed about tobacco, even long after information shocks. Taking this approach, Kenkel (1991) finds that more knowledgeable consumers, as measured by knowledge of the links between smoking and specific diseases, smoke less. Unlike studies using aggregate data, Kenkel's are based on microdata on individuals from the 1985 National Health Interview Survey. The author is able to estimate the effect of information on two outcomes: first, the decision to smoke, or smoking participation; and, second, on how many cigarettes current smokers consume.[5] It should be stressed that the estimated relationship between information and smoking

---

[5] However, the tobit model used in his analysis imposes a restriction on the relationship between the effects of an explanatory variable on the participation decision and its effects on the quantity consumed given participation.

statistically controls for possible differences in observable characteristics such as the person's income and schooling. However, Kenkel suggests that a person who is particularly 'health-minded' might smoke less for any given level of information but also might seek out more health information. This raises the possibility that part of the estimated relationship between information and smoking is spurious and reflects unobservable differences in attitudes towards health. Kenkel adopts a two-stage econometric approach to explore this problem. He concludes that while the pattern of results from this approach is somewhat weaker, it is reasonable to conclude that the relationship between information and smoking is not spurious.

Also using cross-sectional data from surveys of individuals, Viscusi (1990, 1991, 1992) finds that consumers who perceive higher risks are less likely to smoke. As described above in Section 8.3, Viscusi uses quantitative measures of risk perceptions, for example, based on respondents' estimates of the frequency of lung cancer due to a smoking in a group of 100 smokers. Viscusi (1990, 1992) estimates a logit model of the probability that individuals smoke as a function of their perceptions of the risks to their health and a set of socio-economic control variables. He finds that individuals who perceive the risks of lung cancer from smoking to be relatively high are significantly less likely to smoke than individuals who perceive those risks to be relatively low. As one illustration of the magnitude of the estimated effect of information on smoking, Viscusi uses the logit results to simulate the impact of improving the accuracy of people's risk perceptions. The simulation predicts that the societal smoking rate would rise by 6.5% if people believed that the lung cancer risk were 0.1, instead of their own under- and over-estimates. The direction of this result is logical, given Viscusi's somewhat controversial finding that most people in his sample over-estimated the risks of smoking. In other analyses, Viscusi finds that people's smoking decisions are consistent with other risk-taking activities, such as their willingness to accept riskier jobs in return for higher wages.

Viscusi (1991, 1992) also explores the relationship between risk perceptions and smoking for adolescents and young adults. This is central to research, given the important concern that young people in particular fail to internalize and react to hazards to their health. Viscusi finds that the risk assessments of respondents aged between 16 and 21 are higher than those of older respondents. However, risk perceptions appear to influence the smoking behavior of the young in the same way as risk perceptions influence smoking by older adults. The pattern of results leads Viscusi (1992, p. 128) to conclude that: 'There is certainly no evidence of greater neglect of smoking risks by the very young. Indeed, the opposite is the case . . .'. Viscusi suggests that risk perceptions are higher among younger non-smokers and smokers because public anti-smoking campaigns mean that they have been exposed to a very different informational environment than older cohorts.

Liu and Hsieh (1995) estimate the relationship between individual risk perceptions and smoking behavior, using survey data from Taiwan. The risk perception measures and empirical approach are similar to Viscusi (1992). They find that higher risk perceptions reduce the probability of smoking. As Viscusi (1992) finds, the results are robust across several specifications, including one that treats risk perceptions as an endogenous variable.

Jones and Kirigia (1999) have studied the relationship between health knowledge and smoking among South African women. In their sample of about 3500 female respondents, 26% were smokers. Health knowledge was measured by a simple indicator of whether the respondent was aware that smoking has negative health consequences, which was true for 86% of the sample. Jones and Kirigia estimate a bivariate probit model of the determinants of smoking status and health knowledge. Their results yield a negative correlation between the unobserved determinants of smoking and health knowledge. This suggests that unobserved factors that make smoking more likely also make poor health knowledge more likely. Their approach does not provide estimates of the impact of improving health knowledge on smoking, or the impact of specific anti-smoking interventions. However, it provides policy-relevant information. For example, it identifies those women who may be the most likely to respond to health education because they currently smoke but are unaware of the health consequences. Some 7.1% of the total study population of women were unaware of the health consequences; but, among them, smokers were 'over-represented', accounting for 27% of the study population). Furthermore, Jones and Kirigia are able to make these comparisons at a finer level of detail. For example, they find that the proportion of uninformed smokers relative to informed smokers is much greater among Black women.

8.5 The effectiveness of specific health information interventions

This section briefly reviews the evidence for the impact of different types of intervention on smoking prevalence and tobacco consumption.

8.5.1 Mass-media counter-advertising campaigns[6]

Counter-advertising campaigns are another example of public interventions that may improve consumer information about the health and addiction consequences of tobacco. Saffer (Chapter 9) discusses advertising and counter-advertising in more detail. In this section, a few studies of counter-advertising campaigns are highlighted to explore their potential as informational interventions.

   Using microdata on teen smoking in the United States from 1966 to 1970, Lewit *et al.* (1981) explored the impact of the country's first major anti-smoking advertising campaign, during the late 1960s. As explained above, as a result of the Federal Communications Commission's ruling that the Fairness Doctrine applied to cigarette advertising, there was an unprecedented barrage of anti-smoking messages on the US broadcast media from mid-1967 until cigarette broadcast advertisements were banned in 1971 (USDHHS 1989, p.415). The value of the implicit subsidy of donated radio and television time at its peak in 1970 has been estimated at about $200 million in 1985 US dollars (USDHHS 1989) or over $300 million in current dollars. Lewit *et al.* (1981) estimate that the anti-smoking messages required by the Fairness Doctrine had a significant impact on teen smoking participation rates. Their regression results suggest that the 'Fairness Doctrine effect' accounts for about two-thirds of the reduction of 3% to 3.4% in teen smoking participation rates that is predicted by simple trend equations.

   More recently, in 1988, the state of California passed Proposition 99, the *California Tobacco Tax and Health Promotion Act*, increasing the tax on each package of cigarettes from 10 cents to 35 cents beginning from January 1989. In addition, the act

---

[6] Teh Hu contributed to this sub-section of the chapter.

earmarked 20% of the revenue raised by this new tax for health education programs designed to reduce tobacco use. The most visible component of these four programs was the statewide anti-smoking media campaign. According to the California Department of Health Services, between April 1990 and June 1993, the state spent about $26 million on this campaign. Two studies (Hu *et al.* 1995a, 1995b) have empirically examined the effect of California's anti-smoking campaign on cigarette sales. The researchers estimate that every 10% increase in media campaign expenditures has reduced cigarette sales by 0.5%. In absolute terms, the media campaign reduced sales by 7.7 packs per capita during the third-quarter of 1990 through the fourth-quarter of 1992. The reduction of 7.7 packs per capita is about 10% of the average sales (in packs per capita) at the beginning of the campaign in 1990.

A separate analysis was used to examine the effect of the California anti-smoking media campaign on print advertising by the cigarette industry. It was shown that the state media campaign reduced cigarette consumption, while industry advertising increased, as measured in monthly total pages of cigarette advertisement per issue in *Life* magazine. In other words, the industry advertising slightly reduced the absolute magnitude of the effect of state media campaign.

It is notable that the media campaign reduced cigarette consumption in California where, as in the rest of the United States, consumer information about the health and addiction consequences of tobacco use is widespread. Survey evidence suggests that America's young people are less well-informed than older adults, making them a more likely target for the media campaign. However, because cigarette sales are dominated by the choices of adult smokers, it is highly unlikely that the estimated reductions in sales could have come about solely through changing youth smoking behavior. Instead, it seems likely that the California media campaign changed adult smoking behavior. The specific informational content of the campaign for adults could be considered relatively low. In fact, as reviewed by Saffer (Chapter 9), some analysts of the campaign argue that advertisements that emphasized the unhealthiness of cigarettes were the least effective form of counter-advertising.

Mass-media counter-advertising campaigns specifically directed at youth are becoming more prevalent, and preliminary results from several state programs suggest these may be effective in reducing youth smoking. Massachusetts raised its cigarette tax by 25 cents per pack in 1993 and spent about $40 million annually on the Massachusetts Tobacco Control Program (Connolly and Robbins 1998). Connolly and Robbins state that youth smoking rates in Massachusetts were nearly the same in 1996 (31%) as in 1993 (30%), a time when national rates of youth smoking increased, suggesting that Massachusetts' efforts 'worked' to some extent. However, because the tax increase and the anti-smoking media campaign occurred at the same time, it is hard to identify their separate effects. The Florida Youth Tobacco Survey (FYTS) conducted in February 1998 and February 1999, provides data to monitor the impact of the Florida Pilot Program on Tobacco Control (Centers for Disease Control and Prevention 1999). Data from the FYTS suggest that smoking prevalence among Florida high-school students fell from 27.4% in 1998 to 25.2% in 1999, while smoking prevalence in Florida's middle-school students fell from 18.5% to 15%. Florida did not increase its cigarette taxes over this period, but did spend $93 million from its settlement with the tobacco industry on the Pilot Program that included a youth-oriented counter-marketing media campaign. Data to compare Florida's decline in youth smoking to the national experience for 1998–99 are not yet available. It is also important to note that the most recent media campaigns have moved past simply providing information about the health and addiction risks of smoking. Content analysis of these campaigns could shed additional light on the extent to which they should be considered to be interventions to change health information or interventions to change attitudes and perceptions about smoking more broadly.

8.5.2 School health-education programs

Bruvold (1993) reports the results of a meta-analysis of 84 studies published during the 1970s and 1980s that dealt with the prevention of smoking in a school setting. Different programs were classified according to their orientations into four groups:

(1) a 'rational' orientation that focuses on providing factual information about drug use;
(2) a 'developmental' orientation that focuses on affective education (e.g. increasing self-esteem, self-reliance and other skills) and which usually includes minimal or no focus on drug use *per se*;
(3) a 'social norms' orientation that focuses on alternatives (e.g. reducing alienation) and usually includes minimal or no focus on drug use per se; and
(4) a 'social reinforcement' orientation that focuses on developing abilities to recognize and resist social pressures to use drugs.

The results of the meta-analysis suggest that interventions in all four orientation classifications had a significant impact on knowledge or health-information outcomes. However, the results also suggested a clear general pattern: for programs oriented towards social reinforcement and social norms, the impact was positive and significant in encouraging non-smoking behavior; those for programs with developmental orientations were mixed in sign but generally positive and significant; and those for programs with rational orientations were mixed in sign and usually not significant.

Bruvold's (1993) meta-analysis confirms other suggestions that school-based programs with rational information-providing orientations were not as successful as programs with newer orientations, such as social reinforcement and social norms. At least for adolescent smoking decisions, the model that assumes that factual information will shift down consumer demand for tobacco products may be over-simplified, suggesting the need to embed an economic model of adolescent smoking decisions within a broader psychosocial framework. Reid (1996) reviews evidence that even programs with initially favorable behavioral results can delay recruitment to smoking for several years, but not indefinitely. These results suggest that the role of information provision in reducing adolescent smoking may be quite limited.

8.5.3 Warning labels

As noted above in Section 8.2, many countries require health warning labels on tobacco product packages and advertisements. The USDHHS (1987) reviews research on health-warning labels in general. The review concludes that warning labels *can* have an impact on consumers if they are designed to take into account factors that influence consumer response, such as consumers' previous knowledge of the risks and their level of education and reading ability. To be effective, labels should stand out and have a visual impact; have a visible format; and contain specific, rather than general, information. However, the USDHHS (1987) noted that the evidence of the real-world effectiveness of warning labels in some situations cannot be regarded as conclusive evidence that health-warning labels are necessarily effective in all situations.These considerations suggest that, until recently, the warning labels required in many countries were unlikely to be effective, and have prompted some countries to change their policies (Roemer 1993). Past experiences with warning labels may understate the potential for better-designed warning labels to help reduce tobacco consumption.

Nevertheless, past experience with warning labels may give some idea of their potential, as well as for how that potential might be enhanced. For example, the USDHHS (1989) reviews empirical evidence that people did not pay much attention to the warning labels required in US print advertisements before 1984. However, other evidence is somewhat more promising. For example, in a survey conducted 9 months after US policy required rotation of four specific health warnings, 64% of all adult respondents and 77% of cigarette smokers said they recalled seeing one or more of the new warnings. Whether warning labels have met the policy objectives of increasing consumers' knowledge and reducing cigarette consumption is also very difficult to judge and presents a challenge for research. Reviewing US time trends the USDHHS (1989, p. 485) concludes that:

In sum, there are insufficient data to determine either the independent contribution of cigarette warning labels to changes in knowledge or smoking behavior or the precise role played by warning labels as part of a comprehensive antismoking effort.

More recently, the Public Citizen's Health Research Group (1998) provides encouraging evidence on the effect of cigarette-warning labels on reducing cigarette consumption. According to this report, tobacco consumption decreased by 15% in South Africa in 3 years after 1994, when the new warning labels were implemented. Surveys show that 58% of smokers were motivated by the cigarette-warning labels to reduce their tobacco consumption or quit smoking. In Australia, according to a survey conducted in 1997, the strengthened warning labels introduced in 1995 appeared to have a larger effect on inducing smokers to consider quitting than the old labels. Similarly, half of Canadian smokers in 1996 said that cigarette-package warnings had contributed to making them want to quit or cut down their tobacco consumption.

In the preceding section and this one, evidence has been presented that suggests that dissemination of information about the health risks of smoking has decreased demand for tobacco products in many countries and over various time periods. Based on these fairly consistent findings, it seems safe to conclude that new information policies have the potential to decrease tobacco demand in many middle-income and low-income countries. However, predicting the magnitude of the demand response is much more difficult, and will depend upon many factors. The obvious differences between high-income and low-income countries, such as per capita income and varying levels of education and literacy, present challenges for the design of health-information policies. For example, many of the most dramatic decreases in smoking in the United States followed the dissemination of information at a time when when smoking prevalence was high and consumer information was low. Further reductions in smoking in countries where information about the health consequences of smoking is widespread will be more difficult. Two important test cases for information will be China and India. Male smoking prevalence in these countries is about 67% and 40%, respectively. If the patterns seen in the industrialized high-income countries can be generalized, then the recently published and widely disseminated research findings on smoking hazards in China (Liu *et al*. 1998; Niu *et al*. 1998) should start to affect either smoking prevalence or tobacco consumption in the next few years. Similarly, forthcoming research findings on India (see Chapter 2) should also influence behavior in India over the next few years. Monitoring these trends will be crucial to judging the effectiveness of new information.

8.6 Concluding comments

This chapter has discussed two questions: Are consumers well-informed about the consequences of tobacco use? And, can public policies to improve consumer information reduce tobacco use? As is apparent, both questions defy simple answers. Clearly, some consumers are poorly informed about the consequences of tobacco use. This is more likely to be true for consumers in middle-income and low-income countries, and for young people in general, than for adult consumers in the high-income countries. An extrapolation from the experience of countries where information shocks have reduced tobacco consumption suggests that health information is an effective instrument for tobacco control. Moreover, given the continuing accumulation of evidence on the health consequences of tobacco, and the lags in consumers' responses to this information, there is still a role for governments to play in disseminating information, even in high-income countries, as well as in low- and middle-income countries. These conclusions are buttressed by the success of specific interventions to provide consumer information, including mass-media campaigns and warning labels. Disappointingly, however, the evidence suggests that school health-education programs may have less potential.

While there are, therefore, many consumers who are inadequately informed about tobacco and its health risks, it is probably also true that many consumers in high-income countries have been well informed. However, there appear to be gaps in the extent to which these risks are internalized by individuals, in the way that relative risks are understood, and in the way that young people assess the risks of addiction and disease. One of the more controversial issues is whether, on average, consumers over-estimate the risks of smoking. However, this controversy is somewhat irrelevant to the middle-income and low-income countries where most smokers live, and where many still perceive little or no risk from tobacco use. Even where the controversy is relevant, it should be stressed that the arguments refer to what consumers believe 'on average'. In reality, there is great heterogeneity in consumers' risk perceptions, and future research should investigate how to design public information with this heterogeneity in mind. Although in many countries there is still considerable potential for consumer information policies to reduce tobacco use, eventually the law of diminishing returns will come into play and further gains will be much harder. Commenting on the US experience, the USDHHS (1989, p. 221) observes that:

> The fact that in 1985 10% of smokers did not indicate that smoking is harmful to health, despite all efforts designed to impart such information, suggests that this group of smokers may resist accepting any information on the health effects of smoking. This finding . . . implies that other techniques besides providing information (e.g. policy incentives) are necessary to persuade some smokers to quit.

The USDHHS goes on to emphasize the importance of getting smokers to move past simply recognizing a general risk to understanding a personal risk from tobacco use. Weinstein's (1998) more recent review comes to the same conclusion, suggesting that personalizing risks is a critical objective for consumer information campaigns.

References

Abedian, I. (1996). *An Econometric Analysis of the Effect of Advertising on Cigarette Consumption in South Africa: 1970–1995.* Report for the Economics of Tobacco Control Project.

Atkinson, A. B. and Skegg, J. L. (1973). Anti-Smoking Publicity and the Demand for Tobacco in the U.K. *Manchester School of Economic and Social Studies*, **41**, 265–82.

Ayanian J. Z. and Cleary, P. D. (1999). Perceived Risks of Heart Disease and Cancer among Cigarette Smokers. *JAMA*, **281**(11), 1019–21.

Becker, G. S. (1976). The economic approach to human behavior, in *The Economic Approach to Human Behavior* (Chicago: University of Chicago Press).

Becker, G. S. and Murphy, K. M. (1988). A theory of rational addiction. *Journal of Political Economy*, **96**(4), 675–700.

Becker, G. S., Grossman, M., and Murphy, K. M. (1991). Rational addiction and the effect of price on consumption. *American Economic Review Papers and Proceedings*, **81**(2), 237–41.

Becker, G. S., Grossman, M., and Murphy, K. M. (1994). An empirical analysis of cigarette addiction. *American Economic Review*, **84**(3), 396–418.

Benjamin, D. K. and Dougan, W. R. (1997). Individuals estimates of the risks of death: Part I—A reassessment of the previous evidence. *Journal of Risk and Uncertainty*, **15**, 115–33.

Bero L, Galbraith, A., and Rennie, D. (1994). Sponsored symposia on environmental tobacco smoke. *Journal of the American Medical Association*, **271**, 612–7.

Blaine, T. W. and Reed, M. R. (1994). US cigarette smoking and health warnings: new evidence from post-World War II Data. *Journal of Agricultural and Applied Economics*, **26**(2), 535–44.

Bruvold, W. H. (1993). A meta-analysis of adolescent smoking prevention programs. *American Journal of Public Health*, **83**(6), 872–80.

Centers for Disease Control (1999). Tobacco use among middle and high school students—Florida, 1998 and 1999. *Morbidity and Mortality Weekly Report*, **48**(12), 248–53.

Chen, L. (1998). *The Effect of the Presence of Children on Parental Smoking.* Ph.D. Dissertation, Cornell University.

Chinese Academy of Preventive Medicine (1997). Knowledge and attitudes about smoking. In

Smoking and Health in China (1996). *National Prevalence Survey of Smoking Patterns.* Beijing: China Science and Technology Press.

Congressional Budget Office (CBO) (1998). *The Proposed Tobacco Settlement: Issues from a Federal Perspective.* CBO Paper, April.

Connolly, G. and Robbins, H. (1998). Designing an effective statewide tobacco control program—Massachusetts. *Cancer* 83(Supplement 12), 2722–7.

Corti, C. (1931). *The History of Smoking.* Bracken Books, London, UK.

Federal Trade Commison (1988). *Report to Congress Pursuant to the Federal Cigarette Labeling and Advertising Act.* Federal Trade Commission, February.

Gong, Y. L., Koplan, J. P., Feng, W., Chen, C. H. C., Zheng, P., and Harris, J. R. (1995). Cigarette smoking in China: prevalence, characteristics, and attitudes in Minhang district. *JAMA,* 274(15), 1232–4.

Goodin, R. E. (1989). *No Smoking: The Ethical Issues.* Chicago: The University of Chicago Press.

Hakes, J. K. and Viscusi, W. K. (1997). Mortality risk perceptions: a bayesian reassessment. *Journal of Risk and Uncertainty,* 15, 135–50.

Hamilton, J. L. (1972). The demand for cigarettes: Advertising, the health scare, and the cigarette advertising ban. *Review of Economics and Statistics,* 54, 401–11.

Hammond, E. C. and Horn, D. (1958). Smoking and death rates—Report on forty-four months of follow-up of 187,783 men. Paper presented at the American Medical Association, San Francisco, June 21, 1954. *JAMA,* 166, 1159–72; 1294–1308.

Hanson, J. D. and Logue, K. D. (1998). The costs of cigarettes: the economic case for ex post incentive-based regulation. *Yale Law Journal,* 107(5), 1163–361.

Hersch, J. (1998). Teen smoking behavior and the regulatory environment. *Duke Law Journal,* 47(6), 1143–70.

Hu, T. W., Sung, H. Y., and Keeler, T. (1995a). Reducing cigarette consumption in California: tobacco taxes vs. an anti-smoking media campaign. *American Journal of Public Health,* 85(9), 1218–22.

Hu, T. W., Sung, H. Y., and Keeler, T. E. (1995b). The state antismoking campaign and the industry response: The effects of advertising on cigarette consumption in California. *American Economic Review Papers and Proceedings,* 85, 85–90.

Hurd, M. D. and McGarry, K. (1995) Evaluation of the subjective probabilities of survival in the Health and Retirement Study. *Journal of Human Resources,* 30, S268–92.

Jenkins, C. N., Dai, P. X., Ngoc, D. H., Kinh, H. V., Hoang, T. T., Bales, S. *et al.* (1997). Tobacco use in Vietnam: prevalence, predictors, and the role of transnational tobacco corporations. *JAMA,* 277(21), 1726–31.

Jones, A. M. (1999). Adjustment costs, withdrawal effects, and cigarette addiction. *Journal of Health Economics,* 18(1), 125–34.

Jones, A. M. and Kirigia, J. M. (1999). Health knowledge and smoking among South African women. *Health Economics,* 8(2), 165–70.

Kenkel, D. S. (1991). Health behavior, health knowledge, and schooling. *Journal of Political Economy,* 95(2), 287–305.

Kenkel, D. S. and Chen, L. (1999). *Externalities Within the Family: Children and Women's Smoking Decisions.* Working paper, Department of Policy Analysis and Management, Cornell University.

Kennedy, G. and Bero, L. (1996). *Environmental Tobacco Smoke Research in the Lay Press.* American Public Health Association meeting, New York.

Koskowski, W. (1955). *The Habit of Tobacco Smoking.* London: Staples Press.

Leu, R. E. (1984). Anti-smoking publicity, taxation, and the demand for cigarettes. *Journal of Health Economics,* 3, 101–16.

Lewit, E., Coate, D., and Grossman, M. (1981). The effects of government regulation on teenage smoking. *Journal of Law and Economics,* 24, 545–73.

Lichtenstein, S., Slovic, P., Fischhoff, B., Layman, M., and Combs, B. (1978). Judged frequency of lethal events. *Journal of Experimental Psychology: Human Learning and Memory*, **4**(6), 551–78.

Liu, J. T. and Hsieh, C. R. (1995). Risk perception and smoking behavior: empirical evidence from Taiwan. *Journal of Risk and Uncertainty*, **11**, 139–57.

Liu, B. Q., Peto, R., Chen, Z. M., Boreham, J., Wu, Y. P., Li, J. Y. *et al.* (1998). Emerging tobacco hazards in China. I. Retrospective proportional mortality study of one million deaths. *British Medical Journal*, **317**(7170), 1411–22.

Masironi, R. and Rothwell, K. (1988). Smoking trends and effects worldwide. *World Health Statistics Quarterly*, **41**, 228–41.

McNeill, A. D., West, R., Jarvis, M., Jackson, P., and Bryant, A. (1986). Cigarette withdrawal symptoms in adolescent smokers *Psychopharmacology*, **90**, 533–6.

Nayga, R. M., Jr. (1996). Determinants of consumers' use of nutritional information on food packages. *Journal of Agricultural and Applied Economics*, **28**(2), 303–12.

Niu, S. R., Yang, G. H., Chen, Z. M., Wang, J. L., Wang, G. H., He, X. Z. *et al.* (1998). Emerging tobacco hazards in China 2. Early mortality results from a prospective study. *British Medical Journal*, **317**(7170), 1423–24.

Orhpanides, A. and Zervos, D. (1995). Rational addiction with learning and regret. *Journal of Political Economy*, **103**(4), 739–58.

Osler, M. and Kirchhoff, M. (1995). Smoking behaviour in Danish adults from 1982 to 1992. *Public Health*, **109**, 245–50.

Pekurinen, M. (1989). The demand for tobacco products in Finland. *British Journal of Addiction*, **84**, 1183–92.

Public Citizens Health Research Group (1998). Report on web. Web site is: http://www.citizen.org

Reddy, P., Meyer-Weitz, A., and Yach, D. (1996). Smoking status, knowledge of health effects and attitudes towards tobacco control in South Africa. *SAMJ*, **86**(11), 1389–93.

Reid, D. (1996). Tobacco control: overview. *British Medical Bulletin*, **52**(1), 108–20.

Roemer, R. (1993). *Legislative Action to Combat the World Tobacco Epidemic*, 2nd edn. Geneva: World Health Organization.

Royal College of Physicians (1962). *Smoking and Health: Summary and report of the Royal College of Physicians of London on smoking in relation to cancer of the lung and other diseases*. New York: Pitman Pub. Corp.

Royal College of Physicians (1971). *Smoking and Health Now: a new report and summary on smoking and its effects on health, from the Royal College of Physicians of London*. London: Pitman Medical.

Schneider, L., Klein, B., and Murphy, K. M. (1981). Governmental regulation of cigarette health information. *Journal of Law and Economics*, **24**(December), 575–612.

Schoenbaum, M. (1997). Do smokers understand the mortality effects of smoking? Evidence from the Health and Retirement Survey. *Am. J. Public Health*, **87**(5), 755–9.

Sloan, F. A., Taylor, D. H., and Smith, V. K. (1999). *Are Smokers Too Optimistic?* Duke University, Department of Economics, Working Paper.

Slovic, P. (1987). Perception of risk. *Science*, **236**(17 April), 280–5.

Slovic, P., Fischhoff, B., and Lichtenstein, S. (1979). Rating the risks. *Environment*, **21**(3), 14–39.

Slovic, P., Fischhoff, B., and Lichtenstein, S. (1985). Regulation of risk: a psychological perspective. In *Regulatory Policy and the Social Sciences* (ed. R. Noll), pp. 241–78. California Series on Social Choice and Political Economy. Berkeley, California and London: University of California Press.

Smith, V. K., Taylor, D. H., Sloan, F. A., Johnson, F. R., and Desvousges, W.H. (1999). *Do Smokers Respond to Health Shocks?* Duke University, Department of Economics, Working Paper.

Stavrinos, V. G. (1987). The effects of an anti-smoking campaign on cigarette consumption: empirical evidence from Greece. *Applied Economics*, **19**, 323–9.

Tansel, A. (1993). Cigarette demand, health scares and education in Turkey. *Applied Economics*, **25**, 521–9.

Taylor, D. H., Smith, V. K., and Sloan, F. A. (1999). *Rational About Death*. Duke University, Department of Economics, Working Paper.

Townsend, J., Wilkes, H., Haines, A., and Jarvis, M. (1991). Adolescent smokers seen in general practice: lifestyle, physical measurements and response to anti-smoking advice. *BMJ*, **303**, 947–50.

US Department of Health and Human Services (1986). *The Health Consequences of Involuntary Smoking*. A report of the Surgeon General. United States Department of Health and Human Services. DHHS Publication (CDC) 87–8398.

US Department of Health and Human Services (1987). *Review of the Research on the Effects of Health Warning Labels*. A Report to the United States Congress. United States Department of Health and Human Services.

US Department of Health and Human Services (1988). *The Health Consequences of Smoking: Nicotine Addiction*. A Report of the Surgeon General, 1988. US Department of Health and Human Service, Public Health Service, Centers for Disease Control, Center for Health Promotion and Education, Office on Smoking and Health.

US Department of Health and Human Services (1989). *Reducing the Health Consequences of Smoking. 25 Years of Progress*. A Report of the Surgeon General. 1989. US Department of Health and Human Service, Public Health Service, Centers for Disease Control, Center for Chronic Disease Prevention and Health Pro motion, Office on Smoking and Health.

US Department of Health and Human Services (1994). *Preventing Tobacco Use Among Young People*. A Report of the Surgeon General. Atlanta, Georgia: US Department of Health and Human Services, Public Health Service, Centers for Disease Control and Prevention, National Center for Chronic Disease Prevention and Health Promotion, Office on Smoking and Health.

US Department of Health, Education, and Welfare (1964). *Smoking and Health*. Report of the Advisory Committee to the Surgeon General of the Public Health Service. US Department of Health, Education, and Welfare, Public Health Service, Center for Disease Control.

US Department of Health, Education, and Welfare (1972). *Smoking and Health*. Report of the Advisory Committee to the Surgeon General of the Public Health Service. US Depatment of Health, Education, and Welfare, Public Health Service, Center for Disease Control.

Viscusi, W. K. (1990). Do smokers underestimate risks? *Journal of Political Economy*, **98**(6), 1253–69.

Viscusi, W. K. (1991). Age variations in risk perceptions and smoking decisions. *Review of Economics and Statistics*, **73**, 577–88.

Viscusi, W. K. (1992). *Smoking: Making the Risky Decision*. Oxford University Press. New York.

Viscusi, W. K. (1998). *Public Perceptions of Smoking Risks*. Paper prepared for the International Conference on the Social Costs of Tobacco, Lausanne Switzerland, August 21–22, 1998.

Warner, K. E. (1977). The effects of the anti-smoking campaign on cigarette consumption, *American Journal of Public Health*, **67**, 645–50.

Warner, K. E. (1981). Cigarette smoking in the 1970s: The impact of the anti-smoking campaign on consumption. *Science*, **211**, 729–31.

Warner, K. E. (1989). The epidemiology of coffin nails. In *Health Risks and the Press: Perspectives on Media Coverage of Risk Assessment and Health* (ed. M. Moore), pp. 73–88. Washington, DC: Media Institute.

Weinstein, N. D. (1980). Unrealistic optimism about future life events. *Journal of Personality and Social Psychology*, **39**(5), 806–20.

Weinstein, N. D. (1998). Accuracy of smokers' risk perceptions. *Annals of Behavioral Medicine*, **20**(2), 135–40.

9

Tobacco advertising and promotion

Henry Saffer

If tobacco advertising and promotion increase cigarette consumption, they are issues for public health policy. Although public health advocates assert that tobacco advertising does increase cigarette consumption, there is a significant empirical literature that finds little or no effect of tobacco advertising on smoking. In this chapter, these empirical studies are examined more closely with several important insights emerging from the analysis. The chapter also provides new empirical research from 102 countries on the effect of tobacco advertising. The primary conclusion of this research is that a comprehensive set of tobacco advertising bans can reduce tobacco consumption and that a limited set of advertising bans will have little or no effect. The policy options that have been proposed for the control of tobacco advertising include limitations on the content of advertisements, restrictions on the placement of advertising, restrictions on the time that cigarette advertising can be placed on broadcast media, total advertising bans in one or more media, counter-advertising and the taxation of advertising. This analysis concludes that neither restrictions on the content and placement of advertising, nor bans in only one or two media, are effective. However, comprehensive control programs, including comprehensive advertising bans, do reduce cigarette consumption. Counter-advertising, which is the use of media to promote public health, also reduces cigarette consumption. The taxation of advertising also reduces total advertising with the additional advantage of raising revenue that could be used to fund counter-advertising.

9.1 Introduction

If tobacco advertising and promotion increase tobacco consumption, they are public health issues. Although public health advocates (see, for example, Roemer 1993) claim that tobacco advertising and promotion do increase cigarette consumption, there is a significant empirical literature that finds no effect of tobacco advertising on smoking (see, for example, Duffy 1996) and there is very little empirical research on other promotional activities.[1] The empirical literature on advertising provides the basis for the tobacco industry's claim that its advertising only affects market share between various competing brands. This chapter will examine more closely the existing literature on tobacco advertising. Several important guidelines emerge from this analysis. These

---

[1] Since there is little research on the direct effects of these other promotional activities, the literature review emphasizes advertising. Other promotional activities generally either lower the full price of cigarettes or are sponsorships of public events (see Table 9.1). Economists define the full price as the money price, as well as the utility or disutility, of all non-pecuniary aspects of the purchase. Lower full prices result from placement fees paid to retailers, bundling the product with accessories and volume discounts. There are a number of studies (see Chaloupka and Warner, in press) which show that lower full prices increase consumption.

guidelines are used to re-evaluate previous studies, which results in a new and more critical view. This chapter also examines the experience of developing countries with tobacco advertising and promotion controls and reviews the merits and disadvantages of available policy options.

Before examining the prior empirical research on tobacco advertising, it is important to clarify what advertising and promotion are. Advertising can be defined as the use of media to create positive product imagery or positive product associations or to connect the product with desirable personal traits, activities, or outcomes. Promotion, also called marketing, can be defined as the mix of all activities that are designed to increase sales. In the United States, federal law requires that cigarette companies report their 'current practices and methods of cigarette advertising and promotion'. As of 1996, the five major American tobacco companies reported expenditures on 12 categories of advertising and promotion. These categories can be divided into advertising and other promotion activities. The data in Table 9.1 are reported by the Federal Trade Commission (FTC) (1998) and include all categories and the reported spending in each category.

Some additional perspective on the data reported in Table 9.1 is provided by com-

Table 9.1 US tobacco advertising and promotion activities (thousands of 1996 $US)

	1986	1996	Growth rate (%)
Newspapers	140289	14067	−90
Magazines	470874	243046	−48
Outdoor	423446	292261	−31
Transit	58855	28865	−51
Point of sale	294800	252619	−14
Total advertising	**1388265**	**830858**	**−40**
Promotional allowances (expenditures paid to retail outlets for favorable positioning of the product)	1166662	2150838	84
Sampling distributions (the cost of providing free samples to the public)	98816	15945	−84
Specialty item distribution (the cost of consumer accessories with brand names)	251982	544345	116
Public entertainment (the cost of sponsorship of sports ad cultural events)	116801	171177	47
Direct mail	56423	38703	−31
Coupons and retail value added (price reductions, two for the price of one and offers of merchandise)	1159267	1308708	13
All other promotional activities (includes endorsements in 1986 and Internet 1996)	104832	47128	−55
Total other promotional	**2954784**	**4276844**	**45**
Total advertising and other promotional activities (includes a miscellaneous category)	**4343049**	**5107702**	**18**

paring the level of tobacco advertising to advertising expenditures for other products and by examining the time trend in advertising and other promotion activities. Advertising expenditures are typically analyzed as a percentage of sales, which is known as the advertising-to-sales ratio. Schonfeld and Associates (1997) report that advertising-to-sales ratios, at the level of the whole industry (defined as all products, all brands, and all members of brand families sold) are for most industries less than 4%, averaging around 2% to 3%. The advertising-to-sales ratio for cigarettes in 1997 was relatively high at 5.9%. The time-trend in the advertising-to-sales ratio has been relatively stable, with Schonfeld reporting an advertising-to-sales ratio for cigarettes in 1980 of 6.3%. Both advertising expenditure and sales revenue have decreased over time, leaving the advertising-to-sales ratio relatively stable. However, according to the FTC data reported in Table 9.1, other promotional spending has increased over time. For the United States, when advertising and other promotion are added, the total is both high and has been increasing.

9.2 Review of economic issues in advertising[2]

Advertising is an important method of competition in industries that are highly concentrated, such as the cigarette industry. A highly concentrated industry is characterized by a small number of relatively large firms. Firms in industries of this type tend not to compete by price, but try to increase sales with advertising. According to Becker and Murphy (1993), advertising is an information complement to the good itself.[3] Cigarette advertising is not designed to convey information about the physical characteristics of the product. Information about these characteristics is easily obtained. Cigarette advertising is designed to create a fantasy of sophistication, pleasure, and social success. This becomes the product 'personality', which the advertisers expect will appeal to specific segments of the market. In developing countries, this imagery can be designed to associate the product with a glamorous fantasy of American or European life-styles. The relatively small expenditure on tobacco provides a link to this fantasy life-style.

The importance of advertising in opening new foreign markets is understood by the tobacco companies. Bogart (1986) reviews Peckham's rule, which suggests that, for new brands, advertising during the first two years should be 150% of desired sales. After the first two years, advertising should be set at whatever level is required to maintain sales. Philip Morris and British American Tobacco (BAT) are the largest international tobacco companies. *Advertising Age* reports that in 1996, for advertising outside the United States, Philip Morris was the ninth largest advertiser in the world, and BAT was the forty-fourth largest advertiser in the world.[4] In addition, an *Advertising Age* survey of Europe, Asia, and the Middle East finds that tobacco companies are listed in the top 10 advertisers in 21 out of 50 countries. The effectiveness of this advertising is illustrated by Chaloupka and Laixuthai (1996). They found that for four Asian

---

[2] For a discussion of other econometric issues in advertising, see Saffer (1995).
[3] Economists define goods that are often consumed together as complements. An example of complements are cameras and film.

countries, total tobacco advertising increased when US cigarette companies entered and total tobacco use increased by 10%.[5]

Measuring the effect of advertising on consumption can be problematic. Economic theory provides some important insights into how econometric studies of cigarette advertising should be conducted. The most important economic aspect of advertising is the concept of diminishing marginal product.[6] This concept is the basis of the advertising response function. Advertising response functions have been used in brand-level research (that is, research on products that are identifiable by a known name, such as Marlboro) to illustrate the effect of advertising on consumption at various levels of advertising (Ackoff and Ernshoff 1975; Rao and Miller 1975). Economic theory suggests that, due to diminishing marginal product, advertising-response functions flatten out at some point. That is, after a certain point, consumption becomes ever less responsive to increases in advertising. Ultimately consumption is completely unresponsive to additional advertising. One important implication of diminishing marginal product is that, since media are not perfect substitutes, media diversification increases the effect of a given advertising budget.

The same theory that describes the brand-level advertising response function can be applied to the industry level. The industry level is defined as all tobacco products, and includes all brands and all members of brand families sold. The industry-level advertising-response function is similar to the brand-level function and is graphed in Fig. 9.1(a). The vertical axis measures industry-level consumption and the horizontal axis measures industry-level advertising. The industry-level response function is different from the brand-level response function in that advertising-induced sales must come at the expense of sales of products from other industries or savings. Increases in consumption come from new consumers or from increases by existing consumers. In the case of cigarettes, new consumers are often uninformed adolescents. The uptake of smoking by adolescents creates serious health risks for them in adulthood.

A second important aspect of advertising is that its effects linger over time. That is, advertising in period one will have a lingering, although smaller effect, in period two. Although the rate of decline over time remains an arguable issue, research such as Boyd and Seldon (1990) finds that cigarette advertising fully depreciates within a year. The lingering effect of advertising is the basis for a widely used advertising technique known as pulsing. A pulse is a burst of advertising, in a specific market, that lasts for a short time and then stops.[7] After a period of time with no advertising, the market will be exposed to another pulse of advertising. The length and intensity of a pulse will vary due to a number of factors, including the specific media, the specific advertisers, and advertising costs in the specific market.

The two response functions represented in Fig. 9.1(a) and (b) help to illustrate the likely outcome of alternative methods of measuring advertising in econometric studies. There are four methods of measuring advertising used in econometric studies of advertising and industry-level consumption. These four categories are:

---

[4] Under a 1900 agreement BAT is not allowed to sell in the US or in Britain.

[5] A considerable backlash against this advertising developed in Thailand and Taiwan.

[6] The theory that the continued addition of increments of an input to a process will at some point lead to ever smaller increments in output is known as diminishing marginal product.

[7] This practice is also known as flighting and the advertising period is known as a flight.

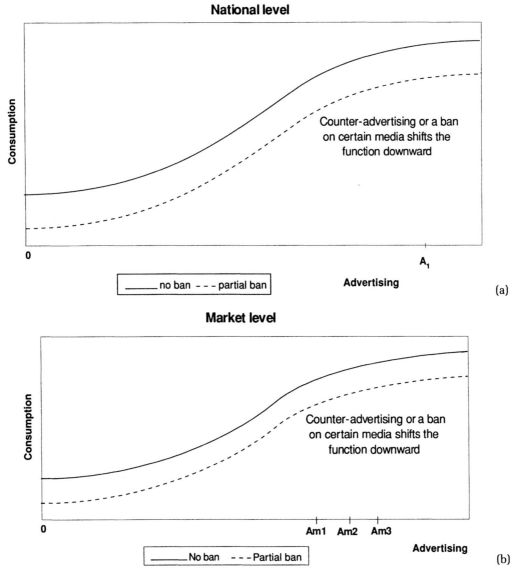

Fig. 9.1 The industry-level advertising-response function at (a) national level and (b) market level.

(1) studies that use annual or quarterly national aggregate expenditures as the measure of advertising;

(2) studies that use cross sectional measures of advertising;

(3) studies of advertising bans; and

(4) studies of counter-advertising.

Consider first, studies that use annual national expenditures as the measure of advertising. Annual national advertising expenditures are the yearly total of all cigarette advertising expenditures, for all advertisers, in all media, for all geographic market areas. This is a high level of aggregation of the advertising data and, as a result, the data have very little variation. Since cigarettes are heavily advertised, the marginal product of advertising may be very low or zero. In Fig. 9.1(a), this is equivalent to measuring advertising in a small range around A_1. The loss of variance due to aggregation leaves little to correlate with consumption and, since the advertising occurs at a level where the marginal effect is small, it is not likely that any effect of advertising will be found.

Consider next, studies that use cross-sectional data as the measure of cigarette advertising. This type of data can differ but would typically be gathered at local level, such as a Metropolitan Statistical Area, for periods of less than a year. This type of data can have greater variation than national-level data for several reasons. One reason for the variation in this type of data is pulsing. The pattern of these pulses varies over local areas. Another reason for variation in advertising levels is that the cost of advertising varies across local areas. This is illustrated in Fig. 9.1(b) by the three data points $Am1, Am2$, and $Am3$. An econometric study that uses monthly or quarterly local-level data would include a relatively larger variation in advertising levels and in consumption data. When the data are measured over a relatively larger range, there is a greater probability that the sample data will fall within an upward-sloping portion of the response function. Local-level advertising data are thus more likely to find a positive relationship between advertising and consumption.

Consider next, studies of advertising bans. The potential effect of a ban on certain media is shown as a downward shift of the response function in Fig. 9.1. An advertising ban may not reduce the total level of advertising but will reduce the effectiveness of the remaining non-banned media. The reason for this is as follows. A ban on one or more media will result in substitution into the remaining media. However, each medium is subject to diminishing marginal product. The increased use of the non-banned media will result in a lower average product for these media. This shifts the response function downward. Firms may or may not respond to this decrease in effectiveness of their advertising expenditures. Some may try to compensate with more advertising, which would be illustrated by moving to a higher level of advertising on a lower advertising response function.[8] Others may increase the use of other promotional techniques such as promotional allowances to retailers.

Finally, consider counter-advertising. Counter-advertising, which is the use of media to promote public health, is subject to the same law of diminishing marginal product as advertising. Figure 9.2 illustrates the effect of counter-advertising on consumption. The vertical axis measures consumption and the horizontal axis measures counter-advertising. The response function is downward sloping, indicating that increases in counter-advertising reduce consumption. Again, the response function flattens out at high levels of counter-advertising due to diminishing marginal product. The level of counter-advertising is usually low and irregular over time. Counter-advertising will,

---

[8] In a simple model, the decrease in marginal product would reduce the use of the input. However, in an oligopoly model, with response to rivals, one reaction to reduced sales is to increase advertising. Recall Peckham's rule that advertising should be set at whatever level is required to maintain sales.

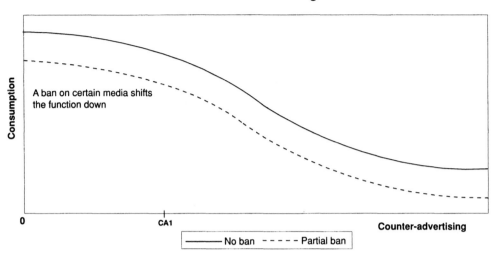

Fig. 9.2 The effect of counter-advertising on consumption.

therefore, be measured over a range that is sufficiently wide to reveal a slope and is measured in an area of the function where the slope is decreasing (see Fig. 9.2). It is likely that a negative relationship between counter-advertising and consumption will be found.

9.3 Prior econometric studies[9]

In this section, the prior econometric studies of the effect of cigarette advertising on cigarette consumption are reviewed. These studies are grouped into the four categories noted above. The four data categories, which are based on the type of data used to measure advertising and consumption, are listed in Table 9.2. They are:

(1) national expenditure data;
(2) cross-sectional data;
(3) advertising bans; and
(4) counter-advertising.

The industry-level response function predicts the likely outcome of these econometric studies based on the type of data used. We will see in this section that the results in each study are very much dependent on the type of data used. A similar conclusion, based on type of data, is found in reviews of alcohol-advertising research (see Saffer 1995).

[9] The 1989 US Surgeon General's report on tobacco reviews various mechanisms by which tobacco advertising and promotion increase tobacco use (USDHHS 1989).

Table 9.2 Prior empirical studies of the effects of advertising on tobacco consumption

Study	Data	Conclusion
Time series studies		
Hamilton (1972)	US 1925–70	No effect of advertising
Grabowski (1976)	US 1956–72	No effect of advertising
Schmalensee (1972)	US 1955–67	No effect of advertising
Schneider et al. (1981)	US 1930–78	No effect of advertising
Baltagi and Levin (1986)	US 1963–80	No effect of advertising
Johnson (1986)	Australian 1961–86	No effect of advertising
Porter (1986)	US 1947–82	No effect of advertising
Wilcox and Vacker (1992)	US quarterly 1961–90	No effect of advertising
Duffy (1995)	UK quarterly 1963–88	No effect of advertising
Bishop and Yoo (1985)	US 1954–80	Small positive effect of advertising
Abernethy and Teel (1986)	US 1949–81	Small positive effect of advertising
Valdes (1993)	Spanish 1964–88	Small positive effect of advertising
Chetwynd et al. (1988)	New Zealand quarterly 1973–85	Small positive effect of advertising
McGuinness and Cowling (1975)	UK quarterly 1957–68	Small positive effect of advertising
Seldon and Doroodian (1989)	US 1952–84	Small positive effect of advertising
Cross-sectional studies		
Lewit et al. (1981)	7000 youths 1966–70	Positive effect of advertising
Goel and Morey (1995)	US States 1959–82	Positive effect of advertising
Roberts and Samuelson (1988)	1971–82 for five firms	Positive effect of advertising
Ban studies		
Hamilton (1975)	11 OECD countries	No effect of a ban
Laugesen and Meads (1991)	22 OECD countries 1960–86	Negative effect of a ban
Stewart (1993)	22 OECD countries 1964–90	No effect of a TV ban
Counter-advertising studies		
Schneider et al. (1981)	US	Negative effect of counter-advertising
Lewit et al. (1981)	US	Negative effect of counter-advertising
Porter (1986)	US	Negative effect of counter-advertising
Hu et al. (1995)	California	Negative effect of counter-advertising
Pierce et al. (1990)	Australia	Negative effect of counter-advertising
Abernethy and Teel (1986)	US	Negative effect of counter-advertising
Pekurinen (1989)	Finland	Negative effect of counter-advertising
Flay (1987)	International review	Negative effect of counter-advertising
Goldman and Glantz (1998)	California	Negative effect of counter-advertising
Baltagi and Levin (1986)	US	Negative effect of counter-advertising

The first category of studies reviewed are those using national-aggregate advertising data as the measure of advertising. The industry-level response function presented above suggests that this type of study will not find any effect of advertising. There will be no effect found since the level of cigarette advertising is relatively high and national-level data may not provide sufficient variance to find any effect.[10] That is, the real expenditure on advertising may not vary enough from year to year to estimate any effect. These studies typically employ annual or quarterly data from one country with between 20 and 90 observations. Advertising is usually measured by expenditures, with control variables, such as price and income, included.

Schmalensee (1972) and Duffy (1996) make the interesting and almost universally ignored point that a study of cigarette advertising should control for changes in the level of advertising in all industries. The level of advertising in all industries is defined as external advertising. The effect of external advertising can be explained with a simple example. Assume that savings are held constant. If all industries, including cigarettes, doubled advertising, cigarette sales would not increase.[11] This is because the effects of spending increases in advertising, in each industry, would be mutually canceling. Cigarette advertising should be measured relative to external advertising.

Table 9.2 lists 15 cigarette advertising expenditure studies that use national, annual, or quarterly time-series data. As expected, all of these studies find either no effect or a small effect of advertising on cigarette demand. Chetwynd *et al.* (1988) find a small effect with quarterly data that is lost when aggregation is increased to the annual level. This supports the theory that annual data have too little variance for effects to be detected. Duffy (1996) reviews these studies and a few more that also use national-level advertising data. He also reports that these studies find either no effect or a small effect and concludes that these studies show that cigarette advertising has no effect on cigarette consumption. An alternative conclusion, as noted by Warner *et al.* (1986), is that studies which use a single time-series of national-level data are inappropriate to measure the effect of advertising on consumption.

The second category of studies includes those that measure advertising at a local cross-sectional level. There are only three studies that use cross-sectional data. The reason for their scarcity is that the data are expensive and difficult to assemble. Cross-sectional data measure advertising over a range, such as that shown in Fig. 9.1(b), which shows an industry-level advertising response function at the market level. Another advantage of cross-sectional data over time-series data is that external advertising does not need to be controlled. The study by Roberts and Samuelson (1988) is somewhat different, but may still be classified as cross-sectional. In this study the cross-sectional unit is the firm. These authors conclude that advertising increases market size, and that market share is related to the number of brands. They show that when advertising is measured over a wide range, such as with cross-sectional data, a significant positive effect of advertising is observed.

The third category of studies examines the effect of advertising bans on various aggregate measures of tobacco use. Advertising bans shift the function in Fig.9.1(a) downward. Three studies of cigarette advertising bans using pooled international data

---

[10] A flat portion of the function has a zero slope, which means a zero regression coefficient, and no relationship between consumption and advertising.
[11] This assumes that there is no change in the relative effectiveness of all advertising.

sets have been published. Hamilton (1975) used data on 11 countries over the period from 1948 to 1973. Hamilton presents a set of regressions using pooled data of countries with bans and countries without bans. The regressions show no effect of a ban. Laugesen and Meads (1991) used data from 22 high-income countries for the period 1960 to 1986. Like Hamilton, these authors also find that, before 1973, cigarette advertising bans had no effect on consumption. However, they find that after 1973, cigarette advertising bans have had a significant negative effect on consumption. Laugesen and Meads argue that, before 1973, manufacturers were able to respond to broadcast advertising restrictions by increasing their marketing efforts in alternative media. These shifts to alternative media are unmeasured in the data set and offset the effect of the broadcast bans. However, after 1972, more comprehensive anti-smoking legislation was enacted in most of the countries. These newer laws restricted advertising efforts to a greater degree and resulted in lower cigarette consumption. The third study of cigarette advertising bans was done by Stewart (1993) who analyzed data from 22 high-income countries for the period 1964 to 1990, and found that a television advertising ban had no effect. This study does not control for other offsetting increases in advertising in other media and does not separately examine the more restrictive period after 1973.

A new study by Saffer and Chaloupka (in press) specifically addresses this issue. The empirical work employs an international data set of 22 high-income countries over the period from 1970 to 1992. Tobacco consumption data from several sources are used. The primary conclusion of this research is that a comprehensive set of tobacco advertising bans can reduce tobacco consumption and that a limited set of advertising bans will have little or no effect. The regression results indicate that a comprehensive set of tobacco advertising bans can reduce consumption by 6.3%. The regression results also indicate that the new European Commission (EC) directive, which will end tobacco advertising in the EU countries, will reduce tobacco consumption by about 6.9% on average in the EU. The regression results also indicate that the ban on outdoor advertising, included in the settlement by the US tobacco industry, will probably not result in much change in advertising expenditures or in tobacco use, since the total number of bans is still relatively limited. However, under the settlement, the tobacco industry would also contribute $1.5 billion over five years for public education on tobacco use. This counter-advertising could reduce tobacco use by about 2%.

The fourth category of advertising studies includes those that examine the effect of counter-advertising on consumption. From 1967 to 1970, broadcasters in the United States were required to donate air time to counter-advertising. At its peak, the ratio of counter-advertising to advertising was one-third. This period, therefore, provides a good opportunity for measuring the impact of counter-advertising. In Fig. 9.2, studies of counter-advertising measure advertising in a range around CA1 (counter-advertising). This type of study is likely to find a significant relationship and, in fact, a considerable number do find that counter-advertising reduces consumption. Warner (1981), Lewit *et al.* (1981), Schneider *et al.*(1981), and Baltagi and Levin (1986), all included measures of counter-advertising, and all concluded that counter-advertising was effective in reducing cigarette consumption. The cigarette companies finally came to the conclusion that the negative effect of counter-advertising on consumption was greater than the positive effect of their advertising. The cigarette companies gave up broadcast advertising so that they would not have to fund more counter-advertising.

A series of local counter-advertising campaigns has also been analyzed. A study by Pierce *et al.* (1990) finds that counter-advertising reduced smoking in two Australian cities. Hu *et al.* (1995) find that counter-advertising reduced smoking in California. Goldman and Glantz (1998) find that counter-advertising in California and Massachusetts reduced smoking. Flay (1987) reviews the results of local counter-advertising campaigns in Finland, Greece, the United Kingdom, Norway, Israel, Austria, and Canada, and concludes that counter-advertising is effective in reducing cigarette consumption.[12]

9.4 Non-economic evidence

Evidence from a number of other disciplines supports the argument that cigarette advertising and promotion directly and indirectly increase cigarette demand (Chaloupka and Warner, in press). A major source of non-economic evidence is survey research and experiments that assess recall of cigarette advertising and smoking behavior, particularly among children. These studies have concluded that cigarette advertising is effective in getting children's attention and that the level of advertising recall is positively correlated with current or anticipated smoking behavior or smoking initiation. However, these studies generally cannot assess the potential endogeneity between an interest in smoking and recall. In other words, such studies cannot rule out the possibility that children who had greater recall of smoking advertisements did so because they were already more interested in smoking anyway, and not because the advertisements stimulated their interest. In addition, Chaloupka and Warner (in press) note that cigarette advertising and promotional activities are not consistent with the tobacco industry's claim that the market for tobacco products is mature and that marketing activities are designed to promote brand share, rather than market expansion. If the industry is a mature or declining one, retaining existing consumers and recruiting new ones would be particularly important in the cigarette market in which about 5% of consumers are lost annually, either through quitting or because they die. Finally, while the overall market may be mature, there are segments of the market that appear to have potential for growth, such as youth in the United States, for whom smoking prevalence rose throughout most of the 1990s, or specific minority groups, such as Hispanic females, for whom smoking rates are well below those of other groups of women.

The content of cigarette advertisements has also been analyzed. Content analysis involves defining a set of coding criteria that are designed to produce numerical data on the visual elements of the advertising. One focus of content analysis is on whether the content of cigarette advertising is designed to appeal to specific demographic groups, such as adolescents. Because most adults who smoke begin to do so as adolescents, and few subsequently switch cigarette brands, this age group forms an important segment of the market and has, therefore, been studied more than other

---

[12] See also Chapter 8.

demographic groups. Pierce *et al.* (1994) studied data from the National Health Interview Surveys and found that after the introduction of cigarette advertising targeted at women, the smoking uptake rates of adolescent girls increased. The Surgeon General's review of advertising content (USDHHS 1994) finds that youth-oriented magazines contained cigarette advertising with themes of adventure and risk. However, McDonald (1993) complains that content studies on advertising and smoking initiation by adolescents do not show causality. Pierce *et al.* (1998) studied a sample of adolescents in California and found that tobacco-promotional activities had a positive effect on the onset of smoking in this group.

9.5 The theory of brand proliferation and market size

Brand proliferation is defined as an increase in the number of brands available to consumers. Brand proliferation, which requires market segmentation, branding, and targeted advertising content, can increase the size of the market. Market segmentation involves dividing the market into a number of segments. These segments can be defined according to four classification systems. The first, geographic segments, are defined by region, size of residential community, etc.. The second, demographic segments, are defined by characteristics such as age, gender, race, and religion. Behavioristic segments are defined by characteristics such as frequency of purchase, the occasion of purchase, and the readiness to purchase. Finally, psychographic segments are defined by values, attitudes, personality, and life-style. Branding consists of creating distinguishable products with unique packaging or with unique product features. Single firms can create separate individual brands, such as *Marlboro* and *Virginia Slims*, which have no association with each other. Branding can also be done with 'brand families'. The brands in a cigarette brand family will all have the same name, but will have different attributes, such as king-sized, filter-tipped, hard pack, menthol, and so on. Wilcox (1991) reports that there was a considerable increase in the number of brands of cigarettes sold in the United States during the 1970s and 1980s. Data from the US Federal Trade Commission indicate that the number of cigarette brands increased from 370 in 1988, to 1249 in 1995. Targeted advertising content refers to the imagery used to create the 'personality' for each brand. These personalities are designed to appeal to specific market segments. For example, *Marlboros* are portrayed through the models in the advertisements as rugged, independent and self-sufficient and by a location that is awesome and unspoiled. Meanwhile, *Virginia Slims* are portrayed through the models in the advertisements as sassy, bold, slim, and exuberantly independent. Use of these products connects the consumer's fantasies to these fantasy images.

A company with a large portfolio of brands can achieve a larger market share than a company with a limited number of brands. Each brand is designed to provide an increased utility to the individuals in a specific market segment and is more likely to be purchased than a less differentiated product.[13] A new brand may take some cus-

---

[13] Knight (1933, p.261), commenting on product branding, writes: 'The morally fastidious (and naïve) may protest that there is a distinction between "real" and "nominal" utilities; but will find it very dangerous to their optimism to attempt to follow the distinction very far. On scrutiny it will be found that most of the things that we spend our incomes for and agonize over, and notably practically all the higher "spiritual"

tomers from an existing brand and may also induce some individuals who are not consumers into the market. In the case of cigarettes, new brands may also induce individuals who might have quit smoking to continue. An increase in the number of brands can, therefore, increase the company's total sales. The theory suggests that the size of the market may increase with the number of brands offered. The brand-proliferation technique may be employed by Western tobacco companies when entering markets in developing countries. The economic feasibility of this strategy is limited by the size of the market, the cost and availability of media to advertise in, and by the cost and creative abilities of the available advertising firms. Also, the cost of launching a new individual brand is larger than the cost of launching a new member of a brand family. In order to justify the cost of creating the new brand and its advertising, a market must be sufficiently large to contain adequate numbers of potential customers in each segment. Also, the media must be available to, and used by, a large number of potential customers in the market segment. The advertising content that is created must also be effective in each market segment.

An interesting example of the industry's use of market segmentation, branding, and targeted advertising content can be seen in Philip Morris's first attempt to enter the Brazilian market. In the early 1980s, Brazil was one of the world's largest tobacco markets. Philip Morris wanted to enter the market but found its competitors well entrenched. Market research by Philip Morris revealed a significant market segment that wanted cigarettes that had less nicotine and that did not irritate the throat. The company created a new brand, which it named *Galaxy* for this market segment. *Galaxy* was launched with heavy advertising that concentrated on the low-nicotine feature. However, *Galaxy* was a failure. Brazilians had perceived it as a 'diet' cigarette and were ashamed to be seen with it. Additional research found that the advertising of the low-nicotine feature was not connected to any outcome: for example, consumers might have experienced some different physical effects, such as reduced throat irritation, from the brand. But because such effects were not made explicit in the advertisements, consumers did not associate the low-nicotine feature with any physical state except dieting. A new advertising campaign was created that repositioned the low-nicotine feature as an intelligent choice for intelligent consumers. After the new campaign, attitudes and sales improved dramatically.

Simonich (1991) finds that the introduction of new brands is associated with increased overall demand for cigarettes but not with an increase in advertising. He estimates that, for every 10 new brands introduced, the market increases by 4%. Roberts and Samuelson (1988) also provide support for the theory of brand proliferation and market size. They studied the competitive behavior of six US tobacco firms from 1971 to 1982. Roberts and Samuelson found that companies increased their market share when they increased the number of brands that they offered. The researchers concluded that an important method of competition for US tobacco firms is through brand proliferation. They also found that advertising which accompanies new brands, increases the size of the total cigarette market. Wilcox (1991) studied the sales of 10 US brand families from 1949 to 1985. He also reported that the number of brands

values, gravitate swiftly into the second class.' What Knight means is that a consumer's satisfaction with a product is subjective. The fantasies associated with the product can provide the consumer with as much satisfaction as any objective product attribute.

increased during this period, and found that advertising and sales were positively related for five brands. Nguyen (1987) studied the effect of advertising by four US tobacco companies. He used data from 1956 to 1979 for 12 brands and concluded that: advertising a brand increased its sales; it had no effect on sales of its brand family, but decreased the sales of other companies' brands. Pollay *et al.* (1996) studied advertising and sales to adults and adolescents for nine brands from 1974 to 1993. They found that brand-level advertising increased market share and that the measured elasticity of market share with respect to advertising was three times larger for adolescents than for adults.

9.6 World data on tobacco advertising bans

A number of countries have successfully passed partial limitations on tobacco advertising. Studies have found that partial bans have no effect on sales. For example, Stewart (1993) found no effect of television advertising bans and concluded that advertising does not affect sales. Alternatively, Stewart's study might be interpreted as evidence that partial advertising bans simply result in substitution to other media or promotional methods. Tobacco companies and advertising agencies have shown great creativity in partial ban situations. For example, a 1976 French law banning tobacco advertising resulted in advertising for matches and cigarette lighters with the company logo. Also, in the United States, after the broadcast ban was adopted, the advertising-to-sales ratio initially fell but climbed back to its 'pre-ban' level within a few years. These data show that advertising bans must be comprehensive to have any effect. The advertising response function shows that partial bans may reduce the effectiveness of a given level of advertising spending. The level of spending is not fixed, however, and may increase if sales fall.

A number of countries have passed comprehensive advertising bans. These countries are listed in Table 9.3.[14] Comprehensive bans include bans on the use of the names, logos, and trademarks of tobacco products in any medium under any circumstances, including advertising for any product or event. These names may be used as part of the product packaging. Games, prizes, and free distribution are also prohibited. The ideal approach to estimating the effects of comprehensive bans is an econometric model, which would hold constant all other factors that affect consumption, such as price, income, and other economic or cultural variables (see Saffer and Chaloupka, in press). In addition, comprehensive bans are most likely to be legislated along with a series of other restrictions on tobacco, such as limitations on places where smoking is allowed, health promotion sponsorship foundations, health education programs, and counter-advertising. However, for many countries these data are not available, thus limiting econometric studies to samples such as the high-income countries. Even within these countries there are limits to the availability of data that can bias econometric studies.

Although econometric modeling of tobacco advertising for a large sample of countries may not be feasible, descriptive statistics of the data from around the world can

---

[14] Roemer (1993) presents time-series charts of per capita tobacco use in Norway and Finland. These charts indicate that following the enactment of advertising restrictions, tobacco consumption declined.

also provide evidence of the effects of comprehensive bans. Descriptive statistics do not control for other factors, but existing econometric studies also do not control for all other factors, and suffer from various other specification problems. Data on advertising bans were taken from WHO (1997) and from Chapman and Wong (1990). The data on advertising bans have been coded as either comprehensive tobacco advertising ban or not. The WHO also provides cigarette consumption data per adult aged 15–64 for 110 countries during 1980–82 and 1990–92. A cigarette consumption growth rate between the two periods was computed with these data.

There are 102 countries that have both advertising ban data and consumption data. These countries are divided into three categories. The three categories are:

(1) countries that have comprehensive bans;
(2) countries without comprehensive bans; and
(3) the former communist countries.

The former communist countries are treated as a separate category since there is an important difference between no advertising in any industry and a ban on tobacco advertising. This is a variant of the external advertising problem discussed by Schmalensee (1972) and Duffy (1996). Advertisers are competing, not only with each other but, with all other industries that advertise. A ban on all advertising might have no effect on the distribution of consumption across all industries. However, a ban on advertising in one industry could reduce sales in that industry in favor of increases in the non-banned industries. Since the link between advertising and consumption for the time period of the data is different for the former communist countries, they are treated as a separate category.

Table 9.3 shows the growth in cigarette consumption for 102 countries. The first four columns show the country name and growth rates for non-communist countries organized by comprehensive ban and no comprehensive ban. The average rate of growth and the population weighted rate of growth for each category are reported.[15] The table shows that per capita cigarette consumption for countries with comprehensive bans has decreased by about 8%, while consumption for countries without comprehensive bans has decreased by only about 1%. Figure 9.3 shows the per capita consumption level, over the sample period, for all countries with a comprehensive ban and without such a ban. The slope of the line indicates that the rate of decrease in consumption for the ban group is higher than the non-ban group. It is interesting that the group with the comprehensive bans starts at a higher consumption level than the non-ban group but ends the period with a lower consumption level. The change is due to the higher negative growth rate in the ban countries.

Table 9.3 also shows the rate of growth of tobacco consumption for the former communist countries. Roemer (1993) reports that in 1990, 27 countries had comprehensive advertising bans. Of the 27 countries, nine were formerly communist and had no advertising at all. Table 9.3 reports only seven countries because of missing consumption data. Table 9.3 shows that the former communist countries increased cigarette consumption over the data period. The weighted average for the communist countries

---

[15] A population weighted average gives a larger weight to countries with a larger population. It is computed by multiplying the country's population divided by the total population of all the countries in the group times the country's growth rate and summing for all countries in the group.

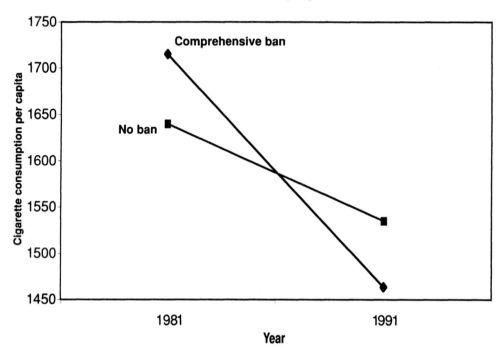

Fig. 9.3 Cigarette consumption per capita, various countries, weighted, ages 15–64.

reflects the large increase in consumption in China and its large population. Only Yugoslavia legislated a tobacco advertising ban during the data period. During this period Yugoslavia had a decrease in cigarette consumption. Also, during the period, these countries were experiencing major changes in economic institutions, which might have affected cigarette consumption. Because of these changes, the data should be interpreted only cautiously as indicating that the abandonment of bans increases consumption.

9.7 Policy options and conclusions

The policy options for the control of tobacco advertising include limitations on the content of advertisements, restrictions on the placement of advertising (such as in certain magazines), restrictions on the time that cigarette advertising can be placed on broadcast media, total advertising bans in one or more media, and counter-advertising. Experience has shown that restrictions on content and placement of advertising, and bans in only one or two media, are not effective. Prior research and the WHO data suggest that comprehensive control programs, including comprehensive advertising bans, reduce cigarette consumption. Usually comprehensive control programs include comprehensive advertising bans. Since they are enacted together, it is difficult to partition the effect of each component of a comprehensive control program. Prior research has shown that counter-advertising can also reduce cigarette consumption.

Table 9.3 Growth in cigarette consumption (per capita growth rate) in adults aged 15–64 during the period 1981–91

Non-communist countries				Former communist countries	
Comprehensive ban		**No ban**		**Country**	**Growth rate**
Country	Growth rate	Country	Growth rate		
Average	−0.082	Average	−0.023	Average	0.033
Weighted average	−0.088	Weighted average	−0.009	Weighted average	0.432
Afghanistan	−0.125	Albania	−0.008	Bulgaria	0.191
Algeria	0.013	Argentina	−0.090	China	0.473
Canada	−0.332	Australia	−0.212	Cuba	−0.133
Finland	−0.033	Austria	−0.156	Hungary	−0.018
Iceland	−0.115	Bangladesh	0.456	Poland	0.065
Iraq	0.174	Belgium	−0.198	Romania	−0.272
Italy	−0.169	Benin	−0.156	Yugoslavia (former)	−0.076
Jordan	−0.087	Bolivia	−0.232		
New Zealand	−0.131	Brazil	−0.143		
Norway	−0.062	Cambodia	−0.032		
Portugal	0.117	Cameroon	0.254		
Singapore	−0.369	Chile	−0.181		
Sudan	0.000	Colombia	−0.022		
Thailand	−0.028	Congo	0.011		
		Costa Rica	−0.118		
		Côte d'Ivoire	−0.123		
		Denmark	−0.054		
		Dominican Rep.	0.000		
		Ecuador	0.048		
		Egypt Arab Rep.	0.025		
		El Salvador	−0.019		
		Ethiopia	0.286		
		France	0.019		
		Germany	−0.025		
		Ghana	−0.432		
		Greece	0.044		
		Guatemala	−0.469		
		Honduras	−0.213		
		India	0.046		
		Indonesia	0.242		
		Iran Islamic Rep.	−0.198		
		Ireland	−0.201		
		Israel	−0.046		
		Jamaica	−0.131		
		Japan	−0.055		
		Kenya	−0.107		
		Korea Rep.	0.095		
		Lao PDR	0.000		

Table 9.3 (*Cont.*)

Non-communist countries				Former communist countries	
Comprehensive ban		No ban		Country	Growth rate
Country	Growth rate	Country	Growth rate		
		Madagascar	−0.021		
		Malawi	0.000		
		Malaysia	−0.205		
		Mauritius	−0.057		
		Mexico	−0.292		
		Morocco	−0.179		
		Mozambique	0.000		
		Myanmar	0.071		
		Nepal	1.000		
		Netherlands	−0.143		
		Nicaragua	0.014		
		Niger	0.700		
		Nigeria	0.057		
		Pakistan	−0.111		
		Panama	0.011		
		Paraguay	0.068		
		Peru	−0.103		
		Philippines	−0.196		
		Saudi Arabia	0.098		
		Senegal	0.382		
		Sierra Leone	0.000		
		South Africa	0.075		
		Spain	0.094		
		Sri Lanka	−0.173		
		Sweden	−0.158		
		Switzerland	−0.049		
		Tanzania	0.000		
		Togo	0.021		
		Trinidad	−0.092		
		Tunisia	0.101		
		Turkey	−0.067		
		Uganda	0.000		
		United Kingdom	−0.193		
		United States	−0.250		
		Uruguay	−0.012		
		Venezuela	−0.131		
		Vietnam	0.000		
		Yemen Rep.	0.421		
		Zambia	0.000		
		Zimbabwe	−0.348		

According to Tobacco Alert (World Health Organization 1996), the World Health Assembly has urged all member states to adopt comprehensive tobacco control programs, including advertising restrictions. Resolution WHA43.16 in 1990 recommends actions to eventually eliminate all direct and indirect advertising, as well as promotion and sponsorships concerning tobacco. While the resolution was adopted without dissent, not many member states have enacted these comprehensive advertising bans.

Two notable new comprehensive advertising ban initiatives were enacted by Thailand (see Chapter 14) and the European Parliament. The European Parliament voted in late 1997 to ban all tobacco advertising and sponsorship in all 15 countries of the EU. The ruling will not go fully into effect until 2006. Print advertising will be phased out over four years, sponsorships over six years, and car racing will have eight years to cease. Tobacco advertising on TV was banned in the EU in 1989.

Four tobacco companies have begun a legal challenge against the European directive banning tobacco advertising and sponsorship. A High Court judge in the United Kingdom has ruled that there is a question over the legal validity of the directive, which should be referred to the European Court of Justice. The tobacco companies are Gallaher, Imperial Tobacco, British American Tobacco, and Rothmans (UK). They challenged the directive on six grounds, each of which was found to be arguable by the court. Although the United Kingdom's courts do not have the power to overturn European legislation, they can refer it back to the European courts for clarification. The tobacco manufacturers claim that the legal question mark hanging over the European directive means that the EU governments should hold back from introducing legislation until the matter is settled in the European courts.

Econometric analyses of counter-advertising have generally concluded that these expenditures significantly reduce cigarette smoking (Chaloupka and Warner, in press). Much of the econometric evidence is based on two major counter-advertising campaigns in the United States. However, econometric evidence from Greece (Stavrinos 1987), Finland (Pekurinen 1989), Turkey (Tansel 1993), and the United Kingdom (Townsend 1998), indicates that the US experience is not unique. In each of these studies, mass-media campaigns aimed at reducing cigarette smoking by providing information on the health consequences of smoking were estimated to have led to significant reductions in smoking prevalence and in cigarette consumption. Saffer and Chaloupka (in press) estimate that counter-advertising messages set at about 15% of the total number of advertising messages can reduce smoking by about 2% each year.

Counter-advertising has been an important part of California's new tobacco control program. An interesting study by Goldman and Glantz (1998) has analyzed the effectiveness of different counter-advertising messages. They find that counter-advertising messages are most effective when they focus on the tobacco industry's manipulation of its customers. In such 'industry-manipulation' messages, tobacco executives are depicted as as deceitful, manipulative, dishonest, and greedy. According to the authors, this type of advertising helps adults to change their self-image of smoking from 'guilty addict' to 'innocent victim'.

The least effective counter-advertising portrays smoking as unhealthy and unromantic. The health messages do not convey any new information and, for people with only a dim view of the future, are meaningless. The romantic-rejection themes do not work because people believe that an individual's smoking status could be overlooked if they were otherwise desirable.

The taxation of advertising is not often included as an advertising control option. However, Erlich and Fisher (1982) and Saffer (1997) show that the demand for advertising is responsive to price changes. The taxation of advertising has the dual advantages of preventing media substitution and raising revenue. Media substitution would not be induced by a tax that applied equally to all media. Revenue would be generated either by a direct tax on advertising or by eliminating the tax deductibility of advertising. While advertising is price-responsive, the level of advertising chosen by individual companies is also dependent on the behavior of rivals. The demand for advertising could increase if sales were to fall. In this case, taxation might not reduce advertising but would raise more revenue than if the demand for advertising did not increase. Cigarette-advertising tax revenue could be used to fund counter-advertising.

References

Abernethy, A. and Teel, J. E. (1986). Advertising for cigarettes. *Journal of Advertising*, **15**(4), 51–5.
Ackoff, R. L. and Ernshoff, J. R. (1975). Advertising research at Anheuser-Busch, Inc. (1963–68). *Sloan Management Review*, **16**(3), 1–15.
Advertising Age. www.adage.com
Baltagi, B. H. and Levin, D. (1986). Estimating dynamic demand for cigarettes using panel data: the effects of bootlegging, taxation, and advertising reconsidered. *Review of Economics and Statistics*, **68**(1), 148B55.
Becker, G. S. and Murphy, K. (1993). A simple theory of advertising as a good or a bad. *Quarterly Journal of Economics* (November 4): 941–64.
Bishop, J. A. and Yoo, J. H. (1985). 'Health scare,' excise taxes and advertising ban in the cigarette demand and supply. *Southern Economic Journal*, **52**(2), 402B11.
Bogart, L. (1986). *Strategy in Advertising*. NTC Business Books: Lincolnwood IL.
Boyd, R. and Seldon, B. (1990). The fleeting effect of advertising. *Economic Letters*, **34**, 375–9.
Chaloupka, F. J. and Laixuthai, A. (1996). *Us Trade Policy and Cigarette Smoking in Asia*. National Bureau of Economic Research Working Paper 5543 1996 National Bureau of Economic Research.
Chaloupka, F. J. and Warner, K. E. The economics of smoking. In *The Handbook of Health Economics*. (ed. A. J. Culyer and J. P. Newhouse), New York: North-Holland (In press.)
Chapman, S. and Wong, W. L. (1990). *Tobacco Control in the Third World: a Resource Atlas*. Penang, Malaysia: International Organization of Consumers Unions.
Chetwynd, J., Coope, P., Brodie, R. J., and Wells, E. (1988). Impact of cigarette advertising on aggregate demand for cigarettes in New Zealand. *British Journal of Addiction*, **83**, 409–14.
Duffy, M. (1995). Advertising in demand systems for alcoholic drinks and tobacco: a comparative study. *Journal of Policy Modeling*, **17**(6), 557–77.
Duffy, M. (1996). Econometric studies of advertising, advertising restrictions, and cigarette demand: a survey. *International Journal of Advertising*, **15**, 1–23.
Erlich, I. and Fisher, L. (1982). The derived demand for advertising: a theoretical and empirical investigation. *American Economic Review*, **72**(3), 366–88.
Federal Trade Commission (1998). *Federal Trade Commission Report to Congress for 1996: Pursuant to the Federal Cigarette Labeling and Advertising Act*. Washington: Federal Trade Commission.

Flay, B. (1987). Mass media and smoking cessation: a critical review. *American Journal of Public Health*, **77**(2), 153–60.

Goel, R. K. and Morey, M. J. (1995). The interdependence of cigarette and liquor demand. *Southern Economic Journal*, **62**(2), 451–9.

Goldman, L. K. and Glantz, S. A. (1998). Evaluation of antismoking advertising campaigns *Journal of the American Medical Association*, **279**(10), 772–7.

Grabowski, H. G. (1976). The effect of advertising on the inter-industry distribution of demand. *Explorations in Economic Research*, **3**, 21–75.

Hamilton, J. L. (1972). Advertising, the health scare, and the cigarette advertising ban. *Review of Economics and Statistics*, **54**: 401–11.

Hamilton, J. L. (1975). *The Effect of Cigarette Advertising Bans on Cigarette Consumption.* Proceedings of the Third World Conference on Smoking and Health, Washington, D.C.: US DHEW.

Hu, T.-W., Sung, H.-Y., and Keeler, T. E. (1995). Reducing cigarette consumption in California: tobacco taxes vs an anti-smoking media campaign. *American Journal of Public Health*, **85**(9), 1218B22.

Johnson, L. W. (1986). Advertising expenditure and the aggregate demand for cigarettes in Australia. *International Journal of Advertising*, **1**, 45–58.

Knight, F. H. (1933). *Risk Uncertainty and Profit.* The London School of Economics: London.

Laugesen, M. and Meads, C. (1991). Tobacco advertising restrictions, price, income, and tobacco consumption in OECD countries 1960–1986. *British Journal of Addiction*, **86**, 1343–54.

Lewit, E. M., Coate, D., and Grossman, M. (1981). The effects of government regulation on teenage smoking. *Journal of Law and Economics*, **24**(3), 545B69.

McDonald, C. (1993). Children, smoking and advertising: what does the research really tell us? *International Journal of Advertising*, **12**, 279–87.

McGuinness, T. and Cowling, K. (1975). Advertising and the aggregate demand for cigarettes. *European Economic Review*, **6**, 311–28.

Nguyen, D. (1987). Advertising, random sales response, and brand competition: Some theoretical and econometric implications. *Journal of Business*, **60**, 259–79.

Pekurinen, M. (1989). The demand for tobacco products in Finland. *British Journal of Addiction*, **84**, 1183–92.

Pierce, J. P., Macaskill, P., and Hill, D. (1990). Long-term effectiveness of mass media led anti-smoking campaigns in Australia. *American Journal of Public Health*, **80**(5), 565–9.

Pierce, J. P., Lee, L., and Gilpin, E. (1944). Smoking initiation by adolescent girls, 1944 through 1988. *Journal of the American Medical Association*, **271**(8), 607–11.

Pierce, J. P., Choi, W. S., Gilpin, E. A. *et al.* (1998). Tobacco industry promotion of cigarettes and adolescent smoking. *Journal of the American Medical Association*, **279**(7), 511–5.

Pollay, R. A. *et al.* (1996). The last straw? Cigarette advertising and realized market shares among youths and adults, 1979–1993. *Journal of Marketing*, **60**, 1–16.

Porter, R. H. (1986). The impact of government policy on the US cigarette industry. In *Empirical Approaches to Consumer Protection Economics* (ed. P. M. Ippolito and D. T. Scheffman DT), pp. 447–84. Washington: US Government Printing Office.

Rao, R. and Miller, P. (1975). Advertising/sales response functions. *Journal of Advertising Research*, **15**, 7–15.

Roberts, M. J. and Samuelson, L. (1988). An empirical analysis of dynamic, nonprice competition in an oligopolistic industry. *RAND Journal of Economics*, **19**(2), 200–20.

Roemer, R. (1993). *Legislative Action to Combat the World Tobacco Epidemic*, 2nd edn. Geneva: World Health Organization.

Saffer, H. (1995). Alcohol advertising and alcohol consumption: Econometric studies. In *The Effects of the Mass Media on the Use and Abuse of Alcohol* (ed. S. E. Martin), pp. 83–99. Bethesda: National Institute on Alcohol Abuse and Alcoholism.

Saffer, H. (1995). Alcohol advertising and highway fatalities. *Review of Economics and Statistics*, **79**(August), 351–25.

Saffer, H. and Chaloupka, F. The effect of tobacco advertising bans on tobacco consumption. *Journal of Health Economic*, in press.

Schmalensee, R. L. (1972). *On the Economics of Advertising*. Amsterdam: North Holland.

Schneider, L., Klein, B., and Murphy, K. (1981). Government regulation of cigarette health information. *Journal of Law and Economics*, **24**, 575–612.

Schonfeld and Associates (1997). *Advertising Ratios and Budgets*. Schonfeld and Associates, Lincolnshire IL.

Seldon, B. J. and Doroodian, K. (1989). A simultaneous model of cigarette advertising: effects on demand and industry response to public policy. *Review of Economics and Statistics*, **71**, 673B7.

Simonich, W. L. (1991). *Government Antismoking Policies*. New York: P. Lang.

Stavrinos, V. G. (1987). The effects of an anti-smoking campaign on cigarette consumption: empirical evidence from Greece. *Applied Economics*, **19**(3), 323–9.

Stewart, M. J. (1993). The effect on tobacco consumption of advertising bans in OECD countries. *International Journal of Advertising*, **12**, 155–80.

Tansel, A. (1993). Cigarette demand, health scares and education in Turkey. *Applied Economics*, **25**(4), 521–9.

Townsend, J. L. (1998). UK smoking targets: policies to attain them and effects on premature mortality. In *The Economics of Tobacco Control: Towards an Optimal Policy Mix* (ed. I. Abedian, R. van der Merwe, N. Wilkins, and P. Jha). Cape Town (South Africa): Applied Fiscal Research Centre, University of Cape Town.

US Department of Health and Human Services (1994). *Preventing Tobacco Use Among Young People*. A Report of the Surgeon General. Office on Smoking and Health. Washington: US Government Printing Office.

Valdes, B. (1993). Cigarette consumption in Spain: empirical evidence and implications for public health policy. *Applied Economics*, **20**, 149–56.

Warner, K. E. (1981). Cigarette smoking in the 1970s: the impact of the antismoking campaign on consumption. *Science*, **211**, 729–31.

Warner, K. E., Ernster, V. L., Holbrook, J.H. *et al.* (1986). Promotion of tobacco products: issues and policy options. *Journal of Health Politics, Policy and Law*, **11**, 367–92.

Wilcox, G. B. (1991). Cigarette brand advertising and consumption in the United States: 1949–1985. *Journal of Advertising Research* (August/September), 61–7.

Wilcox, G. B. and Vacker, B. (1992). Cigarette advertising and consumption in the United States. *International Journal of Advertising*, **11**, 269–78.

World Health Organization (1996). *Tobacco Alert*. Geneva: World Health Organization.

World Health Organization (1997). *Tobacco or Health: a Global Status Report*. Geneva: World Health Organization.

10
The taxation of tobacco products

Frank J. Chaloupka, Teh-wei Hu, Kenneth E. Warner,
Rowena Jacobs, and Ayda Yurekli

This chapter reviews a variety of issues related to the taxation of cigarettes and other tobacco products. The empirical evidence showing that higher cigarette taxes result in higher cigarette prices is reviewed. This is followed by a discussion of the econometric literature examining the impact of prices and taxes on the demands for tobacco products. The small but growing body of research for low-income and middle-income countries clearly shows that higher prices would lead to significant reductions in tobacco use. Similarly, numerous studies from high-income countries reach the same conclusion. The estimated price-elasticities for low-income and middle-income countries are about double those for high-income countries, where estimates center on –0.4. Because of the addictive nature of tobacco use, demand for tobacco products is more elastic in the long-run. In addition, estimates from high-income countries indicate that youth and young adults, less educated persons, and those with lower incomes will be relatively more responsive to price changes. This review is followed by a discussion of the various motives for tobacco taxation, including the use of these taxes to generate revenues and to improve economic efficiency and public health. Finally, several other issues in tobacco taxation, including the earmarking of tobacco tax revenues and barriers to tobacco taxation, are discussed.

Sugar, rum, and **tobacco, are commodities which are no where necessaries of life, which are become objects of almost universal consumption, and which are therefore extremely proper subjects of taxation.** . . . In the mean time the people might be relieved from some of the most burdensome taxes; from those which are imposed either upon the necessaries of life, or upon the materials of manufacture. The labouring poor would thus be enabled to live better, to work cheaper, and to send their goods cheaper to market. The cheapness of their goods would increase the demand for them, and consequently for the labour of those who produced them. This increase in the demand for labour, would both increase the numbers and improve the circumstances of the labouring poor. Their consumption would increase, and together with it the revenue arising from all those articles of their consumption upon which the taxes might be allowed to remain.

(Smith, 1776, Book V, Chapter III, pp. 474–476.) (Emphasis added.)

10.1 Introduction

Shortly after Columbus returned to Europe bringing tobacco from the New World with him, tobacco use was subject to much controversy. Indeed, a number of countries soon adopted laws prohibiting the sale of tobacco and/or its public use, while others described tobacco as a 'social menace'—among the more severe penalties for selling and/or consuming tobacco products were whippings, beheadings, and nose slittings in Russia, China, Turkey, India, and elsewhere (Wagner 1971; Dillow 1981). However, it was not long before these laws were repealed as treasuries realized that significant revenues could be generated from the sale and taxation of tobacco and tobacco products. For centuries, nearly every country in the world has taxed tobacco and/or tobacco products, largely because the relatively inelastic demands for these products make them an easy source of revenues. Over time, however, as the health consequences of cigarette smoking and other tobacco use were discovered, increased taxation of these products has been used, by at least some governments, as a way of reducing the health damage caused by tobacco.

This chapter reviews a variety of issues related to the taxation of cigarettes and other tobacco products, beginning with a review of the economics literature on the impact of tobacco taxation on price and the subsequent effects of prices on the demands for cigarettes and other tobacco products. The various rationales for tobacco taxation, including those related to revenue generation, equity, and as a means to improve public health, are then discussed. Issues related to the design and administration of tobacco taxes are covered elsewhere (Chapter 17).

10.2 The impact of tobacco taxes on the prices of tobacco products

Increases in taxes on cigarettes and other tobacco products are expected to result in higher prices for these products. This is clearly reflected by the data in Table 10.1, which describes cigarette taxes, prices, and taxes as a percentage of price in selected countries. As expected, prices generally rise with taxes. In general, taxes in low- and middle-income countries are well below taxes in high-income countries; consequently cigarette prices in low- and middle-income countries are well below prices in high-income countries. Moreover, the cigarette tax usually accounts for two-thirds or more of price in higher-income countries (with the notable exception of the United States), compared to half or less of the price in many low- and middle-income countries.

When specific excise taxation (based on quantity) is the primary form of taxation, the real value of the tax will fall over time, unless regularly increased to account for inflation. Given that taxes are important components of the prices of tobacco products, one consequence of using specific excise taxes is that the real prices of tobacco products will decline over time as the prices of other goods and services increase more rapidly. In the United States, for example, the relative stability of federal and state cigarette excise taxes in the 1970s contributed to a drop of nearly 40% in real cigarette prices between 1971 and 1981 that was reversed by a series of federal and state tax increases in the 1980s and 1990s. In contrast, under a system that primarily uses *ad valorem* taxation (based on value), the real value of the tax and the real price of tobacco products will likely be stable over time as nominal prices rise with the prices of other goods and services.

Table 10.1 Cigarette prices and taxes, selected countries, by income group

	Price (US$)	Tax (US$)	Tax as percentage of price
Low-income countries			
Armenia	0.20	0.10	50
Bangladesh	0.09	0.03	30
Cambodia	0.05	0.01	20
China	0.20	0.08	38
India (white sticks)	0.37	0.28	75
Pakistan	0.28	0.21	73
Sri Lanka	1.05	0.25	24
Vietnam	0.10	0.04	36
Zambia	0.65	0.20	30
Zimbabwe	0.43	0.34	80
Lower-middle-income countries			
Albania	0.29	0.20	70
Bolivia	0.32	0.20	61
Bulgaria	0.60	0.25	42
Colombia	0.06	0.03	45
El Salvador	0.67	0.28	42
Indonesia	0.0004	0.0001	30
Jamaica	0.37	0.16	42
Philippines	0.22	0.14	63
Thailand	0.60	0.37	62
Turkey	0.51	0.22	42
Venezuela	0.07	0.04	50
Upper-middle-income countries			
Argentina	1.38	0.97	70
Brazil	1.05	0.79	75
Chile	0.88	0.62	70
Czech Republic	0.33	0.0003	0.1
Hungary	0.52	0.22	42
Malaysia	0.68	0.23	33
Mexico	0.63	0.38	60
Poland	0.50	0.20	39
Slovak Republic	0.58	0.20	34
Slovenia	1.08	0.68	63
South Africa	1.32	44	33
High-income countries			
Australia	4.85	3.15	65
Austria	2.96	2.16	73
Belgium	3.32	2.49	75
Canada	3.98	2.04	51
Denmark	5.21	4.38	84
Finland	4.49	3.28	73
France	2.90	2.17	75
Germany	3.38	2.43	72
Greece	1.90	1.39	73
Ireland	1.69	1.27	75

Table 10.1 (*Cont.*)

	Price (US$)	Tax (US$)	Tax as percentage of price
Italy	2.19	1.60	73
Japan	2.43	1.46	60
Korea, Republic of	0.77	0.46	60
Netherlands	2.99	2.15	72
New Zealand	4.69	3.19	68
Norway	7.01	5.47	78
Portugal	1.47	1.19	81
Spain	1.38	0.99	72
Sweden	4.58	3.16	69
Switzerland	2.80	1.45	52
United Kingdom	4.16	3.24	78
United States	1.94	0.58	30

Source: unpublished data, World Bank.

In a perfectly competitive market with constant long-run costs of production, an increase in tobacco taxes would be fully passed on to consumers in the form of an equivalent price increase. At the opposite extreme, a private monopolist would share the burden of the tax increase with smokers, with consumers bearing relatively more of the burden when demand is relatively inelastic. In the past, a single firm dominated the tobacco industry in many countries; in some countries, the government was the monopolist. Over time, however, with increasing trade liberalization and the growth of multinational tobacco companies, this has changed (as described in Chapter 14). As shown by Jacobs *et al.* (Chapter 13), the tobacco industry in nearly every country is at neither extreme, but is instead an oligopoly. The oligopolistic nature of the tobacco industry in most countries has significant implications for the effects of tobacco tax increases on the prices of tobacco products.

Nearly all of the empirical analyses of the relationship between tobacco taxes and prices are based on data for cigarettes from the United States. The earliest studies produced generally inconsistent findings, with some concluding that price increased by less than the amount of a tax increase (consistent with monopoly behavior), while others concluded that the tax increase was fully passed on to consumers (consistent with more competitive behavior) (Barzel 1976; Johnson 1978; Sumner 1981; Sumner and Ward 1981; Bulow and Pfleiderer 1983; Bishop and Yoo 1985; Sullivan 1985; Sumner and Wohlgenant 1985; Ashenfelter and Sullivan 1987). One general weakness of these studies is that they failed to account for the dynamic interaction of firms in an oligopolistic industry, a factor that has become increasingly important in recent years as the growth of multinational tobacco companies has led to greater competition in once monopolized markets and increased consolidation in markets that were once relatively more competitive.

More recent studies have attempted to more formally model the dynamic nature of an oligopolistic industry when estimating the impact of cigarette taxes on cigarette prices. Models of oligopoly behavior, however, have less clear implications for the effects of tax increases on price. Those in which there is relatively little collusion among firms, for example, suggest that increases in taxes would be at least partially borne by tobacco firms. Those where there is more coordinated behavior, however, could result in price increases of the same or greater magnitude than the tax increase. Historically, there is consistent evidence of collusive behavior among tobacco firms (although it falls short of perfectly collusive, or monopoly, behavior). For example, internal industry documents recently uncovered as part of Washington state's lawsuit against US tobacco companies suggest that Philip Morris and British American Tobacco (the two largest multinational tobacco companies) colluded to fix cigarette prices and divide markets in Costa Rica, Argentina, Venezuela, and other Latin American countries (Levin 1998). The collusion was not perfect, however; for example, one British American Tobacco memo suggests that a price war in Venezuela resulted when smuggled cigarettes became more common.

Most of the more recent empirical studies of the tax-price relationship that have modeled the dynamic, oligopolistic behavior of tobacco companies conclude that increases in cigarette taxes lead to significant increases in cigarette prices. Harris (1987), for example, used data on wholesale and retail cigarette prices, as well as data on manufacturing costs and state cigarette taxes, to estimate the impact of the doubling of the US federal cigarette tax (from 8 to 16 cents per pack) in 1983 on US cigarette prices. He concluded that the tax increase led to a price increase that was more than double the size of the tax hike (17 cents), which could not be explained by increases in manufacturing costs. Harris argued that firms in the US cigarette market used the scheduled tax increase as a coordinating mechanism for an oligopolistic price increase, noting that the price increases began shortly after the tax increase was announced, but well before the tax was actually increased.

This issue was re-examined by Barnett and his colleagues (1995), who argued that Harris attributed too much of the price increase to the tax increase, noting that the underlying upward trend in cigarette prices predated the debate over the US tax increase. Instead, they argued that the introduction of generic cigarettes in 1981 was used as the mechanism for coordinated, oligopolistic increases in the prices of premium cigarettes. The lower-priced, lower-quality generic cigarettes kept at least some of the more price-sensitive smokers in the market.

In a series of papers, Keeler and his colleagues (Sung *et al.* 1994; Barnett *et al.* 1995; Keeler *et al.* 1996) explored the relationship between state and federal cigarette tax increases and cigarette prices. Their models accounted for the interaction of supply and demand, the oligopolistic nature of the cigarette industry, and, in some cases, the addictive nature of cigarette smoking. Using annual, state-level data for the period from 1960 through 1990, Keeler *et al.* (1996) estimated that a 1-cent increase in a state's cigarette tax would lead to a 1.11-cent increase in the state's average cigarette prices. Moreover, they estimated that a national tax increase would lead to an even larger increase in price. The relatively smaller increase in state prices was attributed to the potential for cross-border shopping for cigarettes in nearby lower tax and price states. In addition, Keeler and his colleagues concluded that cigarette producers price-discriminate by state. That is, cigarette producers charge relatively low prices in states where there are stronger state and local tobacco control policies than they do in places with weaker policies. However, they noted that the effect of this price discrimination on retail prices was relatively small.

In addition, recent theoretical advances in the modeling of addictive behavior also imply that increases in tobacco taxes will lead to disproportionate increases in the prices of tobacco products. Becker *et al.* (1994) describe the behavior of a monopolist producing an addictive good like cigarettes. They argued that the monopolist will set a price below the short-run profit-maximizing level when consumption is addictive and future prices will exceed future marginal costs because of their monopoly power. The lower price 'hooks' consumers on their addictive product, thus raising the future demand for this product. When cigarette taxes are increased, Becker *et al.* argued that cigarette companies will raise price by more than the amount of the tax increase in order to obtain the maximum profits from current, addicted smokers. The increase in current profits helps them offset the future losses from the reduced smoking initiation that results from the tax and price increase. Becker and his colleagues explained this apparent paradox as follows (1994, p.413):

If smokers are addicted and if the industry is oligopolistic, an expected rise in future taxes and hence in future prices induces a rise in current prices even though current demand falls when future prices are expected to increase.

The key conclusion to draw from both the empirical and theoretical research is that increases in cigarette and other tobacco taxes, because of the addictive nature of consumption and because of the oligopolistic structure of the industry, will lead to increases in the prices of tobacco products that are likely to match or exceed the increase in the tax in most countries. Relatively larger increases in prices will occur in countries where there is less potential for cross-border shopping (i.e. relatively low tax-and-price countries surrounded by relatively high tax-and-price countries).

10.3 Tobacco taxes, prices, and the demands for tobacco products

10.3.1 Theoretical foundations

Perhaps the most fundamental law of economics is that of the downward-sloping demand curve derived from the consumer's constrained utility-maximization process. This law states that as the price of a product rises, the quantity demanded of that product falls. For many years, however, numerous researchers viewed cigarette smoking and other addictive behaviors as exceptions to this most basic law of economics because of the seeming irrationality of these behaviors (i.e. Schelling 1978, 1984; Elster 1979; Winston 1980). A now substantial and rapidly expanding literature, however, clearly indicates that the demands for tobacco products do respond to changes in prices and other factors. This is apparent from the simple descriptive data presented in Figs 10.1–10.3, as well as from the econometric research that has applied both traditional models of demand and the more recent studies that explicitly account for the addictive nature of cigarette smoking and other tobacco use (see Chapter 5 for a detailed discussion of the economics of addiction).

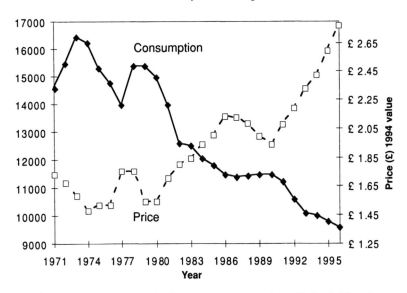

Fig. 10.1 Real cigarette prices and cigarette consumption, United Kingdom, 1971–96. (Source: Townsend 1998.)

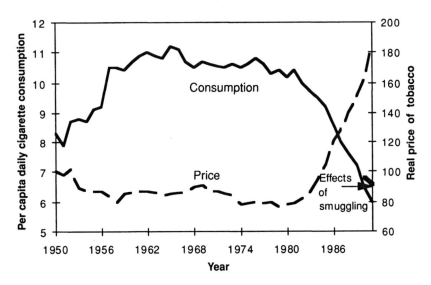

Fig. 10.2 Real cigarette prices and daily per capita cigarette consumption among persons 15 and older, Canada 1950–91. (Source: Townsend 1998.)

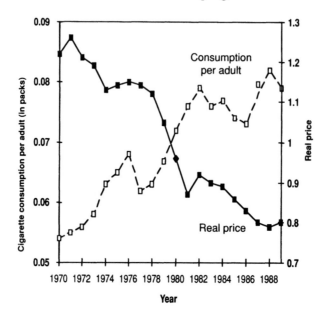

Fig. 10.3 Real cigarette prices and cigarette consumption, South Africa, 1970–89. (Source: Townsend 1998.)

10.3.2 Estimation issues

Over the past several decades, numerous studies have examined the effects of taxes and prices on the demands for cigarettes and other tobacco products. Most of the earliest involved applications of a traditional model of demand, but many of the more recent studies have modeled the addictive nature of tobacco use. These studies have employed diverse econometric and other statistical methods on data from numerous countries. Many have used aggregate time-series data on cigarette sales for a single geographical unit, while others have employed pooled cross-sectional time-series data. Still others have used data on individuals taken from surveys. One clear conclusion emerges from this literature: increases in the prices of cigarettes and other tobacco products significantly reduce cigarette smoking and other tobacco use. Most estimates for the price-elasticity of demand from the large literature on high-income countries fall into the relatively narrow range from – 0.25 to – 0.50, with many clustering around – 0.40. In contrast, estimates from the much smaller literature on low-income and middle-income countries suggest that demand in these countries is more responsive to price than demand in high-income countries, with most estimates in the range from – 0.50 to – 1.00.

Several difficulties are likely to be encountered by researchers when using aggregate data to estimate the demand for cigarettes. In a time-series model, the estimated price and income elasticities of demand will be sensitive to the inclusion of variables controlling for the effects of other important determinants of smoking, including advertising, changes in existing policies for reducing tobacco use, and increased awareness of the health consequences of smoking. High correlations among these variables can lead to unstable estimates for the parameters of interest. However, excluding potentially important variables that are correlated with those that are included can lead to biased estimates of the included variables. Many of the studies discussed below, however, have used state-of-the-art methods for time-series to address these difficulties. In general, the aggregate measures of cigarette consumption reflect tax-paid cigarette sales rather than actual consumption. When cross-border shopping and smuggling are important, sales are likely to understate consumption in relatively high tax-and-price jurisdictions, while overstating consumption in relatively low tax-and-price jurisdictions. If these factors are not controlled for, then estimates of the effects of taxes and prices on demand based on sales data are likely to overstate the impact of price on cigarette smoking. However, many of the recent studies employing aggregate data have made careful efforts to allow for cross-border shopping and organized cigarette smuggling; although imperfect, these efforts should significantly reduce the biases associated with the use of sales data as the measure of consumption. An additional problem in the analysis of aggregate data arises from the fact that cigarette prices are determined by the interaction of supply and demand. Failing to account for this simultaneity leads to biased estimates of the price-elasticity of demand. Again, several recent studies have theoretically and empirically modeled the supply and demand for cigarettes. Alternatively, others have taken advantage of natural experiments (such as large increases in cigarette taxes) to avoid the simultaneity problem. Finally, studies employing aggregate data are limited to estimating the impact of changes in prices and other factors on aggregate or per capita estimates of cigarette consumption. Consequently, these studies cannot provide information on the effects of these factors on the prevalence of tobacco use, initiation, cessation, or quantity and/or type of tobacco product consumed. Similarly, these studies cannot explore differences in responsiveness to changes in price and other factors among different population subgroups, including those defined by age, gender, race/ethnicity, and socio-economic status.

The use of individual data taken from surveys avoids some of the problems associated with the use of the aggregate data. For example, the data collected in the surveys provide measures of the prevalence of tobacco use and consumption of tobacco products, avoiding some of the difficulties associated with using sales data as a proxy for consumption. Similarly, many of the key determinants of tobacco use at the individual level are likely to be much less correlated with one another than comparable aggregate measures, creating fewer estimation problems and likely resulting in more stable parameter estimates. Likewise, because individual smokers' purchase decisions are too small to affect the market price of cigarettes, the use of individual-level data is not as likely to be subject to the simultaneity problems inherent in the use of aggregate data. The use of individual-level data, particularly longitudinal data, also allows researchers to explore issues that are difficult to adequately address with aggregate data, including the separate effects of price and other factors on the prevalence of tobacco use, frequency and level of tobacco consumption, initiation, cessation, and type of product consumed, as well as the differential effects among population subgroups. However, the use of individual-level data is not without its own problems. These data may be subject to a significant ecological bias to the extent that omitted variables affecting tobacco use may be correlated with the included determinants of demand. Excluding these variables will, consequently, produce biased estimates for the included variables.

In addition, the use of individual-level data is subject to potential reporting biases; the potential under-reporting of tobacco consumption can lead to problems in interpreting the estimates that are produced from these data. In general, studies using individual-level data have implicitly assumed that the degree of under-reporting is pro-portional to the actual level of use, implying that the estimated effects of price and other factors will not be systematically biased. Finally, one of the limitations of using survey data is that data on price, availability, advertising, policies, and other important, macro-level determinants of demand, are generally not collected in the surveys. As a result, many relevant variables may be omitted from the analysis, while others added from archival sources may be subject to measurement errors.

10.3.3 Estimates from low-income and middle-income countries

A small but growing number of studies have examined the demands for cigarettes and other tobacco products in a few low- and middle-income countries, while new research is beginning to focus on others. Warner (1990) argued that economic theory suggests that demand in these countries is likely to be more sensitive to price than demand in more affluent countries given the relatively low incomes in these countries. Similarly, the economic models of addiction suggest that the generally lower level of education in lower-income countries is likely to make the demand for tobacco products in these countries relatively more responsive to changes in monetary prices than demand in higher-income countries. In general, the findings from these studies are consistent with these hypotheses, suggesting that cigarette demand in lower-income countries is two or more times as sensitive to price as demand in higher-income countries.

Chapman and Richardson (1990) were the first to empirically estimate the impact of tobacco taxes on the demands for cigarettes and other tobacco products in a devel-oping country. Using annual data on the weight of cigarette and non-cigarette tobacco consumed in Papua New Guinea for the period from 1973 through 1986, they esti-mated excise tax elasticities of –0.71 for cigarettes and –0.50 for other tobacco prod-ucts. Their relatively simple double-log regression analysis modeled each of the measures of tobacco use as a function of the excise tax on cigarettes, the excise tax on other tobacco products, income, and a time trend. In addition to the strong own-tax effects that they estimated, Chapman and Richardson also found significant cross-tax effects. Their estimated cross-tax elasticity of cigarette consumption, with respect to other tobacco taxes, was 0.50, while that for other tobacco consumption with respect to the cigarette tax was 0.62. Their estimates clearly indicate that cigarettes and other tobacco products are substitutes for one another. That is, an increase in the cigarette tax, all else constant, would reduce cigarette smoking in Papua New Guinea, with much of the reduction in cigarette tobacco consumption offset by an increase in other tobacco consumption. In addition, Chapman and Richardson found strong, positive income effects for both types of tobacco products.

As Warner (1990) and the authors note, their tax elasticity will understate the true price-elasticity of demand given that taxes are less than 100% of price. Assuming that the tax is fully passed on to consumers, the price-elasticity of demand will be directly related to the inverse of the share of tax in price. For example, if half of price is accounted for by the tax, then the price-elasticities of cigarette and other tobacco demands in Papua New Guinea would be −1.42 and −1.00, respectively. Unfortunately, the authors' efforts to obtain information on the relationship between taxes and prices were 'fruitless'. Nevertheless, their estimates provided the first evidence that the demand for tobacco products in low-income countries was more responsive to price than demand in high-income countries.

Tansel (1993), however, reached the opposite conclusion for Turkey, a lower-middle income country. Using annual time-series data on cigarette consumption per adult over 15 for the period from 1960 through 1988, Tansel estimates a series of double-log models that include cigarette prices, income, and an indicator for the period when health-warning labels were required on cigarette packages. Additional specifications include an indicator for the years when anti-smoking media campaigns were in place, measures of secondary and higher education enrollment, and/or a measure of lagged consumption (consistent with assuming myopically addictive behavior). He found a negative and significant effect of price on cigarette demand in all specifications. The average short-run price-elasticity of demand implied by the alternative estimates was −0.21. Moreover, lagged cigarette consumption had a positive and significant impact on current consumption, consistent with the assumption of addictive behavior. As expected, the estimated long-run price-elasticity of demand (− 0.37) was well above the short-run estimates. In addition, Tansel found a strong positive effect of income on cigarette demand in Turkey, as well as negative and significant effects for the various indicators for health information and education.

Several recent studies provide some estimates on the price-elasticity of cigarette demand in China (Mao *et al.* 1997; Mao and Xiang 1997; Hsieh and Hu 1997; Xu *et al.* 1998). These estimates, in a range centering on − 0.75, are consistent with the hypothesis that cigarette demand in China is relatively more responsive to price than demand in most developed countries. The first, by Mao and his colleagues (1997), used annual time-series data from the Sichuan province for the period from 1981 to 1993 to estimate the price-elasticity of cigarette demand. Their time-series model included the price of cigarettes, personal disposable income, and per capita alcohol consumption. Two alternative specifications, one including a time-trend variable and one excluding it, were estimated using weighted least squares methods; both produced significant estimates for the cigarette price variable. Based on these results, Mao and his colleagues estimated that the price-elasticity of cigarette demand was in the range from − 0.656 to − 0.803. In contrast to trends in developed countries, the coefficient on their time-trend variable was positive and significant, indicating that cigarette smoking in Sichuan was increasing during the period covered by their data. In addition, Mao *et al.* also estimated models accounting for the addictive nature of cigarette consumption, producing estimated long-run price-elasticities of −1.03 and −1.32 from models that assumed myopic and rational behavior, respectively. Given these estimates, and information on the share of cigarette taxes in price, the authors concluded that raising cigarette taxes in China would lead to both significant reductions in smoking and large increases in cigarette tax revenues.

In a follow-up study, Mao and Xiang (1997) used a cross-sectional survey of 2431 adults in the Sichuan province to estimate a two-part model of cigarette demand. Cigarette price data were collected at the retail level based on the survey respondents' location. They estimated a price-elasticity for smoking participation of − 0.89 and a conditional demand elasticity of − 0.18. These estimates imply that sizable increases in

Chinese cigarette taxes would lead to sharp reductions in smoking prevalence among adults.

Hsieh and Hu (1997) produced similar estimates for Taiwan using annual time-series data for the period from 1966 through 1995. The authors estimated several alternative specifications, including one that allowed for the potential endogeneity of price and another allowing for myopically addictive behavior. In addition to price, their models included income, the market share of low tar cigarettes (which they interpret as reflecting the spread of information about the health consequences of smoking), an indicator for the time when strong health warning labels were required, the female labor force participation rate, and the market share of imported cigarettes (to capture the effects of the opening of the Taiwanese cigarette markets in the late 1980s, described in more detail by Taylor *et al.* in Chapter 14). In addition to estimating overall cigarette demand, Hsieh and Hu separately estimated the demands for domestically produced and imported cigarettes. In all equations, they found strong negative and significant price effects, with estimated price-elasticities of demand from the various specifications in the range from -0.5 to -0.7. In addition, they found that the demand for imported cigarettes was much more price sensitive than the demand for domestic brands, with a price-elasticity for imports of -2.7, and that Taiwanese smokers viewed domestic and imported cigarettes as substitutes for one another. In addition, they conclude that both increased income and the opening of the Taiwanese cigarette markets led to an increase in demand, while new information on the health consequences of smoking reduced demand. Similarly, current smoking was found to be positively related to past consumption, consistent with myopic addiction. Finally, they noted that their estimates clearly imply that higher cigarette taxes (which they point out are low in Taiwan compared to most developed countries) are an important policy tool for reducing cigarette smoking in Taiwan.

Most recently, Xu *et al.*(1998) estimated the demand for cigarettes in China using annual time-series data for the period from 1978 through 1992. As the authors described, the data limitations that are typical for many empirical studies are particularly severe for low-income countries, including China. The authors begin their analysis with 1978, since prior to that government control of the cigarette markets in China was very tight and the price of cigarettes was largely fixed. After 1978, however, cigarette prices were allowed to vary, enabling them to conduct an econometric analysis of demand. In addition to estimating the impact of prices on demand, the authors estimated the effects of cigarette taxes on demand in models that also include a measure of per capita income and a time-trend variable. They found that both higher cigarette taxes and prices lead to a significant reduction in per capita cigarette consumption. They estimate a price-elasticity of demand of -0.987. Their estimate of the tax elasticity of demand, -0.57, is very consistent with this given the share of taxes in cigarette prices in China and the assumption that taxes are fully passed on to smokers. Xu and his colleagues used their estimates to compute the revenue maximizing value of the tax and the optimal tax in China, concluding that the actual tax was well below both of these.

Studies conducted as part of the Economics of Tobacco Control Project (ETCP) at the University of Cape Town's School of Economics project provide estimates of the price-elasticity of cigarette demand for other low-income countries (Maranvanyika

1998; van der Merwe 1998). As part of this project, researchers estimated the demand for cigarettes in South Africa in a series of alternative specifications that modeled the simultaneity of cigarette demand and supply, as well as the addictive nature of cigarette smoking. In addition to price and income, these models included measures of cigarette advertising, an indicator for years when anti-smoking advertising was broadcast, and unemployment and divorce rates. Using sophisticated econometric methods applied to annual time-series data for the period from 1970 through 1994, the ETCP estimated that the short-run price-elasticity of demand for cigarettes in South Africa was – 0.59. In addition, they estimated a long-run price-elasticity of demand of – 0.68 in their empirical application of a rational addiction model; their estimates, however, did not support the hypothesis of rational addiction. Similarly, the ETCP researchers employed a similar approach to estimate the demand for cigarettes in Zimbabwe using annual time series data for the period from 1970 through 1996. Data limitations, however, required them to estimate a relatively lean specification that included cigarette price, income, and lagged consumption. Based on this model, the researchers concluded that the price-elasticity of demand for cigarettes in Zimbabwe was – 0.85, well above most estimates from high-income countries. Costa e Silva (1998) provided similar estimates for Brazil in a study presented at the ETCP's 1998 Cape Town conference. Using the very limited annual data available for the period from 1983 through 1994, she applied the rational addiction model in an econometric examination of cigarette demand in Brazil. Her estimates from these very limited data indicate that higher cigarette prices would lead to significant reductions in cigarette demand, with a long-run price-elasticity of demand of – 0.80, well above the short-run estimate of – 0.11. However, given the rational addiction model's demands on the very limited data, these should be viewed as a suggestive rather than definitive estimates of the magnitude of the effect of price on demand in Brazil.

One clear conclusion emerges from the econometric studies of the effects of prices on the demands for tobacco products in low- and middle-income countries: higher taxes on cigarettes and other tobacco products would lead to significant reductions in cigarette smoking and other tobacco use. This finding is consistent with a fundamental principle of economics—the law of the downward-sloping demand curve—as well as with the substantial body of research from higher income countries discussed in the next section. In addition, the estimates from low- and middle-income countries suggest that demand in these countries is relatively more responsive to price than demand in high-income countries. Estimates of the price-elasticity of demand for China (including Taiwan), Turkey, Papua New Guinea, and South Africa fall in the relatively wide range from – 0.1 to –1.0 (or higher, given the tax elasticity estimated for Papua New Guinea), with most in the range from – 0.5 to –1.0, while those from higher income countries tend to fall in the range from – 0.25 to – 0.5. This difference in relative price sensitivity is consistent with standard economic theory that suggests that price sensitivity will be greater among those with lower incomes as well as the economic theories of addictive behavior that suggest that less educated, lower income persons will be more responsive to changes in monetary prices than those with more education and higher incomes.

In addition, these studies suggest two interesting, policy relevant conclusions. First, they suggest that cigarettes and other tobacco products are substitutes for one another.

Increases in the prices of one type of cigarettes, for example, will lead to reductions in the consumption of that type of cigarettes that will be partially offset by increases in consumption of other types of cigarettes as well as other tobacco products. Second, the estimates that have attempted to account for addiction provide mixed support for the hypothesis of rational addiction, but are more generally supportive of myopic addiction. This implies that the long-run reductions in cigarette smoking and other tobacco use resulting from a price increase will exceed the short-run effects.

10.3.4 Estimates from high-income countries

In contrast to the relatively small number of studies for low- and middle-income countries, there is a large and growing body of research on the demands for cigarettes and other tobacco products in high-income countries, including the US, Canada, the UK, Ireland, Finland, Austria, Switzerland, other Western European countries, Australia, New Zealand, Japan, and others. Many have used aggregate time-series data comparable to that used in the studies from low- and middle-income countries described above, although the time-period covered in the studies for high-income countries is typically much longer than that for the studies of low- and middle-income countries. Many others have employed pooled cross-sectional times-series data for countries (i.e. OECD countries) or political divisions within a country (i.e. the states of the United States). Still others have employed individual-level data taken from surveys within a given country. Most of the early studies ignored the impact of addiction on the demands for tobacco products; several of the more recent studies, however, do account for the addictive nature of smoking and other tobacco use.

In general, the studies from high-income countries are consistent with those from low- and middle-income countries, in that they find strong and consistent evidence that increases in the prices of cigarettes and other tobacco products will lead to significant reductions in cigarette smoking and other tobacco use. The studies from high-income countries produce estimates of the price-elasticity for overall cigarette demand that fall in a relatively wide range, but most fall in the relatively narrow range from -0.25 to -0.5 (for more detailed reviews, see: US Department of Health and Human Services 1989, 1992, in press; and Chaloupka and Warner, in press). In addition, the studies from high-income countries have addressed a number of issues that, to date, it has not been possible to address in the studies for low- and middle-income countries given the limitations of the data on cigarette smoking and other tobacco use in these countries. These findings, and their implications for the effects of tobacco taxes and prices in low- and middle-income countries are the focus of this section.

A relatively small, but growing number of cigarette-demand studies have used data on individuals taken from large-scale surveys (mostly from the US). In general, the price-elasticities of demand estimated in these studies are very consistent with those obtained in studies that employ aggregate data. Because of their use of individual-level data, however, these studies are able to address issues that can not be addressed with aggregate data; most importantly, they can provide separate estimates of the impact of price on the prevalence of cigarette smoking and other tobacco use, and the conditional demands for cigarettes and other tobacco products (the consumption of these products conditional on being a consumer). In general, most of the recent studies that used individual-level data on cigarette smoking have concluded that half or more of the effect of price on cigarette demand is on smoking prevalence; the remainder of the effect is on cigarette consumption by continuing smokers (i.e. Lewit and Coate 1982; Mullahy 1985; Wasserman *et al.* 1991; Chaloupka and Grossman 1996; US Centers for Disease Control and Prevention 1998). For example, a recent study by the US Centers for Disease Control and Prevention (CDC 1998) that used data from 13 large population surveys conducted from 1976 through 1993, estimated a prevalence elasticity of cigarette demand of – 0.15 and an overall demand elasticity of – 0.25. The same pattern is likely to apply in low- and middle-income countries; that is, approximately half of the impact found in the studies using aggregate data described above is likely to be on smoking prevalence. Given the epidemiological evidence on the health consequences of tobacco use and the benefits of cessation (Chapter 2), this implies that significant increases in cigarette and other tobacco taxes would lead to substantial reductions in the morbidity and mortality resulting from tobacco use.

   In addition, a number of studies have employed aggregate and individual-level data from a variety of countries to estimate cigarette demand in the context of myopic and rational addiction models (Young 1983; Mullahy 1985; Baltagi and Levin 1986; Pekurinen 1989, 1991; Chaloupka 1991; Becker *et al.* 1994; Conniffe 1995; Duffy 1996; Cameron 1997; Bardsley and Olekalns 1998). In general, these models provide strong support for the hypothesis that cigarette smoking is an addictive behavior, based on their findings that higher past consumption has a positive and significant impact on current cigarette smoking. In contrast, the estimates from these studies provide mixed support for the hypothesis of rational addiction. In general, estimates from studies for the US (Chaloupka 1991; Keeler *et al.* 1993; Becker *et al.* 1994; Sung *et al.* 1994), Finland (Pekurinen 1991), and Australia (Bardsley and Olekalns 1998) are inconsistent with myopic addiction, although the relatively high discount rates implied by some estimates are not consistent with fully rational behavior. Estimates for the UK (Duffy 1996), Greece (Cameron 1997), and Ireland (Conniffe 1995), however, generally provide little support for the rational addiction model; the relatively small number of observations available for their analyses and the use of several highly correlated regressors, however, generally limit these studies. As discussed above, the key implication of applications of the economic models of addiction to the demands for tobacco products is that demand will adjust slowly to changes in price. These studies consistently produce estimates of the long-run price-elasticity of demand that are about double that obtained for the short-run. The key policy implication of this is that the impact of tax increases that result in sustained increases in the real prices of cigarettes and other tobacco products will grow over time. As a result, the long-run health benefits of higher tobacco taxes will be larger than the more immediate benefits (Townsend 1993).

   Several recent studies from the US have used individual-level data to explore differences in the price-elasticity of cigarette demand by age, with a particular emphasis on youth and young adults given that most smoking initiation takes place during the teenage years and becomes firmly established during young adulthood. Grossman and his colleagues (Lewit *et al.* 1981; Grossman and Chaloupka 1997) have suggested that younger persons would be more sensitive than older persons to changes in cigarette prices for several reasons. First, given the addictive nature of cigarette smoking, they

argued that youth who had been smoking for a relatively short time would be likely
to adjust more quickly to changes in price than long-term, more addicted adult
smokers. Second, peer smoking has a much greater impact on youth smoking than it
does on adult smoking, implying a multiplicative effect of price on youth smoking. That
is, an increase in cigarette price directly reduces a given youth's smoking and then indirectly reduces it by lowering peer smoking. Third, the fraction of disposable income a
young smoker spends on cigarettes is likely to exceed that spent by an adult smoker;
economic theory implies that this will make youth smokers more responsive to price.
Finally, compared to adults, youth are likely to be more present-oriented. In the context
of the economic models of addiction, this implies that a change in the monetary price
of cigarettes will have a greater impact on youth smoking than it will for adults.

The earliest research on this issue supported the hypothesis that younger persons
would be more responsive to changes in cigarette prices than older persons. Lewit and
his colleagues (Lewit *et al.* 1981; Lewit and Coate 1982) concluded that there was an
inverse relationship between price-elasticity and age, with teenagers up to three times
more sensitive to price than adults. A decade later, however, Wasserman and his colleagues (1991), Chaloupka (1991), and Townsend and her colleagues (1994) concluded
that youth and young adults were not significantly more responsive to cigarette price
changes than were older adults. A number of recent US studies, however, based on
several large, nationally representative surveys, have supported Lewit and his colleagues' findings of an inverse relationship between price and age (Chaloupka and
Grossman 1996; Chaloupka and Wechsler 1997; Lewit *et al.* 1997; Evans and Huang
1998; Tauras and Chaloupka 1999; CDC 1998). Chaloupka and Grossman (1996), for
example, used data on over 110 000 eighth-, tenth-, and twelfth-grade students to
examine the effects of price and a variety of tobacco control policies on youth smoking.
They estimated an overall price-elasticity of demand for youth smoking of –1.31, concluding that just over half of the effect of price was on youth smoking prevalence.
Similarly, the CDC's estimated price-elasticity of cigarette demand by young adults
(– 0.58) was more than double their overall estimate (– 0.25). These results have important implications for low- and middle-income countries where youth smoking prevalence has been increasing in recent years (see Chapter 2). Given that tobacco use
among youth is relatively more responsive to price and that most smoking initiation
occurs before age 20, significant increases in tobacco taxes in developing countries
would be effective in producing long-run reductions in smoking in all segments of the
population.

In general, researchers examining the effects of price on smoking prevalence using
individual level data have assumed that the impact of higher prices in reducing
smoking prevalence reflects reduced smoking initiation among youth and increased
smoking cessation among adults. A few recent studies have attempted to address these
issues more directly. Douglas (1998) and Douglas and Hariharan (1994), for example,
applied hazard methods to retrospective data on smoking initiation taken from two
large US surveys to estimate the impact of price on smoking decisions in the context
of the Becker and Murphy (1988) model of rational addiction; Douglas (1998) was able
to do the same for smoking cessation. Both studies found little evidence that higher
prices reduced smoking initiation. However, as the authors noted, the errors-in-
variables problems associated with both the retrospective data on smoking initiation

and the cigarette price data biased their estimates for price towards zero. Two recent studies using data from a longitudinal survey of youth in the US produce mixed evidence on this issue (DeCicca *et al.* 1998; Dee and Evans 1998). DeCicca and his colleagues concluded that higher cigarette prices have little impact on smoking initiation, while Dee and Evans estimated price effects consistent with those obtained in the recent studies based on cross-sectional data described above. Differences in variable construction and the treatment of missing data account for the differences in findings between the two studies. In contrast to the findings for initiation, Douglas (1998) did find strong evidence that higher prices reduced the duration of smoking, with an estimated price-elasticity of –1.0; that is, he concluded that an increase of 10% in price would reduce the duration of smoking by approximately 10%. Clearly, more research using appropriate longitudinal data is needed before rejecting the consistent findings from recent studies based on the cross-sectional survey data.

Several recent studies suggest important differences in the price sensitivity of demand among different socio-economic groups. The US Centers for Disease Control and Prevention (1998), for example, concluded that US Hispanics and Blacks were much more sensitive to price than were White non-Hispanics; Chaloupka and Pacula (1999) found similar differences among black and white youths. To the extent that socio-economic status is correlated with race and ethnicity in the United States, these findings suggest that people on lower incomes may be more sensitive to price. More compelling evidence resulted from the CDC's (1998) separate estimates of cigarette demand by low- and high-income persons in the United States. They estimated that the price-elasticity of cigarette demand by persons at or below the median family income in their sample was over 70% larger than their estimate for persons in families above the median. Chaloupka's (1991) finding, in the context of the rational addiction model, that less educated persons were relatively sensitive to price, while more educated persons were generally insensitive to price, is consistent with the hypothesis that there is an inverse relationship between the price-elasticity of cigarette demand and income. Townsend and her colleagues (1994) provided additional support for this hypothesis. Using data from the British General Household Survey, they concluded that people in the highest socio-economic groups were relatively unresponsive to price, while those in the lowest socio-economic groups were very responsive to price. These findings are consistent with the discussion above comparing the estimates obtained from low- and middle-income countries to those from high-income countries, and provide additional support for the contention that proportionate increases in the prices of tobacco products would have a larger impact on tobacco use in low- and middle-income countries than they would in high-income countries.

Finally, several studies from a variety of countries have examined the impact of taxes and prices on other tobacco products on the demands for these products, generally producing results consistent with the estimates from studies of cigarette demand (Thompson and McLeod 1976; Pekurinen 1989, 1991; Leu 1984; Ohsfeldt and Boyle 1994; Chaloupka *et al.* 1997; Oshfeldt *et al.* 1997, 1999). In addition, these studies generally found evidence that cigarettes and other tobacco products are substitutes for one another, consistent with the conclusion suggested above for developing countries. Similarly, recent work by Evans and Farrelly (1998) concluded that increases in cigarette taxes lead to compensating behavior by smokers. Using data from the United

States, they found that smokers in high-tax states were more likely to smoke longer cigarettes and/or higher tar and nicotine cigarettes, potentially offsetting some of the health benefits of the higher taxes. Similar substitution away from manufactured tobacco products that are more easily subjected to taxation and other regulation towards other more difficult to tax/regulate products (such as *bidis* in SE Asia) might also result from increases in taxes. The main policy implication of these findings is that comparable increases in the taxes on all tobacco products, and differential treatment of products epidemiologically proven to by more harmful, are likely to be needed to maximize the health benefits associated with increased tobacco taxation.

10.4 Motives for tobacco taxation

Cigarettes and other tobacco products have long been taxed in nearly every country around the world. As the introductory quotation highlights, even those who least support government intervention in the marketplace have supported the taxation of tobacco products as an easy source of revenues that imposes relatively few distortions. More recently, as the information on the health consequences of tobacco use has expanded, tobacco taxes have been seen as an appropriate 'user's fee' that covers the social costs of tobacco use, and as a powerful tool for improving public health. Nevertheless, proposed increases in tobacco taxes raise a host of philosophical and practical questions. This section reviews the theoretical and empirical evidence from the economics literature relevant to addressing many of these questions.

10.4.1 Tobacco taxation and revenues

The primary historical motivation, and still the most common rationale for tobacco taxation, is its revenue-generating potential. While tobacco tax revenues have historically accounted for as much as 3–5% of total government revenues in many high-income countries, their importance has generally declined over time. In contrast, tobacco tax revenues account for a significant share of total government revenues in many upper middle-income countries, but are relatively less important in most lower income countries (see Table 10.2).

A fundamental principle related to the efficiency of taxation is that taxes which generate substantial revenues, while minimizing the welfare losses associated with the higher prices resulting from the taxes, are preferable to those that result in greater welfare losses. As the so-called 'Ramsey Rule' dictates for consumption taxes (Ramsey 1927), the level of taxes will be inversely related to the price-elasticity of demand (holding the supply elasticity constant). Thus, goods with relatively inelastic demands should be taxed more heavily, while those with relatively elastic demands should be taxed least.

Given the evidence described above, cigarettes and other tobacco taxes appear to satisfy the Ramsey Rule. In the short-run, at least, the demand for tobacco products is relatively inelastic in most countries. Thus, increases in the taxes on tobacco products, even though they lead to significant reductions in cigarette smoking and other tobacco use, will at the same time lead to significant increases in tax revenues. This is in large

Table 10.2 Tobacco tax revenues as a share of total
government revenues, selected countries

	Percentage of total government revenues accounted for by tobacco taxes
Low-income countries	
China	9.05
India	1.81
Nepal	5.40
Zimbabwe	1.04
Lower-middle-income countries	
Bulgaria	2.80
Colombia	0.73
Costa Rica	1.35
Egypt	0.78
Estonia	1.15
Upper-middle-income countries	
Argentina	4.00
Brazil	4.88
Chile	3.38
Greece	7.72
High-income countries	
Australia	3.04
Denmark	1.73
Finland	1.73
Spain	2.20
United Kingdom	2.98
United States	0.41

Source: World Bank.

part why institutions such as the International Monetary Fund have viewed increased
tobacco taxes favorably (Sunley 1998).

For example, consider South Africa, where the long-run price-elasticity of cigarette
demand was estimated to be -0.68 and where taxes account for almost 40% of price.
Assuming that an increase in cigarette taxes is fully passed on to consumers, and that
the long-run price-elasticity of demand is constant, a permanent doubling of the South
African cigarette tax would reduce cigarette demand by over 27% in the long-run,
while raising cigarette tax revenues by nearly 50%. This positive relationship between
cigarette taxes and cigarette tax revenues is clearly shown in Figs 10.4–10.6 that plot
real cigarette taxes and cigarette tax revenues over time for the United States, South
Africa, and Zimbabwe.

In general, the revenue-generating potential of cigarette and other tobacco taxes will
be highest where the demands for these products is more inelastic and/or where taxes
as percentages of prices are relatively low. Given the available estimates, there is ample

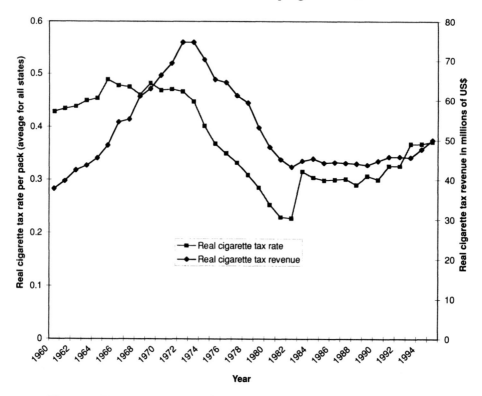

Fig. 10.4 Cigarette tax rate and cigarette tax revenue in the US 1960–95.

room for most countries to raise cigarette and other tobacco taxes, and at the same time generate additional revenues from these taxes. Consider China, for example, where estimates of the short-run price-elasticity of demand for cigarettes range from – 0.65 to –1.00. Assuming the low-end elasticity of – 0.65, a cigarette tax increase that led to a 10% increase in Chinese cigarette prices would result in a 6.5% reduction in cigarette sales, while total sales revenues would rise by 2.9% (Hu 1997). With an effective tax rate of 38% in 1992, these estimates imply that cigarette tax revenues would rise by 18.2%. On the other hand, assuming the price-elasticity of demand was constant at –1.00 and that a tax increase would be fully passed on to smokers, Hu (1997) estimated that a doubling of the Chinese cigarette tax would reduce cigarette consumption by nearly 40%, while raising cigarette tax revenues in China by approximately 20%. Given that cigarette-tax revenues in China account for about 9% of total revenues, Hu concluded that cigarette taxes are a very important government fiscal instrument (see Chapter 17 for a similar exercise for 70 countries and additional discussion).

To summarize, given the relative inelasticity of the demands for cigarettes and other tobacco products, tobacco taxes appear to satisfy the Ramsey Rule. That is, they generate substantial revenues in the short-run, while having a relatively small impact on social welfare. Moreover, given the share of taxes in prices, these taxes are likely to be

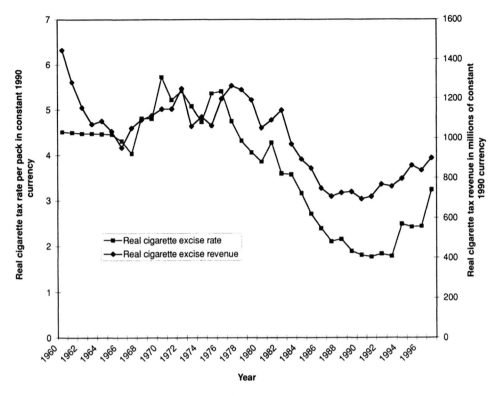

Fig. 10.5 Real cigarette tax rate and real cigarette tax revenue in South Africa 1960–97.

well below their revenue maximizing levels in most countries, including nearly all low- and middle-income countries.

10.4.2 Fairness standards

Debates over the appropriate level of tobacco taxes will necessarily encompass issues of equity and efficiency. With respect to equity, the focus has been on issues related to vertical equity—specifically on the apparent regressivity of cigarette and other tobacco taxes—and the 'benefit principle' of taxation. With respect to efficiency (aside from the efficiency arguments embedded in the Ramsey Rule), the focus has been on the use of tobacco taxes to cover the net social costs of cigarette smoking and other tobacco use. Each of these issues is discussed in more detail below.

Vertical equity

A basic principle of tax policy is the notion of vertical equity, which suggests that individuals with the greatest ability to pay should be taxed more heavily. This notion is reflected, for example, in progressive income tax systems where marginal tax rates rise as incomes rise. Cigarette and other tobacco taxes, however, appear to violate this

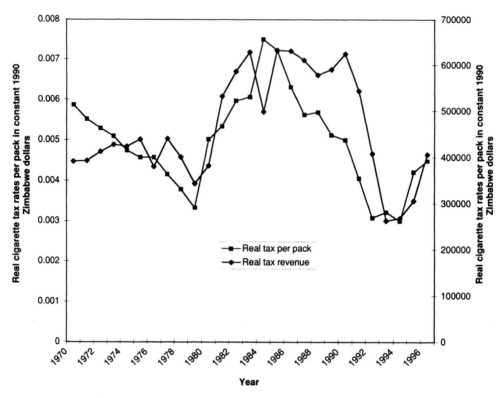

Fig. 10.6 Real cigarette tax rates and real cigarette revenue in Zimbabwe 1960–97.

principle. These taxes would be regressive with respect to income if the consumption of tobacco products was the same for both more affluent and poorer individuals. An additional concern in tax policy is the principle of horizontal equity, which implies that all individuals should be treated equally. Clearly, tobacco taxation violates this principle, since otherwise identical people who consume different quantities of tobacco products will be taxed differently.

In high-income countries, where tobacco use tends to be inversely related to income in recent years, the apparent regressivity of tobacco taxes is exacerbated. In most low- and middle-income countries, where tobacco consumption often rises with income, the regressivity of the taxes is less severe, although tobacco taxes as a share of income or total expenditures generally rises in these countries as income falls (see Chapter 3 for a more detailed discussion of the relationship between tobacco use and income in low-, middle- and high-income countries).

As discussed earlier, several recent studies found an inverse relationship between the price-elasticity of cigarette demand and socio-economic status (Chaloupka 1991; Townsend *et al.* 1994; CDC 1998). These estimates suggest that even though cigarette taxes may fall most heavily on lower income smokers, increases in these taxes may be progressive given the significantly larger reductions in smoking that occur among lower income smokers in response to a tax increase. Consider the following simple example.

Assume there are two smokers consuming the same number of cigarettes (x), one with relatively low income (y) and the second with relatively high income (3y). As implied by estimates of the price-elasticity of demand for different income groups, assume that the low-income smoker is relatively more price-sensitive (elasticity of -0.80), while the high-income smoker is less price-sensitive (elasticity of -0.20). Finally, assume that the cigarette tax is 50% of price (treat price per cigarette as the numeraire; i.e. $p = 1$) and assume that a tax increase is fully passed on to smokers. Given this, both pay x/2 in cigarette taxes; for the low-income person, this is x/2y of income as compared to x/6y for the high-income person. This tax is clearly regressive. However, the same is not true for a tax increase. Doubling the cigarette tax, assuming constant price-elasticities of demand, will reduce both smokers' cigarette consumption, with a relatively larger reduction for the lower income smoker. In addition, the total tax paid by both smokers will rise (to 0.6x/y for the low-income smoker and 0.3x/y for the high-income smoker). However, the increase in the tax paid by the low-income smoker is 0.1x/y, while that for the high-income smoker is 0.133x/y. Thus, while the existing tax may be regressive, a tobacco tax increase may be progressive and the overall regressivity of the tobacco tax will be reduced.

Moreover, given the estimated differences in the price-elasticity of demand by income, the health benefits resulting from tax-induced reductions in smoking would be disproportionately larger in the lowest income populations. Particularly appropriate would be the earmarking of new tobacco tax revenues to subsidize the provision of nicotine-replacement products and other smoking-cessation services for the poor, further reducing the perceived regressivity of a tax increase and increasing the progressivity of the health benefits from a tax increase (see Chapter 12 for more on this issue).

Finally, as has been pointed out by a number of analysts, the tax systems of most countries are a mix of many different taxes, where the overall goal of the taxation and expenditure system is to be progressive or proportional, even though specific elements of the system may be regressive (US Congressional Budget Office 1990; Warner *et al.* 1995). Increased progressivity of other tax and transfer programs could be used to offset the potential regressivity of tobacco tax increases. This is clearly the case when new tobacco tax revenues are earmarked for programs targeting low-income populations, including many of those discussed below that have used tobacco taxes to subsidize the provision of healthcare to low-income individuals.

The 'benefit principle'

The 'benefit principle' of taxation states that individuals should pay for their use of government-provided services in proportion to the benefits they derive from consuming these services. This notion is reflected in petroleum taxes and highway tolls that are then dedicated to financing road maintenance and construction. Thus, the taxes serve as 'user fees' that are paid roughly according to an individual's level of use. For cigarettes and other tobacco products, this concept is tied to the tobacco user's consumption of publicly funded healthcare to treat the consequences of his or her cigarette smoking and/or other tobacco use, as well as the use of other publicly funded services associated with tobacco use.

The direct application of the benefit principle to tobacco taxes will clearly depend on the mix of publicly versus privately provided healthcare and other services and the impact of cigarette smoking and other tobacco use on the costs of these services. These issues are discussed extensively by Lightwood *et al.* in Chapter 4. In addition, the notion of tobacco taxes as user fees is inextricably tied to issues concerning the negative externalities associated with tobacco use. These issues are discussed in the following section on the economic efficiency of tobacco taxes.

10.4.3 Economic efficiency and tobacco taxes

Two notions of economic efficiency are important when discussing the appropriate levels of tobacco taxes. The first, discussed above, is reflected in the Ramsey Rule. That is, given that governments need to generate revenue and that consumption taxes are to be used for this purpose, taxes that are applied to goods and services with relatively inelastic demands will be more efficient than taxes applied to those with more elastic demands (holding the elasticity of supply constant). Given the estimates from the econometric studies of tobacco demand, tobacco taxes appear to be 'efficient' taxes, at least in the short run and in most countries.

A second notion of economic efficiency relates to the issue of externalities. This concept implies that individuals should bear the full costs of their consumption. When one individual's consumption imposes costs on others (a negative externality), others are paying part of the burden of that individual's consumption. Pigou (1962) has suggested that taxes could be used to improve economic efficiency in this situation. The Pigovian tax that would raise the tobacco user's marginal cost to the point where it was equal to the marginal social cost of tobacco use would produce an economically efficient outcome. Consequently, estimates of the net social costs of tobacco use are critical in determining the appropriate level of tobacco taxes. As Cook and Moore (1993) note, however, taxes that equated the user's marginal cost with the social marginal cost, for some goods, could generate tax revenues that exceed the net social cost, since the efficient tax would be based on marginal rather than average external costs.

Estimating the costs of the negative externalities resulting from cigarette smoking and other tobacco use is a highly controversial subject. In general, these externalities fall into two categories:

(1) the financial externalities associated with the impact of tobacco use on the costs of healthcare, group health and life insurance, pensions, and other collectively financed programs; and
(2) the costs associated with the health and other consequences of exposure to environmental tobacco smoke (ETS).

There is an abundance of evidence on the health consequences of tobacco use that clearly implies that the direct medical care costs of preventing, diagnosing, and treating tobacco-related diseases are substantial. (See, for example, the discussion of the health consequences of tobacco use in Chapter 2, as well as that on the impact of tobacco use on health systems costs in Chapter 4.) In addition, some have argued that the indirect morbidity and mortality costs associated with the lost earnings from work loss attributable to tobacco use should also be included when calculating the social costs of tobacco use. In general, these costs are included in most calculations of the costs of smoking. In contrast, there are a number of costs that are typically not included, including the treatment of burn victims from smoking-related fires, the short-term healthcare costs and longer-term developmental costs associated with maternal smoking during pregnancy, the costs of treating illnesses related to exposure to ETS, intangible costs of tobacco-attributable morbidity and mortality (that is, the pain and suffering associated with the illness and the grief experienced by family and friends), and the annoyance costs of exposure to ETS.

Even if all of these costs were included in the calculus, the economist attempting to compute the net social costs of cigarette smoking and other tobacco use would face a number of challenges. First, one must determine an appropriate approach to valuing the life-years lost as a result of tobacco use, as well as which of these should be included in the computations. Most studies have taken a human capital approach to valuing life-years, an approach that critics argue significantly understates the value of a life. Using even relatively conservative figures for the value of a life-year, obtained from a willingness-to-pay approach, will significantly increase the estimates of the indirect costs of tobacco use. In addition, most studies of net social costs treat the indirect morbidity and mortality costs for tobacco users as internal costs, while the comparable costs from exposure to environmental tobacco smoke are more appropriately treated as external costs.

Similarly, only the healthcare and other costs that are not covered privately would be included as social costs in the conventional economist's accounting framework. In most high-income countries, where a substantial portion of healthcare is publicly provided, the social costs from treating tobacco-related illnesses will be substantial. In many low- and middle-income countries, however, where there is less publicly provided healthcare, and where the health consequences of smoking and other tobacco use are only beginning to appear, these costs will be modest. They will, however, grow over time as public insurance programs are adopted and as the health toll from tobacco grows. Moreover, even if there were no changes in public insurance, tobacco use would impose a significant social cost as a result of the increased demand for healthcare to treat tobacco-related illnesses, driving up the costs of all medical care, including that consumed by people who do not consume tobacco products.

A more difficult conceptual issue relates to determining whether or not the effects of an individual's tobacco use on his or her spouse and children should be included as an internal or external cost. Many of the economic studies on the social costs of smoking treat the family as the decision-making unit, with the earliest studies assuming that all of the health consequences of ETS exposure occurred within the family (i.e. Manning *et al.* 1991). Given the assumption that the family is the decision-making unit, the health consequences of a child's exposure to environmental tobacco smoke produced by parents' smoking would be considered an internal rather than external cost. Although many economists would accept treating the health costs of spouses as internal costs, there is considerable debate on applying this approach to fetuses and children who are relatively powerless to alter parents' consumption decisions that affect their health (see Chapter 7 for further discussion). Moreover, the disease and developmental problems associated with fetal and infant exposure to tobacco smoke have support costs that spill over into the broader society, as public institutions in many societies pick up part of the medical, institutional, and other costs related to these problems. Similarly, as information on the health consequences of ETS exposure has increased, it has become clear that many of these costs are external to the family.

A more controversial question concerns the inclusion of transfers in the calculations of external costs. These transfers include the reduction in income taxes and insurance premiums paid by tobacco users because of reduced earnings associated with tobacco-related illnesses, the value of public and private retirement pensions foregone because of tobacco-attributable premature deaths, higher healthcare costs paid by public and private insurance plans that result from treating illnesses related to tobacco use, and the increased sick pay and disability benefits paid during these illnesses. Particularly objectionable to many is the idea that foregone public and private pension benefits should be considered a 'benefit' to non-tobacco users in the computation of the social costs of tobacco use. In high-income countries, where publicly financed retirement programs are important, the inclusion of the 'benefits' from tobacco-attributable premature death significantly reduces the estimates of the net social costs of tobacco use (i.e. Shoven *et al.* 1989; Manning *et al.* 1991; Viscusi 1995). In contrast, in most low- and middle-income countries, where old-age expenses are largely a private matter, the inclusion of these 'benefits' would have little impact on the estimated social costs.

As this discussion clearly demonstrates, the calculation of the 'true' net social costs of tobacco use is an exceedingly difficult challenge that involves difficult conceptual questions, epidemiologic and other data considerations, and moving targets in terms of both knowledge and institutional structures. More research is clearly required, particularly for low-income and middle-income countries, given the relevance of this task to determining economically efficient levels of tobacco taxes.

10.4.4 Public health standards

As the review of the studies on the demands for tobacco products clearly demonstrated, increases in the taxes on and prices of these products lead to substantial reductions in cigarette smoking and other tobacco use. These reductions are not limited to reductions in the frequency or quantity of tobacco products consumed, but also include reduced initiation among youth and young adults, and increased cessation among adults. Given the substantial health consequences of tobacco use and the significant health benefits from cessation (see Chapter 2 and Chapter 12), millions of premature, tobacco-related deaths could be averted by large increases in cigarette and other tobacco taxes.

The econometric evidence on the direct relationship between higher tobacco taxes and the health consequences of tobacco use is limited to two recent studies from the US (Moore 1996; Evans and Ringel, in press). Moore, using state-level data on tobacco-related death rates for the period from 1954 through 1988, concluded that higher cigarette taxes would significantly reduce smoking-related deaths. His estimates imply that a 10% increase in the cigarette tax would result in approximately 6000 fewer premature, smoking-related deaths in the United States each year. Similarly, Evans and Ringel (1999) used data on over 10.5 million births in the United States during the years from 1989 through 1992 to examine the impact of cigarette smoking and cigarette taxes on the incidence of low-birthweight births. They estimated a smoking prevalence elasticity of – 0.5 for pregnant women and, consistent with the medical literature, found a strong positive relationship between cigarette smoking and the probability of a low-birthweight infant, leading them to conclude that increased cigarette taxes would significantly raise birthweight and reduce the adverse health and developmental consequences associated with low birthweight .

Similarly, several researchers in the United States have used estimates of the price-elasticities of smoking prevalence for different age groups to predict the likely impact of increased cigarette taxes, concluding that large tax increases would delay hundreds of thousands of premature, smoking-related deaths (Warner 1986; Harris 1987; US General Accounting Office 1989; Chaloupka 1998). Elsewhere in this volume, Ranson *et al.* employ a similar methodology to estimate the health benefits of global increases in the prices of cigarettes and other tobacco products (Chapter 18). Even under relatively conservative assumptions about the impact of price increases on demand and the impact of tobacco use on health, they conclude that millions of premature deaths could be avoided over the next several decades with even modest increases in tobacco taxes and prices.

10.5 Other issues in tobacco taxation

10.5.1 Tobacco tax earmarking

A significant feature of the tobacco tax structure in a growing number of countries is the hypothecation or earmarking of tobacco tax revenues for spending on specific activities. In part, these earmarked taxes reflect the growing use of increased tobacco taxes as a way to promote public health and/or more directly cover the social costs resulting from cigarette smoking and other tobacco use. For example, governments in several countries, including one of China's largest cities (Chongqing) and several US states (most notably California, Massachusetts, Arizona, and Oregon) earmark a portion of tobacco taxes for tobacco-related education, counter-advertising, and other tobacco-control activities. Still others dedicate a portion of their tobacco tax revenues to funding healthcare for under-insured populations, cancer control research, and other health-related activities, as well as, in others, general education (e.g. Canada, Ecuador, Finland, French Polynesia, Guam, Iceland, Indonesia, Korea, Malaysia, Nepal, Peru, Poland, Portugal, Romania, the United States, and others). Similarly, several Australian states, New Zealand, and others have adopted the 'Vic-Health model', using tobacco tax revenues to fund sporting and artistic events previously funded by the tobacco industry. An often debated, but yet to be adopted, form of earmarked tobacco taxes would dedicate a portion of the taxes to helping tobacco farmers and those employed in the manufacturing of tobacco products move into other crops and industries.

Many public finance economists have long opposed earmarked taxes because of the rigidities they introduce that make it more difficult to allocate general revenues among competing uses, while others have argued that the use of earmarked tobacco taxes to fund health promotion and disease prevention is consistent with the 'benefit principle' of taxation and can reduce the loss of producer and/or consumer surplus resulting from higher taxes (Hu *et al.* 1998). Moreover, given that many publicly provided health insurance programs target lower-income populations, this type of earmarking is consistent with an overall system of taxes and transfers that promotes vertical equity. Similarly, to the extent that tobacco farmers and those employed in tobacco manufacturing bear part of the burden of increased tobacco taxes in the short run (although, as described in Chapter 13, the impact of higher taxes on tobacco-related employment has been overstated by the tobacco industry), earmarking part of the new revenues from tobacco tax increases for crop-substitution and retraining programs can significantly reduce the impact on tobacco growers and producers. As Hu and his colleagues described, many of the activities funded by earmarked tobacco taxes significantly reduce the welfare losses resulting from tobacco tax increases.

Moreover, tobacco tax increases that are earmarked for anti-tobacco media campaigns, prevention programs, subsidization of tobacco cessation products and programs, and other activities to reduce tobacco use, generate even larger reductions in tobacco use and improvements in health than the tax increase alone. As described by Saffer (Chapter 9), Kenkel and Chen (Chapter 8), and Novotny *et al.* (Chapter 12), the variety of anti-tobacco activities funded by earmarked tobacco taxes have led to reductions in cigarette smoking and other tobacco use that exceed those that would have been achieved in the absence of earmarking.

10.5.2 Tobacco tax increases and consumer price indices

Opponents of tobacco tax increases have argued that tax hikes would be inflationary, given that tobacco products are included in the basket of goods and services used in computing price indices in most countries, and given that many wages and salaries, and other public and private expenditures, are tied to these indices. While it is true that large tobacco tax increases would lead to increases in prices as measured by most consumer price indices, the impact of large tax increases on inflation would be very modest. Moreover, relatively modest tax increases would have almost no detectable effect on these indices.

One possible solution to the potential inflationary impact of tobacco tax increases is the construction of multiple price indices that are used for different purposes, as has been done in a number of countries. France, Luxembourg, and Belgium, for example, compute one consumer price index that excludes tobacco products and a second that includes these products. The latter is used for historical and international comparisons, while the former (excluding tobacco products) is used for the indexation of wages and social security allowances (Joossens, personal communication). Sweden did the same with petroleum products in the 1980s (Nordgren, personal communication).

10.5.3 Tobacco taxation and other market failures

As described more fully by Jha *et al.* (Chapter 7) and Kenkel and Chen (Chapter 8), there are other failures in the tobacco markets that justify government intervention in these markets, most notably the imperfect information in these markets. While many of the health consequences of cigarette smoking and other tobacco use are well known, others are continually being discovered. Similarly, while some populations are well aware of these risks (i.e. more educated persons), others are much less informed and/or myopically discount away the future health and other consequences of tobacco use to their later regret. Moreover, even though the risks of tobacco use are generally under-stood in some countries (Viscusi 1992), tobacco users in these countries do not neces-sarily internalize these risks (Schoenbaum 1997). This suggests that the prevalence of tobacco use is much higher than it would be if users were well informed about the risks from tobacco use and appropriately internalized these risks.

Governments could use a variety of policies, including the increased taxation of tobacco products, to correct for these other market failures (see Chapter 7 for a dis-cussion of alternative approaches). While clearly an appropriate tool for correcting for the net social costs of tobacco use, tobacco taxes are, in some respects, a less than ideal approach to correcting for these other market failures. Specifically, tobacco taxation is a blunt policy tool that reduces the welfare of tobacco users who choose to use these products with a clear understanding of the consequences of their addiction. However, in the absence of adequate knowledge, higher taxes can be justified (Cordes *et al.* 1990). This is particularly true when it comes to tobacco use among youth. A group of leading health economists who have studied the economics of tobacco use recently concluded that protecting children from a future of nicotine addiction, with its associated health risks, was the most compelling reason favoring increased tobacco taxation (Warner *et al.* 1995). They perceived higher taxes as an appropriate way to balance children's inad-equate perceptions concerning the addictive nature of tobacco products and their relatively myopic behavior that discounts away the future health consequences of tobacco use, as well as an environment in which tobacco companies' multi-billion dollar advertising and promotion campaigns target youth. Given their relatively more elastic demands for tobacco products, the benefits from the large reductions in youth tobacco use resulting from a tax increase would be substantially larger than the losses incurred by adult tobacco users. Similar arguments could be made for other less-informed popu-lations that are relatively more responsive to price, including less educated and lower income groups.

10.5.4 Barriers to tobacco taxation

There are a number of political, economic, and social arguments that have long been used as arguments against significant increases in cigarette and other tobacco taxes. Upon more careful analysis, however, these arguments are not persuasive and should not be used to discourage governments from raising tobacco taxes. Objections to higher taxes include the following: that higher tobacco taxes will lead to significant increases in smuggling between high-tax and low-tax countries; that tobacco tax increases necessarily place a disproportionate burden on the poor; that higher tobacco taxes will lead to reductions in tobacco tax revenues; and that tobacco tax hikes will lead to significant reductions in employment and macro-economic activity. This section briefly addresses these arguments; more detailed discussions are contained in other sections of this chapter and other chapters in this volume.

Tax increases and smuggling

It has been argued that higher tobacco taxes will lead to increased smuggling and related criminal activity, while not reducing tobacco consumption or increasing tobacco tax revenues. While it is true that cigarette smuggling is a serious problem and that tax increases can lead to increases in smuggling, the scale of the problem has been significantly overstated (see Chapter 15 and Chapter 16). Numerous countries have significantly increased tobacco taxes without experiencing dramatic increases in smuggling. Likewise, sharp, industry-initiated price increases in some countries have not led to a significant rise in smuggling in these countries. Moreover, several relatively easy-to-implement policies, including improved tracking of cigarette consignments and stronger penalties for smugglers who are detected, could be used to address this problem.

Tobacco tax increases and the poor

A second common objection to tobacco tax increases is that they will fall disproportionately on the poor. While it is true that current tobacco taxes are regressive in most countries, given that tobacco use is more prevalent among those with lower incomes, a growing literature suggests that tobacco tax *increases* might be progressive. As described above, several recent studies conclude that lower income persons are more responsive to changes in cigarette prices than higher income persons, implying that increased cigarette taxes would reduce smoking by more in lower income groups than in higher income groups, reducing the relative burden of tobacco taxes on the poor. Moreover, tobacco taxes are but one part of an overall fiscal system that in most countries includes a wide variety of other taxes and transfer programs, suggesting that increased progressivity of other tax and transfer programs could be used to offset the regressivity of tobacco taxes. This is most clearly the case when the new revenues generated from tobacco tax increases are earmarked for programs that target low-income populations.

Tobacco tax increases and revenues

A third frequent misperception, often coupled with the first, is that increases in tobacco taxes will actually lead to reductions in tobacco tax revenues. Those making this argument suggest that the reductions in tobacco sales resulting from the tax increase would be so large as to more than offset the impact of the higher tax rate. Given the relatively inelastic demand for tobacco products and the current share of tobacco taxes in price, nearly every country has substantial room for increasing tobacco tax revenues by increasing tobacco taxes. Estimates described by Sunley *et al.* (Chapter 17) indicate that a relatively modest increase of 10% in cigarette taxes would lead to an increase of almost 7%, on average, in cigarette tax revenues. Moreover, even in countries where demand is relatively more elastic and taxes account for a relatively high share of tobacco prices, increases in these taxes will lead to increases in tax revenues.

Tobacco tax increases and the macro-economy

A final argument that is often employed in the debate over increased cigarette taxes is that these tax increases would lead to significant reductions in employment in tobacco growing and manufacturing, as well as more general wholesaling, retailing, and other sectors. Consequently, opponents argue, the tax increases would have an adverse impact on the macro-economy. While it is true that employment in jobs directly related to tobacco growing and manufacturing would decline as a result of the reductions in tobacco consumption induced by the tax increase, the impact on other sectors is likely to be minimal. Moreover, as described more fully by Jacobs *et al.* (Chapter 13), employment in other areas would likely increase as the money smokers would have spent on tobacco products is spent on other goods and services, with the net macro-economic impact of higher tobacco taxes being negligible or positive in all but a very few countries.

10.6 Conclusions

Several clear conclusions emerge from the review of the economics literature on tobacco taxation contained in this chapter.

Increases in cigarette and other tobacco taxes will significantly reduce both the prevalence and consumption of tobacco products. Estimates from numerous studies indicate that the short-run price-elasticity of cigarette demand in high-income countries is in the range from -0.25 to -0.5 implying that a tax increase that raises prices by 10% will reduce cigarette smoking by up to 5%. Several studies indicate that increased taxes will be particularly effective in reducing tobacco use among youth and young adults, for whom demand is estimated to be up to three times more sensitive to price. The reductions are the result of reduced initiation of tobacco use, increased cessation, and reductions in the consumption of tobacco products by continuing users.

Emerging evidence from low-income and middle-income countries, as well as recent research on different socio-economic groups in high-income countries, implies that the effects of tobacco tax increases in developing countries would be larger than the impact of comparable increases in high-income countries. These recent studies suggest that the short-run price-responsiveness of cigarette demand in low- and middle-income countries is about double that in high-income countries. Thus, a tax increase that raises tobacco product prices by 10% in low-income and middle-income countries would lead to a reduction of approximately 8% in tobacco use in these countries.

Large tobacco tax increases, by significantly reducing the prevalence of tobacco use, would have a major impact on the health and other consequences of tobacco use. Even relatively modest increases in taxes would generate significant health benefits. Estimates indicate that global cigarette tax increases that raised prices by 10% everywhere would reduce premature deaths attributable to smoking by approximately 10 million in the current cohort of smokers (see Chapter 18). Almost 90% of these extended lives would be for persons in low- and middle-income countries.

Given the inelasticity of the demands for tobacco products in most countries, increases in tobacco taxes will result in sizable increases in tobacco tax revenues. Given existing tax levels, nearly every country has significant scope for generating new tax revenues through large tobacco tax increases. Estimates suggest that a 10% cigarette tax increase will lead to an average increase of nearly 7% in cigarette tax revenues in the short-run. Larger increases in revenues are expected in countries where demand is relatively more inelastic, while smaller, but still sizable, increases are expected in counties where demand is more responsive to price.

Significant increases in tobacco taxes can be justified on several grounds, including as a relatively efficient tool for generating tax revenues, as a means to reduce inequity, as an appropriate way to promote economic efficiency, as an effective approach to improving public health, and as a way to correct for the market failures inherent in the markets for tobacco products. Given the relatively low levels of cigarette and other tobacco taxes in many low- and middle-income countries, as well as in several high-income countries, a policy that aimed these taxes to the point where they account for two-thirds to three-quarters of the retail prices of tobacco products appears achievable and appropriate.

Earmarking of revenues from higher tobacco taxes is consistent with many of the principles of appropriate tax policy and is likely to produce larger reductions in tobacco use and greater health benefits than would result from the higher taxes alone. The use of these revenues for mass-media campaigns on the health consequences of tobacco use, increased accessibility to nicotine-replacement products and other approaches to smoking cessation, particularly for low-income smokers, and the public provision of medical care are but a few examples of what many countries are doing and/or can do with earmarked tobacco taxes.

References

Ashenfelter, O. and Sullivan, D. (1987). Nonparametric tests of market structure: an application to the cigarette industry. *Journal of Industrial Economics*, **35**(4), 483–98.

Baltagi, B. H. and Levin, D. (1986). Estimating dynamic demand for cigarettes using panel data: the effects of bootlegging, taxation, and advertising reconsidered. *Review of Economics and Statistics*, **68**(1), 148–55.

Bardsley, P. and Olekalns, N. (1998). *Cigarette and Tobacco Consumption: Have Anti-smoking Policies Made a Difference?* Working Paper. Department of Economics, The University of Melbourne.

Barnett, P. G., Keeler, T. E., and Hu, T.-W. (1995). Oligopoly structure and the incidence of cigarette excise taxes. *Journal of Public Economics*, **57**(3), 457–70.

Barzel, Y. (1976). An alternative approach to the analysis of taxation. *Journal of Political Economy*, **84**(6), 1177–97.

Becker, G. S. and Murphy, K. M. (1988). A theory of rational addiction. *Journal of Political Economy*, **96**(4), 675–700.

Becker, G. S., Grossman, M., and Murphy, K. M. (1994). An empirical analysis of cigarette addiction. *American Economic Review*, **84**(3), 396–418.

Bishop, J. A. and Yoo, J. H. (1985). 'Health scare,' excise taxes and advertising ban in the cigarette demand and supply. *Southern Economic Journal*, **52**(2), 402–11.

Bulow, J. I. and Pfleiderer, P. (1983). A note on the effect of cost changes on prices. *Journal of Political Economy*, **91**(1), 182–5.

Cameron, S. (1997). Are Greek smokers rational addicts? *Applied Economics Letters*, **4**(7), 401–2.

Chaloupka, F. J. (1991). Rational addictive behavior and cigarette smoking. *Journal of Political Economy*, **99**(4), 722–42.

Chaloupka, F. J. (1998). *The Impact of Proposed Cigarette Price Increases*. Policy Analysis No. 9, Health Sciences Analysis Project. Washington: Advocacy Institute.

Chaloupka, F. J. and Grossman, M. (1996). *Price, Tobacco Control Policies and Youth Smoking*. National Bureau of Economic Research Working Paper No. 5740.

Chaloupka, F. J. and Pacula, R. L. (1999). Sex and race differences in young people's responsiveness to price and tobacco control policies. *Tobacco Control*, **8**(4), 373–7.

Chaloupka, F. J. and Warner, K. E. The economics of smoking. In *The Handbook of Health Economics* (ed. J. P. Newhouse and A. J. Culyer). New York: North-Holland. (In press.)

Chaloupka, F. J. and Wechsler, H. (1997). Price, tobacco control policies and smoking among young adults. *Journal of Health Economics*, **16**(3), 359–73.

Chaloupka, F. J., Tauras, J. A., and Grossman, M. (1997). Public policy and youth smokeless tobacco use. *Southern Economic Journal*, **64**(2), 503–16.

Chapman, S. and Richardson, J. (1990). Tobacco excise and declining consumption: The case of Papua New Guinea. *American Journal of Public Health*, **80**(5), 537–40.

Conniffe, D. (1995). Models of Irish tobacco consumption. *Economic and Social Review*, **26**(4), 331–47.

Cook, P. J. and Moore, M. J. (1993). Taxation of alcoholic beverages. In *Economics and the Prevention of Alcohol-Related Problems* (ed. M. E. Hilton and G. Bloss G), pp. 33–58. Research monograph no. 25. Rockville (MD): US Department of Health and Human Services, Public Health Service, National Institutes of Health, National Institute on Alcohol Abuse and Alcoholism. NIH Publication No. 93–3513.

Cordes, J. J., Nicholson, E. M., and Sammartino, F. J. (1990). Raising revenue by taxing activities with social costs. *National Tax Journal*, **43**(3), 343–56.

Costa e Silva, V. L. (1998). The Brazilian cigarette industry: Prospects for consumption reduction. In *The Economics of Tobacco Control: Towards an Optimal Policy Mix* (ed. I. Abedian, R. van der Merwe, N. Wilkins, and P. Jha), pp. 336–49. Cape Town (South Africa): Applied Fiscal Reseach Centre, University of Cape Town.

DeCicca, P., Kenkel, D., and Mathios, A. (1998). *Putting Out the Fires: Will Higher Cigarette Taxes Reduce Youth Smoking?*. Working Paper. Department of Policy Analysis and Management, Cornell University.

Dee, T. S. and Evans, W. N. (1998). *A Comment on DeCicca, Kenkel, and Mathios*. Working Paper. School of Economics, Georgia Institute of Technology.

Dillow, G. L. (1981). Thank you for not smoking: The hundred-year war against the cigarette. *American Heritage*, **32**, 94–107.

Douglas, S. (1998). The duration of the smoking habit. *Economic Inquiry*, **36**(1), 49–64.

Douglas, S. and Hariharan, G. (1994). The hazard of starting smoking: estimates from a split population duration model. *Journal of Health Economics*, **13**(2), 213–30.

Duffy, M. (1996). An econometric study of advertising and cigarette demand in the United Kingdom. *International Journal of Advertising*, **15**, 262–84.

Elster, J. (1979). *Ulysses and the Sirens: Studies in Rationality and Irrationality*. Cambridge: Cambridge University Press.

Evans, W. N. and Farrelly, M. C. (1998). The compensating behavior of smokers: taxes, tar and nicotine. *RAND Journal of Economics*, **29**(3), 578–95.

Evans, W. N. and Huang, L. X. (1998). *Cigarette Taxes and Teen Smoking: New Evidence From Panels of Repeated Cross-Sections*. Working paper. Department of Economics, University of Maryland.

Evans, W. N. and Ringel, J. S. (1999). Can higher cigarette taxes improve birth outcomes? *Journal of Public Economics*, **72**, 135–54.

Grossman, M. and Chaloupka, F. J. (1997). Cigarette taxes: The straw to break the camel's back. *Public Health Reports*, **112**(4), 290–7.

Harris, J. E. (1987). The 1983 increase in the federal cigarette excise tax. In *Tax Policy and the Economy*, Vol. 1 (ed. L. H. Summers), pp. 87–111. Cambridge (MA): MIT Press.

Hsieh, C. R. and Hu, T. W. (1997). *The Demand for Cigarettes in Taiwan: Domestic versus*

Imported Cigarettes. Discussion Paper No. 9701. Nankang, Taipei: The Institute of Economics, Academia Sinica.

Hu, T. W. (1997). Cigarette taxation in China: Lessons from international experiences. *Tobacco Control*, 6(2), 136–40.

Hu, T. W., Xu, X. P., and Keeler, T. (1998). Earmarked tobacco taxes: lessons learned. In *The Economics of Tobacco Control: Towards an Optimal Policy Mix* (ed. I. Abedian, R. van der Merwe, N. Wilkins, and P. Jha), pp. 102–18. Cape Town (South Africa): Applied Fiscal Reseach Centre, University of Cape Town.

Johnson, T. R. (1978). Additional evidence on the effects of alternative taxes on cigarette prices. *Journal of Political Economy*, 86(2, Part 1), 325–8.

Keeler, T. E., Hu, T.-W., Barnett, P. G., and Manning, W. G. (1993). Taxation, regulation and addiction: a demand function for cigarettes based on time-series evidence. *Journal of Health Economics*, 12(1), 1–18.

Keeler, T. E., Hu, T.-W., Barnett, P. G., and Manning, W. G. (1996). Do cigarette producers price-discriminate by state? An empirical analysis of local cigarette pricing and taxation. *Journal of Health Economics*, 15, 499–512.

Leu, R. E. (1984). Anti-smoking publicity, taxation, and the demand for cigarettes. *Journal of Health Economics*, 3(2), 101–16.

Levin, M. (1998). Tobacco memos show overseas price fixing. *Los Angeles Times*, September 17. (On-line.)

Lewit, E. M. and Coate, D. (1982). The potential for using excise taxes to reduce smoking. *Journal of Health Economics*, 1(2), 121–45.

Lewit, E. M., Coate, D., and Grossman, M. (1981). The effects of government regulation on teenage smoking. *Journal of Law and Economics*, 24(3), 545–69.

Lewit, E. M., Hyland, A., Kerrebrock, N., and Cummings, K. M. (1997). Price, public policy and smoking in young people. *Tobacco Control*, 6(S2), 17–24.

Manning, W. G., Keeler, E. B., Newhouse, J. P., Sloss, E. M., and Wasserman, J. (1991). *The Costs of Poor Health Habits*. Cambridge (MA): Harvard University Press.

Mao, Z. Z. and Xiang, J. L. (1997). Demand for cigarettes and factors affecting the demand: a cross-sectional survey. *Chinese Healthcare Industry Management*, 5, 227–9. (In Chinese.)

Mao, Z. Z., Xiang, J. L., and Kon, Z. P. (1997). Demand for cigarette and pricing policy. *Chinese Health Economics*, 16(6), 50–2. (In Chinese.)

Maranvanyika, E. (1998). The search for an optimal tobacco control policy in Zimbabwe. In *The Economics of Tobacco Control: Towards an Optimal Policy Mix* (ed. I. Abedian, R. van der Merwe, N. Wilkins, and P. Jha), pp. 272–81. Cape Town (South Africa): Applied Fiscal Reseach Centre, University of Cape Town.

Moore, M. J. (1996). Death and tobacco taxes. *RAND Journal of Economics*, 27(2), 415–28.

Mullahy, J. (1985). Cigarette smoking: habits, health concerns, and heterogeneous unobservables in a micro-econometric analysis of consumer demand [dissertation]. Charlottesville (VA): University of Virginia.

Ohsfeldt, R. L. and Boyle, R. G. (1994). Tobacco excise taxes and rates of smokeless tobacco use in the US: an exploratory ecological analysis. *Tobacco Control*, 3(4), 316–23.

Ohsfeldt, R. L. and Boyle, R. G. (1997). Capilouto EI. Effects of tobacco excise taxes on the use of smokeless tobacco products. *Health Economics*, 6(5), 525–32.

Ohsfeldt, R. L., Boyle, R. G., and Capilouto, E. I. (1999). Tobacco taxes, smoking restrictions, and tobacco use. In *The Economic Analysis of Substance Use and Abuse: an Integration of Econometric and Behavioral Economic Research* (ed. F. J. Chaloupka, M. Grossman, W. K. Bickel, and H. Saffer), pp. 15–29. Chicago: University of Chicago Press for the National Bureau of Economic Research.

Pekurinen, M. (1989). The demand for tobacco products in Finland. *British Journal of Addiction*, 84, 1183–92.

Pekurinen, M. (1991). *Economic Aspects of Smoking: Is There a Case for Government Intervention in Finland?* Helsinki: Vapk-Publishing.

Pigou, A. C. (1962). *A Study in Public Finance*, 3rd revised edn. London: Macmillan and Co.

Ramsey, F. P. (1927). A contribution to the theory of taxation. *Economic Journal*, **37**, 47–61.

Schelling, T. C. (1978). Egonomics, or the art of self-management. *American Economic Review*, **68**, 290–4.

Schelling, T. C. (1984). Self-command in practice, in policy, and in a theory of rational choice. *American Economic Review*, **74**, 1–11.

Schoenbaum, M. (1997). Do smokers understand the mortality effects of smoking? Evidence from the Health and Retirement Survey. *American Journal of Public Health*, **87**(5), 755–9.

Shoven, J. B., Sundberg, J. O., and Bunker, J. P. (1989). The social security cost of smoking. In *The Economics of Aging* (ed. D. A. Wise), pp. 231–54. Chicago: University of Chicago Press.

Smith, A. (1776). *An Inquiry Into the Nature and Causes of the Wealth of Nations* (ed. E. Canaan). Chicago: University of Chicago Press.

Sullivan, D. (1985). Testing hypotheses about firm behavior in the cigarette industry. *Journal of Political Economy*, **93**(3), 586–98.

Sumner, D. A. (1981). Measurement of monopoly behavior: an application to the cigarette industry. *Journal of Political Economy*, **89**(5), 1010–9.

Sumner, D. A. and Wohlgenant, M. K. (1985). Effects of an increase in the federal excise tax on cigarettes. *American Journal of Agricultural Economics*, **67**(2), 235–42.

Sumner, M. T. and Ward, R. (1981). Tax changes and cigarette prices. *Journal of Political Economy*, **89**(6), 1261–5.

Sung, H.-Y., Hu, T.-W., and Keeler, T. E. (1994). Cigarette taxation and demand: an empirical model. *Contemporary Economic Policy*, **12**(3), 91–100.

Sunley, E. M. (1998). *The Design and Administration of Alcohol, Tobacco and Petroleum Excises: a Guide for Developing and Transition Countries*. Working Paper, Fiscal Affairs Department, International Monetary Fund.

Tansel, A. (1993). Cigarette demand, health scares and education in Turkey. *Applied Economics*, **25**(4), 521–9.

Tauras, J. A. and Chaloupka, F. J. (1999). *Price, Clean Indoor Air Laws, and Cigarette Smoking: Evidence from Longitudinal Data for Young Adults*. National Bureau of Economic Research Working Paper No. 6937.

Thompson, M. E. and McLeod, I. (1976). The effects of economic variables upon the demand for cigarettes in Canada. *Mathematical Scientist*, **1**, 121–32.

Townsend, J. L. (1993). Policies to halve smoking deaths. *Addiction*, **88**, 43–52.

Townsend, J. L. (1998). The role of taxation policy in tobacco control. In *The Economics of Tobacco Control: Towards an Optimal Policy Mix* (ed. I. Abedian, R. van der Merwe, N. Wilkins, and P. Jha), pp. 85–101. Cape Town (South Africa): Applied Fiscal Reseach Centre, University of Cape Town.

Townsend, J. L., Roderick, P., and Cooper, J. (1994). Cigarette smoking by socio-economic group, sex, and age: effects of price, income, and health publicity. *British Medical Journal*, **309**(6959), 923–6.

US Centers for Disease Control and Prevention (1998). Response to increases in cigarette prices by race/ethnicity, income, and age groups—United States 1976–1993. *Morbidity and Mortality Weekly Report*, **47**(29), 605–9.

US Congressional Budget Office (1990). *Federal Taxation of Tobacco, Alcoholic Beverages, and Motor Fuels*. Washington: US Government Printing Office.

US Department of Health and Human Services (989). *Reducing the Health Consequences of Smoking: 25 Years of Progress. A Report of the Surgeon General*. Atlanta: US Department of Health and Human Services, Public Health Service, Centers for Disease Control, National Center for Chronic Disease Prevention and Health Promotion, Office of Smoking and Health. DHHS Publication No. (CDC) 89–8411.

US Department of Health and Human Services (1992). *Smoking and Health in the Americas: a 1992 Report of the Surgeon General in Collaboration with the Pan American Health Organi-*

zation. Atlanta: US Department of Health and Human Services, Public Health Service, Centers for Disease Control, National Center for Chronic Disease Prevention and Health Promotion, Office of Smoking and Health.. DHHS Publication No. (CDC) 92–8419.

US Department of Health and Human Services. *Reducing Tobacco Use: a Report of the Surgeon General*. Atlanta: US Department of Health and Human Services, Public Health Service, Centers for Disease Control, National Center for Chronic Disease Prevention and Health Promotion, Office of Smoking and Health. (In press.)

US General Accounting Office (1989). *Teenage Smoking: Higher Excise Tax Should Significantly Reduce the Number of Smokers*. Washington: General Accounting Office.

van der Merwe, R. (1998). The economics of tobacco control in South Africa. In *The Economics of Tobacco Control: Towards an Optimal Policy Mix* (ed. I. Abedian, R. van der Merwe, N. Wilkins, and P. Jha), pp. 251–71. Cape Town (South Africa): Applied Fiscal Reseach Centre, University of Cape Town.

Viscusi, W. K. (1992). *Smoking: Making the Risky Decision*. New York, Oxford University Press.

Viscusi, W. K. (1995). Cigarette taxation and the social consequences of smoking. In *Tax Policy and the Economy* (ed. J. M. Poterba), pp. 51–101. Cambridge (MA): Massachusetts Institute of Technology Press.

Wagner, S. (1971). *Cigarette Country: Tobacco in America, History and Politics*. New York: Praeger Publishers.

Warner, K. E. (1986). Smoking and health implications of a change in the federal cigarette excise tax. *Journal of the American Medical Association*, **255**(8), 1028–32.

Warner, K. E. (1990). Tobacco taxation as health policy in the Third World. *American Journal of Public Health*, **80**, 529–31.

Warner, K. E., Chaloupka, F. J., Cook, P. J. *et al.* (1995). Criteria for determining an optimal cigarette tax. *Tobacco Control*, **4**, 380–6.

Wasserman, J., Manning, W. G., Newhouse, J. P., and Winkler, J. D. (1991). The effects of excise taxes and regulations on cigarette smoking. *Journal of Health Economics*, **10**(1), 43–64.

Winston, G. C. (1980). Addiction and backsliding: a theory of compulsive consumption. *Journal of Economic Behavior and Organization*, **1**(4), 295–324.

Xu, X., Hu, T.-W., and Keeler, T. E. (1998). *Optimal Cigarette Taxation: Theory and Estimation*. Working Paper. Department of Economics, University of California, Berkeley.

Young, T. (1983). The demand for cigarettes: alternative specifications of Fujii's model. *Applied Economics*, **15**, 203–11.

11

Clean indoor-air laws and youth access restrictions

Trevor Woollery, Samira Asma, and Donald Sharp

The development of public policy on tobacco is incomplete without the consideration of clean indoor air and youth access policies. Clean indoor-air laws protect non-smokers from the dangers of environmental tobacco smoke and implicitly transfer property rights to ambient air from smokers to non-smokers, but also have economic costs for individuals and businesses. Numerous studies conclude that comprehensive clean indoor-air policies lead to significant reductions in smoking prevalence and average cigarette consumption among continuing smokers. Youth access laws limit the supply of tobacco products to adolescents, who are deemed too young to fully comprehend the risks of consuming tobacco products. The existing empirical evidence on the impact of limits on youth smoking is mixed. For both clean-air laws and youth access restrictions, economic theory justifies government intervention in an inefficient tobacco market. The laws work best when drafted comprehensively without pre-emptive provisions. Clean indoor-air policies can, in some instances, be self-enforcing, while youth access policies depend crucially on aggressive enforcement to ensure compliance. Overall, the global coverage of clean indoor air and youth access policies is minimal. While high-income countries as a group have histories of clean indoor air and, to a lesser extent, youth access laws, low-income and middle-income countries are in the nascent stages of developing such policies.

11.1 Introduction

In addition to measures that raise prices and increase information, governments that seek to reduce demand for tobacco may consider policies for clean indoor air and youth access restrictions. Both policies are justified on economic efficiency grounds (see Chapter 7). Clean indoor-air policies are important because they partly address the external physical costs that are borne by non-smokers exposed to environmental tobacco smoke (ETS). Youth access policies are salient because young people do not know how to assess or accurately appreciate the risks of consuming tobacco products and becoming addicted to nicotine.

Clean-air laws explicitly transfer 'ambient air' property rights from smokers to non-smokers (US Department of Health and Human Services (USDHHS) 1986; California Environmental Protection Agency (California EPA) 1997; National Cancer Institute (NCI 1999). As clean-air laws become more restrictive and comprehensive, however, they impose additional costs on smokers. For some smokers, these higher costs will result in reduced cigarette consumption or cessation. In contrast, youth access restrictions assume that minors should be protected from the inherent dangers of tobacco, since they do not know how to assess or accurately appreciate the risks of becoming addicted to nicotine (USDHHS 1994). Youth access restrictions aim, in effect, to raise the costs of smoking for adolescents to such high levels that few children would begin to smoke, and so that young smokers would find it difficult to continue.

This chapter is in four parts. First, the effectiveness of clean indoor-air laws and their costs are reviewed. Second, the impact of youth access restrictions and the associated costs of ensuring compliance are described. Third, the relevance of these tobacco-control policies to low-income and middle-income countries is discussed. Finally, con-clusions are presented and research priorities are discussed. It is important to note that this chapter draws heavily on studies in North America. Clean-air laws and youth restrictions have been the focus of many of the tobacco-control efforts in North America, and specifically the United States. North American settings tend to have higher levels of general awareness about the risks of tobacco use, more spending on tobacco control programs, and greater administrative capacity than their counterparts in other countries. Consequently, there may be some difficulty in exporting the policy lessons from these countries to low-income and middle-income countries. Nonetheless, the lessons learned in North America could be instructive in drafting tobacco-control policies in low-income and middle-income countries, and in spurring research.

11.2 Clean air policies

11.2.1 Definition

Clean indoor-air laws are inextricably linked to the growing scientific evidence on the health risks faced by non-smokers exposed to second-hand or environmental tobacco smoke (ETS) (USDHHS 1986; California EPA 1997; NCI 1999). Clean indoor-air laws protect the public from ETS by transferring rights to ambient airspace from smokers to non-smokers, and they serve to reduce the social desirability of smoking. These laws typically prohibit smoking in one or more of the following locations: elevators, health-care facilities, public transportation, indoor cultural and recreational facilities, govern-ment buildings, public meeting rooms, schools, shopping malls, retail stores, and, in some jurisdictions, restaurants, bars, and private workplaces.

11.2.2 The effectiveness of clean-air laws

The evidence evaluating the effectiveness of smoking restrictions is considerable (see, for example, Warner 1981a, 1981b; Borland *et al.* 1990; Wasserman *et al.* 1991; Chaloupka 1992; Chaloupka and Saffer 1992; Evans *et al.* 1999; Yurekli and Zhang, 2000). On the whole, solid support is found for the hypotheses that restrictions on smoking in public places and private workplaces will reduce both smoking prevalence and average daily cigarette consumption among smokers. Wasserman *et al.* (1991), for example, in one of the earliest studies, found that overall per capita smoking was reduced by approximately 6% as a result of relatively restrictive clean indoor air policies.

Chaloupka and Saffer (1992) similarly explored the effect of clean indoor-air laws on the demand for cigarettes over time. The authors examined whether laws that prohibited cigarette smoking in a number of public places and restaurants, and laws that additionally regulated smoking in private work places, had different effects on demand. Estimating single-equation and simultaneous-equation econometric models, they concluded that the enactment of clean-air laws is a function of cigarette demand, implying that localities with low levels of cigarette sales are more likely to have adopted relatively comprehensive clean indoor-air laws (in particular, those that restrict smoking in private workplaces). This result is consistent with the conclusions of Warner (1981a, 1981b), who reported that regions where smoking is less prevalent are more likely to pass clean-air laws. Chaloupka and Saffer concluded that laws restricting smoking in public places and restaurants had a negative and significant impact on cigarette demand but, after accounting for the reverse causality, they concluded that laws restricting smoking in private workplaces had no additional impact. The authors noted that the weak effect of restricting smoking in private workplaces did not imply that smoking would not be reduced if such laws were more widespread. Rather, the results suggested that only US states with low levels of smoking due to strong anti-smoking sentiment had passed private workplace clean-air laws during the period covered by their data.

Using data from a large national US survey, Chaloupka (1992) explored the impact of clean-air laws on individuals' cigarette smoking in the context of an economic model of addiction. His analyses indicated that clean-air laws produced a statistically significant reduction in the demand for cigarettes. However, it did not appear that more restrictive laws had an increasingly large impact on cigarette consumption. It should be noted, however, that the apparent lack of a marginal effect of more extensive laws was likely due to the very small number of individuals (about 2.4% of the sample) living in states with very extensive clean indoor-air laws during the time period covered by his data.

More recent research by Yurekli and Zhang (2000), using more recent annual data for US states, reached the opposite conclusion. They created an index for clean indoor-air laws that assumes that the laws have a gradually growing impact on smoking over time. The index takes into account whether or not there are laws restricting smoking in the places where people spend most of their time. It also takes account of the level of smoking restrictions, such as whether there is a complete smoking ban or whether the restrictions allow for smoking in specific areas. They concluded that clean indoor-air laws significantly reduced per capita cigarette consumption, with greater reductions resulting from more comprehensive restrictions. Using their estimates, the authors predicted that consumption decreased by 4.8 packs per person per year in states that had adopted clean indoor-air laws.

In a critical review of evaluations of workplace health-promotion programs, published between 1968 and 1994, Eriksen and Gottlieb (1998) concluded that workplace smoking restrictions reduced smoking in these locations and, consequently, exposure to ETS. However, they found that the restrictions did not reduce smoking prevalence among workers. This is consistent with the findings of Borland *et al.* (1990) in Australia. They concluded that a smoking ban across the entire Australian Civil Service reduced cigarette consumption among smokers by 5.2 cigarettes per day but did not significantly affect smoking prevalence.

In contrast, Glasgow *et al.* (1997) used data from the Community Intervention Trial for Smoking Cessation (COMMIT) to examine the relationship between workplace smoking restrictions and changes in smoking behavior in a cohort of smokers. Their results revealed that employees who worked in a smoke-free workplace in 1988 were over 25% more likely to make a serious quit-attempt by 1993, and over 25% more likely to quit smoking, than those who worked where smoking was permitted. Among continuing smokers, those in smoke-free workplaces consumed an average of 2.75 fewer cigarettes per day than those who worked in places with a non-restrictive smoking policy. Based on these results, the authors estimated that if all workplaces in the United States were smoke-free, 178 000 smokers would quit.

In the most recent analysis of the impact of workplace smoking bans, Evans *et al.* (1999) developed a sophisticated simultaneous-equations econometric model that allowed for worker self-selection (i.e. the model allowed smokers and non-smokers to choose the type of clean-air environment they worked in). Estimates from their models indicated that workplace smoking bans reduced smoking prevalence by 4–6% and also reduced average daily cigarette consumption among smokers by 10%. Furthermore, they found that workplace smoking bans had the largest impact on workers who worked longer hours, and the smallest impact on part-time workers.

In addition, Evans and his colleagues examined the possibility that workplace smoking bans might impose economic costs on firms, if talented smokers (both current workers and new job applicants) strongly preferred employers with weak workplace smoking policies. If their empirical results were driven purely by worker self-selection or by the movement of smokers away from firms with smoking bans, then the effect of smoking bans would have been present only for new or recently hired workers. Their estimates, however, showed that smoking bans had the smallest effect on workers with the shortest length of service, and no systematic difference in service length was noted between workers from firms with smoking bans and firms without bans. Thus, they concluded that smoking bans did not result in the self-selection of workers at any significant level.

Finally, in addition to reducing overall smoking, clean indoor-air policies alter the smoking behavior of adolescents and young adults. Chaloupka and Wechsler (1997), for example, found that relatively strong restrictions, at state or local level, on smoking in public places resulted in reduced smoking prevalence in college students. Additionally, they found that some restrictions on public smoking led to further reductions in smoking by lowering average cigarette consumption among smokers. Chaloupka and Grossman (1996) found similar effects of strong restrictions on US adolescents.

11.2.3 Costs of clean-air laws

The costs of clean-air laws fall on smokers, firms, and society at large. The largest cost, and the hardest to quantify, is the extra cost imposed on smokers from having fewer opportunities to smoke and having to go elsewhere to smoke. These costs include the discomfort experienced from standing outside to smoke in the cold or heat, or of congregating in a room full of smokers to smoke, possibly exposing smokers to more smoke than they care to inhale. These extra costs to smokers are offset, however, by increased access to smoke-free places and reduced costs for non-smokers from ETS, nuisance, dry cleaning, and so on.

As arguments to counter the enactment of smoking restrictions, the tobacco and restaurant industries often present the possibility that substantial economic losses arise from these restrictions. For example, the National Smokers' Alliance in the United States, an organization funded by Philip Morris and other tobacco companies, claimed that restaurants and bars suffered a 15% loss of business from the enactment of the California law banning smoking in their premises in 1998. Furthermore, the American Beverage Institute reported that 60% of Californian bartenders surveyed suggested that they lost business and tips, and that 30% said there were layoffs or shorter workweeks for bar employees following the ban. These claims, however, have not been independently verified.

In contrast, several studies that use data from the receipts of taxable meals as a measure of business (Glantz and Smith 1994, 1997; Bartosch and Pope 1999; Hyland and Cummings 1999a, 1999b) found that there were no adverse economic effects of smoking restrictions. Similarly, other studies that considered effects on employment in the restaurant industry and the number of surviving operations showed that employment and the number of businesses increased after the implementation of smoking restrictions (Hyland and Cummings 1999a, 1999b).

More recently, concerns have been voiced by opponents of clean-air laws about their potential negative impacts on tourism. Empirical studies, however, find that clean-air laws have not harmed tourism revenues. Hyland *et al.* (1999), for example, analyzed taxable sales receipts in New York before and after the passage of New York City's smoke-free air law, and found that restaurant business grew after the law went into effect. In a broader study, Glantz and Charlesworth (1999) analyzed hotel revenues and tourism rates in areas that had passed laws requiring 100% smoke-free restaurants and compared these with figures from the United States overall. The authors found that international tourism was either unaffected or increased following the implementation of smoke-free laws. Specifically, a smoke-free restaurant law was associated with a statistically significant increase in hotel revenues in four localities and no significant change in four others.

In theory, a workplace smoking ban could reduce health and fire insurance premiums, reduce worker absenteeism, increase productivity, and reduce property damage and maintenance costs (Rice *et al.* 1986). The Office of Technology Assessment estimated that US smokers cost their employers between $2000 and $5000 annually, in increased healthcare and fire insurance premiums, absenteeism, lost productivity, and property damage (Warner 1994). Dow Chemical Company revealed that one of its divisions was losing about $600 000 annually from the absenteeism of ill smokers (Sculco 1992). Non-smokers work longer hours per day compared to their smoking peers because smokers take smoking breaks. In an effort to level the playing field, Thurrock council in Essex, England announced that smokers would be asked to sign a contract extending their working hours from 37 to 39 hours a week to make up for their cigarette breaks. This difference is based on the assumption that smokers take two

15-minute breaks per day to leave the office and light up. This policy was passed osten-sibly to safeguard the health and safety of all employees and to minimize legal liabil-ity (resulting from damages claims for injuries caused by passive smoking). Despite these examples, it is important to note that definitive studies on the net savings or costs to employers from smoking restrictions have not yet been done.

Clean-air laws are among the most controversial topics in public policy at all levels of government. On the one hand, smokers have individual liberties and legal rights to consume a lethal good without undue government interference. On the other hand, non-smokers have implicit rights to clean air and full information. Extending protec-tive rights to one group compromises the freedom and satisfaction of the other. A detailed discussion of the political economy issues, including tactics by the tobacco industry to thwart public policy initiatives, is beyond the scope of this chapter (for dis-cussions of these issues see: Jacobson and Wasserman 1997; Jacobson and Wu 2000).

11.3 Youth access policies

11.3.1 Definition

Youth access laws are designed to limit the availability of tobacco from commercial sources to minors. Conceptually, this type of supply-reduction policy can work if all suppliers are effectively regulated. Jurisdictions attempt to limit the sale of cigarettes to minors by prohibiting vendors from selling to under-age adolescents, establishing minimum age-at-sale laws, banning self-service displays and limiting vending machines to locations restricted to adults, banning the sale of loose cigarettes, and outlawing the distribution of free tobacco samples to minors. Additionally, some jurisdictions require retail vendors to be licensed to sell tobacco products and some include revocation of the license for retailers who repeatedly violate the law.

11.3.2 The effectiveness of youth access restrictions

The existing empirical literature provides mixed evidence on the effectiveness of youth access laws in reducing youth smoking. Wasserman *et al.* (1991) explored the impact of state laws that restricted the sale or distribution of cigarettes to minors. They found that these laws reduced a teenager's probability of being a smoker but did not affect average cigarette consumption by young smokers. More recently, Chaloupka and Grossman (1996) examined the impact of several policies, implemented by US state and local authorities, that limited youth access to tobacco on youth smoking. They found little impact of these policies, including minimum age-at-sale laws, the posting of 'minimum-age' signs where tobacco products are sold, limits on the distribution of free samples to adolescents, restrictions on vending machine sales, and retailer licens-ing provisions on youth smoking. They attributed these findings to the relatively weak enforcement of these laws and retailers' poor compliance with them.

The issue of retailers' compliance with limits on cigarette sales to youth has received much attention (Jason *et al.* 1991,1996; Lynch and Bonnie 1994; USDHHS 1994; Rigotti *et al.* 1997; Forster *et al.* 1998). In general, the evidence suggests that retailer compliance is relatively low. The US Centers for Disease Control and Prevention (CDC 1997), for example, summarized the results of a survey conducted as part of the Mexican national program to reduce the prevalence of smoking among children and adolescents. The survey found that 443 of 561 (79%) of retailers sold cigarettes to minors, and that older minors and female minors were more likely to be able to purchase cigarettes than younger minors and male minors. Furthermore, very few retailers asked the minor's age, or asked for proof of age. The presence of a warning sign was not associated with lower sales rates. In a follow-up study, the CDC (1999b) compared illegal sales of cigarettes to minors on both sides of the Mexican border with the United States. Results showed that illegal sales rates to minors were higher in Ciudad Juarez, Mexico (98.1%) than in El Paso, Texas (18.0%) or Las Cruces, New Mexico (6.1%). The CDC noted that differences in the percentage of retailers willing to sell tobacco to minors between Ciudad Juarez and the two US border cities may reflect the efforts in the United States to enforce minors' access laws and to provide comprehensive retailer education programs.

Even in situations where the laws exist and are enforced, if the risk of prosecution is minimal or the fines are substantially less than the benefits from breaking the law, retailers will not comply with the law (Carruthers and McDonald 1995). In general, however, it appears that retailer compliance with laws prohibiting sales to minors can be increased through active enforcement, including fines or the threat of fines for violators (Jason *et al.* 1991; Difranza *et al.* 1992; Cummings *et al.* 1998; Forster and Wolfson 1998), educational interventions (Altman *et al.* 1991; Feighery *et al.* 1991; Gemson *et al.*1998), and community involvement (Forster *et al.* 1998). The evidence on the impact of higher compliance on youth smoking, however, is more mixed.

Jason *et al.* (1991), for example, found that vendors' compliance in Woodridge, Illinois, was substantially improved by various measures, including: informing vendors of the law; conducting regular compliance checks with stiff fines and license suspensions for violations; fining youth smokers; enlisting strong community support; and attracting the attention of the news media. Using 12- and 13-year-olds for compliance checks, they found a 93% reduction in illegal over-the-counter sales 18 months after their intervention. In a follow-up study (Jason *et al.* 1996), they found that compliance was demonstrated 80% of the time for sales to adolescents under the age of 17, and 75% of the time to 17-year-olds. In addition, they found that there were significant reductions in youth smoking prevalence as a result of the retailers' increased compliance.

In contrast, in a 2-year controlled study in six Massachusetts communities, Rigotti *et al.* (1997) found that regular compliance checks with an escalating series of warnings and penalties significantly raised vendor compliance but did not affect youth smoking. Using 16-year-old girls for compliance checks, they found that average compliance rates rose from 35% to 82% in three experimental communities in Massachusetts, significantly more than the increase from 28% to 45% observed in three control sites. However, there was no difference in perceived access by youth to commercial sources of tobacco between the control and the intervention communities. Consequently, the researchers found that adolescent smoking was not reduced in the intervention communities.

More recently, however, Forster *et al.* (1998) found that minimum-age laws, active community support for reducing illegal sales to youth, and ongoing enforcement of these laws, coupled with graduated fines for violators, resulted in a significantly slower rate of increase in youth smoking prevalence in intervention communities compared to control communities. Similarly, a recent longitudinal analysis of adolescents in Massachusetts by Siegel *et al.* (1999) examined the impact of limits on youth access to tobacco on the uptake of smoking by young people. They found little evidence that adolescents in communities with local tobacco sales ordinances perceived that cigarettes were less available than those living in communities with no policies. They did find, however, that adolescents in communities with a local tobacco sales ordinance at baseline were less likely to become regular smokers, suggesting that these policies may be effective in preventing adolescents from starting smoking. Similarly, Chaloupka and Pacula (1998), using nationally representative data on youth smoking in the United States, concluded that comprehensive state-wide efforts to enforce youth access laws that resulted in increased retailer compliance would significantly reduce youth smoking prevalence. In addition, they found that when states pre-empted more restrictive local policies, a higher proportion of adolescents were likely to smoke.

Forster and Wolfson (1998) summarized workable policies to restrict youth access to tobacco. They argued that strong limits on youth access should include the following provisions:

(1) complete restrictions on promotional distribution through bans on free samples and coupons;
(2) regulation of the means of sale through bans or locks on vending machines, placement of tobacco products behind service counters, and prohibitions on the sale of single/loose cigarettes; and
(3) regulation of the seller through licensing requirements on tobacco products that include possible revocation and the passage of minimum age-at-sale laws whose violation results in stiff penalties and fines.

As youth access to commercial sources of tobacco grows more limited, non-commercial sources of tobacco—such as other adolescents, parents, older friends, and strangers—will become more important and pose greater intervention challenges (Forster and Wolfson 1998; Forster *et al.* 1998; Wolfson *et al.* 1997). Research shows that older adolescents are more likely than their younger peers to purchase tobacco products from commercial sources and that older adolescents are willing to share tobacco products with their younger peers (Wolfson *et al.* 1997). Eliminating illegal sales to under-age adolescents would, therefore, reduce access from this particular non-commercial source (Forster *et al.* 1997). However, other strategies to address the social availability of tobacco products would also need to be developed to close all avenues for under-age youth to acquire tobacco products.

11.3.3 The costs of youth access restrictions

Youth-restriction policies are relatively inexpensive to legislate, but costly to enforce. For example, based on their experiences assisting city inspectors, Radecki and Zdunich (1993) estimated the cost of quarterly tobacco compliance checks at $35 per establishment per year. An annual licensing fee for retailers, they noted, could easily cover this cost. The CDC (1999a) recommended that US states should plan on spending between $0.43 and $0.80 per capita for the enforcement of youth access restrictions, retailer licensure provisions, and non-sales policy areas. State costs vary depending upon the number of retail outlets selling tobacco, the proportion of outlets in rural areas, and the proportion of outlets found to be non-compliant and requiring follow-up visits.

11.4 Implications for low-income and middle-income countries

Both within and between regions around the world, there is considerable variation in the prevalence and comprehensiveness of clean indoor-air policies and youth access restrictions, as Table 11.1 shows. The table summarizes the results from a recent World Health Organization survey of tobacco control policies in 134 countries (WHO 1997). The vast majority of countries now have some form of restriction on smoking in public places, while relatively few have laws limiting youth access to tobacco products. High-income countries are more likely than low-income and middle-income countries to have enacted both types of laws. Among high-income countries, most have some provision for smoke-free public places, health establishments, and work-sites; however, fewer have laws creating smoke-free restaurants and cafes. Similarly, relatively fewer high-income countries have laws limiting youth access to tobacco products, with only a few countries, notably Ireland, the United Kingdom, Canada, Australia, and the United States, having any history of enforcing their age-at-sale laws.

Among low-income and middle-income countries, laws requiring smoke-free public places are most prevalent, although the coverage of these laws is limited in restaurants, cafes, worksites, and healthcare establishments. Youth access is minimally covered in the low-income and middle-income countries included in the survey, implying that the ability of minors to purchase tobacco products in most of these countries is unlimited. Table 11.1 is not comprehensive. A Medline search for missing countries and contacts with control programs and researchers in these countries generally found that they did not have any laws.

Several factors can influence the effectiveness of clean-air laws and youth access restrictions in low-income or middle-income countries. These include: the cultural acceptability of tobacco; the degree of enforcement or self-enforcement associated with the laws; the presence or absence of an informal economy; and youth involvement in selling tobacco products.

The evidence from high-income countries suggests that clean-air laws can be self-enforcing. This may not, however, be universally true. For example, the prevalence of smoking in males is about the same in New Delhi as it is in California, and both have a law banning smoking in public places. Whereas the California laws are self-enforced, the law in Delhi is largely ignored. The two key conditions for effective self-enforcement appear to be a sufficient demand for clean-air laws (arising, possibly, from information on the health consequences of smoking and ETS) and the comprehensiveness of the laws. Partial laws are not likely to be self-enforcing.

In contrast, the empirical evidence indicates that youth access policies must be enforced in order to be successful in all countries. This implies that compliance checks must be carried out to ensure that laws are being followed, thus requiring funding to

Table 11.1 Distribution of youth access restrictions and smoke-free air policies, selected countries

	Smoke-free public places	Smoke-free restaurants	Smoke-free cafes	Workplace smoking restrictions	Smoke-free health establishments	Ban on sales to minors	Ban on vending machines	Minimum age restriction
High-income-OECD (27)	24	9	9	18	20	13	11	14
Low/middle income (81)	74	19	11	32	23	30	6	15
Africa (17)	17	0	0	2	4	4	1	1
Asia (15)	12	5	3	8	3	3	2	4
Europe (19)	15	7	6	9	4	11	1	5
Latin America & Caribbean (19)	19	3	2	10	8	8	0	3
Middle East (6)	6	1	0	2	1	1	0	0
Pacific Islands (5)	5	3	0	1	3	3	2	2

High Income-OECD: Australia, Austria, Belgium, Canada, Czech Republic, Denmark, Finland, France, Germany, Greece, Hungary, Ireland, Italy, Japan, Korea, Luxembourg, Mexico, The Netherlands, New Zealand, Norway, Poland, Portugal, Spain, Sweden, Turkey, United Kingdom, United States.

Low/middle income:
Africa: Algeria, Benin, Botswana, Cote d'Ivoire, Egypt, Ghana, Kenya, Mauritius, Morocco, Namibia, Nigeria, Senegal, South Africa, Tunisia, Uganda, Zambia, Zimbabwe.
Asia: Bangladesh, Cambodia, China, Hong Kong, India, Japan, Republic of Korea, Lao PDR, Mongolia, Myanmar (Burma), Nepal, Pakistan, Sri Lanka, Thailand, Vietnam.
Europe: Albania, Armenia, Belarus, Bulgaria, Croatia, Estonia, Kazakhstan, Kyrgyz Republic, Latvia, Lithuania, Moldova, Romania, Russian Federation, Slovak Republic, Slovenia, Tajikistan, Turkmenistan, Ukraine, Uzbekistan.
Latin America & Caribbean: Argentina, Bolivia, Brazil, Chile, Colombia, Costa Rica, Dominican Republic, Ecuador, El Salvador, Guatemala, Honduras, Jamaica, Panama, Paraguay, Peru, Puerto Rico, Trinidad & Tobago, Uruguay, Venezuela.
Middle East: Iran, Israel, Jordan, Kuwait, Oman, Saudi Arabia.
Pacific Islands: Indonesia, Malaysia, Papua New Guinea, Philippines, Singapore.

Source: based on WHO 1997, and World Bank data 1998; total number of countries in parentheses.

ensure the success of youth access policies. In low-income countries, the necessary systems, infrastructure, and resources for implementing such restrictions and enforcing them are likely to be less widely available than in the high-income countries. It may be possible to finance compliance checks with licensing fees received from vendors and retailers, although the distortionary effects of such financing are not well studied. Finally, like clean-air laws, comprehensive legislation to restrict youth access is more likely to succeed than would be partial restrictions on access.

11.5 Conclusions and research priorities

Low-income and middle-income countries should include clean-air and youth access laws as integral components of a comprehensive strategy of tobacco control. Experience from the high-income countries suggests that comprehensive clean-air policies, which restrict smoking in public and private places, do protect the health of non-smokers and also lead to reductions in smoking prevalence and cigarette consumption among continuing smokers. Clean-air laws impose some costs on continuing smokers, but do not appear to cause economic harm to tourism, restaurants, bars, and employers in smoke-free workplaces.

Like clean-air policies, youth access laws are most effective when administered in a comprehensive manner. This means banning vending-machine sales, banning sales of single cigarettes, mandating minimum age-at-sale laws, limiting self-service, requiring vendor licensing, and imposing graduated fines on retailers who violate the law. However, the key condition needed to ensure the effectiveness of youth restrictions in reducing youth smoking appears to be strict enforcement. These enforcement costs can be substantial. In lower-income countries, the necessary systems, infrastructure, and resources for implementing such restrictions and enforcing them are likely to be less widely available than in the high-income countries. Despite the low effectiveness and high costs of intervening, however, youth access restrictions are valuable in any event, partly to ensure broad interventions, to build political support, and to refute arguments from the tobacco industry and others who argue that limits on youth access should be adopted before stronger policies, such as tax increases and limits on advertising.

Research priorities for the development of laws for clean air and youth restrictions on access to tobacco begin with the ongoing evaluation of the success of existing policies. Specific research topics include:

(1) an assessment of the current tobacco-control environment in specific countries as this relates to clean indoor air and youth access regulation and laws; the number and type of laws, and pre-emption provisions, if any;
(2) an assessment of the level of sales to adolescents in specific countries, of the degree of active enforcement, and consumers' and vendors' compliance with tobacco control laws;
(3) a continuing assessment of the effectiveness of clean indoor air and youth access legislation in reducing the uptake of and prevalence of smoking, and in reducing average tobacco consumed by continuing users; and

(4) an evaluation of the economic effects of clean-air laws on business revenue and survival and industry employment.

References

Altman, D. G., Rasenick-Douss, L., Foster, V., and Tye, J. B. (1991). Sustained effects of an educational program to reduce sales of cigarettes to minors. *American Journal of Public Health*, **81**(7), 891–3.

Bartosch, W. J. and Pope, G. C. (1999). The economic effect of smoke-free restaurant policies on restaurant policies on restaurant business in Massachusetts. *Journal of Public Health Management and Practice*, **5**(1), 53–62.

Borland, R., Chapman, S., Owen, N., and Hill, D. (1990). Effects of workplace smoking bans on cigarette consumption. *American Journal of Public Health*, **80**(2), 178–80.

California Environmental Protection Agency (California EPA) (1997). *Health Effects of Exposure to Environmental Tobacco Smoke*. Office of Environmental Health Hazard Assessment. Sacramento, California Environmental Protection Agency.

Carruthers, S. and McDonald, C. (1995). The availability of cigarettes to minors in Perth, Western Australia. *Tobacco Control*, **4**, 49–52.

Centers for Disease Control and Prevention (CDC) (1997). Illegal sales of cigarettes to minors: Mexico City, Mexico, 1997. *Morbidity and Mortality Weekly Report*, **46**(20), 440–4.

Centers for Disease Control and Prevention (CDC) (1999a). *Best Practices for Comprehensive Tobacco Control Programs—August 1999*. Atlanta GA: US Department of Health and Human Services, Centers for Disease Control and Prevention, National Center for Chronic Disease Prevention and Health Promotion, Office on Smoking and Health.

Centers for Disease Control and Prevention (CDC) (1999b). Illegal sales of cigarettes to minors: Ciudad Juarez, Mexico; El Paso, Texas; Las Cruces, New Mexico, 1999. *Morbidity and Mortality Weekly Report*, **48**(19), 394–8.

Chaloupka, F. (1992). Clean indoor-air laws, addiction and cigarette smoking. *Applied Economics*, **24**, 193–205.

Chaloupka, F. J. and Grossman, M. (1996). *Price Tobacco Control Policies and Youth Smoking*. National Bureau of Economic Research Working Paper No. 5740.

Chaloupka, F. J. and Pacula, R. L. (1998). *Limiting Youth Access to Tobacco: The Early Impact of the Synar Amendment on Youth Smoking*. NBER.

Chaloupka, F. J. and Saffer, H. (1992). Clean indoor-air laws and the demand for cigarettes. *Contemporary Policy Issues*, **X**, 72–83.

Chaloupka, F. J. and Wechsler, H. (1997). Price, tobacco control policies and smoking among young adults. *Journal of Health Economics*, **16**(3), 359–73.

Cummings, K. M., Hyland, A., Saunders-Martin, T., Perla, J., Coppola, P. R., and Pechacek, T. F. (1998). Evaluation of an enforcement program to reduce tobacco sales to minors. *American Journal of Public Health*, **88**(6), 932–6.

Difranza, J. R., Carlson, R. R., and Caisse, R. E. Jr. (1992). Reducing youth access to tobacco. *Tobacco Control*, **1**(1), 58.

Eriksen, M. P. and Gottlieb, N. H. (1998). A review of the health impact of smoking control at the workplace. *American Journal of Health Promotion*, **13**(2), 83–104.

Evans, W. N., Farrelly, M. C., and Montgomery, E. (1999). Do workplace smoking bans reduce smoking? *American Economic Review*, **89**(4), 728–47.

Feighery, E., Altman, D. G., and Shaffer, G. (1991). The effects of combining education and enforcement to reduce tobacco sales to minors. *Journal of the American Medical Association*, **266**(22), 3168–71.

Forster, J. L. and Wolfson, M. (1998). Youth access to tobacco: policies and politics. *Annual Review of Public Health*, **19**, 203–35.

Forster, J. L., Wolfson, M., Murray, D. M., Blaine, T. M., Wagenaar, A. C., and Claxton, A. J. (1997). Perceived and measured availability of tobacco to youths in 14 Minnesota communities: the TPOP study. *American Journal of Preventive Medicine*, **13**(3), 167–74.

Forster, J. L., Murray, D. M., Wolfson, M., Blaine, T. M., Wagenaar, A. C., and Hennrikus, D. J. (1998). The effects of community policies to reduce youth access to tobacco. *American Journal of Public Healt*, **88**(8), 1193–8.

Gemson, D. H., Moats, H. L., Watkins, B. X., Ganz, M. L., Robinson, S., and Healton, E. (1998). Laying down the law: reducing illegal tobacco sales to minors in Central Harlem. *American Journal of Public Health*, **88**(6), 936–9.

Glantz, S. A. and Charlesworth, A. (1999). Tourism and hotel revenues before and after passage of smoke-free restaurant ordinances. *JAMA*, **281**(20), 1911–8.

Glantz, S. and Smith, L. R. A. (1994). The effect of ordinances requiring smoke-free restaurants on restaurant sales. *American Journal of Public Health*, **84**, 1081–5.

Glantz, S. and Smith, L. R. A. (1997). The effect of ordinances requiring smoke-free restaurants and bars on revenues: a follow-up. *American Journal of Public Health*, **87**, 1687–3.

Glasgow, R. E., Cummings, K. M., and Hyland, A. (1997). Relationship of worksite smoking policy to changes in employee tobacco use: findings from COMMIT. *Tobacco Control*, **6**(supplement 2), S44–S8.

Hyland, A. and Cummings, K. M. (1999a). Restaurant employment before and after the New York City smoke-free air act. *Journal of Public Health Management and Practice*, **5**(1), 22–7.

Hyland, A. and Cummings, K. M. (1999b). Restaurateur reports of the economic impact of the New York City smoke-free air act. *Journal of Public Health Management and Practice*, **5**(1), 37–42.

Hyland, A., Cummings, K. M., and Nauenberg, E. (1999). Analysis of taxable sales receipts: was New York City's smoke-free air act bad for restaurant business? *Journal of Public Health Management and Practice*, **5**(1), 14–21.

Jacobson, P. D. and Wasserman, J. (1997). *Tobacco Control Laws: Implementation and Enforcement*. Santa Monica (CA): RAND.

Jacobson, P. D. and Wu, L. Clean indoor air restrictions: progress and promise. Working paper, Department of Health Management and Policy, School of Public Health, University of Michigan.

Jason, L. A., Ji, P. Y., Anes, M. D., and Birkhead, S. H. (1991). Active enforcementof cigarette control laws in the prevention of cigarette sales to minors. *Journal of the American Medical Association*, **266**(22), 3159–61.

Jason, L. A., Billows, W. D., Schnopp-Wyatt, D. L., and King, C. (1996). Long-term findings from Woodridge in reducing illegal cigarette sales to older minors. *Evaluation and the Health Professions*, **19**, 3–13.

Lynch, B. and Bonnie, R. (ed.) (1994). *Growing Up Tobacco Free: Preventing Nicotine Addiction in Children and Youths*. Washington, DC: Institute of Medicine, Committee on Preventing Nicotine Addiction in Children and Youth.

National Cancer Institute (NCI) (1999). *Health Effects of Exposure to Environmental Tobacco Smoke*. The Report of the California Environmental Protection Agency. Smoking and Tobacco Control Monograph no. 10. Bethesda, MD. US Department of Health and Human Services, National Institutes of Health, National Cancer Institute, NIH Pub. No. 99–4645.

Radecki, T. E. and Zdunich, C. D. (1993). Tobacco sales to minors in 97 US and Canadian communities. *Tobacco Control*, **2**, 300–5.

Rigotti, N. A., Difranza, J. R., Chang, Y. C., Tisdale, T., Kemp, B., and Singer, D. (1997). The effect of enforcing tobacco-sales laws on adolescents' access to tobacco and smoking behavior. *New England Journal of Medicine*, **337**(15), 1044–51.

Rice, D. P., Hodgson, T. A., Sinsheimer, P., Browner, W., and Kopstein, A. N. (1986). The economic costs of the health effects of smoking. *Milbank Quarterly*, **64**, 489–546.

Sculco, T. W. (1992). Smokers' rights legislation: should the state butt out of the workplace? *Boston College Law Review*, **33**, 879–902.

Siegel, M., Biener, L., and Rigotti, N. A. (1999). The effect of local tobacco sales laws on ado-
    lescent smoking initiation. *Preventive Medicine*, **29**, 334–42.
US Department of Health and Human Services (1986). *The Health Consequences of Involun-
    tary Smoking*. A report of the Surgeon General. Rockville MD: US Department of Health
    and Human Services, Public Health Services, Centers for Disease Control, Center for Health
    Promotion and Education, Office on Smoking and Health. (DHS Publication No (CDC)
    87–8398.)
US Department of Health and Human Services (1994). *Preventing Tobacco Use Among Young
    People*. A Report of the Surgeon General, Atlanta, Georgia: US Department of Health and
    Human Services, Public Health Service, Centers for Disease Control and Prevention, National
    Center for Chronic Disease Prevention and Health Promotion, Office on Smoking and Health.
Warner, K. E. (1981a). State legislation on smoking and health: a comparison of two policies.
    Policy Sciences, **13**, 139–52.
Warner, K. E. (1981b). Cigarette smoking in the 1970's: the impact of the anti-smoking campaign
    on consumption. *Science*, **221**, 729–31.
Warner, D. (1994). 'We do not hire smokers': may employers discriminate against smokers?
    Employee Responsibilities Rights Journal, **7**, 129–40.
Wasserman, J., Manning, W. G., Newhouse, J. P., and Winkler, J. D. (1991). The effects of excise
    taxes and regulations on cigarette smoking. *Journal of Health Economics*, **10**(1), 43–64.
Wolfson, M., Forster, J. L., Claxton, A. J., and Murray, D. M. (1997). Adolescent smokers' provi-
    sion of tobacco to other adolescents. *American Journal of Public Health*, **87**(4), 649–51.
World Health Organization (1997). *Tobacco or Health:aA Global Status Report*. Geneva: World
    Health Organization.
Yurekli, A. and Zhang, P. (2000). The impact of clean indoor-air laws and cigarette smuggling on
    demand for cigarettes: an empirical model. *Health Economics*.

12

Smoking cessation and nicotine-replacement therapies

Thomas E. Novotny, Jillian Clare Cohen, Ayda Yurekli,
David Sweanor, and Joy de Beyer

Initiatives that help smokers to quit are key components in an effective tobacco-control program. Unaided, individuals' chances of quitting are low, but success rates are higher when smokers use nicotine-replacement therapies (NRTs) and other pharmacological therapies. The current market for NRTs worldwide is small compared with the market for cigarettes, and is mostly concentrated in high-income countries. The small market largely reflects low levels of demand, especially in low-income and middle-income countries. However, the regulation of NRTs, for example through conditions of sale, also reduces access to them. Public policy options for increasing access to NRTs include the deregulation of conditions of sale. In addition, increased public information about the hazards of smoking and the benefits of cessation appear to be important for increasing demand for NRTs. Where studied, NRTs have been found to be cost-effective. Theoretically, these therapies could be publicly financed for the poorest smokers. In practice, however, it would be difficult to target those on the lowest incomes.

12.1 Introduction

Support for smoking cessation is an important component of comprehensive population-based tobacco-control programs (Novotny *et al.* 1992). Given current patterns of smoking, 100 million adults who currently smoke will be killed prematurely by tobacco over the next 20 years (Peto *et al.* 1999). Smokers who quit before the onset of major illnesses, especially those who quit at earlier ages, avoid most of the excess risk accrued by continuing smokers (Doll *et al.* 1994). The benefits of quitting have been extensively documented and include reduction of risk for all major forms of tobacco-attributable disease and improved life expectancy (Chapter 2; USDHHS 1990).

This chapter reviews cessation methods, focusing on nicotine-replacement therapy (NRT), and, to a lesser extent, on other pharmacological adjuncts to cessation, such as bupropion. The chapter has three parts. First, we review briefly the effectiveness of various types of cessation. (More details of cessation methods can be found elsewhere: Fiore *et al.* 1996; USDHHS 1988, 1990; American Psychiatric Association 1996). Second, we discuss issues concerning the price of NRTs, public information about them, and regulations on their sale. Because NRT markets can only be understood in the context of the cigarette market, we compare the two products. Third, we explore public policy options, including deregulation of NRT products and conditions of sale, and public or insurance financing for NRT.

12.2 Smoking cessation

In countries where there is relatively widespread knowledge about the risks of smoking and the benefits of quitting, a significant proportion of smokers will try to stop smoking each year. In the United States, for example, an estimated 16 million current daily smokers in 1997 had stopped smoking at least one day during the preceding year (US Centers for Disease Control and Prevention 1999a). Widespread quitting has contributed to reduced levels of lung cancer and cardiovascular disease in males in several high-income countries (Chapter 2).

Quitting smoking is well described by a 'stages of change' model (Prochaska and DiClemente 1983). According to this model, smokers move along a continuum of behavior, from pre-contemplation (not thinking of quitting), to contemplation (preparing to quit), action (cessation), and finally maintenance. Many factors may influence movement along this continuum. Kenkel and Chen (Chapter 8) and Saffer (Chapter 9) expand, respectively, on the effectiveness in reducing tobacco consumption of widespread public information about the risks of smoking and bans on advertising and promotion. Information will move some smokers from pre-contemplation to contemplation of quitting. Advertising and promotion bans may reduce the environmental cues that support smoking. Similarly, higher taxes may encourage some smokers to try quitting, as discussed by Chaloupka *et al.* (Chapter 10). The availability of effective cessation therapy might also help move smokers from pre-contemplation and contemplation stages to action and maintenance.

The success of unaided smoking cessation is low in relative terms, although it is the most common method used. Unaided cessation is common enough to have contributed to the accumulation, over time, of substantial numbers of male smokers quitting in high-income countries (USDHHS 1990). However, even where there is a high level of public awareness of the health dangers of smoking, only 3–5% of all smokers who try to quit by themselves are permanently successful on any given attempt. We summarize the effectiveness of three types of interventions that could increase the proportion of smokers who succeed in quitting: community cessation programs; specific advice from a health provider; and NRT or adjunct non-NRT pharmacological treatment. Most studies of efficacy for these interventions have been performed in high-income countries. Wherever possible, we discuss the applicability of these approaches to low-income and middle-income countries.

12.2.1 Community cessation programs

Community or population-based smoking-cessation projects aim to increase the number of quitters in a given community. These projects involve mass communications to raise public awareness, encouragement of health professionals to improve their efforts with individual patients, widespread provision of self-help materials through medical and non-medical channels, and smoking cessation events such as 'Quit and Win' contests (Foulds 1996). Some of these programs in the United States, notably in

California and Massachusetts, have been financed through a specific, one-time increase in cigarette tax (Bal *et al.* 1990). Few have used subsidies for cessation therapy.

Large-scale community cessation efforts in high-income countries have shown modest efficacy at best (Foulds 1996). In the United States, the Community Intervention Trial for Smoking Cessation (COMMIT) was a randomized controlled trial over 4 years that focused on quitting among heavy smokers in large communities (defined as those with populations between 50 000 and 250 000). This intervention included public information, interventions by health professionals, work-site activities, and the development of community cessation resources. There were no differences in quit rates for heavy smokers between the control and intervention communities, and there was only a 3% improvement in quitting among light-moderate smokers (COMMIT Research Group 1995). Somewhat more encouraging results were noted in the North Karelia project in Finland. In this non-randomized, community-based cardiovascular disease prevention program, the percentage of men currently smoking declined during the first 10 years of the program (from 50% to 37%), and this decline was sustained over the next 10 years (Vartiainen *et al.*1998). This study found that 50% of those who could not stop smoking indicated a desire to do so. The authors suggested that NRT availability might improve the success of a community-based strategy. In the Netherlands, a non-randomized smoking cessation campaign involving the mass media included television shows, a television clinic, a quit line, local group programs, and a publicity campaign (Mudde and De Vries 1999). It produced high levels of program awareness and the number of smokers who abstained for a significant period increased by 4.5% over and above the baseline level. This success was probably reduced by a massive rise in tobacco promotion during the campaign. The cost per long-term quitter was $12.

Well-evaluated community approaches to smoking cessation are rare in low-income or middle-income countries. Gupta *et al.* (1986) conducted a non-randomized trial among 36 471 tobacco smokers and chewers in three rural districts of India. Interventions included health professionals' advice, information campaigns in the mass media, and cessation camps. At the end of 5 years, the quit rates ranged from 9% to 17% in the intervention cohorts, and from 3% to 9% in the control cohorts, with the difference being statistically significant in two districts. However, community cessation programs are not likely to yield high *absolute* numbers of quitters in low-income and middle-income countries because, at present, these countries have lower overall quitting rates than high-income countries (Chapter 2). Also, some components of cessation programs in high-income countries (such as telephone help-lines) are less feasible or affordable in low or middle-income countries.

12.2.2 Advice from health providers

In many high-income countries, effective cessation treatment protocols are widely available to individual smokers as part of a medical approach. The US Agency for Health Care Policy and Research (AHCPR) published a thorough review of the literature and a discussion of these guidelines (Fiore *et al.* 1996). Briefly, the recommendations include screening all patients for tobacco use, advising patients who use tobacco to quit, setting a specific quit date, and providing NRTs. These treatments include minimal counseling by health providers, brief or more extensive counseling by specially trained providers, and group-intensive counseling. All interventions will be more effective against a social milieu in which tobacco cessation and non-smoking are the norm (Novotny 1988). The AHCPR guidelines also call for infrastructure changes and reimbursement as ways to increase the availability and accessibility of treatment services and products.

Health providers can enhance individual cessation efforts through social support and other proactive interventions (Orleans *et al.* 1991). Individual or group counseling increases cessation rates substantially, but this approach also requires motivation for smokers to participate. Further disadvantages include the direct costs, and the opportunity costs (such as lost work time). Anthonisen *et al.* (1994) showed that a combination of intensive, specialized care, NRTs, behavioral modification, and relapse prevention training achieved the highest rates of cessation success, with 35% of the intervention group succeeding versus 9% of the controls. However, this intervention was in a group of adults with early signs of lung disease. The program was resource-intensive, expensive, and not applicable to general populations. Even with such intensive therapy, 65% of smokers did not quit, and of those that did, 37% had relapsed within 5 years.

In the United Kingdom, trained pharmacists provide information and support for smokers who seek NRT; interventions provided through pharmacists have increased counseling and improved cessation rates (Sinclair *et al.* 1998). In developing countries, where there is extensive self-medication and use of pharmacists for medical advice (Kamat and Nichter 1998), pharmacists could play a valuable role by advising clients of the benefits of cessation.

Overall, medically-based cessation interventions are unlikely to be accessible to individual smokers in low-income and middle-income countries. Smokers are unlikely even to seek treatment from physicians. Moreover, we are not aware of any studies of the effectiveness or cost-effectiveness of cessation advice provided by healthcare providers in a developing country.

12.2.3 Non-NRT therapies

Mood, or affect, appears to influence the likelihood of addiction. Bupropion hydrochloride, a widely used anti-depressant, has recently been marketed in the United States and Canada as an effective smoking cessation treatment (Hurt *et al.* 1997). Bupropion is not an addictive drug and can be used for longer periods for maintenance in appropriate patients (Miller and Griffith 1983). Some consumers may prefer non-nicotine products, such as bupropion, as a way of helping to end their addiction. A randomized trial comparing NRT patches and bupropion reported that cigarette abstinence at 12 months was 16.4% in the NRT patch group, 30.3% in the bupropion group, and 35.5% in the group treated with NRT patch and bupropion combined (Jorenby *et al.* 1999). Data on the population-wide efficacy or cost-effectiveness of this drug are not yet available. More research is needed to show whether anti-depressants or similar therapies can increase cessation rates among smokers in low- and middle-income countries. The market for these non-NRT therapies has not been extensively studied.

12.2.4 Nicotine and nicotine-replacement therapy

Nicotine is the primary active ingredient in cigarettes that reinforces individual smoking behavior (USDHHS 1990). However, it is other constituents of tobacco, and not nicotine, that cause widespread mortality and morbidity. Tobacco use can be classified as a 'dependence' within the criteria of the International Classification of Diseases (WHO 1994). The criteria include *use despite damage*, *physical* and *psychological dependence*. Knowledge of the addictive nature of nicotine provides a rationale for substituting a less-harmful source of nicotine for cigarettes.

NRT products take a number of forms: gum, transdermal patch, nasal spray, oral inhaler, and tablet. All of these products have different levels of efficacy and variable rates of nicotine absorption, and they are most effective when the consumer also receives parallel cessation-counseling, but nevertheless are effective even without accessory behavioral therapy (Fiore *et al.* 1996).

A number of studies have demonstrated the efficacy, safety, and utility of NRT (Silagy *et al.* 1994; Cromwell *et al.* 1997; Shiffman *et al.* 1997; Shiffman *et al.* 1998). Of smokers who use a pharmacological aid, such as NRT, 10–30% are able to stop smoking for at least six months (Fiore *et al.* 1996). This represents a significant improvement over the success of self-help and brief advice from a physician. NRT, in fact, has been found consistently to double a smoker's chances of successful quitting with or without concomitant behavioral therapy (Fowler 1998; Raw *et al.* 1999). Table 12.1 summarizes the evidence.

NRT products are used primarily to quit smoking and effectively treat the symptoms of nicotine withdrawal and are not prescribed or recommended for any other purpose (Silagy 1994). Other issues to consider are the health implications of long-term use of NRT alone (Fagerstrom *et al.* 1997), and the implications of the mixed use of NRT and cigarettes. A recent review of the risks and benefits of NRT reported several significant pieces of evidence regarding these products (Benowitz 1998). If used appropriately, NRTs are comparatively safe products. They emit no tar or carbon monoxide, and they produce lower blood nicotine levels than cigarettes. The use of nicotine products in individuals who are tolerant is not likely to be associated with any acute behavioral toxicity.

Table 12.1 Effectiveness of various cessation interventions

Intervention and comparison	Increase in percentage of smokers abstaining for 6 months or more
Brief advice to stop (3 to 10 minutes) by clinician versus no advice.	2 to 3
Adding NRT to brief advice versus brief advice alone or brief advice plus placebo.	6
Intensive support (e.g., smokers' clinic) plus NRT versus intensive support or intensive support plus placebo.	8

Sources: Fiore *et al.* 1996; Raw *et al.* 1999.

Table 12.2 Annual smoking cessation among 50 million smokers in the United States: utilization, efficacy and impact of different cessation interventions

Intervention	Utilization (number of smokers using the method annually)	Efficacy (percentage sustained quitting at 6 months)	Impact (number of sustained successful quitters annually)
None	22 800 000	3	684 000
NRT by prescription, 1995	2 500 000	14	350 000
Over-the-counter NRT, 1996	6 300 000	14	882 000
Behavioral counseling	395 000	24	94 800

Source: Shiffman *et al.* 1997; Shiffman *et al.* 1998.

Some smokers may need long-term nicotine maintenance therapy, which these products can offer. Exposure to nicotine with NRT use is generally no greater than the exposure during cigarette smoking, and because NRT products do not contain the toxic chemicals found in cigarettes, the benefits of nicotine maintenance therapy almost certainly outweigh the risks of NRT. Use of nicotine in pregnancy may be associated with spontaneous abortion, low birthweight, and neonatal toxicity. NRT will certainly be less hazardous than cigarettes, but should only be used by pregnant women to completely cease cigarette smoking. Controlled clinical trials of NRT in smokers with documented cardiovascular disease have found no evidence that NRT products are harmful, even if used for as long as 5 years. Finally, limited data suggests that use of NRTs by smokers—for example, in non-smoking situations such as air travel or workplaces—reduces the overall amount of smoking, and thus confers health benefits. However, more research is required in this area.

Table 12.2 provides estimates of the population impact of cessation with or without NRT, based on data from the United States (Schiffman *et al.* 1997; Schiffman *et al.* 1998). The authors estimated that adding pharmacological therapy to other cessation methods could increase the quitting rate from 3% to 14%.

With increasing restrictions on smoking in workplaces and public transportation in most of the world (WHO 1997), demand for NRT products could increase. The availability of pharmacotherapy for nicotine-dependent smokers may even make it easier to implement health policies aimed at smoking cessation and establishing smoke-free environments because affected employees now have alternatives that could help them avoid nicotine withdrawal symptoms.

In sum, NRTs appear to be effective and feasible for use in high-income countries. We now describe the NRT market.

12.3 Key issues in the nicotine market

Currently, NRT products compete with large legal and illegal markets in cigarettes. In many countries, the cigarette industry is a duopoly or oligopoly. In India and some other countries, however, there are also significant sales of other nicotine-containing products (snuff, chew, etc.) that are not controlled by the same companies. In order to understand how NRT and other pharmacological cessation products compete with the established nicotine market, it is important to understand some dynamics of this market. Key factors include: market size and relative market shares, product characteristics (including effectiveness), public information, and cost.

12.3.1 Market size and shares

NRT products represent only a tiny fraction (less than half of 1%) of the global pharmaceutical market, which was around $300 billion in 1998 (*Scrip* Magazine 1999). The global market for NRT products was estimated to be only $725 million in 1998, about $553 million of which was in the United States. Nicotine gum accounts for almost half of this, with the patch second. In contrast, cigarettes comprise a world retail market of some US$300 billion (WHO, 1999), more than 440 times larger than NRT sales. The future growth of the NRT market depends on several factors, some of which are discussed below.

In comparison with cigarettes, NRT products are much less widely available worldwide. Figures for NRT availability have been compiled by the Medical Information Database (MIDAS), which contains data on international and national pharmaceutical products, such as average ex-manufacturing price, average price for consumer, sales in US dollars, sales in terms of standard dose unit, and the number of sales packages (IMS Global Services 1998). MIDAS excludes some major European countries such as Denmark, Sweden, and Switzerland. MIDAS expenditure data for 1996 reveals that, of 63 countries assessed, NRT products were available in 21 high-income, 27 middle-income, and only 2 low-income countries. In most countries, patches account for over 95% of the NRT market. Almost 70% of global NRT product sales are in the United States, nearly 20% of sales are in Europe, and 10% in other industrialized countries. Middle-income countries have less than 1% of the NRT market share, while NRT sales are almost non-existent in low-income countries.

12.3.2 Product characteristics

Tobacco products are designed to encourage long-term nicotine maintenance with maximum consumer utility. They also deliver other products that are harmful to health. NRT products, on the other hand, are produced to assist nicotine-dependent smokers who want to quit. They provide users with a small amount of nicotine to reduce withdrawal symptoms. Tobacco products and NRT products are substantially different, not only in their components, but also in their effectiveness as nicotine delivery devices and the way in which they are sold. Table 12.3 summarizes these differences.

Smoking results in rapid peak nicotine levels. Nicotine from cigarettes is quickly absorbed via the lungs of smokers and reaches the brain within seconds. NRT products, on the other hand, are designed to deliver more gradual increases in blood levels of nicotine without the peaks and valleys associated with cigarettes. With nicotine gum, patches, and inhalers, nicotine is absorbed gradually through the mouth, skin, or respiratory passages (Schneider *et al.* 1996; Shiffman *et al.* 1998). Nicotine nasal spray provides a rather rapid absorption, and hence may be more like the dosing experience of smoking cigarettes.

Table 12.3 Differences between pharmaceutical NRT products and cigarettes

Pharmaceutical NRT products	Cigarettes
Subject to strict regulations including safety standards for use.	Limited regulatory control with no safety standards for use.
Lower abuse potential.	Maximize pleasurable/reinforcing effects of addiction.
Appeal and acceptability targeted to consumers for indicated use, minimizing youth appeal.	High sensory and packaging appeal targeted to susceptible youth.
Slow nicotine absorption rates.	Fast nicotine absorption rates.
Rigorous manufacturing standards.	Non-rigorous manufacturing standards.
Safe if used as intended.	Hazardous if used as intended; risks minimized by manufacturers.
Select distribution points.	Wide distribution networks.
May increase quit rates among smokers.	Significant population health risk.
Designed for short-term use and treatment of nicotine dependence.	Designed for long-term use, creation, and maintenance of nicotine dependence.
Costly in up-front costs, but comparable to cigarettes on daily cost.	Inexpensive, sold in small less costly units.

Source: Based on Warner *et al.* 1997, 1998.

12.3.3 Consumer information about NRT products

Compared with cigarettes, there have been only minor initiatives to inform consumers about NRT products or to market them. Moreover, NRT advertising campaigns have had a rather narrow focus, presenting a product for use by committed quitters and not acting as a cue to all smokers to quit. Although comprehensive global information on the regulation of advertising or distribution of NRT products is not available, the existing evidence suggests that many governments treat NRTs like other pharmaceutical products and prevent their manufacturers from advertising them directly to consumers. A few high-income countries are exceptions to this pattern.

Among the public, knowledge about NRT is poor, and misinformation about nicotine is widespread. Even health professionals commonly confuse the effects of nicotine with the effects of its main delivery vehicle, the cigarette. Surveys in several countries find that high percentages of the public, and of physicians, erroneously believe that nicotine itself causes cancer. For example, a survey of five high-income countries found that 43% of respondents believed that nicotine causes cancer and 33% were not sure.[1] In the United States, a 1997 survey of perceptions about the effects

[1] Based on unpublished survey data provided by Pharmacia and Upjohn 1996, 1997.

of tar and nicotine found that more than 80% of smokers mistakenly believed that the nicotine in cigarettes causes emphysema, cancer, and cardiovascular disease (Porter Novelli 1997). A recent Gallup poll confirmed that consumers do not understand the characteristics of nicotine, the benefits of NRT, or the risks of continuing to smoke so-called 'light' cigarettes. In this survey, 40% believed that NRT could cause or worsen health problems (Gallup Organization 1998). These findings indicate a clear need for better information about nicotine and NRTs for policy-makers, health professionals, and the public. Health providers trained in the use of NRT and in protocols to assist smokers could be a useful additional source of information to their patients.

Better publicity about NRTs may motivate quit attempts among smokers who would not have otherwise tried. Within the Prochaska model of stages of quitting, it is reasoned that smokers may move along the continuum of quitting, from contemplation to action, if they have access to both information about NRT products and the products themselves. A recent poll in the United States found that about 30% of current smokers were more motivated to think about quitting, or would actually quit smoking, if NRT products or other proven treatments were more readily available (Gallup Organization 1998). It is not clear whether this is a result of NRT advertising or due to the better availability of the NRT products. However, the survey reported that a large majority (86% of smokers and 89% of former smokers) felt that clinically proven cessation treatment should be as readily available as cigarettes.

12.3.4 Regulation

There are three broad and overlapping categories of consumer regulation (Room 1997) with respect to nicotine-containing products. We outline these, contrasting NRTs with cigarettes.

Regulation of the product

Tobacco products are not generally regulated in terms of health or manufacturing standards. Labeling for tar and nicotine content is required in only 36 countries (WHO 1997). Trade in tobacco products is less strictly regulated than NRT (see Chapter 14). On the other hand, NRT products are classified as pharmaceuticals, and must undergo various phases of approval in many countries before they are able to enter into a market. For example, a new drug requires a license, which is only granted after the product has had clinical trials and has been tested for safety, quality, and veracity and completeness of packaging information.

Modifications in cigarettes (e.g. toward lower tar levels) are permitted without regulation. In contrast, if a pharmaceutical company decides to modify a previously approved NRT product, it is obliged to seek further approval from the relevant regulatory authority. If a product is approved for consumption in one market, it must pass again through regulatory procedures if it is to enter another market.

Regulation of the provider or seller or the conditions of sale

In some countries, a license is required to sell tobacco, but throughout the developing world, tobacco is widely sold by small, unlicensed vendors. Like other pharmaceuticals, NRT products are generally sold only in pharmacies, either over the counter (OTC) or on prescription only. The exceptions are OTC NRT products in the United States, which may also be sold in grocery and general stores, and in the United Kingdom and Canada, where general retailers may also sell nicotine patches. These regulations would be difficult to enforce in many developing countries, where most pharmaceuticals are widely sold by vendors who are not pharmacists, with or without prescriptions, and few pharmacies have trained pharmacists in attendance. But to the extent that NRT products are sold only in pharmacies, the supply of physicians, pharmacies and pharmacists, and other bottlenecks in the distribution system, will constrain access in many developing countries. In addition, the advertising and promotion of cigarettes tends to be less restricted than that for NRTs in many countries.

Regulation of the consumer

Prescription requirements for NRT products are a significant effective restriction on consumers. In 7 out of 24 countries in Europe for which data are available, prescriptions are required for nicotine patches, and are required everywhere for nasal spray (IMS Global Services 1998). An extreme form of consumer regulation is in Japan, where NRT products may be sold only to smokers who suffer a tobacco-related disease. Currently, regulations prohibiting the sales of tobacco products to minors exist in only 43 of 134 countries surveyed by the WHO in 1995 (WHO 1997). But these regulations are usually ineffective or not enforced, as discussed by Woollery *et al.* in Chapter 11. Youth sales of NRTs are limited because, even where they are sold OTC, purchase by under-age consumers is prohibited.

12.3.5 Affordability: the cost of using NRT to quit

Most spending on NRT products is out-of-pocket. Insurance programs rarely cover the costs of NRT products, even in high-income countries. So household income and NRT prices are important determinants of access to NRT.

NRT expenditures vary widely across countries by income group. Based on data from IMS Global Services (1998) we calculate that in the United States, consumers spent $10.88 per smoker on NRT products in 1996. In other high-income countries, consumers spent on average $1.63 per smoker. Consumers in upper-middle-income countries spent $0.03 per smoker. NRT prices in the United States tend to be considerably higher than elsewhere, except in Japan,[2] where NRT products cost nearly twice as much as in the United States. Figure 12.1 compares the weighted average prices of a standard NRT unit (one patch or one piece of gum) in 14 countries, using a

---

[2] For more information about Japan's unique pharmaceutical policy, see: Thomas III 1994.

NRT Products Per Standard Unit in Selected Countries, Relative to the United States, 1996

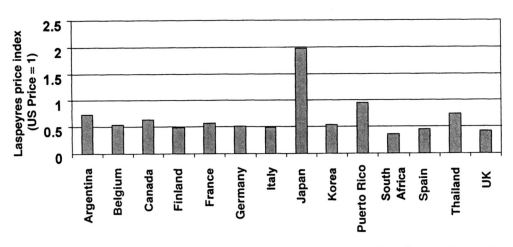

Fig. 12.1 Relative price of NRT products per standard unit in selected countries, 1996 (United States price = 1). Source: authors' calculations from World Bank data and IMS 1998.

Note: Laspeyres price index uses US NRT consumption as weights to estimate this index.

Laspeyres index, with the US price set to 1. NRT prices in several developing countries were between 25% and 35% lower than in the United States.

Whereas cigarette purchase is a long-term expense, the cost of NRTs is borne, at least in theory, over a limited period of a few months as smokers try to quit. We compared average annual spending on cigarettes per smoker (using average annual consumption and average price per pack) with the cost of a 3-month supply of NRT in 30 countries for which data were available. We assumed that 3 months' consumption would be the maximum usage of NRT products, given the usual recommendation that patches be used for up to 10 weeks. We assumed that consumers use one patch or 10 pieces of gum a day (well within the recommendation that no more than 20 pieces of gum be used per day). The costs are estimated for minimum and maximum prices of gums and patches.

For most industrialized countries, a 3-month supply of NRT products costs about half as much as a 1-year supply of cigarettes (Table 12.4). In developing countries, where cigarette prices are much lower, the cost of NRT for 3 months was equivalent to between one year's worth and four years' worth of cigarettes. In Argentina, it was 1.6 years, in Brazil 3.6–3.8 years, and in Indonesia, 7 years. However, these comparative figures probably do not capture very well the decision that the consumer makes. Even if consumers consider cigarettes and NRTs as substitutes to choose between at some point, their decision horizon may be relatively short, comparing the price of a pack or carton of cigarettes with a package or 1-week supply of NRTs. NRT gum is

Table 12.4 Costs of NRTs and cigarettes in selected countries, 1996

Countries	Annual cost of cigarettes in US$	Cost of 3 months of NRT		Number of years of cigarette costs that are equivalent to 3 months of NRT	
		Patches	Gum	Patches	Gum
Argentina	191	316	358	1.7	1.9
Australia	1200	200–356	168	0.2–0.3	0.1
Austria	451	341–351	242	0.8	0.5
Belgium	881	367–385	186	0.4	0.2
Brazil	135	492–517		3.6–3.9	
Canada	613	328–377	248–518	0.5–0.6	0.4–0.8
Czech Rep	52	199	176	3.8	3.4
Finland	652	155–169	144–162	0.2–0.3	0.2
France	447	327–330	330	0.7	0.7
Germany	664	282–316	345	0.4–0.5	0.5
Greece	463	65–231	127–144	0.1–0.5	0.3
HongKong	211	352	270	1.7	1.3
Hungary	128		151		1.2
Indonesia	38		273	7.1	
Ireland	339	260–264	253	1.5–1.6	1.5
Italy	339	256–275	193–214	0.8	0.7
Japan	502		976–1010		1.9–2.0
Malaysia	127	271	287	2.1	2.3
Mexico	61	179–257		3.0–4.2	
Netherlands	474	271–288	228–287	0.6	0.5–0.6
New Zeal.	686	182–192	229	0.3	0.3
Norway	358	266–271	218	0.7–0.8	0.6
Poland	84	195		2.3	
Portugal	301	247–348	272	0.8–1.2	0.9
Singapore	475	240		0.5	
S. Africa	151	215–217	193	1.4	1.3
Spain	233	263–359	140–193	1.1–1.5	0.6–0.8
Thailand	64	412	222		3.4
UK	770	213–235	163–175	0.3	0.2
US	479	400–472	441–745	0.8–1.0	0.9–1.6

Source: authors' calculations from IMS Global Services (1998) Medical Information Database.

usually sold in packs of 32–120 pieces, and patches in packs of 7–32. Their price ranges across countries from $7 in the Netherlands to $65 in Puerto Rico per pack of gums, and from $11 in Venezuela to $65 in France per pack of patches. In contrast, average cigarette pack prices range from a few cents to $1.50 in low-income and middle-income countries, and, even where prices are highest in some Scandinavian countries, rarely exceed about $7 (see Chapter 10). In many low-income countries, single cigarettes are sold on the street.

12.4 Policy options for governments

Given the currently limited market for NRT products, what are the implications for possible government intervention? Three broad areas of intervention are possible. They are: providing better information; changing the regulatory environment; and the financing of NRT products.

12.4.1 Information

The quantity of NRTs demanded appears small in the low-income and middle-income countries compared with the high-income countries. This is probably because fewer smokers in the low-income and middle-income countries are trying to quit, and because of the high prices and limited availability of the products. Government efforts to inform consumers better about the risks of smoking and the benefits of cessation are warranted on purely public goods criteria (see Chapter 8 for more detailed discussion on consumer information). There may be little justification for governments to intervene to publicize the benefits of NRT *per se*. However, many economists consider that there is a justification for publicizing the benefits of quitting (see Chapter 7).

12.4.2 Changes in regulations

As we have shown, the regulation of pharmaceutical nicotine products is considerably more extensive than the regulation of cigarettes. This gives cigarettes market advantages. Cigarettes are liberally marketed and harmful, while NRTs are more regulated but can reduce health damage from smoking. The tobacco industry has long-standing knowledge of the role of nicotine in initiating and sustaining cigarette consumption (Hurt and Robertson 1998). Given these imbalances, some analysts have argued that a consistent and integrated regulatory environment should in future be applied to all nicotine products. There is debate about whether NRT products should be deregulated so that they can compete more effectively with cigarettes and other tobacco products, or whether, instead, cigarettes ought to be more regulated or restricted (Kessler *et al.* 1997). The debate, however, is largely academic. If existing pharmaceuticals safety standards were applied to tobacco products, they would likely have to be removed completely from the market, or strictly regulated, because they are so hazardous. But market and political realities make such strict regulation impossible. Deregulating nicotine may be easier to implement and is more justifiable in economic terms (Sweanor 1998).

The liberalization of NRT markets could have significant health benefits if it resulted in increased cessation rates. However, opening the nicotine market without additional controls on tobacco marketing could potentially have significant adverse impacts on health behavior. These include the following:

(1) NRT products could become gateway products for tobacco use;
(2) they might be viewed as a substitute for cigarettes;
(3) they might reassure smokers that they can delay cessation, and suggest to children that their risk of long-term addiction is reduced;
(4) they could encourage lapsed smokers to start again;
(5) they might not be effective among non-addicted smokers and could, thus, be perceived as generally ineffective in supporting cessation; and
(6) ineffective or harmful products might become available with resultant adverse consequences.

To help limit some of these negative potential consequences, effective policies for pricing, regulation and information dissemination, both on tobacco use and NRT products, would be essential accompaniments to any increased availability of alternative pharmaceutical products. In addition, it could be beneficial to liberalize the criteria for marketing these products. Below we discuss several changes to NRT regulation that could increase the use of these products.

12.4.3 Reducing barriers to entry

Within overall trade policies, trade and non-trade barriers to NRT products can be reduced. One specific effort involves international harmonization of national pharmaceutical registration procedures, so that countries adopt consistent standards. Such harmonization could help make NRT products and other pharmaceutical products more widely available in the global market. Efforts at pharmaceutical harmonization are already underway regionally and inter-regionally. The European Union is the first region to harmonize pharmaceutical registration as part of its efforts to create a single market that allows for free trade in pharmaceuticals (IFPMA 1997). Mercosul (Argentina, Brazil, Paraguay, and Uruguay) countries have also taken steps to harmonize their drug registration procedures.

The International Conference on Harmonization of Technical Requirements for the Registration of Pharmaceutical Products for Human Use (ICH) is another international effort to standardize drug registration procedures. The ICH is focused on drug-registration procedures in Japan, the United States, and member countries of the European Union, but it is likely that its procedures will be extended to other countries as well. The ICH is working towards the harmonization of drug registration procedures for new products that demonstrate safety, efficacy, and quality. The potential benefits include cost savings through the elimination of duplicated registration procedures, more rapid entry of new products, and greater certainty of quality and safety standards.

Equally important, the harmonization of drug regulations may lower costs for pharmaceutical companies and make market entry more attractive. This, in turn, may provide incentives for further product development. Harmonization may be particularly useful for many low-income and middle-income countries where the burden of smoking is highest, financial resources are limited, and institutional capacity may be weak.

12.4.4 Reducing regulation of the provider, seller, or the conditions of sale

As discussed above, the regulation of NRT sales is often strict. There is evidence that deregulation, such as making sales available OTC, increases the use of NRT products in high-income countries. In 1986, the US Food and Drug Administration gave OTC approval to the nicotine transdermal patch and gum. As a result, NRT use increased dramatically. In 1995, an estimated 2.5 million quit attempts were made using prescription NRT products. In 1997, there were about half a million quit attempts using prescription NRT, and on conservative estimates, 5.8 million quit attempts used OTC NRT. Shiffman *et al.* (1997) suggest that, in addition to those who would have quit on baseline levels, between 114 000 and 304 000 Americans successfully quit smoking in 1997, due to the greater availability of NRT OTC range. In California, sales of NRT, both under prescription and OTC, are statistically associated with reduced cigarette consumption (Hu *et al.* in press).

12.4.5 Financing NRT

A priori, there is little government justification for paying for or subsidizing NRT products, because they are largely private goods. However, as noted in Chapter 7, there may be an argument for governments to directly fund pharmaceutical quitting aids for the poor in order to reduce price constraints that limit access. In the United Kingdom, for example, the government has introduced limited free NRT treatment under its National Health Service, with the goal of targeting the poorest (United Kingdom Department of Health 1998). There are theoretical gains in efficiency and equity if cigarette taxes are used to finance NRT for the poorest smokers.

We have estimated the number of smokers for whom governments could subsidize cessation aids by using the revenues generated from a 10% tax increase. We used a price elasticity of –0.4 for developed countries and –0.8 for developing countries. Estimating the revenue effect of changes in excise rates is reasonably straightforward (see Chapter 10 and Chapter 17). Based on the costs of gums and patches per smoker estimated above, we found that the additional revenues could subsidize between 3% and 30% of smokers in developed countries (Table 12.5). In the developing countries for which estimates were possible, fewer than 2% of smokers could be subsidized because tax rates and cigarette prices are low and NRT product prices are relatively high. In addition, the difficulties of targeting NRT subsidies to the poorest are considerable, as they are with many health interventions (World Bank 1993).

12.4.6 The cost-effectiveness of NRT

To consider including NRT in a basic universal package of clinical services in low-income and middle-income countries available to poor *and* non-poor smokers (World Bank 1993), governments would need to consider the burden addressed by smoking,

Table 12.5 Proportion of smokers who could receive subsidized NRT with an excise tax increase of 10%, selected countries, 1999

	Percentage of smokers that could be subsidized
High-income countries	
Greece	32.0
Australia	25.0
Finland	18.5
New Zealand	17.3
United Kingdom	15.6
Germany	10.3
Singapore	9.8
Canada	9.4
Belgium	8.6
Norway	7.1
Austria	6.8
Ireland	6.7
France	6.5
Italy	6.1
Portugal	6.1
Netherlands	5.5
Spain	4.7
United States	3.1
Low- and middle-income countries	
Czech Republic	1.8
Argentina	1.7
Poland	1.5
South Africa	1.3
Malaysia	1.0
Mexico	0.9
Brazil	0.6
Thailand	0.4

These estimates are based on expected revenue increase from a 10% increase in cigarette excise tax (see Chapter 17 for details), and the average cost of NRT in these countries if used for 3 months.

Source: authors' calculations from World Bank data and IMS Global Services (1998) Medical Information Database.

which is considerable, and the cost-effectiveness of the intervention. There have been few cost-effectiveness studies of NRT in low-income and middle-income countries. Ranson *et al.* (Chapter 18) have made some estimates. These suggest that, assuming public finance and an effectiveness of 2.5%, NRTs could cost about $276 per disability-adjusted life-year (DALY) in low-income and middle-income countries. This would be regarded as broadly cost-effective; the World Bank suggests that health interventions that can be delivered for less than the average per capita GDP of a country are cost-effective (low-income countries are defined as those with a per capita GDP of $765 or less). In high-income countries, the cost-effectiveness of smoking cessation has been established (USDHHS 1990; Curry *et al.* 1995; Fischle and Franks 1996; Cromwell *et al.* 1997; Wasley *et al.* 1997). Although the cost-effectiveness of short, provider-assisted smoking cessation has also been established (Cummins *et al.* 1989), such interventions still depend on physician action and patient access to medical care. Cromwell *et al.* (1997) determined that implementing the AHCPR guidelines on smoking cessation across the United States, which include costs of physician advice, counseling, NRT, and other therapies costs, would cost approximately $3 500 per additional quality-adjusted life-year (QALY) saved. Greater cost-effectiveness was found in the interventions using NRT. The authors compared this cost to the cost of mammography screening (which exceeds $61 000 per QALY) and hypertension screening (which exceeds $23 000 per QALY).[3]

Cost-effectiveness studies of cessation therapies are complicated because there are many different pharmaceutical cessation treatments sold in different package configurations, through different distribution networks, with different concomitant counseling or treatment, and in countries with varied regulatory regimes for such products. In addition, those seeking to quit smoking do not necessarily use cessation products appropriately.

Analyses of the cost-effectiveness of NRTs often fail to take into account two key factors. First is the total cost of cigarette consumption. This is important since consumers are substituting one good (cessation products) for another, inferior, good (Warner *et al.* 1997, 1998). If the savings on tobacco products (and the other costs associated with the use of these products) are not taken into account, opportunity costs are missed out of the assessment. Second, some of the costs associated with cessation therapies can be attributed to government-induced regulation, such as restrictions on sales outlets and promotional activities. It should be noted, however, that if health insurers do not cover OTC products, and NRT products are not available by prescription, patients face higher out-of-pocket costs (Smeeth and Fowler 1998).

12.4.7 Mandating insurance coverage of NRT

Aside from direct finance, governments may also be able to mandate the coverage of key items through public or private insurance schemes (Musgrove 1999). Most insurers, with the exception of a few companies in the United States, do not reimburse for NRT products. Only 6 of the 51 state-funded insurance programs for the poor in the United States cover smoking-cessation programs (CDC 1999b). One report found that general smoking-cessation services were available in two-thirds of HMO health-financing plans sampled. The nicotine transdermal patch was covered by 64% of the plans, and nicotine gum by 44%. These programs usually required members to enroll

---

[3] The cost per QALY reflects attributable doctor and patient time at US wage rates, and is not representative of such costs in lower wage economies.

in or complete a smoking cessation class as a condition of coverage, or to make out-of-pocket payments for NRT (Pinney Associates 1995).

In Australia in 1995, the federal government rejected a recommendation made by the Pharmaceutical Benefits Advisory Committee that NRT qualify for a (capped) subsidy under the Pharmaceutical Benefits Scheme (PBS). As the health minister explained at the time, the cost would have been prohibitively expensive, both in terms of the PBS and the impact of increased prescription costs under the Medicare program (Scollo 1995). By comparison, a recent study in the United States of the use and costs of cessation services among fully insured persons estimated the average cost at $328 per user. This one-time cost compares favorably with the annual cost of treating heart disease ($6 941) or hypertension ($5 921), which persist over the life of the patient (Curry *et al.* 1998).

In sum, the arguments in favor of direct public finance for NRT, or the mandating of insurance coverage for it, are less clear than the case for deregulating access to these therapies and their use. Further cost-effectiveness studies are required to inform national policy.

12.5 Conclusions

Tobacco products are a major cause of ill health and premature death. Smoking cessation is a critical element of tobacco control, but information about the benefits of smoking cessation aids, their effectiveness, and their cost-effectiveness, is generally deficient in low-income and middle-income countries. Although nicotine is the addictive agent in tobacco products, it is the delivery vehicle rather than the nicotine in these products that causes the harm. Thus, cessation and reduction of tobacco use, using approved pharmacotherapy for continuing smokers, is a reasonable objective for public health. Yet these products are often not available at all in developing countries, are not competitively priced, or face regulatory limitations on availability and indications for use. The market for nicotine is largely deregulated for cigarettes, but regulated for NRTs.

NRT and other pharmacological treatments for nicotine addiction are comparatively safe if used as directed, and they are unlikely to cause adverse behavioral, cardiovascular, or other health effects. Although additional research is necessary, the benefits of long-term NRT use among smokers who are unable to quit should be considered. In addition, more pharmacological products that assist cessation should be developed.

Governments may be able to improve the success of tobacco control efforts by helping to increase the availability and affordability of NRT and other devices. This could be done by deregulating the conditions for the sales of these products, and through regional and global harmonization of registration and regulation. However, the prospects for government financing of NRTs, even for the poor, appears limited. This is due to the relatively high cost of the products, the fact that they are a private good, and difficulties in targeting NRT subsidies to the poor.

NRTs are not solutions in themselves to the public health problem of cigarette use. Rather, their use must be considered as part of comprehensive prevention and cessation programs.

References

American Psychiatric Association (APA) (1996). Practice guidelines for the treatment of patients with nicotine dependence. *Am. J. Psychiatr.*, **153**(10 Supplement), 1–31.

Anthonisen, N. R., Connett, J. E., Kiley, J. P., Altose, M. D., Bailey, W. C., Buist, A.S. *et al.* (1994). Effects of smoking intervention and the use of an inhaled anticholinergic bronchodilator on the rate of decline of FEV1. The Lung Health Study. *JAMA*, **272**(19), 1497–505.

Bal, D. G., Kizer, K. W., Felten, P. G., Mozar, H. N., and Niemeyer, D. (1990). Reducing tobacco consumption in California. Development of a statewide anti-tobacco use campaign. *JAMA*, **264**(12), 1570–4.

Benowitz, N. L. 1998. *Nicotine Safety and Toxicity*. New York: Oxford University Press.

COMMIT Research Group (1995). Community intervention trial for smoking cessation (COMMIT): I. Cohort results from a four-year community intervention. *Am. J. Public Health*, **85**, 183–92.

Cromwell, J., Bartosch, W. J., Fiore, M. C., Hasselblad, V., and Baker, T. (1997). Cost-effectiveness of the clinical practice recommendations in the AHCPR guideline for smoking cessation. *JAMA*, **278**, 1759–66.

Cummins, S. R., Rubin, S. M., and Oster, G. (1989). The cost-effectiveness of counseling smokers to quit. *JAMA*, **261**, 75–9.

Curry, S. J., McBride, C. M., Grothaus, L. C., Louie, D., and Wagner, E. H. (1995). A randomization trial of self-help materials, personalized feedback, and telephone counseling with non-volunteer smokers. *J. Consult. Clin. Psychol.*, **63**, 1005–14.

Curry, S. J., Grothaus, L. C., McAfee, T., and Pabiniak, C. (1998). Use and cost effectiveness of smoking-cessation services under four insurance plans in a health maintenance organization. *New Engl. J. Med.*, **339**, 673–9.

Doll, R., Peto, R., Wheatley, K. *et al.* (1994). Mortality in relation to smoking: 40 years' observations on male British doctors. *BMJ*, **309**, 901–11.

Fagerstrom, K. O., Tejding, R., Westin, A., and Lunell, E. (1997). Aiding reduction of smoking with nicotine replacement medications: hope for the recalcitrant smoker. *Tobacco Control*, **6**, 311–6.

Fiore, M. C., Bailey, W. C., Cohen, S. J. *et al.* (1996). *Smoking Cessation*. Clin Pract. Guideline No. 18. Rockville, MD: AHCPR Publ. No. 96–0692 and www.ahcpr.gov/clinic/smoview.htm

Fischle, K. and Franks, P. (1996). Cost-effectiveness of the transdermal nicotine patch as an adjunct to physicians' smoking cessation counseling. *JAMA*, **275**, 1247–51.

Foulds, J. (1996). Strategies for smoking cessation. *British Med. Bull.*, **52**, 157–73.

Fowler, G. (1998). Nicotine replacement therapy for a healthier nation. *BMJ*, **317**, 1266–7.

Gallup Organization (1998). New Gallup survey reveals smokers' increased desire to kick the habit. *Press Release*. Princeton, NJ: Gallup Organization, October 20.

Gupta, P. C., Mehta, F. S., Pindborg, J. J., Aghi, M. B., Bhonsle, R. B., Daftary, D. K. *et al.* (1986). Intervention study for primary prevention of oral cancer among 36 000 Indian tobacco users. *Lancet*, **1**(8492), 1235–9.

Hurt, R. D., Sachs, D. P., Glover, E. D., Offord, K. D., Johnston, J. A., Dale, L. C. *et al.* (1997). A comparison of sustained-release bupropion and placebo for smoking cessation. *New Engl. J. Med.*, **337**, 1195–202.

Hurt, R. D. and Robertson, C. R. (1998). Prying open the door to the tobacco industry's secrets about nicotine. *JAMA*, **280**, 1173–81.

Hu, T., Sung, H., Keeler, T., Marciniak, M., Keith, A., and Manning, R. (in press). *Cigarette Consumption and Sales of Nicotine Replacement Products*.

IMS Global Services (1998). Medical Information Database (MIDAS)

International Federation of Pharmaceutical Manufacturers Association (IFPMA) (1997). *Issues Handbook: Registration of Medicines and Harmonization*. Geneva: IFPMA.

Jorenby, D. E., Leischow, S. J., Nides, M. A., Rennar, S. I., Johnston, J. A., Hughes, A. R. *et al.*

(1999). A controlled trial of sustained-release bupropion, a nicotine patch, or both for smoking cessation. *New Engl. J. Med.*, **340**, 685–91.

Kamat, V. R. and Nichter, M. (1998). Pharmacies, self-medication and pharmaceutical marketing in Bombay, India. *Soc. Sci. Med.*, **47**, 779–94.

Kessler, D. A., Barnett, P. S., Witt, A. *et al.* (1997). Legal and scientific basis for FDA's assertion of Jurisdiction over cigarettes and smokeless tobacco. *JAMA*, **277**, 405–9.

Miller, L. and Griffith, J. (1983). A comparison of bupropion, dextroamphetamine, and placebo in mixed-substance abusers. *Psychopharmacology*, **80**, 199–205.

Mudde, A. N. and De Vries, H. (1999). The reach and effectiveness of a national mass media-led smoking cessation campaign in The Netherlands. *Am. J. Public Health*, **89**(3), 346–50.

Musgrove, P. (1999). Public spending on health care: how are different criteria related? *Health Policy*, **47**(3), 207–23.

Novotny, T. E. (1988). Cessation of smoking and the social milieu. (Editorial.) *Mayo Clin. Proc.*, **63** 729–31.

Novotny, T. E., Romano, R. A., Davis, R. M., and Mills, S. L. (1992). The public health practice of tobacco control: lessons learned and directions for the states in the 1990s. *Ann. Rev. Public Health*, **13**, 287–318.

Orleans, C. T., Schoenbach, V. J., Wagner, E. H. *et al.* (1991). Self-help quit smoking interventions: effects of self-help materials, social support instructions, and telephone counseling. *J. Consul. Clin. Psychol.* **59**, 439–48.

Peto, R., Chen, Z. M., and Boreham, J. (1999). Tobacco: the growing epidemic. *Nature Medicine*, **5**(1), 15–17.

Pinney Associates (1995). *Smoking Cessation and Managed Care.* Bethesda, MD: Pinney Associates.

Porter Novelli Associates (1997). *Perceptions About the Effects of Tar and Nicotine. April 2, 1997.* Survey sponsored by SmithKline Beecham.

Prochaska, J. O. and DiClemente, C. C. (1983). Stages and processes of self-change of smoking: toward an integrative model of change. *J. Consult. Clin. Psychol.*, **51**(3), 390–5.

Raw, M., McNeill, A., and West, R. (1999). Smoking cessation: evidence-based recommendations for the healthcare system. *BMJ*, **318**(7177), 182–85.

Room, R. (1997). Control systems for psychoactive substances. 1997. Workshop Presentation: *Alternative Nicotine Delivery Systems–Harm Reduction and Public Health.* Toronto, March 21–23, 1997.

Schneider, N., Olmstead, R., Nilsson, F. *et al.* (1996). Efficacy of a nicotine inhaler in smoking cessation: a double-blind, placebo controlled trail. *Addiction*, **91**, 1293–1306.

Scollo, M. (1995). *Statement of Rejection of PBAC Recommendation on Nicotine Patches.* Commonwealth Government. Canberra: Memo.

Scrip Magazine, 1999, 75, 29–32. Anon. 'World Market Data: Slow but steady for world pharma sales.'

Shiffman, S., Gitchell, J., Pinney, J. M., Burton, S. L., Kemper, K. E., and Lara, E. A. (1997). The public health benefit of over-the-counter nicotine medications. *Tobacco Control*, **6**, 306–10.

Shiffman, S., Mason, K. M., and Henningfield, J. E. (1998). Tobacco dependence treatments: Review and prospectus. *Ann. Rev. Public Health*, **19**, 335–58.

Silagy, C. (1994). Nicotine replacement therapies in smoking cessation. *Biomedicine and Pharmacotherapy*, **48**, 407.

Silagy, C., Mant, D., Fowler, G., and Lodge, M. (1994). Meta-analysis on efficacy of nicotine replacement therapies in smoking cessation. *Lancet*, **343**, 139–142.

Sinclair, H. K., Bond, C. M., Lennox, A. S. *et al.* (1998). Training pharmacists and pharmacy assistants in the stage-of change model of smoking cessation: a randomised controlled trial in Scotland. *Tobacco Control*, **7**, 253–61.

Smeeth, L. and Fowler, G. (1998). Nicotine replacement therapy for a healthier nation—nicotine replacement is cost effective and should be prescribed on the NHS. *BMJ*, **317**, 1266–7.

Sweanor, D. T. (1998). The regulation of tobacco and nicotine: the creation, and potential for resolution, of a public health disaster. *Drugs: Education, Prevention, and Policy*, **5**.

Thomas III, L. G. (1994). Pricing, regulation, and competitiveness: lessons for the US from the Japanese pharmaceutical industry. *Pharmacoeconomics*, **6**, Suppl. 1, 67–70.

United Kindgom Department of Health (1998). *Smoking Kills: a white paper on tobacco*. London: the Stationary Office. (http://www.official-documents.co.uk/document/cm41/4177/4177.htm)

US Centers for Disease Control and Prevention (1999a). Cigarette smoking among adults–United States, 1997. *Morb. Mortal Wkly Rep.*, Nov. 5, **48**(43), 993–6.

US Centers for Disease Control and Prevention (1999b). *Best Practices for Comprehensive Tobacco Control Programs*. Atlanta GA: US Department of Health and Human Services, Centers for Disease Control and Prevention, National Center for Chronic Disease Prevention and Health Promotion, Office on Smoking and Health.

US Dept of Health and Human Services (1988). *The Health Consequences of Smoking–Nicotine Addiction*. A Report of the Surgeon General. Rockville, Maryland: US Dept of Health and Human Services, Public Health Service, Centers for Disease Control, Center for Health Promotion and Disease Prevention, Office on Smoking and Health; DHHS publication no. (CDC)88–8406.

US Dept of Health and Human Services (1990). *The Health Benefits of Smoking Cessation*. A Report of the Surgeon General. Rockville, Maryland: Office on Smoking and Health; DHHS publication no. (CDC) 90–8416.

Vartiainen, E., Korhonen, H. G., Koskela, K., and Puska, P. (1998). Twenty year smoking trends in a community-based cardiovascular diseases prevention programme—results from the North Karelia Project. *Eur. J. Public Health*, **8**, 154–9.

Warner, K. E., Slade, J., and Sweanor, D. T. (1997). The emerging market for long-term nicotine maintenance. *JAMA*, **278**, 1087–92.

Warner, K. E., Peck, C. C., Woosley, R. L. *et al.* (1998). Treatment of tobacco dependence: innovative regulatory approaches to reduce death and disease. *Food and Drug Law J.*, **58**, 1–8.

Wasley, M. A., McNagny, S. E., Phillips, V. L., and Ahluwalia, J. S. (1997). The cost-effectiveness of the nicotine transdermal patch for smoking cessation. *Prev. Med.*, **26**(2), 264–70.

World Bank (1993). *World Development Report 1993: Investing in Health*. Washington, DC: World Bank Publications.

World Health Organization (1994). *International Statistical Classification of Diseases and Related Health Problems, Volume 3*, Geneva: World Health Organization.

World Health Organization (1997). *Tobacco or Health: A Global Status Report*. Geneva: World Health Organization.

World Health Organization (1999). *World Health Report: Making a Difference*. Geneva: World Health Organization.

Section IV
Supply of tobacco

13

The supply-side effects of tobacco-control policies

Rowena Jacobs, H. Frederick Gale, Thomas C. Capehart,
Ping Zhang, and Prabhat Jha

This chapter examines whether tobacco-control policies will have a detrimental effect on countries' economies, in particular on employment, and examines the impact of supply-side interventions. For the majority of countries, even stringent tobacco-control policies will have either a minimal impact or no net impact on total employment, as money that would formerly have been spent on tobacco tends to be spent on other goods and services. However, for a handful of tobacco-exporting countries that are not diversified, falling demand for tobacco would result in job losses, although such transitions would be gradual. Supply-side policies, such as price supports and quotas, provide incentives to grow tobacco, but their net impact on retail price, and hence consumption, is small. Given high demand and the presence of alternative suppliers, policies such as crop diversification or buy-outs are largely ineffective in reducing the supply of tobacco or its consumption. Nevertheless diversification, placed within broader rural development programs, can help meet the transition costs of the poorest farmers. Ultimately, the most effective supply-side policy may be to focus on reducing the demand for tobacco, and to allow supply to respond to slow changes in demand.

13.1 Introduction

This chapter addresses the supply-side impact of tobacco-control policies, specifically the macro-economic, employment, and agricultural issues. These are important political issues, given that supply-side stakeholders, mainly farmers and manufacturers of tobacco products, tend to form a political and emotional lobby to resist control policies that jeopardize their interests. Consequently, policy-makers are likely to be required to balance the public health imperative of reducing smoking against the economic interests of their tobacco-producing or tobacco-manufacturing constituents.

We address some commonly-held concerns about the macro-economic impact of tobacco-control measures. For example, the discussion examines the view, frequently voiced by the tobacco industry, that measures such as raising tobacco taxes would cause large and precipitate job losses, reduce total tax revenue, or alter the trade balance. We also address the question of how policy-makers who decide to implement tobacco-control measures can strategize the transition in agriculture to reduced dependency on tobacco crops. Are supply-side measures effective in reducing consumption? What is the impact of farmer subsidies or price-support measures? Should policy-makers encourage substitution from tobacco to alternative crops, or even buy-out tobacco producers altogether?

The chapter is in four sections. First, we describe tobacco farming and manufacturing, including the shift in tobacco production to low-income countries, and the size of the tobacco industry. Second, we examine whether tobacco-control policies have any detrimental impact on economies. We analyze studies, both independent and industry-sponsored, on this topic and revisit some of their conclusions. We also examine differences in the impact of control policies in countries that are net importers or exporters of tobacco, and go on to describe job losses stemming from improvements in the tobacco industry's manufacturing technology. Third, we examine the effectiveness of a range of supply-side interventions, such as subsidies, diversification, 'buy-out' efforts or attempts at outright bans on production. Finally, in the conclusion we briefly discuss research priorities.

13.2 Tobacco farming and the tobacco-manufacturing industry

One of the chief obstacles to tobacco-control measures is the economic and political importance of tobacco farming in many countries around the world (Altman *et al.* 1996). Understanding the tobacco industry and agricultural sector is essential, therefore, to the formation of a tobacco-control policy. The following sections examine the key players in tobacco production and trade, and the size of the global industry in terms of the amount of employment it creates, so as to assess how many people would be potentially affected by control policies. We focus on tobacco farming as it has attracted the most debate (ITGA 1996a, 1996b), and because it contributes far more to jobs than does cigarette production.

13.2.1 The top tobacco-producing countries

Tobacco is grown in more than 100 countries, including about 80 developing countries. Given its hardiness, tobacco grows well in a variety of climates and topographies. The largest producer of tobacco, as shown in Table 13.1, is China, which has been increasing its share of production rapidly. The United States is the second-largest producer, but its share is currently falling. India and Brazil follow the United States, and they have also been increasing their share of global production. These four countries account for about two-thirds of production world-wide. The top 20 countries, with their diverse mix of income levels, account for approximately 90% of production.

Table 13.1 reveals that many of the tobacco-growing countries export a large share of their tobacco production. Zimbabwe, Italy, and Kyrgyzstan export around three-quarters or more of theirs. Other countries with high export shares are Brazil, Turkey, Malawi, Greece, Argentina, and Spain. Many of these countries use a considerable amount of tobacco leaf domestically in cigarette manufacturing. Of the top 20 producing countries, only Zimbabwe and Malawi do not have a significant cigarette manufacturing industry. There is considerable 'cross-hauling' (Gale *et al.* in press) in Spain, where exports and imports are both large. Japan is the largest net importer. China is essentially self-sufficient in tobacco, as are Indonesia, Pakistan, and Bulgaria. Despite a projected increase in tobacco production for the future, the total area of land

Table 13.1 The top tobacco-growing countries, the area cultivated, and import and export ratios

Country	Area (1000 hectares)	Share of total world area (%)	Production of leaf (1000 metric tons)	Production change	Share of world total volume (%)	Export ratio[a] (%)	Import ratio[b] (%)	Tobacco export revenue as % of total export
	1997	1997	1997	1975–97	1997			1995
China	2353.0	43.9	3920.0	308.3	45.6	2.3	0.4	0.68
USA	328.4	6.1	810.1	−18.2	9.4	28.3	37.9	0.55
India	420.2	7.8	623.7	71.8	7.2	6.1	0.0	0.44
Brazil	346.2	6.5	619.8	116.7	7.2	51.5	3.1	2.55
Turkey	294.7	5.5	286.0	43.0	3.3	56.8	19.0	1.17
Zimbabwe	99.3	1.9	215.3	148.4	2.5	76.6	4.8	23.05
Malawi	114.8	2.1	158.1	352.7	1.8	59.5	0.8	60.64
Indonesia	219.9	4.1	139.7	46.1	1.6	30.2	33.7	0.42
Greece	65.9	1.2	136.9	15.0	1.6	69.5	10.9	2.05
Italy	48.0	0.9	133.0	17.3	1.5	74.4	25.9	0.04
Argentina	69.7	1.3	123.2	26.0	1.4	52.4	4.6	0.59
Pakistan	48.9	0.9	91.6	19.5	1.1	0.3	0.0	0.08
Thailand	49.7	0.9	74.2	18.3	0.9	25.6	12.8	0.11
Canada	26.0	0.5	70.3	−33.7	0.8	44.8	26.4	0.04
Japan	26.5	0.5	68.0	−59.0	0.8	9.1	144.7	0.04
Philippines	57.8	1.1	65.0	13.8	0.8	26.3	33.7	0.17
South Korea	27.2	0.5	54.3	−47.8	0.6	6.1	23.8	0.02
Bulgaria	38.0	0.7	51.8	−68.0	0.6	24.9	22.2	5.40
Spain	17.0	0.3	43.0	66.0	0.5	51.2	129.3	0.06
Dominican Rep.	18.8	0.4	39.2	13.3	0.5	48.4	0.0	5.26
Bangladesh	34.8	0.7	38.1	−5.6	0.4	1.7	4.5	0.03
Poland	16.7	0.3	32.3	−68.4	0.4	17.4	137.6	0.12
Cuba	41.5	0.8	31.4	−25.6	0.4	25.4	14.9	N/A
Colombia	15.8	0.3	28.7	−50.1	0.3	29.5	6.4	N/A
Vietnam	28.3	0.5	28.3	112.8	0.3	1.8	13.8	0.04
South Africa	15.0	0.3	26.4	−3.9	0.3	28.7	56.6	0.31
Kyrgyzstan	8.5	0.2	25.7	N/A	0.3	74.2	0.0	6.96
Tanzania	32.5	0.6	25.0	77.2	0.3	24.9	0.0	4.53
World Total	5358.9	100.0	8603.4	58.7	100.0	21.8	23.0	

[a] Ratio of exports to domestic production.
[b] Ratio of imports to domestic production.
N/A = not available.

Source: USDA (1998); FAO (1998); IEC (1998).

under tobacco is falling, as better cultivation methods lead to higher productivity. The 5.3 million hectares under tobacco account for less than 1% of the world's arable crop area (approximately half the area devoted to coffee) (Food and Agriculture Organization 1989, 1998).

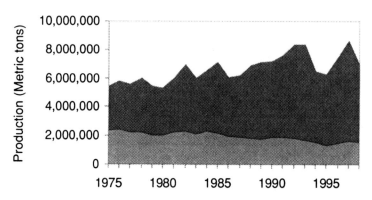

Fig. 13.1 Tobacco production by developed and developing countries, 1975–98.

Source: FAO (1998).

In most countries, tobacco export revenue, as a share of total export, is below 1%. A few countries receive a more significant share of foreign exchange earnings— between 2% and 5%—from tobacco; they include Tanzania, Kyrgyzstan, the Dominican Republic, and Bulgaria. Only Zimbabwe and Malawi are highly dependent on tobacco for export earnings, with tobacco accounting for 23% and 61% of total exports, respectively.

13.2.2 The shift of tobacco farming to developing countries

In recent decades, the growth in world tobacco production has come primarily from low-income and middle-income countries. Between 1975 and 1998, production in developed countries fell by 31%, while production in developing countries rose by 128%, as shown in Fig. 13.1.

As shown in Fig. 13.2, Asia (including the Middle East) increased its share of world tobacco production from 40% to 60% during the period 1977–97, while the total share of the high-income countries fell from 30% to 15%. Africa's share rose from 4% to 6%. The share of tobacco grown in Eastern Europe and the states of the former Soviet Union fell during the 1990s.

In many developing countries, there has been considerable emphasis on agricultural research to increase the efficiency of tobacco farms. The aims have included raising farmers' income and exports, reducing reliance on imported tobacco, and earning or conserving foreign exchange. An additional factor is the growth in demand for tobacco products in developing countries, as incomes and purchasing power have grown. In some countries, farmers have been encouraged to plant tobacco to supply new processing plants built to expand local cigarette production. Many developing countries are attempting to increase cigarette exports or substitute domestic products for imported cigarettes. Increasing taste for Western-style cigarettes has spurred demand for flue-cured Virginia tobacco (Joossens and Raw 1996).

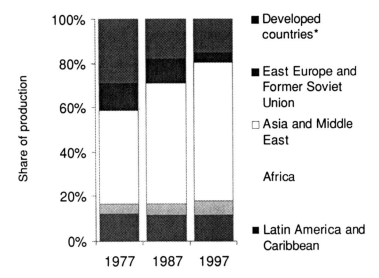

Fig. 13.2 Shares of world tobacco production, by region, 1977–97. Developed countries* include North America, Western Europe, and Japan.

Source: FAO (1998).

13.2.3 The size of the tobacco farming and manufacturing industries

Few reliable estimates are available on the current size of either the farming industry or the manufacturing industry. Tobacco-industry estimates suggest that worldwide, some 33 million people are employed in tobacco growing, usually part-time, counting family members, seasonal workers, and other laborers. It is estimated that approximately 15 million people are employed in tobacco farming in China alone (Skolnick 1996), 3 million in India (Patel 1992), 488 000 in the Philippines (Ernst and Young 1991), and nearly 100 000 in Zimbabwe (Maravanyika 1997). In the European Union there are 135 000 tobacco farms and an estimated 170 000 laborers located largely in Italy, Greece, Spain, and France. The United States has about 120 000 farms. There are no reliable independent estimates of the number of seasonal laborers.

However, from a macro-economic perspective, the important statistic is the *percentage* of those employed in any country that are dependent on tobacco products for their livelihood, and not the absolute numbers of people employed. Thus, even in Malawi, the percentage of people employed in tobacco relative to other agricultural products is small. There are also several conceptual difficulties in estimating the absolute numbers. Tobacco labor on farms and in primary processing is seasonal, and its contribution to the formal economy is unclear. Laborers include migrants, unpaid family members, and casual laborers from the community. Few hired workers work full-time in tobacco farming or primary processing (Gale 1998). It is therefore misleading to compare employment figures in these sectors of the tobacco industry with employment from sectors where jobs are full-time and year-round. As Table 13.2 indicates, in developing countries when full-time equivalent (FTE) figures are used,

Table 13.2 Employment in tobacco growing in various developing countries, 1990, ranked by the share of tobacco-growing jobs in total labor force

	Share of agriculture in total GDP (%)	Number employed in growing tobacco ('000)	FTE employed in growing tobacco ('000)	Tobacco FTE as % of agricultural labor force (%)	Tobacco FTE as % of total labor force (%)
Malawi	33	157	93	2.34	2.03
Turkey	18	560	313	2.41	1.29
Philippines	22	488	301	2.71	1.24
China	27	15 998	6152	1.25	0.90
Zimbabwe	13	92	39	1.25	0.85
Sri Lanka	26	150	50	1.50	0.73
Colombia	17	302	101	2.73	0.73
Thailand	12	1 362	213	1.05	0.67
Iraq	18[a]	57	29	3.90	0.63
Indonesia	22	1 466	454	1.02	0.57
Malaysia	2[a]	100	39	1.96	0.54
Myanmar	N/A	350	114	0.73	0.53
Brazil	10	600	289	1.90	0.44
Bangladesh	38	409	205	0.61	0.40
Argentina	13	105	44	2.97	0.36
Tanzania	59	178	47	0.43	0.36
Cuba	N/A	20	17	1.95	0.35
Venezuela	6	95	23	2.63	0.32
India	31	3 500	1108	0.48	0.31
Syria	28	54	10	0.87	0.29
Tunisia	16	15	7	0.87	0.24
Guatemala	26	24	7	0.45	0.23
Pakistan	26	205	86	0.39	0.20
Nigeria	36	217	42	0.28	0.12
Congo	30	21	13	0.12	0.08
Morocco	16	15	7	0.17	0.08
Kenya	28	11	5	0.06	0.04
Chile	9	4	2	0.21	0.04
Average[b]	26	NA	NA	1.01	0.63

FTE = full-time equivalent; [a] 1965 values; [b] average is weighted by total labor force.

Source: Chapman and Wong (1990); Ernst and Young (1991); Patel (1992); World Bank (1992); Skolnick (1996); FAO (1998); ILO (1998).

the average FTE is typically about one-third of the total absolute number reported by the tobacco industry (Chapman and Wong 1990).

Many farms that grow tobacco grow only a small amount, and most tobacco operations are extremely small, averaging less than 1 hectare in many developing countries. Only in parts of the United States and Zimbabwe are large-scale tobacco operations common, due to the difficulties involved in mechanization and the predominance of smallholders. In the United States the allotment system, discussed below, has served to keep many farms small.

In certain low-income and middle-income countries, tobacco growing is important for several reasons, chiefly because of its labor intensity and its ability to generate dependable cashflow for poor small farmers. Tobacco is among the more labor-intensive crops (and an additional reason why farms are small). Seasonal labor is required for transplanting young plants from seedbeds or greenhouses to fields, and for removing tops when plants begin to flower and suckers that grow out from the stalk (to maximize growth and quality of leaves). Flue-cured tobacco is harvested by removing a few leaves at a time, a very labor-intensive process. Machines are available for flue-cured harvesting and have been adopted in some areas, but there is no mechanization for burley tobacco. Curing is also often done on the farm to ensure the correct moisture, nicotine, and sugar content, which affect the quality and taste. Mechanization has been difficult to achieve in tobacco farming, due to the complexity of these tasks. Additionally, much tobacco is grown on hilly or mountainous land that is unsuitable for mechanised equipment (Chapman and Wong 1990).

Many of the developing countries, shown in Table 13.2, that grow tobacco, have highly agrarian economies with large proportions of the total labor force in agriculture. Most of these economies are, however, diversified in that they produce various agricultural products. The relative contribution of agriculture to gross domestic product (GDP) is falling: between 1965 and 1990, the contribution of agriculture shrank from 29% to 17% in low-income and middle-income countries (World Bank 1993).

In contrast to farming, tobacco manufacturing is a mechanized production process and generates few jobs. Table 13.3 below shows employment in tobacco manufacturing for selected countries for 1990. In very few countries does tobacco manufacturing make up more than 1% of total manufacturing employment. The nature and size of the multinational tobacco industry has been discussed elsewhere (Johnson 1984; WHO 1999).

We now examine the impact of control policies on key economic variables, chiefly employment.

13.3 Do tobacco-control policies have a detrimental effect on the economy?

To combat tobacco-control policies, the tobacco industry has long argued that nations are economically dependent on tobacco for employment and incomes. The argument is usually put forward that measures that threaten tobacco sales bring serious political risks because of damage to the economy. We review studies that have estimated the impact of tobacco-control policies on employment, tax revenue, and incomes. These studies have been commissioned by the tobacco industry and also by independent researchers.

13.3.1 Industry-commissioned studies on the economic contribution of tobacco

A large number of industry-sponsored studies have suggested that tobacco-control policies would have a detrimental impact on the economies of high-income countries

Table 13.3 Employment in cigarette manufacturing as a proportion of total manufacturing employment for selected countries, 1990, ranked in absolute numbers

Country	Employment in tobacco manufacturing	Proportion of total manufacturing employment
China	265 000	N/A
Indonesia	241 126	5.32
United States	41 000	0.19
Russia	33 000	N/A
Turkey	32 142	1.56
Bangladesh	27 155	1.6
Egypt	17 513	1.24
Italy	15 845	0.39
Bulgaria	15 300	N/A
Philippines	13 941	0.88
United Kingdom	13 000	0.25
Japan	12 000	0.09
Thailand	10 500	0.55
Iran	10 500	1.28
Poland	10 000	0.25
Pakistan	9 400	0.60
Spain	8 607	0.32
Korea Republic	7 200	0.17
Netherlands	7 000	0.61
Romania	6 200	0.18
Zimbabwe	5 414	N/A
Mexico	5 240	0.14
France	5 100	0.12
Canada	5 000	0.23
Hungary	5 000	0.43

N/A = not available.

Source: UNIDO (1998).

(for the United States: Wharton Applied Research Center 1979; Chase Econometrics 1985; Price Waterhouse 1990, 1992; Tobacco Merchants Association 1995; American Economics Group 1996; for Europe: PEIDA 1985; Agro-Economics Services Ltd. and Tabacosmos Ltd. 1987; for Canada, Deloitte & Touche 1995; for Hong Kong: Coopers & Lybrand 1996). Economic consulting firms typically estimate the employment attributable to the growing of tobacco as well as to the manufacture, distribution, and sale of tobacco products. They also calculate the incomes associated with this employment, tax revenues generated by the sale of tobacco products, and, where relevant, the contribution to a country's trade balance.

Generally, these studies estimate *gross* employment and do not consider that the decline of one economic activity (tobacco) would be replaced by alternative spending and economic activity that would generate alternative employment. The tobacco industry uses the gross estimates made in these studies to indicate the significance of tobacco in the economies and to make gross projections of jobs and tax revenues that will be lost on adoption of tobacco control policy measures. Further, based on these estimates, multipliers then establish the indirect effects of the industry's employment contribution to other sectors. The multipliers used in these studies are useful insofar as they estimate the effect of one type of economic activity in stimulating additional economic activity (output multipliers), but not the actual number of jobs dependent on tobacco spending (Arthur Andersen Economic Consulting 1993). In general, the industry-commissioned estimates use generous multipliers.

13.3.2 Independent studies on the economic contribution of tobacco

In recent years, macro-economic research in several countries has challenged the conclusions of the industry studies. Unlike the industry-commissioned studies that stop with the gross economic contribution of tobacco, the numbers of jobs, earnings, and taxes paid, the independent studies estimate the *net* impact by comparing tobacco-related economic activity with assumed production after the redistribution of the resources that would be freed from tobacco consumption to alternative uses (Warner 1987). Table 13.4 provides the results of these quantitative independent studies, and some qualitative studies.

Most of the independent studies simulate the net impact on economic activity from eliminating or reducing expenditure on tobacco, and make certain assumptions about how the alternative expenditure will take place in the economy. Their basic underlying assumption is usually that of zero or greatly reduced expenditure on cigarettes. This is obviously an extreme assumption. However, since the input–output models used are essentially linear, the resource reallocations following specified reductions or elimination of tobacco can be approximately interpolated from the results.

The results of most of the studies show that job losses occur in the sectors that are immediately associated with cigarette production: tobacco manufacturing and farming, and the cigarette retail, wholesale and distribution sectors. In some cases, jobs would also be lost in government if there were a loss in government revenue. However, these losses are outweighed in most studies by increases in employment in all other industries (services, manufacturing, transport, communication, public utilities, finance, construction, and mining). The increase in jobs is most marked in the service industries, which are labor-intensive. Jobs lost in retailing tobacco are likely to replaced by jobs retailing other products that people purchase with the money formerly spent on tobacco. As noted by Sunley *et al.* (Chapter 17), tax increases on tobacco products would increase revenues in the short to medium term.

In most studies net gains in activity would be realized in every broad economic sector, which suggests that, in general terms, the required degree of readjustment to the economy without tobacco would be limited. Most independent studies assume that income not spent on tobacco will be spent on other goods and services according to consumers' existing (average) expenditure patterns. Some studies (Buck *et al.* 1995; van der Merwe 1998a) have, however, tested alternative expenditure patterns following evidence that consumers' cessation of smoking leads to new spending patterns. For

Table 13.4 Independent studies on the contribution of tobacco to various countries' economies

Study	Dynamic or static model	Assumption of reduction or elimination of domestic consumption expenditures or production	Assumption of alternative expenditure patterns	Assumption of government reaction	Results
Quantitative studies					
Scotland (McNicoll and Boyle 1992)	Static	Elimination of domestic consumption expenditures in 1989.	According to 'average' expenditure patterns.	No change in government expenditure.	Net gain of 7869 jobs in 1989.
Michigan (Warner and Fulton 1994)	Dynamic	Scenarios: elimination of domestic consumption expenditures, and doubling the rate of decline in consumption over the period 1992–2005.	According to 'average' expenditure patterns.	Increases in other government taxes, and/or reduced government spending.	Net gain of 5600 jobs in 1992 up to an additional 1500 jobs by 2005.
United States (Warner et al. 1996)	Dynamic	Scenarios: elimination of domestic consumption expenditures, and doubling the rate of decline in consumption over the period 1993–2000.	According to 'average' expenditure patterns.	Increases in other government taxes, and/or reduced government spending.	Net gain of 47 jobs in 1993 and 133 000 jobs by 2000, 19719 net jobs with doubling consumption decline.
United Kingdom (Buck et al. 1995)	Static	40% decline in domestic consumption expenditures in 1990.	Scenarios: according to 'recent stoppers', to non-smokers, all former smokers, and 'average' expenditure patterns.	Increases in other government taxes or reduced government spending.	Net gain of 155542 jobs or 115688 full-time equivalent jobs in 1990 with 'recent stopper' expenditures and government increasing other consumer taxes.
Canada (Irvine and Sims 1997)	Static	20% decline in domestic demand for cigarettes in 1995.	According to 'average' expenditure patterns.	Reduced government spending.	Net loss of 6120 jobs in 1995.

Study		Assumptions			Conclusions
South Africa (van der Merwe 1998a)	Static	Scenarios: elimination of domestic consumption expenditures, and doubling the rate of decline in consumption in 1995.	Scenarios: according to 'recent stoppers', and 'average' expenditure patterns.	Increases in other government taxes, and/or reduced government spending.	Net gain of 50236 jobs in 1995 with elimination of tobacco and 'recent stopper' expenditures.
Zimbabwe (van der Merwe 1998b)	Static	Elimination of domestic consumption expenditures and all tobacco production in 1980.	Scenarios: according to 'average' input–output patterns and all production shifted to alternatives in agriculture.	No change in government expenditure.	Net loss of 87798 jobs in 1980 and 47463 jobs when all output goes to alternatives in agriculture.
Bangladesh (van der Merwe 1998c)	Static	Elimination of domestic consumption expenditures and all tobacco production for cigarettes and bidis in 1994.	According to 'average' expenditure patterns.	No change in government expenditure.	Net gain of 10989192 jobs in 1994.

Study	Assumptions	Conclusions
Qualitative studies Canada (Allen 1993)	1. Jobs could be subsumed through normal workforce attrition. 2. Technological changes caused many job losses. 3. Increased public revenues could be spent to maintain services and create jobs. 4. Cost savings in shifting Canadian production abroad. 5. Distribution jobs would remain. 6. Economy would self-correct.	Control policies, primarily taxes, would have negligible adverse effect on employment.
Pacific Islands (Collins and Lapsley 1997)	1. Alternative cash crops are likely available on islands that grow tobacco. 2. Freed expenditure resources directed to goods and services with higher labor content. 3. Improvement in balance of payments on current account from reduced tobacco imports.	Reduction in consumption would probably produce small increase in employment.

example, some studies assumed that former smokers would use their marginal increase in income, in the short-term, to increase expenditure on luxury items such as recreational goods and services, while expenditure on essential items such as housing would change very little (Buck *et al.* 1995). Studies in the United Kingdom and South Africa examining the expenditure of people who had recently quit smoking showed that they made increased use of labor-intensive services such as recreation, education, and communications (van der Merwe 1998d). If this behavior pattern were seen on a national scale, there would be larger structural adjustments and transition costs in the economy, but there would also be larger net gains.

The results also show that the tobacco-producing regions or countries, for example the south-eastern part of the United States, Zimbabwe, and Canada, would have suffered job losses (Warner *et al.* 1996; van der Merwe 1998b; Irvine and Sims 1997). However, in the United States (Warner *et al.* 1996), with every non-tobacco producing region enjoying a net gain in jobs, all non-tobacco regions collectively would have gained enough employment to offset the losses.

Most studies are also based on the use of input–output tables, which show the interdependencies between industrial sectors and sub-sectors in the economy (Miernyk 1957), and how the changes in one industry affect the level of output in other industries. This static approach usually compares two alternative situations in a given base year, one with and one without (or with reduced) tobacco expenditures taking place. Alternatively, dynamic models (Warner and Fulton 1994), allow one to simulate trade flows and feedback effects.

Even where it is assumed that a portion of the reallocated resources would go to saving rather than spending, the studies show that there could still be employment gains. If the money consumers once spent on tobacco were saved instead of spent, this would also be expected to generate jobs because of incremental investment demand, assuming people use their savings to acquire financial assets other than cash.

Finally, certain assumptions are made as to how governments may react to a possible loss in revenue from a fall in consumption in the long run. These usually include alternatives such as reduced government expenditure, and hence employment (Allen 1993) or the collection of consumer taxes on alternative goods and services (Warner *et al.* 1996). If the fall in consumption is brought about not by excise taxes, but by other regulatory actions such as an advertising ban, then consumers would have the additional money to spend on goods and services besides cigarettes. Alternatively, if the fall in consumption is brought about by tax increases, then new jobs will also be created, as long as the government spends the additional tax revenues. Even in the unlikely case of governments using all extra income for deficit reduction, reduced interest rates would result in increased employment. Taken together, the evidence suggests that the economy, at a macro-level, can respond to the decline in cigarette consumption by generating at least as many jobs in other industries as were lost in tobacco growing or manufacturing (Allen 1993). As others (Chapter 17) show, tax increases on cigarettes would cause an increase in government revenues in the short- to medium-term. In the long run, excise tax revenues may be reduced as a result of lower consumption levels. Any reduction in revenue would either need to be replaced from other sources, or could alternatively also result in employment loss in government. It might be assumed that government would react to the loss in revenue in this transition by increasing taxes from other goods and services. This would naturally occur as consumer expenditure switched to other goods and taxes were collected on these items. The studies therefore usually test one or more ways in which government may react to possible long-run revenue losses, usually including the assumption that a natural shift to alternative tax bases will take place (Allen 1993).

Finally, these studies estimate dramatic declines in tobacco use, or even its complete elimination. In reality, however, there is little prospect of a sharp and sudden reduction in tobacco production. If demand for tobacco falls, it will fall slowly. Others in this volume describe how control policies such as taxes (Chapter 10) and information (Chapter 8) yield modest but gradual reductions in demand. This allows for an equally slow process of transition for those most directly affected. For example, total cigarette sales have fallen in the United Kingdom from 138 billion to 50 billion over three decades (Nicolaides-Bouman *et al.* 1990). Similarly, in the United States, the decline in smoking prevalence among men has taken place over three decades (USDHHS 1989). This means that the costs of adjusting supply as demand diminishes will also be stretched out over decades. Thus, the transition costs would also be spread over a long period.

13.3.3 The impact of control policies on trade in tobacco

In principle, control policies will have both negative and positive economic impacts on trade in tobacco, particularly with respect to jobs. However, employment losses are expected to be greater for countries that are net exporters of *unprocessed or total tobacco* (Table 13.5), than for countries that are net exporters of *cigarettes* (Table 13.6). We focus on trade in unprocessed and total tobacco below.

Countries may be divided into five possible generic categories with respect to tobacco production:

(1) the country produces but does not consume tobacco, making it a *full exporter*;
(2) the country produces more tobacco than it consumes; in other words it is a *net exporter*;
(3) the country produces and consumes the same amount of tobacco—this is a case of a '*self-contained*' industry with respect to tobacco;
(4) the country produces less than it consumes, in other words it is a *net importer*;
(5) the country does not produce tobacco but consumes it, in other words it is a *full importer* of the product.

The impact of control measures would differ in each of these categories. Countries in Category 1 are a theoretical possibility but in practice rare. Zimbabwe would probably be the country closest to this, where in 1996, 99% of tobacco production went for export (Maravanyika 1997). Most countries fall into Categories 2–4. In general, as one moves from Category 5 through to Category 1, the transition costs of tobacco control rise. For instance, for a full importer economy, there would be no production loss (or associated employment loss) even if demand fell dramatically. The full burden of transition would fall on the consumption side and its related elements, including import taxes, sales taxes, and trade-related employment. In general, countries that are net importers would be less affected by control policies than net exporters. There are only

Table 13.5 Net exporters and net importers of tobacco, 1995

Income	Net exporters Category 1 and 2	'Self-contained' Category 3	Net importers Category 4 and 5	
Low-income	India Kenya Malawi Tanzania Zimbabwe	China Pakistan Sri Lanka Zambia	Bangladesh Bosnia and Herzegovina Cote d'Ivoire	Nepal Nigeria Vietnam
Lower middle-income	Colombia Guatemala Macedonia Thailand Turkey	Bulgaria Egypt Philippines	Algeria Bolivia Botswana Estonia Indonesia Iraq Kazakhstan Lithuania Morocco	Papua New Guinea Peru Poland Romania Russia Slovakia South Korea Ukraine Venezuela
Upper middle-income	Argentina Brazil Chile Greece Mexico	South Africa	Croatia Czech Rep. Hungary Malaysia Saudi Arabia Slovenia	
High-income	Canada Italy United States	United Arab Emirates	Australia Austria Belgium Luxembourg Cyprus Denmark Finland France Germany Hong Kong Ireland Israel	Japan Netherlands New Zealand Norway Portugal Qatar Singapore Spain Sweden Switzerland United Kingdom

Source: Market File (1998); UNIDO (1998); World Bank (1997).

a few major producers and exporters of tobacco that fall into Category 2. They include: the United States, Canada, India, Brazil, Zimbabwe, Turkey, and Malawi. These major producers and net exporters, as shown in Table 13.5, would have higher transition costs if global demand falls.

Even in net exporting countries, control policies that reduce *domestic* tobacco consumption will have negligible effects on output in the economy and employment. Only when the control policies directly impact on their export markets do they face poss-

Table 13.6 Net exporters and net importers of cigarettes, 1995

Income	Net exporters Category 1 and 2	'Self-contained' Category 3	Net importers Category 4 and 5
Low-income			Afghanistan Albania Myanmar
Lower middle-income	Bolivia Venezuela	Slovakia	Iran Lebanon Paraguay
Upper middle-income	Croatia Hungary	Czech Rep. Greece Malaysia	
High-income	Austria Denmark Finland Germany Ireland Netherlands Switzerland United Kingdom	Australia Cyprus Hong Kong New Zealand Singapore	Guam Iceland Kuwait Macao

Source: Market File (1998); UNIDO (1998); World Bank (1997).

ible job losses. In addition, these countries would be the hardest hit by attempts to restrict global supply, or supply from these countries. For example, bans on importing tobacco from these countries would yield significant short-term job losses, particularly in Zimbabwe and Malawi.

Several of the countries that appear in Categories 1 and 2 are not major exporters or producers of tobacco, and hence control policies would have smaller repercussions in their economies. In fact, many countries, particularly in Europe, import tobacco leaf and are then exporters of manufactured cigarettes. Control policies will thus affect their manufacturing industries, which generally employ fewer people than the primary production side, and are less labor-intensive.

The number of countries falling into Category 3—neither net importers nor net exporters—is also relatively limited. A few prominent members, some already shown in Table 13.5, are China, the Philippines, Pakistan, Bulgaria, and South Africa. The 'self-contained' category would expect to see no job losses or modest gains with reduced demand. For example, studies in South Africa and Scotland concluded that there would be a net increase in employment (Table 13.4).

Generally, the elimination of the tobacco industry in net importer countries is expected to create jobs overall. One study in Bangladesh, a net importer, found increases in employment with reduced demand (van der Merwe 1998b). In addition, a reduction in imports should also improve the trade balance and have positive economic effects through reduced foreign exchange losses (Collins and Lapsley 1997). It should be noted that Tables 13.5 and 13.6 are based on 1995 data and that, over time, some categorization shifts may take place.

13.3.4 Industry-generated employment losses

Often overlooked in the debate over tobacco control and jobs is the fact that several countries have simultaneously increased tobacco production and decreased employment in tobacco manufacturing. This is a consequence of productivity improvements and technological changes rather than imposed tobacco-control policies (Connolly 1992).

A study in the United Kingdom (PEIDA 1991) showed that much of the employment loss in manufacturing between 1980 and 1990 was due to productivity improvements. In the United States, manufacturing jobs fell by 29% between 1982 and 1992, despite the fact that US cigarette output actually increased during that period due to increased exports (Allen 1993). In Colombia, output increased by 26% over the first half of the 1980s, yet the number of jobs dropped by 25% to 2973 in 1985. Similarly, in Spain in the 1980s, output increased by 14% and employment fell over the same period, by 14% to 10 200 in 1986. In Malaysia, output increased by 15% in the 1980s and tobacco manufacturing employment fell over the same period by 62% to 4300 in 1987. In Pakistan, output increased 23% and employment fell 8% over the same period in the 1980s. Similarly in the Philippines, production increased in the 1980s by 17% and employment over the same period fell by 28% to 13 000 by 1987 (UNIDO 1998).

Finally, domestic sales of US leaf tobacco have fallen over the past several years despite the increase in domestic cigarette production. This decline in demand, and the corresponding drop in tobacco farm employment, is due primarily to increasing reliance by major manufacturers on imported tobacco (Arthur Andersen Economic Consulting 1993).

We now turn to a discussion of the incentives to grow tobacco, and review the role of supply-side interventions such as subsidies, diversification, buy-outs or bans on production.

13.4 The effectiveness of supply-side instruments such as subsidies and tobacco farm diversification

While tobacco growers account for a small share of the total income generated by the tobacco industry, they are a key source of opposition to tobacco control. Therefore, knowledge of the incentives to grow tobacco, and the operation of world tobacco markets, are critical to the design of workable tobacco control policy and strategies.

13.4.1 The incentives for producing tobacco

The chief incentive for tobacco farming is that it is more profitable than many other crops. In the United States, for example, net returns of roughly US$2000 per acre of tobacco far exceed the net returns from most other crops (Gale *et al.* in press). In Zimbabwe, tobacco is roughly six times more profitable than the next-best alternative crop (Maravanyika 1997). An industry-sponsored study that attempted to identify alternative crops and compare their returns with those of tobacco in seven developing countries concluded that there are few profitable, sustainable alternatives to tobacco production that could be widely adopted (ITGA 1996b). For many people who grow tobacco in developing countries, tobacco is their only cash crop, and these people are often poor. Tobacco growers in high-income countries are not poor by the standards of Africa or South Asia, but they tend to be concentrated in relatively impoverished regions of their countries.

The indirect benefits of tobacco cultivation to farmers are also considerable. Tobacco cash income enables the purchase of farm equipment and household goods, and supports other farm enterprises, including food crops that are consumed by the household. In the Philippines, tobacco is grown as a dry-season crop, while palay is grown in the wet season (Ernst and Young 1991). In some developing countries, tobacco production has generated improvement in farming practices that not only increase tobacco yields but also increase the production of other crops (Maravanyika 1998). For example, Zimbabwean tobacco farmers also produce large proportions of the country's maize, cotton, beef, wheat, and soybeans (Chapman and Wong 1990). In Malawi, the tobacco crop finances the bulk of marketed maize and virtually all paprika production. In Ghana and India, it was found that farmers who grew tobacco were more likely to use improved, modern technology in producing their non-tobacco crops. In addition, the cultivation of tobacco may attract investment by multinational companies in low-income or middle-income countries, thus raising overall income levels (Lewit 1987).

In contrast to developing countries, tobacco farmers in high-income countries usually have other cash-generating farm enterprises, though tobacco generates most of the net returns to the farm. However, many, if not most, tobacco-farming families in these countries do not rely solely on farm income (Gale 1998). Off-farm work provides the bulk of income for many tobacco-growing households. In the United States, farms that produce flue-cured tobacco are likely to grow soybeans, corn, cotton, and wheat as well. On smaller US farms typical of burley tobacco, beef cattle are common.

13.4.2 Taxation of tobacco producers in low- and middle-income countries

Many low-income countries rely on revenue from export taxes and industry excise taxes, since income taxes are difficult to administer without an adequate infrastructure (Pena and Norton 1993; Beghin *et al.* 1996). Argentina, Brazil, Turkey, and recently Zimbabwe all have export taxes on tobacco products. In low-income and middle-income countries, marketing boards or state-approved tobacco monopolies often purchase tobacco leaf at low prices, indirectly taxing tobacco growers. In some countries, governments try to offset these taxes with subsidies for credit, electricity, and other production inputs. Other ways of extracting revenue from tobacco include over-valued exchange rates. The taxation of producers discourages tobacco production by pushing land, labor, and capital out of tobacco production into other types of farming, urban non-farm employment, work in the informal sector, or unemployment. However, despite the taxation, tobacco is still more profitable than available alternatives in most countries where it is grown. Where alternatives to tobacco are poor, producer taxation can succeed in raising revenue since growers cannot respond to lower returns to tobacco (or farming in general) by switching to other activities. In such a situation, governments have incentives to encourage tobacco production. Peng (1996) describes how a lack of economic development and a poorly functioning tax system in the transition to a decentralized economy created fiscal dependence on tobacco in a poor region of China. Peng goes on to describe how local governments may pressurize farmers to plant tobacco in order to increase tobacco tax revenue.

13.4.3 Subsidies, quotas and supply control

In the high-income countries, stagnant or falling domestic demand, pessimistic pronouncements about the future of tobacco farming, attractive non-farm opportunities, and rising farm productivity have contributed to a slow, but substantial, movement of people out of all types of farming, including tobacco (Gale 1998). The number of tobacco farms in the United States and Canada fell by nearly two-thirds from the early 1960s to the 1990s. However, structural adjustments would have been even more dramatic without the incentives provided by tobacco subsidies, which have preserved the structure of small farms and prevented regional shifts in production (Sumner and Alston 1985; Industry Commission 1994; Brown 1998).

Governments in many countries have introduced price supports, subsidies or credit for fuel and transport, export subsidies, marketing programs, and national or regional policies that benefit the sector. These policies increase the profitability of tobacco and induce farmers to plant tobacco that would not otherwise be grown (Beghin *et al.* 1996). In high-income countries, tobacco price supports were introduced for two reasons. First, there were concerns that tobacco prices are not set by free markets, because cigarette manufacturers are few in number and it is believed that they have power to set prices that are disadvantageous to farmers. Second, there were concerns about potential instability in the tobacco markets, and resulting uncertainty in prices from year to year, due to weather, disasters, overplanting, or other economic fluctuations. Therefore, unlike many other cash crops, the producer price of tobacco does not fluctuate substantially. Growers negotiate sales prices in advance of planting so they are protected from unexpected price changes and they are paid in cash immediately upon sale of the crop. Therefore much of the risk of tobacco growing is shifted from the farmer to the purchaser (Lewit 1987). Even though in the United States, many of the reasons for implementing the initial price supports are no longer valid, the federal government still maintains the program mainly for political reasons (Tweeten 1995).

Governments in several high-income countries set prices above world market levels, while restraining production through supply controls. In the United States, Canada and Western Europe, governments set minimum prices for each type of tobacco, based largely on the costs of producing it, which are significantly higher than prices in world markets (Coady *et al.* 1991; Joossens and Raw 1996; Irvine and Sims 1997). These high, stable prices would draw resources into tobacco production (or prevent them from exiting). But these price support schemes also include strict quotas on production and marketing that limit the quantity grown. Tobacco growing is limited to those possessing production rights assigned by the government (acreage allotments and marketing quotas). Due to these limitations on supply, production levels are lower than would occur in an unregulated market (Sumner and Alston 1985; Brown 1998). Informal estimates indicate that flue-cured tobacco production might be tripled if quotas were not in place. Therefore, the United States's tobacco subsidy reduces the US share of the world tobacco market, despite the incentive to produce provided by high prices. Nevertheless, US tobacco has maintained a large world market share due to its high quality. High prices have not only reduced foreign demand, but have also encouraged US cigarette manufacturers to increase their use of cheaper foreign tobacco. Some European countries have also restrained production through quotas, but historically European subsidies have encouraged the production of low-quality/high-tar tobacco varieties that are not in demand in their own markets. Much of this European tobacco was exported, often with the help of export subsidies, to Central and Eastern Europe and the Middle East, while most tobacco used in European cigarette manufactures was imported (Townsend 1991; Joossens and Raw 1996). Some of the larger tobacco-producing countries that give subsidies for tobacco growing include Argentina, Bulgaria, Columbia, Germany, Greece, Italy, Spain, Turkey, and also Brazil, Hungary, and Uruguay, which have general agricultural subsidy programs that include tobacco.

These price supports introduce certain distortions in the market. In particular, quotas and allotments make tobacco growing more profitable to the farmer (or allotment holder) than it would be if market forces determined prices. This encourages a shift of resources from other crops to tobacco. In competitive markets, this resource shift leads to an expansion of supply and an equilibrating fall in price. Where supply is controlled, price does not fall and as a result excess profits, called 'economic rents', are created, which make the government-assigned right to produce and sell tobacco a valuable asset. Excess profits encourage producers to organize politically to protect their rents against falling prices, imports, and government tobacco-control policies designed to decrease demand. Such 'rent-seeking' behavior could be considered a likely consequence of regulatory and subsidy policies (Lewit 1987).

Tobacco is far from unique among various agricultural markets in having a history of supply controls and quotas. These systems were created largely before the health effects of tobacco were understood. Now, however, the protection of economic rents has motivated growers to unite in opposition to tobacco control efforts. In the United States, transferability of production quotas has created a class of 300 000 quota owners, many of whom rent out their quota and do not grow tobacco themselves. This large number of individuals, each with a small stake in maintaining the tobacco subsidy, further strengthens opposition to its elimination (Warner 1988).

Tobacco subsidies have often been criticized as a form of government hypocrisy. A common public perception is that tobacco subsidies directly encourage smoking by encouraging tobacco cultivation. More recently, however, it has become more widely recognized that the reality is more complex. In high-income countries, subsidy schemes may actually discourage consumption slightly by restricting the amount of leaf produced and thus raising the price. Higher tobacco prices raise the cost of cigarettes, thus discouraging smoking. But the effect is small since tobacco leaf accounts for less than 5% of retail cigarette prices (Zhang and Husten 1998) and prices in high-income countries are primarily determined by taxation.

In order to conserve foreign exchange, many low-income and middle-income countries may attempt to discourage imports of both tobacco leaf and cigarettes, particularly if the countries have domestic tobacco industries. Imports are discouraged by restricting the availability of foreign exchange for tobacco imports, and by differential taxation. These interventions result in substantial price differences between domestically-produced cigarettes that contain foreign tobacco and those that do not. As a result of import duties and other import restrictions, prices received by tobacco growers in these countries are likely to be higher than they would be otherwise, because domestic production is stimulated and tobacco farmers' incomes increased (Lewit 1987).

Tobacco production for farmers may, therefore, appear to be desirable because it allows participation in a subsidized market. In addition, policies within low-income and middle-income countries that limit tobacco imports also benefit domestic producers at the expense of consumers. Accordingly, the subsidies may cause policy-makers and farmers to mis-value the crop. In the short-run, therefore, tobacco production may prove very profitable and raise national incomes in low-income and middle-income countries. However, it will induce self-protective behavior by its participants, which may make it very difficult for governments to mount effective programs for control of tobacco use.

13.4.4 Tobacco-farm diversification

There is much discussion of tobacco-farm 'diversification' or 'crop substitution', which entails farmers switching from tobacco to other crops (Aberg and Tedla 1979; Al-Sadat and Zain 1997; Altman *et al.* 1998). Such supply-side efforts, often driven by a desire to move production toward crops with less negative health implications, are not likely to be effective as a means of controlling tobacco use. A basic observation in markets is that, if one supplier of a commodity is prevented from operating, another will quickly emerge to take its place, as long as there is a strong incentive to do so. 'Diversification' is actually a misnomer since, as discussed above, most tobacco-growing households are already quite diversified. In countries of all income levels, however, tobacco usually provides an important share of cash income (Lewit 1987).

Large-scale efforts to encourage tobacco farmers to diversify and substitute alternative crops have occurred in only a few countries. In the United States, farmers have expended considerable effort in searching for alternatives to tobacco, motivated in part by the US market's uncertain prospects. A recent survey of US tobacco farmers showed that 70% had attempted supplemental enterprises in the previous five years (Altman *et al.* 1996). Efforts, however, have been scattered and piecemeal, and farmers have not been offered financial incentives to switch crops. There have been attempts to grow familiar crops like broccoli, as well as more exotic enterprises, such as llamas and ginseng. Several alternative crop programs could succeed. Labor-intensive speciality crops and value-added activities are viewed as the most promising alternatives, pri-

Table 13.7 Economic returns of alternative crops to flue-cured Virginia tobacco in India, 1989

Crop	Yield (kg/ha)	Cost of cultivation (Rs./ha)	Gross income (Rs./ha)	Cost–benefit ratio
Safflower	1800	3661	14 400	1:4.0
Mustard	1500	3196	12 000	1:3.3
Flue-cured Virginia tobacco	1417	8464	17 620	1:2.0

Source: Chari and Kameswara Rao (1992).

marily fruit, vegetables, tree crops, and flowers. In the United States, farmers and agricultural specialists are exploring Asian vegetables, greenhouse crops, organic vegetable production, aquaculture, and on-farm recreation.

For developing countries, a number of alternative crops have also been identified. These include cassava in Brazil, sugar cane in Kenya, and chillies, soya beans, cotton, and mustard in India. Rose blooms have been identified as a more profitable alternative to tobacco in Zimbabwe, but obstacles to adoption include the large net investment, a lack of cashflow in initial years, and transportation problems in getting fresh flowers to markets in Western Europe (Maravanyika 1998). Eggplant has been recommended as an alternative or supplemental crop in the Philippines (Campos and Alejandro 1994). Yach (1996) reported that, worldwide, more than 50 alternative crops and land uses for tobacco have been identified, but acknowledged that several obstacles prevented implementation.

When examined on a cost–benefit basis, tobacco may not always ultimately produce the best economic returns, as shown in India in Table 13.7. The highest gross revenue per acre is not always synonymous with highest returns to labor. Moreover, tobacco farming is labor-intensive with high labor costs that reduce the net returns to land. Therefore, with higher cultivation and labor costs in tobacco, alternative crops can sometimes yield greater cost-benefit ratios, despite earning a lower gross income. Table 13.7 shows returns from tobacco and non-tobacco crops from one study in India.

One important barrier for farmers contemplating a switch of crop may be a lack of credit with which to purchase new seeds or other inputs. In many countries, tobacco growers obtain production loans from processors or marketing boards that are repaid when the tobacco crop is sold. Strong logistical support offered by the tobacco industry with technical advice and packages that include seeds, fertilisers, and pesticides, comes with the production loans. In some cases the loans are sufficiently large that small farmers may be unable to repay them (Kweyuh 1998). Another problem is an apparent lack of markets for tobacco alternatives. Other crops often suffer from post-harvest perishability in delivery, where tobacco is generally drought-resistant and its storability can reduce year-to-year fluctuations in prices.

The available evidence suggests that diversification plans are more likely to succeed if their impact on all relevant markets has been carefully considered. Some speciality crops are able to provide competitive returns for a few farms, but widespread adoption would drive prices down, thus eliminating any profitability advantage. For example, in the United States, there are relatively few vegetable growers in tobacco-growing areas. A large increase in production resulting from tobacco farmers entering the vegetable market would have a large downward impact on vegetable prices, with negative effects on current vegetable growers as well as diversifying tobacco farmers. Careful market analysis must also be conducted before recommending substitutes for tobacco (Ernst and Young 1991). The analysis must consider the size of the potential market (domestically and overseas), elasticity of demand (sensitivity of price changes to quantity), inter-regional and international competition, and the relative advantage of the tobacco-growing region (in terms of production costs, soils, and access to markets) compared with competing regions.

Diversification should be viewed as a broad process, with crop substitution being only one component of the whole (see Box 13.1). Analyses suggest that diversification programs have a greater chance of success if they are designed in terms of broad economic development in tobacco-growing areas to provide non-farm employment opportunities, sources of tax revenue, and foreign exchange. A non-farm job may be the best alternative to tobacco growing in many places, as suggested by Table 13.2. Rural economic development, including value-added enterprises, should be encouraged in order to provide additional job opportunities. This may require investment in transportation and other infrastructure, education and job training, and access to credit for small businesses (Altman *et al.* 1998).

Farmers are likely to need compensation and assistance to make the transition to other crops, retirement, or non-farm employment. Informational databases that include soil characteristics, topography, rainfall patterns, field size configurations, machinery complements, and any requirement for managerial expertise, would help farmers to evaluate the prospects for successful adoption of alternatives. Geographic information systems could also be used to identify suitable areas for various alternatives (Bonoan 1994).

Box 13.1 Help for poorer farmers in tobacco production

An accurate assessment of the way in which gradually falling demand will affect tobacco-farming communities is clearly critical for policymakers. Studies in most high-income countries suggest that the economies of these countries' tobacco-growing are already diversified. A survey of tobacco farmers in the United States indicates, for example, that half of those questioned were at least aware of profitable alternative agricultural activities (Altman *et al.* 1998). Younger and more educated farmers were more likely than older farmers to be interested in diversification and would see fewer obstacles. Likewise, a sizeable minority of farmers questioned in the survey were aware of the prospect of change, but recognized that it would be slow. Although more than eight out of ten said that they personally expected to remain in tobacco farming, one in three said they would advise their children not to remain in the same business.

Farmers have invested considerable amounts of time and effort in gaining knowledge and skill in growing tobacco. Learning to grow and market a new crop, perform a non-farm job, or operate a business requires new capital, knowledge, and experience for success. For many older farmers, such investments are not worthwhile, since they have relatively few working years remaining in their life-cycle to recoup the investment of time and financial resources needed to succeed in an alternative activity. Older farmers also have the highest economic rents in tobacco production and, therefore, the highest opportunity costs in switching to alternatives. For this reason, shifting from farming to other sectors is usually undertaken by younger generations entering alternative occupations. Younger tobacco farm operators are also more inclined to experiment with on-farm alternatives to tobacco and are less likely to report lack of skills as a barrier to engaging in other activities (Altman *et al.* 1996). Movement of people out of tobacco production requires investments in education and development of skills that will equip members of younger generations to seek alternative opportunities to tobacco and this investment necessarily has a long payback period.

The education of farmers about the hazards of smoking and availability of alternative crops may have some impact on decisions to grow tobacco, but most farmers are likely to continue growing tobacco as long as it is more profitable than other activities and demand is there. Setting prices that reflect the true marginal social costs of allocating resources to tobacco production is difficult and complex, considering the complexity of tobacco policy and variability from one country to the next (Zhang and Husten 1998).

Nonetheless, there are several reasons why governments would want to provide assistance to meet the transition costs for their poorest farmers. Farms are a major source of rural employment, and often are viewed as socially important by many societies. In addition, farmers can represent significant political opposition to tobacco control. Appropriate action for governments would involve a number of different efforts, such as encouraging sound agricultural and trade policies, the provision of broad rural development programs, assistance with crop diversification, rural training, and other 'safety-net' systems. Some governments have proposed that such support could be financed out of tobacco taxes. Governments may also learn from the success of local efforts. In the United States, for instance, some rural communities that are traditionally dependent on tobacco have formed coalitions with public health constituencies to agree core principles for policies that will reduce tobacco consumption and also promote sustainable rural communities (Altman *et al.* 1998).

13.4.5 Inducements to leave tobacco farming

Since tobacco provides much higher returns than alternative crops, farmers would require some financial inducement to switch crops. However, such inducements would be costly and are unlikely to be effective in reducing demand. High buy-out costs reflect the high-opportunity cost attached to switching to an alternative use of productive resources that are currently deployed for tobacco production in countries such as Malawi, Zimbabwe, and China.

A few governments have offered, or have proposed offering, farmers inducements to leave tobacco farming, but none have clearly succeeded in significantly cutting tobacco production. Canada's Tobacco Diversification Plan provided incentives to stop growing tobacco and develop alternatives to assist the orderly downsizing of the Canadian tobacco industry in the 1980s (PAHO 1992). Significant numbers of farmers ceased production through this program, but many participants acknowledged that they would have quit tobacco farming without it. The program's success is further qualified by the finding that 24% of participants continued to work in tobacco farming as employees, rather than as entrepreneurs. Australia eliminated production subsidies, domestic content rules for cigarette manufactures, and lowered tariffs, while at the same time offering a buy-out of tobacco quotas (Australian Financial Review 1998). As a result of the Australian deregulation and buy-out, many growers left the tobacco sector, but they tended to be less-efficient producers of low-grade leaf; those remaining tended to expand the scale of their operations to increase efficiency. In the United States, officials drafting comprehensive tobacco legislation in 1997 and 1998 discussed a buy-out quota of US$ 8 per pound of tobacco payments to tenant farmers, as well as job training, education, and rural development grants. However, nothing was enacted at that time. The US proposals involved buying out the government-assigned right to produce for subsidies, not the right to grow tobacco at all. Because the buy-out would also lift production quotas, a US buy-out could actually result in greater production of flue-cured tobacco and little change in burley production.

If a buy-out or other scheme were successful in reducing production in a particular country or region, there will be little effect on the world supply of tobacco. As Fig. 13.2 demonstrates, world production is already shifting to lower income countries. Developed countries have restricted their production (albeit for producer-welfare rather than tobacco-control objectives) over the last several decades. At the same time, developing countries have rapidly expanded production to fill the void and meet world demand, so that world production has continued to grow. It is likely that new buy-out policies would merely create huge profits for other tobacco suppliers, and a rapid increase in 'replacement' production.

13.4.6 Outright bans on tobacco production

Given tobacco's unprecedented capacity to damage health, some public health advocates have called for it to be prohibited, arguing that the problem of tobacco is not in its consumption, but its production (Beaglehole and Bonita 1997). Advocates of tobacco prohibition point to the marked reduction in alcohol-related diseases when alcohol supply was restricted earlier in the twentieth century. For example, when alcohol supplies were restricted during the Second World War, alcohol consumption in Paris fell by 80% per capita. Deaths from liver disease in men were halved within one year, and fell by four-fifths after five years. After the war ended, mortality from liver disease returned to pre-war levels. Restrictions during the US prohibition were less effective, and prohibition did not significantly stem alcohol use or abuse; indeed, it created its own problems (Berkelman and Buehler 1990).

However, the prohibition of tobacco is unlikely to be either feasible or effective, for a number of reasons. First, even when substances are prohibited, they continue to be widely used, as is the case with many illicit drugs. Second, prohibition creates its own sets of problems: it is likely to increase criminal activity and entail costly police enforcement. Third, the prohibition of tobacco is unlikely to be politically acceptable in most countries. In India, recent attempts to ban a chewed type of tobacco known as *gutka* failed, largely for political reasons (George 1998). Fourth, from an economic (as opposed to public health) perspective, optimal consumption is not zero, given that some fully informed adults would still be interested in smoking (Chapter 7; Pekurinen 1991). Finally, as noted above, drastic supply reductions would lead to significant welfare losses for the poorest farmers in countries highly dependent on tobacco as a source of cash income.

Additional lessons can be taken from experience in some of the draconian attempts to control the supply of illicit narcotics through eradication of crops such as coca, hemp, and opium poppies. Eradication efforts reduce the total area under cultivation, but do not eliminate production completely. Attempts to promote adoption of alternative crops have been unsuccessful, due largely to the profitability of growing illicit crops. Outlawing crops raises the cost of production by forcing production into less accessible areas and raises marginal returns to compensate producers for greater risks of incurring penalties, other sanctions, or having crops destroyed by law enforcement officials. By raising marginal returns and pushing production into less-accessible areas where alternative opportunities are poor, the difference in income between growing illicit crops and alternatives becomes even more pronounced, making crop substitution more unlikely. There have been attempts to accompany crop eradication with promotion of alternative crops and rural development efforts, but these have been hampered by lack of technical assistance to advise farmers growing the new crops, expense of administration (Crooker 1988; Crooker and Martin 1992), and lack of long-term commitment.

13.4.7 The impact of lower producer prices

Overall, because economic incentives remain strong for supplying tobacco as long as demand persists, it is unlikely that most supply-side interventions will be effective at reducing consumption. In fact, the key factor that would tend to lower the tobacco supply would be lower producer prices, translating to a lower incentive to grow tobacco. Tax increases, which already determine much of the retail price of cigarettes, would be used to offset any marginal decrease in retail price from lower producer prices.

The trend since 1960 has indeed been a slow eroding of the world tobacco price, such that for the period 1960–89 the world price for flue-cured tobacco declined in real terms between 1.1% and 1.7% per year. Thus, while the nominal price of tobacco is expected to increase from the 1985 base year of US$1950 per ton to US$2521 per ton by 2000, the real value will decline to about US$1221 (World Bank 1992). However, tobacco prices have been more stable than many other agricultural commodities over the 10-year period prior to 1993, which is why tobacco remains a popular crop. Tobacco prices declined by 29% between 1985 and 1993. However, real prices of most agricultural and other basic commodities have fallen even more in recent years (ITGA 1996c). Thus, growers have little incentive to switch to alternatives.

As noted above, it is not clear how the removal of price supports and subsidies would affect global price. Higher domestic prices in the United States may help to raise the global price of raw tobacco leaf, offering better returns to farmers in low-income countries. On the other hand, there would be mixed effects for farmers in low-income countries if both subsidies and trade restrictions were removed. If, for example, the price of domestically produced tobacco in the United States were to fall because of the removal of subsidies, cigarette manufacturers there might use more of it, in turn reducing their imports of lower quality imports from low-income countries. But at the same time, with freer trade, imports of such tobacco could increase. Regardless of their minimal impact on consumption, price supports and subsidies for most agricultural products make little sense in a framework of sound agricultural and trade policies (World Bank 1991). Rather than attempts to influence global price through supply-side measures, gradual reductions in the number of farmers are far more likely to occur with falling demand and hence lower producers' prices. It is unlikely that such falling demand could be augmented with even more extensive supply-side efforts.

13.5 Conclusions and research priorities

This examination leads to some fundamental conclusions. First, in the majority of countries, and in the medium- and long-run, even very stringent tobacco-control policies would be expected to have minimal negative impact on long-run GNP, employment, tax revenue, and the foreign trade balance, as expenditure switches and reallocations in the economy take place.

Second, a country's reliance on tobacco exports and its stage of development are key factors in determining the economic consequences for its economy of tobacco-control measures. For the majority of countries that import and consume, or produce and consume, tobacco in a self-sufficient way, policies that reduce their demand for tobacco will probably have little or no net impact on the jobs, revenues, and on the trade balance (which may, in fact, improve by reducing tobacco imports). In many countries, there will be macro-economic benefits to reducing tobacco use. For the few countries that export tobacco and are not diversified in their economies, falling tobacco demand globally would result in some income and employment losses, particularly among farmers. Domestic tobacco control efforts in these countries, however, would have little or no impact. Effects would be greatest for the few countries that earn a significant share of foreign earnings from tobacco (chiefly Malawi and Zimbabwe).

Third, though some sectors will experience economic losses, realistic reductions in tobacco demand will take place very gradually. Thus supply-side responses to lower demand will also be very gradual, reducing transition costs.

Fourth, as long as global demand continues, supply-side policies such as crop diversification or buy-outs result in very limited or zero reductions in the supply of tobacco. Specific diversification programs, placed within broader development programs, can help to meet the transition costs of poorest farmers in low-income countries that are now substantially dependent on tobacco production

Thus, this chapter concludes that the global supply of tobacco is most likely to fall if demand for tobacco falls, rather than as a result of supply-side interventions. Reductions in the world price of tobacco and in subsidies, price supports, quotas, and other supply-control measures, may reduce tobacco production to some extent. Elimination of the tobacco subsidy and other controls will cause a modest decline in the price of tobacco leaf, and—assuming no offsetting tax increases—a small decrease in the cigarette retail price. However, removal of such subsidies is justified on the basis of sound agricultural and trade policy.

Research priorities for the future include continued research into the macro-economic effects of tobacco-control policies at individual country levels, stakeholder analyses at the country level, and an assessment of the transitional costs from reduced tobacco production. Basic data requirements in many developing countries are paramount and include employment data, output data, and cost data with a rudimentary assessment of the producer surplus in producing countries. Continued investment in the search for viable alternatives for the tobacco crop at a country and regional level also remains important.

References

Aberg, E. and Tedla, G. (1979). *Tobacco and Alternative Crops.* Report 77, Upsala: Swedish University of Agricultural Sciences, Department of Plant Husbandry.

Agro-Economic Services Ltd. And Tabacosmos Ltd. (1987). *The Employment, Tax Revenue and Wealth that the Tobacco Industry Creates.* London: Agro-Economic Services.

Allen, R. C. (1993). *The False Dilemma: The Impact of Tobacco-control Policies on Employment in Canada.* National Campaign for Action on Tobacco: Ottawa, Ontario.

Al-Sadat, N. and Zain, Z. (1997). *Diversification of Tobacco Farming in Malaysia.* Paper presented at Tenth World Conference on Tobacco or Health, 24–28 August, 1997, Beijing, China.

Altman, D. G., Levine, D. W., Howard, G., and Hamilton, H. (1996). Tobacco farmers and diversification: opportunities and barriers. *Tobacco Control,* **5,** 192–8.

Altman, D. G., Zaccaro, D. J., Levine, D. W., Austin, D., Woodell, C., Bailey, B. *et al.* (1998). Predictors of crop diversification: a survey of tobacco farmers in North Carolina. *Tobacco Control,* **7**(4), 376–82.

American Economics Group (1996). *The US Tobacco Industry in 1994: Its Economic Impact on the States.* Washington: American Economics Group, March 1996.

Arthur Andersen Economic Consulting (1993). *Tobacco Industry Employment: A Review of the Price Waterhouse Economic Impact Report and Tobacco Institute Estimates of Economic Losses from Increasing the Federal Excise Tax.* Los Angeles, CA: Arthur Andersen Economic Consulting.

Australian Financial Review (1998). *Australia: Total Tobacco Deregulation Has Brought New Lease of Life to Industry and Local Content Rules are Abolished Too.* 19 Jan 1998, 6.

Beaglehole, R. and Bonita, R. (1997). *Public Health at the Crossroads: Achievements and Prospects*. New York: Cambridge University Press.

Beghin, J. C., Foster, W. E., and Kherallah, M. (1996). Institutions and market distortions: international evidence for tobacco. *Journal of Agricultural Economics*, **47**(3), 355–65.

Berkelman, R. L. and Buehler, J. W. (1990). Public health surveillance of non-infectious chronic diseases: the potential to detect rapid changes in disease burden. *Int. J. Epidemiol.*, **19**(3), 628–35.

Bonoan, R. R. (1994). Rezonification of tobacco-growing areas. *Philippine Journal of Crop Science*, **19**, 56.

Brown, A. B. (1998). *Farm Level Effects an Increase in Federal Cigarette Taxes under Two Scenarios: Keep vs. Eliminate the Tobacco Program*. USDA Outlook Forum: Washington DC.

Buck, D., Godfrey, C., Raw, M., and Sutton, M. (1995). *Tobacco and Jobs, Society for the Study of Addiction and Centre for Health Economics*. York: University of York.

Campos, F. F. and Alejandro, I. G. (1994). Eggplant: an alternate or alternative crop to tobacco. *Philippine Tobacco News*, **12**, 13.

Chapman, S. and Wong, W. L. (1990). *Tobacco Control in the Third World: A Resource Atlas*. Penang, Malaysia: International Organization of Consumers Unions.

Chari, M. S. and Kameswara Rao, B. V. (1992). Role of tobacco in the national economy: past and present. In *Control of Tobacco-related Cancers and Other Diseases: International Symposium 1990* (ed. P. C. Gupta, J. E. Hamner, and P. R. Murti). Oxford University Press: Bombay.

Chase Econometrics (1985). *The Economic Impact of the Tobacco Industry on the United States Economy in 1983*. Bala Cynwyd, PA: Chase Econometrics.

Coady, S., Pompelli, G., and Grise, V. N. (1991). Government policies and programs affecting tobacco production and trade in major tobacco trading nations. *Tobacco Situation and Outlook*, US Dept. Agriculture, TS-216, September 1991, 33–7.

Collins, D. and Lapsley, H. (1997). *The Economic Impact of Tobacco Smoking in Pacific Islands*. Pacific Tobacco and Health Project, Adventist Development and Relief Agency, Australian International Development Assistance Bureau, Australia, May 1997.

Connolly, G. N. (1992). Worldwide expansion of transnational tobacco industry. *Journal of the National Cancer Institute*, **12**, 29–35.

Coopers and Lybrand (1996). *A Study of the Economic Impact of a Ban on Cigarette Advertising in Hong Kong*. Association of Accredited Advertising Agencies, 3 June 1996.

Crooker, R. A. (1988). Forces of change in the Thailand opium zone. *The Geographical Review*, **78**(3), 241–56.

Crooker, R. A. and Martin, R. N. (1992). Accessibility and illicit drug crop production: lessons from Northern Thailand. *Journal of Rural Studies*, **8**(4), 423–9.

Deloitte and Touche (1995). *Economic Contributions of the Tobacco Industry in the Tobacco Growing Region of Ontario*. Guelph: Resource Assessment and Planning Committee.

Ernst and Young (1991). *Strategic Directions for the Philippine Tobacco Industry*. Washington, DC: Ernst and Young, November 1991.

FAO (1989). *The Economic Significance of Tobacco*. Committee on Commodity Problems, February 1989.

FAO (1998). *Food and Agriculture Organization of the United Nations Database*. Rome:

Gale, F. (1998). *The Economic Structure of Tobacco Growing Areas, Tobacco Situation and Outlook*. US Department of Agriculture, Economic Research Service, April 1998, 40–7.

Gale, H. F., Foreman, L., and Capehart, T. *Tobacco and the Economy: Farms, Jobs, and Communities*. US Department of Agriculture, Agricultural Economics Report. (In press.)

George, N. (1998). Health ministry isolated on gutka ban. *The Indian Express*, May 9, p. 1.

IEC (1998). *IEC Foreign Trade Statistics, World Bank Economic and Social Database*. World Bank: Washington DC, USA.

ILO (1998). *International Labor Organization Database*. Geneva: ILO.

Industry Commission (1994). *The Tobacco Growing and Manufacturing Industries*. Canberra: Australian Government Publishing Service.

Irvine, I. J. and Sims, W. A. (1997). Tobacco control legislation and resource allocation effects. *Canadian Public Policy*, **23**(3), 259–73.

ITGA (1996a). *Tobacco in Africa: ITGAs Response*. International Tobacco Growers Association, Tobacco Growers: Issues Papers, April 1996, East Grinstead: ITGA.

ITGA (1996b). *Are There Alternatives to Tobacco?* International Tobacco Growers Association, Tobacco Growers: Issues Papers, April 1996, East Grinstead: ITGA.

ITGA (1996c). *Tobacco—a Major World Crop?* International Tobacco Growers Association, Tobacco Growers: Issues Papers, April 1996, East Grinstead: ITGA.

Johnson, P. R. (1984). *The Economics of the Tobacco Industry*. New York: Praeger.

Joossens, L. and Raw, M. (1996). Are tobacco subsidies a misuse of public funds? *BMJ*, **312**, 832–5.

Kweyuh, P. H. M. (1998). Does tobacco growing pay? The case of Kenya. In *The Economics of Tobacco Control: Towards an Optimal Policy Mix* (ed. I. Abedian, R. van der Merwe, N. Wilkins, and P. Jha), pp. 245–50. Cape Town: Medical Association of South Africa Press.

Lewit, E. M. (1987). *Tobacco in Developing Countries: An Economic Approach to Policy Formulation*. Population, Health and Nutrition Department, World Bank, June 1987.

Maravanyika, E. (1997). *The Economics of Tobacco in Zimbabwe*. The Economics of Tobacco Control Project Update 9, University of Cape Town: Cape Town.

Maravanyika, E. (1998). *Do Financially Viable Alternatives to Tobacco Growing Exist in Zimbabwe?* The Economics of Tobacco Control Project Update 12, University of Cape Town, Cape Town.

Market File (1998). *World Tobacco Market File Database*. London: Market Tracking International Ltd.

McNicoll, I. H. and Boyle, S. (1992). Regional economic impact of a reduction of resident expenditure on cigarettes: a case study of Glasgow. *Applied Economics*, **24**, 291–6.

Miernyk, W. H. (1957). *The Elements of Input–output Analysis*. Random House: New York.

Nicolaides-Bouman, A., Wald, N., Forey, B., and Lee, P. (1993). *International Smoking Statistics: a Collection of Historical Data From 22 Economically Developed Countries*. New York: Oxford University Press.

Pan American Health Organization (PAHO) (1992). *Tobacco or Health: Status in the Americas*. Scientific Publication Number 536.

Patel, S. K. (1992). *Production and Marketing of Tobacco in India*. New Delhi: Mittal Publications.

PEIDA (1985). *The Tobacco Industry in the European Community, Including Portugal and Spain*. Edinburgh, September 1985.

PEIDA (1991). *The Economic Significance of the UK Tobacco Industry*. London: PEIDA.

Pekurinen, M. (1991). *Economic Aspects of Smoking: Is There a Case for Government Intervention in Finland?* Helsinki: Vapk-Publishing.

Pena, P. P. and Norton, G. (1993). The effects of sectoral and economic-wide policies on tobacco production in the Dominican Republic. *Journal of Agricultural and Applied Economics*, **25**, 151–64.

Peng, Y. (1996). The politics of tobacco: relations between farmers and local governments in Chinas Southwest. *The China Journal*, **36**, 67–82.

Price Waterhouse (1990). *The Economic Impact of the Tobacco Industry on the United States Economy*. Arlington VA: Price Waterhouse.

Price Waterhouse (1992). *The Economic Impact of the Tobacco Industry on the United States Economy*. Arlington VA: Price Waterhouse.

Skolnick, A. A. (1996). Answer sought for tobacco giant Chinas problems. *Journal of the American Medical Association*, **275**, 1220–1.

Sumner, D. A. and Alston, J. M. (1985). *Removal of Price Supports and Supply Controls for*

US Tobacco: An Economic Analysis of the Impact. Washington, DC: National Planning Association.

Tobacco Merchants Association (1995). *Tobaccos Contribution to the National Economy.* Princeton, NJ: Tobacco Merchants Association.

Townsend, J. (1991). Tobacco and the European Common Agricultural Policy. *BMJ*, **303**, 1008–9.

Tweeten, L. (1995). The twelve best reasons for a commodity program: why none stand scrutiny, *Choices*, 2nd quarter, 4–7.

United Nations International Development Organization (UNIDO) (1998). *United Nations International Development Organization Database.* Vienna: UNIDO.

US Department of Agriculture (USDA) (1998). *US Department of Agriculture Database.* USDA: Washington DC, USA.

US Department of Health and Human Services (1989). *Reducing the Health Consequences of Smoking: 25 Years of Progress.* A Report of the Surgeon General. Rockville, Maryland: US Department of Health and Human Services, Public Health Service, Centers for Disease Control, Center for Chronic Disease Prevention and Health Promotion, Office on Smoking and Health. DHHS Publication No. (CDC)89–8411.

Van der Merwe, R. (1998a). The economics of tobacco control in South Africa. In *The Economics of Tobacco Control: Towards an Optimal Policy Mix* (ed. I. Abedian, R. van der Merwe, N. Wilkins, and P. Jha), pp. 251–71. Cape Town: Medical Association of South Africa Press.

Van der Merwe, R. (1998b). *Employment and Output Effects for Zimbabwe with the Elimination of Tobacco Consumption and Production.* Population, Health and Nutrition Department, World Bank, August 1998.

Van der Merwe, R. (1998c). *Employment and Output Effects for Bangladesh following a Decline in Tobacco Consumption.* Population, Health and Nutrition Department, World Bank, August 1998.

Van der Merwe, R. (1998d). Employment issues in tobacco control. In *The Economics of Tobacco Control: Towards an Optimal Policy Mix* (ed. I. Abedian, R. van der Merwe, N. Wilkins, and P. Jha), pp. 199–209. Cape Town: Medical Association of South Africa Press.

Warner, K. E. (1987). Health and economic implications of a tobacco-free society. *Journal of the American Medical Association*, **258**, 2080–6.

Warner, K. E. (1988). The tobacco subsidy: does it matter? *Journal of the National Cancer Institute*, **80**(2), 81–3.

Warner, K. E. and Fulton, G. A. (1994). The *economic implications of tobacco product sales in a non-tobacco state. Journal of the American Medical Association*, **271**(10), 771–6.

Warner, K. E., Fulton, G. A., Nicolas, P., and Grimes, D. R. (1996). Employment implications of declining tobacco product sales for the regional economies of the United States. *Journal of the American Medical Association*, **275**, 1241–6.

Wharton Applied Research Center (1979). *A Study of the Tobacco Industrys Economic Contribution to the Nation, Its Fifty States, and the District of Columbia.* Philadelphia: Wharton Applied Research Center and Wharton Econometrics Forecasting Associates, Inc., University of Pennsylvania.

The World Bank (1991). *World Development Report 1991: The Challenge of Development.* New York: Oxford University Press.

The World Bank (1992). *Revision of Primary Commodity Forecasts and Quarterly Review of Commodity Markets.* December 1991, Prepared by the International Trade Division, International Economics Department, 5 February 1992.

The World Bank (1993). *Investing in Health.* World Development Report. Washington: Oxford University Press.

The World Bank (1997). *The State in a Changing World.* World Development Report. Washington: Oxford University Press.

World Health Organization (1999). *Making a Difference.* World Health Report. WHO, Geneva, Switzerland.

Yach, D. (1996). Tobacco in Africa. *World Health Forum,* **17,** 29–36.

Zhang, P. and Husten, C. (1998). The impact of the tobacco price support program on tobacco control in the United States. *Tobacco Control: An International Journal,* **7,** 176–82.

14

The impact of trade liberalization on tobacco consumption

Allyn Taylor, Frank J. Chaloupka, Emmanuel Guindon, and Michaelyn Corbett

Over the past two decades, trade in tobacco and tobacco products has expanded dramatically as a result of a variety of bilateral, regional, and international trade agreements that have significantly reduced trade barriers. This chapter provides a brief discussion of arguments derived from economic theory suggesting that the reductions in trade barriers will lead to greater competition, lower prices, and increased advertising and promotion in tobacco-product markets. This is followed by a review of recent trade agreements, highlighting features particularly relevant to tobacco. The limited empirical evidence on the impact of liberalized trade in tobacco products on their consumption is then discussed, followed by a new empirical analysis using data on 42 countries over the period from 1970 through 1995. This new analysis clearly demonstrates that trade liberalization has led to increases in cigarette smoking, with the most significant impact in low-income and middle-income countries. Finally, the globalization of the tobacco industry and global tobacco-control responses are briefly described.

14.1 Introduction

The recent trend towards the increased liberalization of trade in most goods and services has significantly reduced high-tariff and non-tariff barriers to trade in tobacco and tobacco products and contributed to the sharp increase in tobacco use in many low-income and middle-income countries. Over the past two decades, the various bilateral, regional, and multilateral trade agreements that many nations have adopted have led to significantly greater competition in domestic tobacco markets. This increased competition has almost certainly been accompanied by reduced prices for tobacco products and dramatic increases in the advertising and promotion of these products.

This chapter reviews the theoretical and empirical evidence on the impact of trade liberalization on trade in tobacco and tobacco products, and on tobacco consumption. Section 14.2 contains a brief review of the relevant economic theory on the impact of trade barriers and trade liberalization. Section 14.3 describes how recent and proposed bilateral, regional, and multilateral agreements treat tobacco and tobacco products. Section 14.4 presents descriptive information on recent trends in tobacco-related trade and reviews the limited econometric evidence on the impact of trade liberalization on tobacco consumption. This is followed in Section 14.5 by a discussion of the findings from a new empirical analysis of trade and tobacco use. Finally, Section 14.6 discusses the implications of trade liberalization for tobacco control.

14.2 Theoretical foundations

There are several basic reasons why international trade in tobacco and tobacco products has arisen. Grise (1990) and Chaloupka and Corbett (1998), for example, suggest the following:

(1) a country's inability to domestically produce tobacco and tobacco products in sufficient quantity to satisfy domestic demand for these products;
(2) a country's inability to domestically produce tobacco and tobacco products of sufficiently high quality to satisfy domestic demand;
(3) differences in prices among countries for different types and qualities of tobacco and tobacco products; and
(4) the importing of unmanufactured tobacco for use in producing tobacco products for exports.

   In addition, in some countries, tobacco and/or tobacco products are an important source of foreign currency. In recent years, for example, Zimbabwe exported nearly all of its tobacco crop, with these exports accounting for nearly one-quarter of its total export earnings (Maravanyika 1998).
   Global trade in tobacco and tobacco products, while not insignificant, would have been much higher in the past had there not been a variety of restrictive trade policies and other policies protecting domestic tobacco growers and producers of tobacco products from foreign competition (Grise 1990). These barriers include high tariffs on imported tobacco and/or tobacco products, quotas or complete bans on imports, domestic price-support programs, marketing restrictions, licensing requirements, restricted product lists, exchange controls, domestic content requirements, and subsidies on cultivation or production (Grise 1990).
   There are few rationales for trade barriers that are economically justifiable, including the temporary protection of an 'infant' industry and the use of protectionistic interventions as a temporary strategy for promoting economic development. As evidence on the health consequences of smoking has accumulated, some have argued for restricting tobacco-related trade as a way to reduce the death and disease resulting from tobacco use. (While the World Bank does not seek to restrict trade, it does restrict the use of Bank funds (see Box 14.1)). Similar arguments have been used to defend trade restrictions in the case of other goods with negative externalities. These arguments are most well developed in the area of environmental policies (see, for example, Anderson and Blackhurst 1992), with recent research adapting these arguments to consider the negative externalities associated with tobacco use (Shi and Hsieh 1998). In practice, however, trade restrictions have often been used to protect state-owned monopolies on tobacco production and distribution that generate a significant share of total government revenues in these countries. Moreover, the arguments that health concerns are a justification for limiting trade have typically not been accompanied by

Box 14.1 The World Bank's policy on tobacco

The World Bank's activities in the health sector—including sector work, policy dialogue, and lending—discourage the use of tobacco products.

The World Bank does not lend directly for, invest in, or guarantee investments or loans for, tobacco production, processing, or marketing. Exceptions, which must be approved, may be allowed for countries that are heavily dependent on tobacco as a source of income (especially for poor farmers and farm workers) and foreign exchange earnings (i.e. those where tobacco accounts for more than 10% of exports). The World Bank seeks to help these countries diversify away from tobacco.

To the extent practicable, the World Bank does not lend indirectly for tobacco production activities, although some indirect support of the tobacco economy may occur as an inseparable part of a project that has a broader set of objectives and outcomes (e.g. rural roads).

Unmanufactured and manufactured tobacco, tobacco processing machinery and equipment, and related services are included in the negative list of imports in World Bank Loan Agreements.

Tobacco and tobacco-related producer or consumer imports may be exempt from borrowers' agreements with the World Bank to liberalize trade and reduce tariff levels.

Source: the World Bank (1991).

strong efforts to reduce the consumption of domestically produced cigarettes and other tobacco products.

In general, economic theory predicts that barriers to trade in tobacco and tobacco products will reduce the total supply of these products while raising the quantity supplied by domestic growers and producers. Consequently, the prices for raw tobacco, cigarettes, and other tobacco products are likely to be higher under this scenario than they would in the absence of the trade barriers. Given the well-documented evidence on the effects of price on tobacco use (see Chapter 10), higher prices will lead to reduced cigarette smoking and lower use of other tobacco products. Given the clear links between tobacco use and adverse health outcomes (see Chapter 2), the reduced consumption will lead in the long-term to improved health. Domestic suppliers will generally benefit from their higher levels of growing and production and from the higher prices they receive. Foreign suppliers, however, will usually be worse off as a result of their reduced access to protected markets.

In contrast, increasing trade liberalization, as a result of bilateral, regional, and multilateral trade agreements, is likely to have the opposite effect. Reductions in the barriers to tobacco-related trade will likely lead to greater competition in the markets for tobacco and tobacco products, reductions in the prices for tobacco products, and increased advertising and promotion of these products. The increases in advertising and promotion will not only result from the efforts of entrants to gain a foothold in the newly opened markets, but are also likely to reflect increased activity by existing firms attempting to maintain their market shares in the more competitive environment. Given the inverse relationship between price and consumption, as well as the positive relationship between advertising/promotion and demand (see Chapter 9), cigarette smoking and other tobacco use will likely increase under this scenario as tobacco markets become more open. As a result, the death and disease resulting from tobacco use will also increase.

However, the liberalization of trade in other goods and services is expected to have substantial economic benefits, including increased incomes, greater employment, more stable prices, greater innovation, and more rapid economic growth (World Trade Organization 1998a; Yellen 1998), with perhaps the greatest impact in developing countries (Edwards 1992). Edwards, for example, in a sample of 30 developing countries, found strong evidence that growth was higher in countries with more liberal trade policies. There is strong evidence on the link between income and health, particularly at lower income levels, suggesting that overall trade liberalization can lead to improved health outcomes (Preston 1976; Chaloupka and Corbett 1998). However, the increased tobacco use in developing countries that results from increased incomes is likely to, at least partially, offset the health benefits of liberalized trade in other goods and services.

14.3 Review of recent history of trade liberalization

The recent explosion in global trade in tobacco and tobacco products has been due, in part, to a variety of multilateral, regional, and bilateral trade agreements that have significantly reduced trade barriers for numerous goods and services, including unmanufactured tobacco, cigarettes, and other tobacco products. This section reviews existing international, regional, and bilateral agreements that have appreciably reduced tariff and non-tariff barriers to trade in tobacco and tobacco products. In addition, it discusses the implications for national tobacco control efforts of the Multilateral Agreement on Investments, a draft agreement that has been side-lined for the time being but for which negotiations may eventually resume.

14.3.1 multilateral treaties

World Trade Organization multilateral agreements

The World Trade Organization (WTO), formed at the conclusion of the Uruguay Round of the General Agreement on Tariffs and Trade (GATT) in 1994, is the primary international institution governing international trade; approximately 90% of world trade is conducted pursuant to its rules (Dunoff 1994). The initial round of the GATT in 1947 called for the formation of the International Trade Organization to administer the multilateral agreement, but that organization was never formally established. The organizational features of GATT (1947) were, therefore, rudimentary and it functioned primarily as a forum for negotiation. With the conclusion of the Uruguay Round in 1994, the GATT contracting parties took a major step toward strengthening the international trade regime by formalizing the institutional status of the WTO, strengthening the trade dispute mechanisms, and broadening the WTO's jurisdiction.

The Uruguay round brought about an overhaul of the international trade regime by the conclusion of a number of agreements addressing contemporary trade issues. The WTO Agreement has four annexes that contain the agreements reached in the Uruguay Round. GATT (1947) was amended and incorporated into the new WTO agreement, including the case law and interpretive decisions. As a condition of membership in the WTO, members must agree to 24 different agreements, located in Annexes 1–3 to the Marrakesh Agreement. Now known as GATT (1994), the amended agreement and other agreements addressing non-tariff barriers to trade and trade in services are contained in the first Annex. Other WTO agreements, covering trade in intellectual property, as well as dispute settlement rules, are contained in the second and third Annexes. These three sets of multilateral agreements were accepted by member states as a single package during the Uruguay round and, therefore, impose binding obligations on all member states. Only the fourth Annex, which contains the plurilateral agreements, is binding only on the WTO members who have accepted it.

Trade in all tobacco, raw or manufactured, is regulated primarily under the agreements in Annex 1A to the Marrakesh Agreement. For example, the Agreement on Agriculture concerns tariffs, subsidies and domestic supports for all agricultural products, including tobacco. Other key agreements for trade in tobacco, including GATT 1994 and the Agreement on Technical Barriers to Trade, are described below.

The principal aim of the WTO is the reduction of barriers to trade. The general principles of the WTO include: a commitment to achieving free trade and fair competition; limits on, and eventual elimination of, tariff and non-tariff barriers to trade; non-discriminatory treatment of all trading partners; the non-discriminatory treatment of domestically produced and foreign products; predictability by ensuring that trade barriers are not erected arbitrarily; negotiated elimination of trade barriers; the settlement of disputes; and opposition to retaliatory sanctions (WTO 1998a).

The WTO multilateral agreements significantly expanded global trade in tobacco products by mandating sizable reductions in tariff and non-tariff barriers to trade in tobacco products (Chaloupka and Corbett 1998). For example, GATT (1994) calls upon the European Union to reduce its tariff on cigars by 50%, on cigarettes and other manufactured tobacco products by 36%, and on unmanufactured tobacco by 20% (USDA 1997). Similarly, it calls upon the United States to eliminate its tariffs on cigar wrappers and reduce its tariffs on cigar filler and binder tobacco, cigars and most cigarettes by 55%, on tobacco stems and refuse by 20% and on other manufactured and smoking tobacco by 15% (USDA 1997). Furthermore, the new WTO regime has led to the elimination of legislation that required that all cigarettes produced in the United States contain at least 75% domestically grown tobacco (USDA 1997b). It has also led to the elimination of or reduction in tariff and non-tariff barriers to trade in tobacco and tobacco products in numerous other countries.

A number of the binding multilateral agreements may have important implications for global health efforts. The remainder of this section will briefly discuss the impact of some of the more significant WTO multilateral agreements on national and international tobacco control regulatory efforts.

GATT (1994)

The most significant of the WTO multilateral agreements, with respect to international tobacco trade, is GATT (1994). GATT (1994) provides detailed rules and standards for determining what measures are permitted. Article One of the Agreement establishes the principle of most favored nation that, with several exceptions, requires that products from one member country be given no less favorable treatment than 'like' products from any other member country. Article Three establishes the principle of national treatment that, subject to some exceptions, mandates that products imported into a country cannot be treated differently from 'like' domestic products with respect to laws and regulations. Collectively, these principles are designed to prevent members of GATT (1994) from using internal law to favor domestic products over imported goods. These rules thus enshrine the core principle that members are generally entitled to non-discriminatory treatment of their products in other states that are members of the organization.

Article XX of the text of the Agreement provides a critical and highly limited exception for national measures designed to protect public health that would otherwise violate GATT (1994) obligations. Article XX, in relevant part, states (emphasis added):

Subject to the requirement that such measures are not applied in a manner which would constitute a means of arbitrary and unjustifiable discrimination between countries where the same conditions prevail, or a disguised restriction on international trade, *nothing in this Agreement shall be construed to prevent the adoption or enforcement by any contracting party of measures. . . . necessary to protect human. . . . health (or) necessary to secure compliance with the laws or regulations which are not inconsistent with the provisions of this agreement. . . .*

Article XX is a limited and conditional exception from obligations under other provisions of the Agreement. In other words, Article XX exceptions are only relevant if a trade violation is found. In addition, dispute resolution practice establishes that:

(1) GATT panels examine Article XX only if it has been expressly invoked by the party to a dispute;
(2) Article XX is narrowly interpreted; and
(3) the party invoking the Article XX exception has the burden of proof (WTO 1998).

GATT has elaborated on the implications of Article XX in the context of national tobacco control regulations in a 1990 case involving Thailand's ban on cigarette imports and advertising (GATT 1990; Roemer 1993; Chaloupka and Laixuthai 1996; Taylor and Roemer 1996; Chaloupka and Corbett 1998). In this case, American tobacco companies challenged Thailand's ban on advertising and imports, prompting an investigation by the United States Trade Representative who referred the matter to GATT. Article XI:1 of GATT (1947) provides that:

No prohibitions or restrictions . . . made effective through . . . import licenses . . . shall be instituted or maintained by any contracting party on the importation of any product of the territory of any other contracting party. . . .

Although inconsistent with Article XX:1, Thailand contended that the prohibition on imports was justified by the objective of public health policy and was therefore covered under Article XX.

The GATT panel found that Thailand could 'give priority to human health over trade liberalization' as long as the proposed measures were 'necessary'. The panel concluded that Thailand's restrictions on imports could be considered 'necessary' in terms of Article XX, only if there were no alternative measure consistent with the General Agreement—or less inconsistent with it—that Thailand could reasonably be expected to employ to achieve its health policy objectives. Based on its analysis of the 'necessity' of the Thai measures, the panel concluded that Thailand's practice of permitting the sales of domestic cigarettes, while banning the importation of foreign cigarettes, was not 'necessary' and, therefore, not justifiable under Article XX(b), since alternatives to banning the importation of cigarettes were available to protect public health.

The panel further found, however, that requiring foreign tobacco companies to abide by tobacco-control regulations that applied equally to domestic and foreign tobacco products was appropriate and consistent with GATT obligations. GATT upheld the advertising ban and went on to state that various tobacco-control measures could be adopted and applied to both domestic and imported tobacco, in lieu of an import ban, and still be consistent with GATT obligations. Given this decision, Thailand could have banned the sale of all cigarettes, domestic and imported, and remained consistent with GATT. The panel also noted that a ban on advertising applying to both domestic and imported cigarettes would be justified under the Agreement, even if it created unequal competitive opportunities between domestic and foreign firms, because advertising may stimulate demand for cigarettes.

This was the first GATT-case decision on manufactured tobacco products. As such, it has set a critical precedent for other countries. The case sends a message that member nations can adopt strong tobacco-control legislation, as long as the measures are aimed at protecting health and do not discriminate between domestic and imported tobacco. The decision by the GATT Council thus indicates that it is possible to design stringent tobacco-control policies aimed at reducing the death and disease associated with tobacco use that may be adopted and implemented without violating international trade commitments.

As other scholars have noted, however, it cannot be assumed that GATT (1994) will be applied in a manner that supports the protection of public health in future decisions (Bettcher *et al.* in press). The WTO regime is primarily aimed at the limitation of health-based restrictions to those that are necessary and minimally burdensome to trade. In addition, the GATT panel's interpretation of the necessary requirement under Article XX unduly restricts the capacity of countries to adopt standards to protect public health (Schoenbaum 1997). The standard employed by the GATT panel when considering Thailand's import ban requires countries to adopt the least trade-restrictive policy possible. This standard inordinately favors the expansion of free trade over national authority to protect public health.

Notably, the Thai case was handled under the dispute resolution process applicable to GATT (1947). Resolutions of disputes concerning the substantive rights and obligations of WTO member states under the new multilateral agreements are now governed by the Understanding on Rules and Procedures Governing the Settlement of Disputes. These new dispute-resolution procedures are producing a new body of GATT jurisprudence, which differs in significant respects from the rules governing the

Thai case—although not, thus far, in ways that would appear to change the Thai result (Palmeter and Mavroidis 1998, WTO 1998d). In addition, the text of Article XX has been modified in GATT (1994) from the way it originally appeared in GATT (1947), although not in a way that appears relevant to the Thai decision.

The GATT decision in the Thai case has been mistakenly viewed by some as an important victory for public health forces. Although the GATT decision upheld strong, non-discriminatory public health measures as consistent with international trade commitments, the liberalization of the tobacco trade in Thailand, as well as other Asian nations, significantly altered the market structure, expanding imports of cigarettes considered qualitatively superior to those produced by national tobacco monopolies and leading to an overall increase in tobacco consumption in these nations. The global impact of the liberalization of tobacco trade has increased the need to adopt and implement broad tobacco control regulatory measures at the national and international level (Taylor 1996).

To the extent of any conflict between GATT (1994) obligations and the national implementation of the provisions of binding international tobacco control instruments, a tobacco treaty can override GATT (1994) via a rule of international law known as the 'later in time' rule between countries that are parties to both treaties (Taylor and Roemer 1996). Article 30 of the Vienna Convention of the Law of Treaties provides general rules governing the relationship of successive treaties. Under Paragraph 3 of Article 30:

[w]hen all the parties to the earlier treaty are parties also to the later treaty . . . the earlier treaty applies only to the extent that its provisions are compatible with those of the later treaty.

Hence, when the provisions of two treaties are in conflict, the later in time prevails, as between the parties to both, unless one treaty specifies otherwise. If a state is a party to only one of the treaties, under Article 30(4)(b), only that treaty governs. Problems arise, however, if both states are parties to GATT (1994) and only one is a party to a subsequent international instrument on tobacco control.

Trade-related aspects of intellectual property rights (TRIPS)
The World Trade Organization's (1994) Agreement on Trade-Related Aspects of Intellectual Property Rights may have some impact on the capacity of countries to regulate tobacco through the introduction of labeling restrictions and plain or generic packaging. Article 15, the basic rule of the trademarks section in TRIPS, requires that any sign, or combination of signs, capable of distinguishing the goods and services of one undertaking from those of others, must be eligible for registration as a trademark, provided that such a trademark is visually perceptible. Article 20 of TRIPS provides:

The use of a trademark in the course of trade shall not be unjustifiably encumbered by special requirements, such as use with another trademark, use in a special form or use in a manner detrimental to its capability to distinguish the goods or services of one undertaking from those of other undertakings.

The tobacco industry has argued that labeling restrictions are an unjustified encumbrance on the rights of the tobacco companies to use their trademarks and thereby violate Article 20 of TRIPS.

There are, however, strong counter-arguments to the claim of the tobacco industry. TRIPS, like GATT, contains an exception for measures necessary to protect public health. Notably, no TRIPS challenge has been initiated by a member state to date against either Australia or South Africa, both of which require health warnings that take up 25% of the tobacco packet (Allen, personal communication). Whether plain packaging, which would involve displacement of all tobacco company labeling and the removal of trademarks entirely, would violate TRIPS remains an open question. Importantly, tobacco industry lawyers have alleged that plain-packaging requirements would breach state party substantive trademark obligations under the Paris Convention for the Protection of Industrial Property and the North American Free Trade Agreement (NAFTA). Although no legal cases have addressed these issues, authorities suggest that plain-packaging requirements may not violate either agreement (Hertz 1997).

WTO agreements related to non-tariff barriers
With the conclusion of the Uruguay Round, trade ministers adopted a number of agreements that deal with various non-tariff barriers designed by countries to protect domestic industries from foreign competition. Although no case has addressed the issue thus far, such agreements may have some important implications for future tobacco control regulatory efforts.

Countries use non-tariff barriers to treat similar imported goods differently than domestic products. Collectively, the non-tariff barrier agreements are designed to promote free competition by controlling technical and bureaucratic measures that involve hindrances to trade (WTO 1998b). Although it is beyond the scope of this paper to analyze the impact of such agreements in depth, a brief review of some of the more significant agreements is in order. For example, the Agreement on Technical Barriers to Trade (TBT) is intended to ensure that national regulations, standards, testing, and certification procedures for imports do not create unnecessary obstacles to trade. Although the scope of the coverage of the TBT Agreement is not clear, it may have wide-ranging implications for tobacco control efforts, including the regulation of tobacco product constituents, labelling of tobacco product packages, and tobacco package design and marking. An array of regulatory provisions concerning tobacco have been notified to the WTO under the TBT Agreement (Plotkin 2000). The TBT agreement, like GATT (1994), provides an exception for public health. In addition, the Agreement on Import Licensing Procedures requires that import licensing systems should not be used as disguised protectionist measures.

As a further example, the Rules of Origin Agreement requires WTO members to ensure that their rules of origin—the criteria used to define where a good is made— are transparent; that they do not have a restricting, distorting, or disruptive effect on international trade; and that they are administered in a consistent, uniform, impartial, and reasonable manner. Rules of origin are a critical part of trade rules because a number of countries have used rules of origin to protect domestic industries. With the rise of preferential trading arrangements, rules of origin have become increasingly important because the benefit of being determined to be from a certain country or trading group has increased. The Rules of Origin Agreement has already had important implications for countries seeking to protect domestic tobacco production. As described above, it has led to the elimination of domestic content legislation that required that all cigarettes produced in the United States contain at least 75% domestically grown tobacco (USDA 1997b). In addition, the new WTO Agreement on Subsidies and Countervailing Measures (SCM Agreement) addresses two closely related topics: export subsidies and the use of countervailing measures to offset the injury caused by subsidized imports. The new SCM Agreement divides specific subsidies into one of three categories: prohibited, actionable, and non-actionable, and establishes the substantive and procedural requirements that must be fulfilled before a state may apply a countervailing measure (WTO 1998c).

At present, no trade-restrictive measures enacted by countries to protect public health from the international tobacco trade have been challenged as inconsistent with these new multilateral agreements, and the implications of these agreements for national and international efforts to address the adverse impacts of tobacco trade remain unclear. In fact, the relationship of many of the agreements and GATT (1994) is not always clear.

Multilateral agreement on investment (MAI)

Although the negotiations of the MAI came to a standstill in late 1998, it is useful to discuss the implications of the last draft of the treaty since negotiations on the MAI may eventually recommence in some form. The proposed MAI was a new international economic treaty designed and negotiated under the auspices of the OECD but open to signature by all nations. The draft agreement contained a set of rules designed to ease the flow of assets across international borders by restricting the legal authority of nations to regulate foreign investment (Vallianatos 1997; Sforza-Roderick *et al.* 1998). These rules, to some extent, also limited national regulatory authority over both domestic and foreign corporations that do business within its sovereign borders (Preamble Center for Public Policy 1998).

Some draft MAI rules, including national treatment and most favored nation, are familiar concepts well established by GATT and WTO. The draft treaty contained other provisions calculated to remove obstacles to economic integration. For example, the proposed agreement included a ban on restrictions on the repatriation of profits or the movement of capital; empowered private investors and corporations to sue governments and seek monetary compensation in the event that a law, practice, or policy violated investor rights under the treaty; and banned uncompensated expropriation of assets, including governmental actions that are 'tantamount to expropriation'. Other notable aspects of the draft treaty included rollback and standstill provisions that would require governments to eliminate laws that violate MAI rules and to refrain from passing any such laws in the future. The treaty would also place limits on governments' ability to employ performance requirements, which are laws that require investors to invest in the local economy or meet social or environmental goals in exchange for market access.

Proponents of the MAI argued that such an agreement was a necessary step to promote international investment and that the treaty would have limited impact on the capacity of countries to adopt and implement national and international regulatory policies to protect public health, including tobacco control (Dymond 1997). In particular, some argued that the MAI was designed to be consistent with GATT and WTO, and that nations could adopt a wide variety of non-discriminatory tobacco control measures without violating MAI obligations. Further, nations may adopt country-specific reservations and exceptions to the proposed treaty in order to protect public health.

Many public health professionals contend, to the contrary, that the draft MAI could have extremely negative implications for international tobacco control efforts (Clarke 1998). Indeed, the health policy impact of the draft MAI is subject to significant criticism from tobacco-control advocates (Sforza-Roderick *et al.* 1998). Most importantly, the draft MAI, unlike GATT (1994), did not contain exceptions for regulations imposed on public health grounds. Consequently, some have suggested that national regulations regarding tobacco imports, advertising, ingredient disclosure, and other measures could come under attack if the treaty is ever adopted. Furthermore, the draft treaty's provision that gave private investors the same legal standing as governments to enforce the terms of the agreement is a radical departure from the WTO regime, where the right to pursue legal action over perceived trade violations is the sole province of governments. Moreover, the investor–state dispute-settlement mechanism of the draft MAI empowered investors—corporations or individuals—to sue, not only national governments but also, provincial, territorial, and local governments, for monetary damages. Consequently, the tobacco industry could use the MAI, if it enters into force, to threaten important local and national laws that protect public health by arguing that such laws are discriminatory against foreign investors, that they constitute expropriation of investor assets, or that they are illegal performance requirements.

Commentators suggest that, even if tobacco companies lose in court, the mere threat of litigation could chill local and national tobacco-control efforts, particularly in developing nations that are just beginning efforts to pass tobacco-control laws. The draft MAI incorporated a broad definition of expropriation applying it to any action that results in a denial of an investor of some benefit of property ownership. Although the expropriation provisions under NAFTA are not as comprehensive as those under the draft MAI, the MAI's dispute-resolution provisions were explicitly modeled on those of NAFTA. The cases currently being litigated under NAFTA are the first where foreign investors have attacked public health and environmental laws as expropriatory. The outcome of these cases may set a critical example for the MAI. For example, the recently settled *Ethyl Corporation v. Government of Canada,* in which Ethyl claimed that Canada's ban of the gasoline additive MMT violated provisions of NAFTA and sought restitution of $251 million, demonstrates the potential impact of such an agreement (Bettcher, personal communication).

Although the OECD originally intended to complete negotiations on the MAI by May 1997, the timetable was twice extended in an effort to iron out differences (OECD 1998; Preamble Center for Public Policy 1998). With no scheduled deadline to adopt the agreement, negotiations fell through in 1998 and, at the time of this writing, there are no plans to resume negotiation. It is uncertain whether or not talks will resume and, if they do, whether or not the treaty will enter into force in its current form or at all.

14.3.2 Regional agreements

There are a number of regional trade agreements aimed at liberalizing trade among countries. The WTO reports that nearly all of its members have entered into regional trade agreements, with more than 80 of these agreements currently in force (WTO 1998a). Many of these agreements have significantly reduced barriers to trade in a wide variety of goods and services, including tobacco and tobacco products. Major agreements and/or regional trade associations include: NAFTA, the European Union (EU), the Association of SE Asian Nations (ASEAN), the Common Market of East and Southern Africa (COMESA), the Economic Community of Western African States (ECOWAS), and the Organization of American States (OAS) (Chaloupka and Corbett 1998).

The conclusion of NAFTA, for example, created the opportunity for significantly increased tobacco trade in North America. NAFTA is a comprehensive trade agreement that calls for dramatic market opening through the elimination of all tariff and non-tariff barriers to trade between Canada, Mexico, and the United States. The agreement has significant implications for the United States and its tobacco trade in the region (USDA 1998). With the implementation of NAFTA in 1994, nearly one-half of US farm exports, including tobacco, now enter Mexico duty-free. By the tenth year, approximately 95% of agricultural trade in the region will be duty-free. In addition, the largest barrier to US farm exports to Mexico was a restrictive licensing system for some US agricultural products, including tobacco. Upon NAFTA's entry into force, all non-tariff barriers, including Mexico's import licensing requirements, were eliminated (US Department of Commerce 1998). Furthermore, NAFTA obligations include rules of origin designed to prevent free riders from benefiting through minor processing or trans-shipment of non-NAFTA goods with only goods made in North America qualifying for preferential tariff treatment.

The EU has also addressed the production and use of tobacco within the European Community. The EU has heavily subsidized tobacco products pursuant to its Common Agricultural Policy, promoting the sale of tobacco at 'giveaway' prices in Northern Africa and Eastern Europe (Roemer 1993). However, the EU also regulates tobacco products in order to protect public health within the region. Article 129 of the Treaty of Rome provides that the European Commission may take any useful initiative to promote coordination of the member states' policies in order to ensure a high level of human health protection. One example of these initiatives is the recently adopted directive that requires all EU member states to ban almost all tobacco advertising by 2006 (EU 1998). Another is an earlier directive on tobacco-product labeling that specifies the nature of the warning labels, including their content, size, placement, and print, that must appear on tobacco packages in the official language of the country of final marketing, as well as the disclosure of tar and nicotine content and other toxic tobacco additives.

14.3.3 Bilateral treaties

In addition to the regional and international trade agreements, there are numerous bilateral agreements reducing tariff and non-tariff barriers to trade, some of which specifically address trade in tobacco products. As described in Section 14.4 below, among the most notable of the tobacco-related bilateral treaties are the agreements between the United States, Japan, South Korea, Taiwan, and Thailand, resulting from actions take by the United States Representative under Section 301 of the US Trade Act of 1974 (Roemer 1993; Bello and Holmer 1994; Chaloupka and Laixuthai 1996; Chaloupka and Corbett 1998).

Section 301 of the Trade Act of 1974, as amended, is the US legislative device designed to open foreign markets to American exports of goods and services, and to achieve improved protection of intellectual property rights and equitable rules for investment abroad. Section 301 authorized the US President to investigate cases where trade and other practices of foreign countries were considered unjustifiable, unreasonable, or discriminatory, in that they limited the ability of US firms to sell their goods and services in foreign markets. Further, it expanded presidential authority to include trade in all American goods and services, and allowed the investigation of practices that were unreasonable, but that did not necessarily violate GATT. If negotiations were unsuccessful in reducing the limits on trade, Section 301 authorized the president to impose retaliatory trade sanctions.

Section 301 was strengthened by the Omnibus Trade and Competitiveness Act of 1988. Known as 'Super 301', these amendments require the US Trade Representative to annually identify countries whose practices consistently limit market access to US firms. If negotiations fail to eliminate the unfair trading practices, the amendments make retaliatory action under Section 301 'mandatory', unless the President deems these measures harmful to US economic interests. Section 301 has been described as the most important 'crowbar' used by American trade negotiators to enhance their leverage and persuade an otherwise recalcitrant trading partner to agree to open up its markets (Bello and Holmer 1994). This crowbar has been exerted with dramatic effect to open up Asian markets to US tobacco companies.

Between 1986 and 1990, as extensively described by Chaloupka *et al.*, the Reagan and Bush administrations successfully used the threat of retaliatory trade sanctions under Section 301 to pressure Japan, Taiwan, South Korea, and Thailand to establish bilateral trade agreements to open up their closed markets to American cigarette exports (Chaloupka and Laixuthai 1996; Chaloupka and Corbett 1998). As described above, when Thailand resisted, the United States took the matter to GATT, which ruled that Thailand must open its markets to American cigarettes.

Unlike its predecessors, the Clinton administration has not utilized Section 301 to force open foreign markets to American tobacco products (Chaloupka and Corbett 1998). Further, the US government has begun to address public health concerns and tobacco trade policy. The US has agreed not to oppose 'non-discriminatory' tobacco control laws in other countries (Bloom 1998). This position also has been adopted by the US Congress though the Doggett Amendment to the FY98 Appropriations Act for the Departments of Commerce, State and Justice, the Judiciary, and related agencies. The Doggett Amendment mandates that:

None of the funds provided by this Act shall be available to promote the sale or export of tobacco or tobacco products, or to seek the reduction or removal by any foreign country or restrictions on the marketing of tobacco or tobacco products, except for restrictions which are not applied equally to all tobacco or tobacco products of the same type.

The amendment is limited, however, in that it does not cover all federal agencies and is subject to renewal (Weissman and Hammond 1998). On February 17, 1998, the Clinton administration issued a directive to all diplomatic posts with guidelines largely similar to those articulated in the Doggett Amendment (Bloom 1998). As a further example, US health officials are now included in all trade policy deliberations involving tobacco products, and commentators report that public health concerns carry significant weight in tobacco trade policy deliberations (Wildavsky 1995).

Although there has been a notable shift in tobacco trade policy under the Clinton administration, the US government still supports the efforts of the American tobacco industry to export tobacco products in numerous ways (Nagy 1994; Taylor 1996). In general, tobacco products that are sold domestically or exported from the United States are specifically exempted from federal laws and regulations applicable to harmful products, including the Federal Hazardous Substances Act, the Toxic Substances Control Act, and the Controlled Substances Act. Furthermore, although federal regulations require that all cigarette packaging and advertising in the United States contain health warning labels and prohibit television and radio advertising, such regulations do not apply to tobacco exports.

14.4 Existing empirical evidence

As described in the previous section, a variety of agreements have significantly reduced tariff and non-tariff barriers to trade in tobacco and tobacco products. As described in Section 14.2, economic theory suggests that trade in tobacco and tobacco products should be rapidly increasing as tobacco-related trade becomes increasingly liberalized. Descriptive data on global trade in tobacco and tobacco products is consistent with this hypothesis. For example, the agreements reached in the most recently completed round of the GATT appear to have had a dramatic impact on global trade in tobacco and tobacco products. From 1994 through 1997, there was a 12.5% increase in unmanufactured tobacco exports globally, after a decade of virtually no growth (USDA 1994, 1997a). Similarly, cigarette exports, which had been relatively stable over the period from 1975 through 1985, began rising at an increasing rate in the mid-1980s, and have accelerated since GATT (1994), with global cigarette exports rising by 42% from 1993 to 1996 (see Fig. 14.1). The increased trade in tobacco products is likely to have contributed to the 5% growth in global cigarette consumption during this same period (Chaloupka and Corbett 1998).

Relatively few formal econometric analyses have been conducted to examine the impact of trade liberalization on tobacco use. Chaloupka and Laixuthai (1996) were the first to consider this issue by examining the impact of the Section 301 agreements described above on cigarette smoking in Asian countries. They used annual data for the period from 1970 through 1991 for 10 countries: the four affected by the Section 301 agreements (Japan, Taiwan, South Korea, and Thailand) and, as a control group, six others where foreign tobacco firms have historically had limited access to tobacco markets (China, India, Indonesia, Malaysia, Pakistan, and the Philippines). Their outcome variables were per capita cigarette consumption and the market share for US cigarettes. Key independent variables included an indicator for the years in which the Section 301 agreements applied and per capita GDP. Given the lack of consistent data

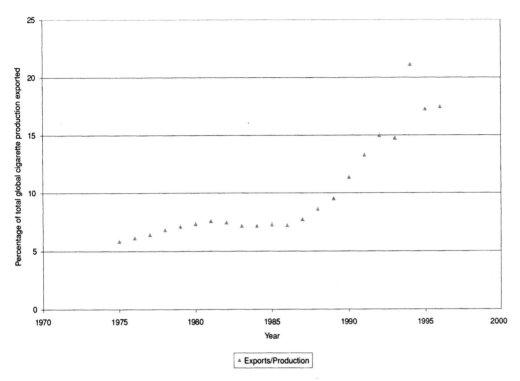

Fig. 14.1 Share of total cigarette production exported globally.

across countries and over time on other important determinants of cigarette demand, they estimated fixed-effects models to control for other unmeasured country- and time-specific influences on demand.

As expected, Chaloupka and Laixuthai found that the market share of US cigarettes in countries affected by the Section 301 agreements rose sharply after their tobacco markets were opened. Their estimates imply that US market shares were 600% higher, on average, in 1991 than they would have been had these markets remained closed. More importantly, Chaloupka and Laixuthai found that the opening of the Japanese, Taiwanese, South Korean, and Thai cigarette markets led to a significant increase in cigarette smoking in these countries. They estimated that per capita cigarette consumption, by 1991, was 10% higher, on average, in the four countries than it would have been in the absence of the bilateral agreements.

As described above, economic theory and extensive empirical research on the determinants of cigarette demand suggest at least two reasons for increased cigarette smoking in response to the liberalization of tobacco-related trade. Before the Section 301 agreements, the tobacco product markets in Japan, Taiwan, South Korea, and Thailand were effectively monopolized, with the state-run monopolist controlling well over 90% of the markets. The monopolies were protected by tariff and non-tariff barriers that would have made imported cigarettes prohibitively expensive for most current or potential smokers. The elimination of the trade barriers and the subsequent entry of US firms made these markets more competitive which, theory predicts, would lead to reduced cigarette prices. Recent evidence from Taiwan supports this hypothesis (Hsieh and Hu 1997). Before the Taiwanese cigarette markets were opened to US firms in 1987, the average price of imported cigarettes in Taiwan was NT$46 per pack, more than double the price of domestically produced cigarettes. Given the large price differences, imported cigarettes comprised less than 2% of total cigarette consumption. In the first year after the Section 301 agreement, inflation-adjusted prices for both domestic and imported cigarettes fell sharply.

Hsieh and Hu (1997) examined the impact of these reductions in cigarette prices on cigarette smoking in Taiwan, decomposing the impact of the opening of the cigarette markets into two effects: a 'switching' effect and a 'market expansion' effect. With respect to the first, Hsieh and Hu noted that the ratio of imported cigarette prices to domestic cigarette prices fell from 2.08 in 1986 to 1.64 in 1987. The decline in the relative price of imported cigarettes resulted in some current smokers switching from domestically produced brands to imported brands. Hsieh and Hu estimated that this switching accounted for a reduction of approximately 10 packs per capita in the consumption of domestic cigarettes. In addition, as a result of the overall decline in all cigarette prices, they estimated that overall cigarette demand rose by about 10 packs per capita—the 'market expansion' effect. As suggested by Hsieh and Lin (1998), this effect induced the Taiwanese government to adopt strong tobacco control policies that, over time, have reduced per capita cigarette consumption below its 1986 level.

A second factor that almost certainly contributed to the increase in smoking that followed the Section 301 agreements is the increased cigarette advertising and promotion that occurred. In Japan, for example, total cigarette advertising by US cigarette companies nearly doubled between 1987 and 1990, while the Japan Tobacco Company responded by increasing its advertising as well. As a result, cigarettes went from being the fortieth most-advertised product on Japanese television to being the second most advertised (Sesser 1993). Hagihara and Takeshita (1995) concluded that US cigarette advertising significantly increased the market share of US cigarettes in Osaka, and suggested that this advertising may explain the increased smoking prevalence observed among young Japanese women in the late 1980s. Similarly, prior to the opening of the Taiwanese cigarette markets, the Taiwan Tobacco and Wine Monopoly Bureau rarely advertised. Its advertisements were limited to new product announcements and a few billboards near the Bureau's branch offices and distribution centers. As part of the Section 301 agreement, however, advertising spread to magazines, with each cigarette producer allowed 120 annual magazine advertisements (Hsieh and Lin 1998).

14.5 New empirical evidence

14.5.1 Data and methods

In order to explore the impact of trade liberalization on tobacco consumption in a larger group of countries, a variant of the model used by Chaloupka and Laixuthai (1996) was estimated using annual data for 42 countries over the period from 1970 through 1995. In the Chaloupka and Laixuthai model, the opening of the cigarette markets was a discrete event that was relatively easy to capture empirically. It is more difficult to do this when trying to develop a measure of 'openness' for most countries. One option would be to construct an objective measure based on tariffs on tobacco and tobacco products. However, the relative importance on non-tariff barriers would render a measure based solely on tariffs suspect (Leamer 1988). Developing an objective measure of non-tariff barriers, however, is a daunting task. Many of these barriers are inherently difficult to quantify, they are not all equally restrictive, and it is not clear how they should be combined with data on tariffs (Leamer 1988). To add to these complications, the necessary data are not readily available for most countries.

An alternative approach is to employ tobacco-related import and export data as an indicator of barriers to trade in tobacco and tobacco products. However, this approach is problematic if the other determinants of trade, including relative prices, technology, and natural barriers to trade, are not constant over time (Leamer 1988). Similarly, the ratio of cigarette imports to domestic cigarette consumption (or production) could be used as a proxy for openness of tobacco-related trade. However, in addition to problems in obtaining the necessary data, the use of this variable as a determinant of cigarette demand would introduce a mechanical relationship between the explanatory variable of interest and the dependent variable. An alternative to this narrowly defined measure of openness would be to use a broader measure of trade intensity, such as total trade (exports plus imports) as a share of GDP. This type of measure, or some variant of it, is commonly used in macro-economic growth models (e.g. Sheehey 1995). This general measure of trade intensity will be a good proxy for tobacco-related trade barriers, if these barriers are highly correlated with barriers to trade in other goods and services. Similar approaches could be used for measuring a country's openness to tobacco-related investment.

Per capita cigarette consumption, based on data from the USDA's tobacco database and the United Nations (UN) Population Division, is the dependent variable in all estimated models. Key independent variables include real per capita GDP, obtained from the United Nations Statistics Division, 'trade openness', based on data from the UN Comtrade database, and lagged cigarette consumption. Lagged consumption is included to account for the addictive nature of cigarette smoking.[1] Following Chaloupka and Laixuthai (1996), fixed-effects models are estimated to account for unmeasured country- and time-specific influences on demand. Finally, because of the correlation between the lagged dependent variable and the error term in this type of dynamic model, the model is first differenced and estimated using instrumental variables methods (Anderson and Hsiao 1981; Greene 1997).

All models are estimated separately for low-income, middle-income, and high-income countries. Low-income countries are defined as those with real average per capita GDP of US$1000 over the 1970–95 period, and include: Bangladesh, China, Egypt, India, Indonesia, Morocco, Nigeria, and the Philippines. Middle-income countries are defined as those with average real per capita GDP in the range from US$1000 to US$3000, and include: Argentina, Brazil, Bulgaria, Colombia, Chile, (former) Czechoslovakia, Hungary, Malaysia, Mexico, Poland, Romania, the (former) Soviet Union, Thailand, and Venezuela. Finally, high-income countries are those with average

---

[1] Given the lack of data on other determinants of cigarette demand, estimating a 'rational addiction' model of cigarette demand was not possible.

real per capita GDP of over US$3000, and include: Australia, Austria, Belgium-Luxembourg, Canada, Denmark, Greece, Taiwan, Turkey, France, Italy, Japan, Netherlands, Portugal, South Korea, Spain, Sweden, Switzerland, the United Kingdom, and the United States.

14.5.2 Results and discussion

The estimates are presented in Table 14. 1. As expected, the estimated coefficient on the 'openness' measure is positive, implying that trade liberalization leads to increased cigarette smoking. This variable is highly significant in models estimated for low-income and middle-income countries, but is insignificant in high-income countries, while the magnitude of the coefficient is largest in low-income countries. This implies that trade liberalization has a large and significant impact on smoking in low-income countries, and a smaller, but still important effect on smoking in middle-income countries, while having no effect on higher income countries. As expected, past cigarette consumption has a strong positive impact on current consumption, consistent with the hypothesis that smoking is an addictive behavior. Finally, smoking is found to be positively related to income in all three groups of countries, with the magnitude of the effect greatest in low-income countries.

There is a plausible explanation for the finding that trade liberalization has its greatest impact on cigarette consumption in low-income countries. In general, openness is higher in high-income countries, consistent with the evidence on the positive relationship between trade and economic growth. If there is a positive but diminishing marginal effect of openness as openness rises, then one would expect to find the greatest marginal effect in low-income countries, which have historically been less open, and the smallest effect in high-income countries, where there have been relatively fewer barriers to trade. Existing empirical evidence supports the hypothesis that the mar-

Table 14.1 Trade liberalization and cigarette consumption, 1970–75

Explanatory variables	Low-income countries	Middle-income countries	High-income countries
Lagged cigarette consumption	0.292[a] (0.072)	0.749[a] (0.161)	0.964[a] (0.146)
'Openness' measure	0.130[a] (0.054)	0.057[b] (0.034)	0.010 (0.042)
Per capita GDP	1.561[a] (0.172)	0.239[a] (0.056)	0.126[a] (0.043)
Intercept	0.134 (0.108)	0.346[a] (0.069)	0.184[a] (0.057)
F statistic	5.44	1.81	1.52

Standard errors are in parentheses.
[a] Indicates significance at the 99% level.
[b] Indicates significance at the 90% level.
All equations include year and country dummy variables, which are not reported here.

ginal impact of trade on development falls as a country's income rises: Baldwin (1984), for example, concluded that the economic effects of trade liberalization in developed countries were very small.

These findings are consistent with the earlier empirical work by Hsieh and Hu (1997) for Taiwan, and Chaloupka and Laixuthai (1996) for several Asian countries, which concluded that liberalization of trade in tobacco products led to significant increases in cigarette smoking. It is important to keep in mind that this analysis does not examine the overall benefits and costs of trade liberalization, but simply that it points out one of the potentially harmful effects of the recent dramatic increases in global trade in tobacco and tobacco products. The key message from this is that, given increasing globalization and the strong positive relationship between globalization and cigarette smoking in low-income and middle-income countries, these countries need to be more proactive in adopting strong tobacco control policies if reducing the health consequences of tobacco use is a priority. As discussed in other chapters in this volume, (see Chapter 10, Chapter 8, Chapter 9, Chapter 11, and Chapter 12), there are a number of policies and other approaches that governments can adopt to discourage tobacco use.

14.6 Conclusions

Controlling the rapid globalization of the tobacco epidemic is an extraordinary public health challenge. The recent liberalization of tobacco-related trade through bilateral, regional, and international trade agreements has significantly reduced tariff and non-tariff trade barriers. The elimination or reduction of these barriers has almost certainly increased competition in tobacco-product markets leading to reductions in the relative prices of these products and increases in their advertising and promotion. Economic theory, and a small but growing body of empirical research, clearly indicate that the liberalization of tobacco-related trade has contributed to global increases in cigarette smoking and other tobacco use, particularly in low-income and middle-income countries. In the absence of strong tobacco-control activities, the long-term consequences of this will be a significant increase in the burden of death and disease caused by tobacco.

Tobacco-related international trade is, however, only one element of the globalization of tobacco growing, production, and use. The globalization of tobacco through trade, investment, advertising, promotion, smuggling, and other means, necessitates prompt and effective national, regional, and global action, including the adoption and implementation of strong tobacco-control regulation, particularly in low-income and middle-income nations where globalization has its greatest impact on tobacco use. Increased trade liberalization and other aspects of globalization, however, do not preclude strong national, regional, and global tobacco control activities. The GATT decision in the Thai case described above suggests that strong-tobacco control policies aimed at reducing the health consequences of tobacco use are consistent with international trade agreements, as long as they are applied in a non-discriminatory fashion. Indeed, the decision implies that a country could ban the sale of all cigarettes and other tobacco products—domestic and foreign—and still be consistent with the GATT.

Since many of the challenges of tobacco control increasingly transcend national boundaries, effectively stemming global tobacco use requires that countries address tobacco control not only within their own borders, but also collectively through the development and implementation of multilateral instruments on tobacco control (Taylor 1996). The increasing transnationalization of the tobacco epidemic restricts the capacity of nations to regulate tobacco effectively through unilateral action. Depending upon the political will of states, these international tobacco-control instruments could promote the harmonization of national measures on aspects of tobacco control that transcend national boundaries, including checks on smuggling, pricing policies, advertising restrictions, the regulation and disclosure of toxic ingredients, and information sharing, as well as the establishment of comprehensive national tobacco control regulatory policies. Moreover, multilateral tobacco-control instruments could incorporate institutional mechanisms and resources to assist developing countries to build sustainable national capacity in tobacco control regulation.

Given global trends toward freer trade, future multilateral instruments for tobacco control could also address tobacco trade issues (Bettcher *et al.* in press). As Bettcher *et al.* have pointed out, it cannot be assumed that GATT (1994) will be applied in a manner that supports the protection of public health in future decisions. Under GATT (1994), the central criterion for resolving trade disputes is the promotion of free trade, not the protection of public health. International legal scholars have frequently and consistently noted the trade bias of the WTO in cross-border disputes relating to the environmental consequences of trade; the same is likely to apply to disputes where trade may have consequences for public health. Moreover, the implications of several new WTO multilateral agreements for tobacco regulation remain uncertain and may leave governments unsure as to their ability to establish and enforce tobacco-related regulations where these regulations have an impact on trade. Finally, future international agreements, such as the for-now side-lined Multilateral Agreement on Investments, may severely restrict the capacity of countries to regulate tobacco to protect public health.

As described further by Jha *et al.* (Chapter 19) and Taylor (1996), the proposed World Health Organization Framework Convention on Tobacco Control offers a long-term approach to global cooperation and coordination on tobacco control. The Convention is likely to be an important mechanism for ensuring that tobacco control moves into a new phase where domestic policies/actions are harmonized with global action and national foreign policies (Yach 1998, Taylor and Bettcher 2000).

References

Anderson, T. W. and Hsiao, C. (1981). Estimation of dynamic models with error components. *Journal of American Statistical Association,* **76**, 598–606.

Baldwin, R. E. (1984). Trade policies in developed countries. In *Handbook of International Economics* (ed. R. W. Jones and P. B. Kener), pp. 571–619. North-Holland, Amsterdam.

Bello, J. and Holmer, A. (1994). The post-Uruguay round future of Section 301 of the Trade Act of 1974. *Law and Policy in International Business,* **25**, 1297.

Bettcher, D., Yach, D., and Guindon, E. Global trade and health: key linkages and future challenges. *Bulletin of the World Health Organization.* (In press).

Bloom, J. (1998). *International Interests in US Tobacco Legislation*. Advocacy Institute, Health Science Analysis Project: Policy Analysis No. 3. http://scarcnet.org/hsap/interanational.htm

Chaloupka, F. J. and Corbett, M. (1998). Trade policy and tobacco: towards an optimal policy mix. In *The Economics of Tobacco Control: Towards an Optimal Policy Mix* (ed. I. Abedian, R. van der Merwe, N. Wilkins, and P. Jha), pp. 129–45. Applied Fiscal Research Centre, University of Cape Town, Cape Town (South Africa).

Chaloupka, F. J. and Laixuthai, A. (1996). *US Trade Policy and Cigarette Smoking in Asia*. National Bureau of Economic Research Working Paper No. 5543, 1996.

Clarke, T. (1998). *License to Loot, Friends of the Earth*. http://www.foe.org/ga/mai/html

Dunoff, J. (1994). Institutional misfits: the GATT, the ICJ & trade-environment disputes. *Michigan Journal of International Law*, **15**, 1043.

Dymond, W. (1997). *MAI Briefing for Non-OECD Countries*. OECD, Paris, France. http://www.oecd.org/daf/cmis/mai/dymond.htm

Edwards, S. (1992). Trade orientation, distortions and growth in developing countries. *Journal of Development Economics*, **39**, 31–57.

European Union (1998). *Policies of the European Union: Advertising of Tobacco Products*. http://europa.eu.int/comm/sg/scadplus/leg/en/cha/c11509.htm

General Agreement on Tariffs and Trade (GATT) (1990). *Thailand—Restriction on Importation of and Internal Taxes on Cigarettes*. Report of the Panel. GATT, Geneva.

Greene, W. H. (1997). *Econometric Analysis*. Prentice-Hall, Englewood Cliffs (New Jersey).

Grise, A. N. (1990). *The World Tobacco Markets—Government Intervention and multilateral Policy Reform*. Staff Report No. AGES 9014. Commodity Economics Division, Economic Research Service, US Department of Agriculture, Washington, DC.

Hagihara, A. and Takeshita, Y. J. (1995). Impact of American cigarette advertising on imported cigarette consumption in Osaka, Japan. *Tobacco Control*, **4**, 239–44.

Hertz, A. (1997). Shaping the trident: Intellectual property under NAFTA, investment protection agreements, and at the World Trade Organization. *Canada–United States Law Journal*, **23**, 261.

Hsieh, C. R. and Hu, T. W. (1997). *The Demand for Cigarettes in Taiwan: Domestic versus Imported Cigarettes*. Discussion Paper No. 9701. The Institute of Economics, Academia Sinica, Nankang, Taipei.

Hsieh, C. R. and Lin, Y. S. (1998). The economics of tobacco control in Taiwan. In *The Economics of Tobacco Control: Towards an Optimal Policy Mix* (ed. I. Abedian, R. van der Merwe, N. Wilkins, and P. Jha), pp. 306–29. Applied Fiscal Research Centre, University of Cape Town, Cape Town (South Africa).

Leamer, K. E. (1988). Measures of openness. In *Trade Policy Issues and Empirical Analysis* (ed. H. Baldwin), pp. 147–200. University of Chicago Press for the National Bureau of Economic Research, Chicago.

Maranvanyika, E. (1998). The search for an optimal tobacco control policy in Zimbabwe. In *The Economics of Tobacco Control: Towards an Optimal Policy Mix* (ed. I. Abedian, R. van der Merwe, N. Wilkins, and P. Jha), pp. 272–81. Applied Fiscal Research Centre, University of Cape Town, Cape Town (South Africa).

Nagy, K. (1994). Farming tobacco overseas: international trade of US tobacco. *Journal of the National Cancer Institute*, **86**, 417.

Organization for Economic Cooperation and Development (1998). http://www.oecd.org/daf/cmis/mai//maindex.html

Palmeter, D. and Mavroidis, P. (1998). The WTO legal system: Sources of law. *American Journal of International Law*, **92**, 398.

Plotkin, B. (2000). Implications of the World Trade Organization Agreement for the Framework Convention on Tobacco Control and Related Possible Protocols. World Health Organization: Geneva. (In press).

Preamble Center for Public Policy (1998). *The multilateral Agreement on Investment: A 'Bill of Rights' for International Investors?* http://www.rtk.net/preamble/mai/maioverv.html

Preston, S. H. (1976). *Mortality Patterns in National Populations.* Academic Press, New York.

Roemer, R. (1993). *Legislative Action to Combat the World Tobacco Epidemic.* World Health Organization, Geneva.

Schoenbaum, T. J. (1997). International trade and the protection of the environment: the continuing search for reconciliation. *American Journal of International Law,* **91**, 268.

Sforza-Roderick, M., Nova, S., and Weisbrot, M. (1998). *Writing the Constitution of a Single Global Economy: a Concise Guide to the Multilateral Agreement on Investment—Supporters' and Opponents' Views.* Preamble Center for Public Policy. http://www.rtk.net/preamble/mai/maioverv.html

Sesser, S. (1993). Opium war redux. *The New Yorker,* **69**, 78–89.

Sheehey, E. J. (1995). Trade, efficiency and growth in a cross section of countries. *Weltwirtschaftliches Archiv,* **131**, 723–36.

Shi, M. S. and Hsieh, C. R. (1998). *Cigarette Import, Welfare and Optimal Taxation.* Presented at the 3rd Biennial Conference of Pacific Rim Allied Economic Organizations, Bangkok, Thailand, January, 1998.

Taylor, A. L. and Bettcher, D. W. (2000). The WHO Framework Convention on Tobacco Control: A global good for public health. *Bulletin of the World Health Organization.* (In press).

Taylor, A. (1996). An international regulatory strategy for global tobacco control. *Yale Journal of International Law,* **21**, 257.

Taylor, A. and Roemer, R. (1996). *International Strategy for Tobacco Control.* Geneva: World Health Organization WHO/PSA/96.6.

United States Department of Agriculture (1994). *US Tobacco Statistics, 1935–1992.* United States Department of Agriculture, Economic Research Service, Washington, DC.

United States Department of Agriculture (1997a). *Tobacco: World Markets and Trade.* United States Department of Agriculture, Foreign Agricultural Service, Washington, DC.

United States Department of Agriculture (1997b). *GATT/WTO and Tobacco.* http://www.fas.usda.gov/itp/policy/gatt/tobacco/html

United States Department of Agriculture (1998). *NAFTA Agricultural Fact Sheet: Tobacco.* http://ffas.usda.gov/itp/policy/nafta/tobacco.html

United States Department of Commerce (1998). *Key NAFTA Sector Specific Provisions* International Trade Administration. http://www.itaiep.doc.gov/nafta/3002.htm

Vallianatos, M. (1997). Multilateral agreement on investment. *Foreign Policy in Focus,* **2**, 39.

Weissman, R. and Hammond, R. (1998). International tobacco sales. *The Progressive Response,* **2**, 20.

Wildavsky, B. (1995). Smoke screens. *National Journal,* **27**(40), 2476–80.

World Bank (1991). *Policy on Tobacco* (R91-225). The World Bank, Washington D.C.

World Trade Organization (1998a). *Development, Regionalism, and Multilateral Tradings.* http://www.wto.org/wto/develop/regional.htm

World Trade Organization (1998b). *Non-Tariff Barriers—Technicalities, Red Tape, etc.* http://www.wto.org/wto/about/agmnts8.htm

World Trade Organization (1998c). *Agreement on Subsidies and Countervailing Measures.* http://www.wto.org/wto/goods/scm.htm

World Trade Organization (1998d). Note by the Secreatariat: GATT/WTO Dispute Settlement Practice Relation to Article XX, Paragraphs (b), (d) and (g) of GATT, WTO Doc, WT/CTE/W/53/Rev.1. Committee on Trade and Environment

Yellen, J. L. (1998). The continuing importance of trade liberalization. *Business Economics,* **33**(1), 23–6.

Yach, D. (1998). *Progress Towards Global Tobacco Control.* Presented at the Joint PAHO-WHO-NHLBI-FIC 50th Anniversary Conference on Global Shifts in Disease Burden: The Cardiovascular Pandemic, Pan American Health Organization Headquarters, Washington D.C., 26–28 May 1998.

15

How big is the worldwide cigarette-smuggling problem?[1]

David Merriman, Ayda Yurekli, and Frank J. Chaloupka

Cigarettes have particular appeal to potential smugglers because taxes often account for a large share of their price, making them a highly profitable product to smuggle. Economic models of smuggling are used to develop techniques for measuring the extent and nature of the worldwide cigarette smuggling problem.

We conduct three separate empirical analyses. Our estimates indicate that between 6% and 8.5% of global cigarette consumption is smuggled. The perceived level of corruption, as measured on a published 'transparency index' ranging from 0 (highly corrupt) to 10 (highly clean), statistically explains more of the variance in experts' estimates of cigarette smuggling than do cigarette prices. Using data on relative cigarette prices and travel between European countries, we estimate the extent of bootlegging (the legal purchase of cigarettes in one country for consumption or resale in another country without paying applicable taxes or duties) in Europe. Simulations show that even when the potential for increased smuggling is taken into account, increases in cigarette tax rates result in increased tax revenue. Coordinated multilateral increases in cigarette taxes would result in significantly more tax revenue and less smuggling than unilateral tax increases.

Smuggling is sometimes perceived to be an insurmountable obstacle to higher cigarette tax rates. Our results suggest that countries need not make a choice between higher cigarette tax revenues and lower cigarette consumption. Higher tax rates will achieve both objectives.

15.1 Introduction

The theory of comparative advantage teaches us that unfettered voluntary trade enhances social welfare. Exceptions to this conclusion may occur if there is imperfect information about the traded good or if the good is associated with negative externalities. In this case, optimal policy may require governments to impose taxes that discourage use of the good. Unfortunately, whenever taxes are imposed, an incentive to evade them arises. Evasion of excise taxes on goods by circumvention of border controls is smuggling. Goods may also be smuggled to evade rules prohibiting their sale.

---

[1] We thank Luk Joossens and other reviewers for useful comments.

A prohibition on sale can be thought of as an infinite tax. Because taxes on cigarettes often account for a large share of their price they are especially appealing to potential smugglers.

The presence of smuggling constrains the use of higher taxes as one element of a comprehensive tobacco-control policy in at least three important ways. First, smuggling reduces the maximum revenue that can be raised by cigarette taxes since, as tax rates increase, the quantity of smuggled cigarettes is also likely to increase. Second, attempts to control smuggling may absorb both private and law-enforcement resources. Third, smuggling may present opportunities for corruption that lower the legitimacy of law enforcement authorities. Estimates of the magnitude and determinants of cigarette smuggling are, therefore, important inputs to the design of tobacco-tax policy.

Two general types of cigarette smuggling may be distinguished. Bootlegging is the legal purchase of cigarettes in one country but consumption or resale in another country without paying applicable taxes or duties. Wholesale smuggling occurs when cigarettes are sold without the payment of taxes or duties, even in the country of their origin. In this paper we use the term 'smuggling' to refer to both bootlegging and wholesale smuggling. A more in-depth discussion of this terminology is found in Chapter 16. Price differentials among countries create incentives for bootlegging, while high cigarette taxes create an incentive for wholesale smuggling—even when tax systems are harmonized.

In 1995, for example, the retail price of a pack of 20 cigarettes in Germany was $3.38.[2] In neighboring Poland and the Czech Republic, cigarette prices were about one-tenth as high (33–37 cents per pack). Disparities in price of more than 100% between neighbor and near-neighbor countries are not unique to Germany and Eastern Europe. Within Western Europe, Scandinavian countries have cigarette prices two to three times as high as those in southern European countries (Italy, Portugal, and Spain). Even more extreme price disparities are found in Latin America and East Asia. Similar disparities exist within some countries (e.g. between states in the United States).

Price disparities create a large incentive for bootlegging. One source estimates that a single truckload of smuggled cigarettes could evade $1.2 million of taxes in the European Union (Joossens 1998, p. 150). Econometric estimates of cigarette smuggling in the United States, discussed in Section 15.3, generally show a low level of smuggling. However, there is reason to believe that the very large price disparities described above may lead to greater smuggling elsewhere, especially in low-income countries where fewer resources may be available to enforce tight smuggling controls. Estimates by experts in the field, discussed in more detail in Section 15.4, suggest that there are many countries in which smuggled cigarettes account for 20% or more of consumption.

Retail price differentials between neighboring countries alone cannot account for the cross-country variance in smuggling. Smuggling requires evasion of border controls or bribery of border guards. A retail network must be available to distribute smug-

---

[2] Throughout this paper local prices are converted to US dollars using prevailing exchange rates. See Section 15.4 for data sources and methods of adjustment.

gled cigarettes. Conditions that contribute to smuggling include high levels of government corruption, an established informal market for cigarettes (sales of cigarettes by street vendors), and a well-organized criminal establishment.

15.2 Theoretical considerations

Several key questions must be addressed. What determines the total value of smuggling? Why is there more smuggling in some countries than in others? Why do legal trade and smuggling of cigarettes persist simultaneously? If the expected return on smuggled cigarettes is greater than the expected return on legal trade, why do not smugglers out-compete legal sellers and dominate the market? We apply Desmond Norton's (1988) model of bootlegging to the cigarette trade to answer these questions.

Norton considers a firm located abroad at a distance d from home. The firm has a fixed quantity of cigarettes $\bar{q}$ that can be sold abroad, legally exported to home or illegally bootlegged into home. For each pack of cigarettes sold abroad, the firm earns a price p (denominated in dollars for convenience). Home levies a tax t on cigarettes that is not levied abroad (this assumption effectively rules out the possibility of wholesale smuggling). The firm earns $(p + pt + \theta)$ for each pack sold at home. θ may be greater than, equal to or less than zero depending upon whether the local tax is fully embodied in the local price. Hence, the model allows for less-than-perfect competition in the cigarette industry. Norton assumes an 'iceberg' specification of transport costs—some portion of shipped cargo evaporates in transport. He designates the cost per smuggled cigarette as s(d) and the cost per legally exported cigarette as L(d) and assumes that s'(d) and L'(d) > 0.

Smugglers face a risk of detection of $(1 - \mu)$ and, if detected, pay a penalty that is proportional to the amount of smuggled cigarettes that are seized. The probability of non-detection, μ, is postulated to be a decreasing function of the amount smuggled and an increasing function of the amount legally exported. That is, Norton assumes that legal exports camouflage bootlegging (see Thursby *et al.* (1991) for a related model of cigarette smuggling).

In Norton's model the firm's objective function is given by:

$$\pi(d) = \mu(q^s, q^L)(p + pt + \theta)(1 - s)q^s$$
$$-(1 - \mu)\alpha(1 - s)pq^s$$
$$+(p + \theta)(1 - L)q^L$$
$$-p(q^s + q^L), \tag{15.1}$$

where q^s = the quantity of cigarettes smuggled into home, q^L = the quantity of cigarettes legally imported to home, and α is the share of revenue from intercepted smuggled cigarettes that offenders must pay as a penalty. The firm's problem is to choose q^s and q^L subject to the constraints that: $q^s + q^L \leq \bar{q}$ and $q^s, q^L \geq 0$.

The first term on the right-hand side of eqn 15.1 is expected revenue from successful bootlegging, the second term is the expected penalty from smuggled cigarettes that are intercepted, the third term is revenue from legal exports, and the fourth term is revenue foregone as a result of reduced sales abroad.

Norton shows that, depending upon the parameters, there are several possible kinds of optimal allocations by the firm. In particular, Norton shows that optimal solutions in which both $q^s > 0$ and $q^L > 0$ are possible. Furthermore, he shows that an increase in the tax rate t will increase the optimal choice of q^s among existing smugglers and increase the number of firms that smuggle, resulting in an increase in the aggregate amount of bootlegging. Norton's model also shows that an increase in the fine paid by smugglers if they are detected (α) reduces the profit-maximizing level of smuggling. In Appendix 15.1 (at the end of the chapter), we extend Norton's model in a straight-forward way and show that an increase in the probability of detection reduces the optimal quantity smuggled. Norton's model has clear empirical implications: we should find higher levels of bootlegging into countries with high taxes and low levels of enforcement.

What are the welfare implications of cigarette smuggling? Bhagwati and Hansen (1974) note that, for goods that carry no negative externalities, optimal economic policy requires that small countries impose no tariffs. They go on to say:

... [i]t is commonly argued that smuggling must improve economic welfare since it constitutes (partial or total) evasion of the tariffs (or quantity restrictions)

However, Bhagwati and Hansen reason that, because smugglers must take action to evade detection, smuggling increases transportation costs. They show that if smuggling occurs under conditions of perfect competition and constant costs then, in any circumstances where smuggling and legal trade coexist, 'smuggling must be a welfare-reducing activity' (p. 13).

Cigarette smoking imposes significant negative externalities (see Chapter 4 and Chapter 7; Chaloupka and Warner, in press). If so, taxation of cigarettes, so that consumers internalize negative externalities, is appropriate. Although there has been no formal theoretical welfare analysis of the smuggling of 'bads' (as distinct from 'goods'), which impose negative externalities, it is clear that Bhagwati and Hansen's results can be extended to cover this case. If smuggling of goods reduces welfare, then smuggling of bads must reduce welfare even further, since it circumvents a tax that would otherwise improve national well-being. Smuggling may reduce retail prices below the social cost of the bad.

15.3 Previous empirical literature

Most of the direct evidence about cigarette smuggling comes from high-income countries. However, the general theoretical model of smuggling is applicable to a broad range of societies. Further, as shown elsewhere in this volume, we have considerable direct evidence that the smoking behavior of individuals in middle-income and low-income countries responds to changes in economic incentives. Therefore, it is reasonable to believe that the lessons about cigarette smuggling learned in high-income countries will be more or less applicable to middle-income and low-income countries.

A number of empirical studies have demonstrated that despite its addictive nature, cigarette smoking—like other consumption activities—responds to economic variables. There is clear evidence that increases in price decrease smoking, but there are mixed empirical results about whether increases in income increase smoking (see Chaloupka and Warner, in press).

Smuggling is inherently difficult to study with econometric methodology. Because of its illegal nature the dependent variable, cigarette smuggling, generally has to be inferred rather than be directly observed. Inferences about smuggling require some confidence about what variables influence the demand for cigarettes in the absence of smuggling and whether illegal behavior, like smuggling, may be influenced by economic incentives. In recent years, economists have reached something approaching consensus on both issues.

In contrast to the difficulty in observing smuggling directly, it is often possible to observe the level of 'tax-paid sales', i.e. the level of cigarette sales on which the government collected excise taxes. The level of smuggling can be inferred by calculating the difference between the demand for cigarettes predicted by econometric models and the observed level of tax paid sales. Furthermore, we may study how sensitive smuggling is to changes in variables that are believed to influence smuggling.

The higher the rewards of smuggling, and the lower the costs, the greater the probability that individuals will engage in it. The reward for smuggling is closely related to the probability of detection, the magnitude of punishment, and the difference in profits from legally sold versus smuggled cigarettes. The costs of smuggling include ordinary economic costs like foregone salaries from other employment and the cost of the capital employed in smuggling. Other costs may also arise, including the cost of bribery or the potential cost of going to jail if the smuggling is discovered.

A number of recent studies that have used this methodology to econometrically measure the degree of cigarette smuggling are briefly outlined in Table 15.1 below. Baltagi and Levin (1986, 1992) studied cigarette bootlegging and legal cross-border shopping between US states. They found that cigarette sales varied inversely with price and that higher prices in neighboring states increased cigarette sales in the state of residence. They reasoned that such price increases reduced the incentive for consumers to cross into neighboring states to make purchases. In their 1992 paper, Baltagi and Levin found that each 10% increase in a neighboring state's price caused an increase of 0.8% in home state sales.

Saba *et al.* (1995) also found significant evidence of citizens crossing US state borders to purchase lower-priced cigarettes. Where many citizens reside in high-tax jurisdictions in close proximity to low-tax jurisdictions (most importantly the District of Columbia and New Hampshire), border-crossing accounted for a substantial portion of sales. However, in most states border-crossing accounted for less than 2% of sales.

A sophisticated study by Thursby and Thursby (2000) allowed for wholesale smuggling, as well as bootlegging and cross-border shopping. Using data from 39 US states, and the District of Columbia from 1972 to 1990, they found that in most years between 3% and 5% of US consumption results from cross-border shopping or smuggling.

Galbraith and Kaiserman (1997) studied smuggling in Canada. They noted that 'virtually all cigarettes smuggled into Canada . . . were previously exported from Canada' (pp. 288–9). Using this insight, they measured the responsiveness of smuggling to changes in taxes. Beginning in the early 1980s, Canada steadily increased its cigarette taxes so that, by 1991, there was a large price differential between US and Canadian cigarettes. In 1994, Canada reduced cigarette taxes due to a perception that smuggling had increased. Galbraith and Kaiserman found that there was a large

Table 15.1 Econometric studies of cigarette smuggling

Study	Geography and period	Results	Notes
Baltagi and Levin (1992)	46 US states 1963–88	10% increase in price in neighboring state causes 0.8% increase in taxed sales of home state	Results largely confirm Baltagi and Levin (1986)
Saba *et al.* (1995)	48 continental US states and DC 1960–86	Excluding DC no state lost more than 2% of sales as a result of purchases in neighboring states in 1986	In many states cross-border sales declined between 1960 and 1986
Thursby and Thursby (1998)	40 US states 1972–90	0.69–7.8% of consumption is smuggled	In most years smuggling is between 3% and 5% of total sales
Galbraith and Kaiserman (1997)	Aggregate Canadian monthly consumption 1980–94	Total consumption is much less responsive to price increases (short-run elasticity of –0.40) than taxed consumption (short-run elasticity of –1.01)	Canada's 1991 cigarette tax increase was rolled-back in 1994 due to belief that high taxes encouraged smuggling

increase in untaxed sales following the increase in Canadian taxes. They estimated a unitary elasticity of taxed cigarette consumption with respect to price: each 1% increase in Canadian taxes causes taxed sales to fall by about 1%. However, Galbraith and Kaiserman found that total consumption (taxed plus smuggled sales) fell by only 0.4%, with smuggled sales increasing by 0.6%. Gailbraith and Kaiserman's estimates suggest that, despite the increase in smuggling, total Canadian tax revenues were not diminished by the tax rate increase, and that total consumption was reduced.

In summary, existing evidence suggests that in the United States interstate smuggling has been, in most cases, a relatively minor annoyance, rather than a major barrier to cigarette taxation. In Canada, cigarette smuggling may be a larger impediment. This difference may stem from the relatively small inter-state price differentials induced by US cigarette taxation compared to the relatively large price differentials brought about by increases in Canadian taxation.

To what extent the experiences of Canada and the US can be extended to other regions of the world is open to debate. Although there are no econometric studies of cigarette smuggling outside North America one careful observer (Joossens 1998, p. 146) notes that:

... it is not always true that the incentive for smuggling is linked to the level of taxes. For example, in countries with the highest taxes in Europe, such as the Scandinavian countries, there is little evidence of smuggling, while in Spain, Italy and many Central and Eastern European countries, where taxes and prices are much lower, the illegal sale of international cigarette brands is widespread.

There is a small empirical literature on smuggling of contraband into and out of low-income and middle-income countries. This literature finds that there is substantial contraband smuggling and that smuggling increases with the level of tariffs and taxes (Bhagwati 1974; Simkin 1974; Norton 1988). In the next section we discuss three empirical exercises in an attempt to quantify more accurately the worldwide cigarette smuggling problem.

15.4 Quantitative analysis of cigarette smuggling

As noted above, it is difficult to study smuggling activities because of the scarcity of data. We approach this problem by discussing three separate empirical exercises, each of which we believe sheds some light on the extent and nature of the worldwide cigarette smuggling problem.

15.4.1 Comparing recorded imports and exports of cigarettes

One method of assessing the amount of illegal trade in a product is to compare recorded exports and imports. This methodology was pioneered by Bhagwati (1974b), who noted that under-recording of imports may be used as a technique to avoid payment of tariffs; and Simkin (1974) who noted that under-recording of exports may be used to avoid payment of export taxes. Bhagwati (1974b) studied Turkey's recorded imports from several trade partners and each of those trade partners' recorded exports to Turkey. Bhagwati cautioned that there are a number of reasons why the levels of recorded imports may be less than those of recorded exports, including: errors of commodity classification; time lags; misallocation of country-of-origin by the receiving country; and over-invoicing by the exporting country. After careful scrutiny of the data, Bhagwati (p. 145) concludes that there are 'significant discrepancies for which the only explanation appears to be the under-invoicing [of goods received from Turkey's trade partners]'. Simkin conducted a similar analysis of Indonesia's exports and reached 'an estimate of $127 million a year for Indonesia's unrecorded exports . . . against a figure of $435 million for their recorded exports' (p. 169).

It is possible to conduct a similar analysis of the world cigarette market. Table 15.2 (reproduced from Joossens 1998) reports aggregates of world-wide recorded exports and imports of cigarettes. Recorded exports are consistently about 1.3 times as great as imports. While recorded cigarette exports grew about five-fold between 1975 and 1996, recorded imports grew only slightly more than four-fold. In 1996, recorded exports exceeded recorded imports by about 400 billion cigarettes, suggesting that perhaps one-third of all recorded exports were smuggled. Chaloupka and Corbett (1998) estimate that in 1996, nearly 17.5% of all global cigarette production was exported (p. 134). If one-third of all exports were smuggled, this would account for about 6% of world cigarette consumption. To this total may be added both unrecorded exports and wholesale-smuggled cigarettes that do not cross national boundaries.

However, cautious interpretation of these results is advisable. As both Bhagwati (1974b) and Simkin (1974) noted, many factors may explain a discrepancy between

Table 15.2 World cigarette imports and exports (billions of sticks)

Year	Imports	Exports	Ratio exports to imports
1975	171	223	1.30
1980	254	323	1.27
1985	313	356	1.14
1990	418	543	1.30
1991	526	712	1.35
1992	568	804	1.42
1993	600	780	1.30
1994	886	1156	1.30
1995	668	987	1.48
1996	707	1107	1.57

Source: US Department of Agriculture (1997), as quoted in Joossens (1998).

recorded exports and imports. An analysis of data from the United Nations Comtrade databank shows large discrepancies between total reported imports and exports of many products (these data may be accessed at http://www.intracen.org/itc/infobase).

We found that manufactured tobacco (SITC 122) trade follows a pattern similar to that described by Joossens (1998). However, there are also large discrepancies between the total recorded imports and exports of rice (SITC 42) and coca (SITC 72). Between 1992 and 1996 manufactured-tobacco exports were between 133% and 147% of manufactured tobacco imports. Coca exports were between 53% and 62% of coca imports and rice exports were between 78% and 119% of rice imports.

Smuggling is not the only possible explanation for these statistical discrepancies (see Feenstra *et al.* 1999). What makes cigarettes different from other commodities is the consistency with which exports greatly exceed imports. Statistical discrepancies alone would not necessarily lead to any consistent relationship between cigarette imports and exports. The most reasonable explanation for the observed data is that a large and growing fraction of international trade in cigarettes is smuggled.

15.4.2 Analysis of experts' estimates of cigarette smuggling

Offical estimates of cigarette smuggling are not available for most countries. We obtained experts' estimates of the amount of smuggling from several sources. Joossens (1998) compiled quantitative estimates for 11 European countries from a variety of official and non-official sources. A private company, Market Tracking International (MTI), published estimates of smuggling as a percentage of total cigarette sales for many countries in its serial publication *World Tobacco File*. When the two sources conflict we have used data from Joossens (1998). Data compiled from these sources is given in column 3 of Table 15.3.

MTI does not publish information about the methodology used to obtain their estimates of smuggling. In communications with the MTI staff we were told that the estimates were obtained by consultation with local experts, government officials and through review of media coverage of local market conditions. In some cases, MTI's

Table 15.3 Estimates of price, smuggling and transparency

Country	Price/pack US$ (1995)[a]	Estimate of smuggling as a percentage of 1995 domestic sales by expert sources	Source of smuggling estimate	Transparency index[b]
Argentina	1.38	14%	2	3.0
Australia	4.85	na	na	8.7
Austria	2.96	15%	4	7.5
Azerbaijan	na	13%	1	na
Bangladesh	0.09	38%	3	na
Belgium-Lux	3.32	7%	4	5.4
Belarus	na	23%	1	3.9
Brazil	1.05	15%	2	4.0
Bulgaria	0.31	15%	1	2.9
Cambodia	0.05	37%	3	na
Canada	3.98	na	na	9.2
China	0.10	4%	2	3.5
Colombia	0.06	30%	2	2.2
Czech Rep	0.33	7%	1	4.8
Denmark	5.21	na	na	10.0
Ecuador	0.15	na	na	2.3
Estonia	na	16%	1	5.7
Finland	4.49	na	na	9.6
France	2.90	2%	4	6.7
Germany	3.38	10%	4	7.9
Greece	1.90	8%	4	4.9
Hong Kong	1.58	10%	3	7.8
Hungary	0.52	5%	1	5.0
India	0.37	1%	2	2.9
Indonesia	0.00	5%	3	2.0
Ireland	1.69	4%	4	8.2
Italy	2.19	12%	4	4.6
Jamaica	0.37	na	na	3.8
Japan	2.43	na	na	5.8
Kazakhstan	na	17%	1	na
Lao	0.43	na	na	na
Latvia	na	39%	1	2.7
Lithuania	na	30%	1	na
Malaysia	0.68	18%	3	5.3
Mexico	0.62	na	na	3.3
Myanmar	0.56	53%	3	na
Nepal	0.08	1%	2	na
Netherlands	2.99	8%	4	9.0
New Zealand	4.69	na	na	9.4
Norway	7.01	na	na	9.0
Pakistan	0.28	30%	2	2.7
Philippines	0.22	19%	3	3.3
Poland	0.37	15%	1	4.6
Portugal	1.47	na	na	6.5
Romania	0.04	20%	1	3.0

Table 15.3 (*cont.*)

Country	Price/pack US$ (1995)[a]	Estimate of smuggling as a percentage of 1995 domestic sales by expert sources	Source of smuggling estimate	Transparency index[b]
Russia	0.03	6%	1	2.4
Korea Rep.	0.77	9%	3	4.2
Singapore	2.24	2%	3	9.1
Slovakia	0.38	3%	1	3.9
South Africa	1.32	na	na	5.2
Spain	1.38	15%	4	6.1
Sri Lanka	1.05	10%	3	na
Sweden	4.58	2%	4	9.5
Switzerland	2.80	na	na	8.9
Taiwan	0.88	14%	2	5.3
Thailand	0.60	11%	3	3.0
Turkey	0.51	na	na	3.4
UK	4.16	2%	4	8.7
United States	1.94	na	na	7.5
Ukraine	na	5%	1	2.8
Uzbekistan	na	11%	1	na
Venezuela	0.07	na	na	2.3
Vietnam	0.10	28%	3	2.5
Zimbabwe	0.43	na	na	4.2

[1] Source is *World Tobacco File* (1997) Emerging markets in Central and Eastern Europe table 6.1.
[2] Source is *World Tobacco File* (1996) **2**, table 10.4.
[3] Source is *World Tobacco File* (1997) Emerging Asian markets table 6.2.
[4] Source is Joossens (1998) p. 150.
na = not available.
Note: When a source gives a range of smuggling estimates (e.g. 5–10%) we use the midpoint of the range (e.g. 7.5%).
[a] Sources: Unpublished data, World Bank, and Marketfile.
[b] Source: Tranparency International 1998.

reports of the share of smuggling in a country vary a great deal from year to year. For example, its estimate of smuggling in Russia increased from 6% of the market in 1995 to 25–30% of the market in 1996 (Market Tracking International 1997). While we are somewhat skeptical of the accuracy of these estimates, we believe that they represent the most comprehensive compilation of experts' estimates of cigarette smuggling available.

The population-weighted average figure for smuggling as a percentage of the total cigarette consumption is about 8.5%; the unweighted average is 13.3%. The experts' population-weighted estimate of cigarette smuggling is remarkably consistent with our estimate from recorded cigarette imports and exports above. Are the experts' estimates of smuggling consistent with the predictions of economic theory?

Norton's (1988) theoretical model implies that the share of bootlegged cigarettes in the local market should be positively associated with the relative price of cigarettes and inversely correlated with enforcement activities in that market. Although we did not have direct estimates of local enforcement activities, we obtained a measure of the perception of corruption in a large number of countries.[3]

Transparency International (1998), a non-governmental organization dedicated to increasing government accountability, compiled surveys of perceptions of the degree of corruption as seen by business-people, risk analysts, and the general public. Among other questions, the surveys asked about respondents' perceptions of illegal payments to public officials and policemen, and those monitoring imports and exports. On the basis of these surveys, Transparency International used a 'poll-of-polls' approach to assign each country a composite corruption perception index ranging between 10 (highly clean) and 0 (highly corrupt). We used this index as a measure of the ease with which illegal cigarettes could be imported and distributed. Transparency International's index for countries on which we have cigarette price or smuggling data is shown in column 5 of Table 15.3.

We estimated local cigarette prices by comparing total quantities of cigarettes sold in the legal market with total expenditures on legal cigarettes. The sales data were obtained from Marketfile, which provided data on millions of cigarettes sold. Domestic per capita cigarette sales were estimated by dividing of the total number of cigarettes by 20 and by the total population. Marketfile was also the source for data on the total value of sales in local currency. This value was adjusted to US dollars using the current US market exchange rate. The nominal price per pack of 20 cigarettes was estimated by dividing the total value of sales by the total number of cigarettes and multiplying by 20. Price estimates for 1995 are shown in column 2 of Table 15.3.

In this sample, we do not have sufficient data to control for prices in neighboring countries. We attempt to do this for a sample of European countries in a subsequent subsection. The amount of bootlegging, i.e. the legal purchase of cigarettes in one country but sale in another country without paying applicable taxes or duties, may depend on the price in neighboring countries. Wholesale smuggling, that is, sale without paying applicable taxes even in the country of origin, may be correlated with the absolute price in a country. We expect to observe little bootlegging among countries with high prices if all neighboring countries also have high prices. However, these countries might be attractive destinations for wholesale smugglers with much lower home-country prices. If the price of cigarettes in neighboring countries is correlated with home-country cigarette price (as, for example, in Western Europe where all countries have relatively high prices), the ratio of home-to-neighboring countries' prices may be uncorrelated with home-country price. If so, our estimates of wholesale smuggling may be unbiased. Hence we interpret the coefficient on cigarette price as an estimate of the change in wholesale smuggling with increases in cigarette prices.

Income was represented by the gross domestic product (GDP) per capita, evaluated at the current US exchange rate. We obtained this data from the World Development Indicators (World Bank 1997). A few former socialist countries (such as Russia, the former German Democratic Republic, Slovakia, and the Czech Republic) have missing values. Germany's data is missing after reunification. The missing income data for these countries were estimated using earlier years of data by the exponential end-point method. Using these data we estimated the regressions shown in Table 15.4.

---

[3] See World Bank (1997) for a discussion of the causes and consequences of government corruption.

Table 15.4 Regressions on experts' estimates of smuggling around the world (t statistics in parentheses)

Specification	1	2	3	4	5
Price per pack in US dollars in 1995	−0.04			−0.002	−0.01
	(2.50)			(0.08)	(0.53)
Transparency index		−0.02		−0.02	−0.02
		(3.38)		(1.76)	(1.88)
GDP per capita 1995			−4.31E-06		2.61E-06
			(2.48)		(0.73)
Constant	0.18	0.22	0.17	0.22	0.23
	(7.12)	(6.74)	(7.13)	(5.63)	(5.48)
Adjusted r-squared	0.124	0.246	0.122	0.221	0.208
N	38	33	38	33	33

Specifications 1, 2, and 3 include price, the transparency index and GDP per capita, respectively, as independent variables. Price and GDP per capita have counter-intuitive negative signs, suggesting that smuggling falls as price and income increase. The transparency index has the expected negative sign—the less corrupt the government is, the less cigarette smuggling is perceived by experts to occur. As shown in specifications 4 and 5, when the transparency index is included along with price and GDP per capita, these variables become insignificantly different from zero while the transparency index maintains its expected negative and significant sign. Apparently, the inverse relationship between price (income) and smuggling is illusory. The negative correlation of smuggling and income comes about because poorer countries tend to have more corruption. The negative correlation between smuggling and price comes about because high-income countries tend to be countries with higher prices.

A 95% confidence interval around the coefficient on price includes both positive and negative values. Consistent with the arguments made in Joossens and Raw (1998) we cannot definitively reject Norton's hypothesis that high-price countries have some wholesale smuggling. However, the empirical results suggest that factors other than price, and particularly transparency, are very important.

According to the empirical results, each 1-point increase in a country's transparency index is associated with a 2%-point decrease in experts' estimates of cigarette smuggling. This means that if Pakistan could increase its transparency index from its current level of 2.7 to 4.9 (the level attained in Greece and the median level for countries on which we have data), we would expect experts' estimates of the proportion of cigarettes smuggled in Pakistan to drop from 30% to about 26%.

15.4.3 Analysis of links between recorded cigarette sales and price in neighboring European countries

Our analysis of recorded imports and exports of cigarettes focused on wholesale smuggling. Our analysis of experts' estimates of cigarette smuggling suggested that transparency had a more important influence on wholesale smuggling than the absolute price of cigarettes but shed little light on the causes or magnitude of bootlegging (legal purchase of cigarettes in one country with resale in a higher-tax country). Most previous econometric analyses of smuggling (see Section 15.3) have focused on North America, where bootlegging is believed to be the primary problem. In this section we turn our attention to bootlegging in Europe.

We analyzed data on European cigarette prices, sales, international travel, and other variables in order to obtain quantitative estimates of the extent of bootlegging during the period 1989–95. We provide a brief description of our procedures and discuss the interpretation of our results. (Appendix 15.2 gives more technical details of our econometric procedures.)

We estimated a statistical equation to explain per capita cigarette sales between 1989 and 1995. In this analysis we restricted our investigations to 23 countries in Europe, where we have fairly complete data on consumption and prices (see Table 15.6 for a list of countries). We also explicitly modeled and attempted to empirically measure the extent of bootlegging among these countries.

Specifically, we assume that cigarette sales depend upon domestic price (P), income (Y), and other variables, such as the degree of corruption in the country, (X). From this total we subtract the quantity of cigarettes purchased by citizens while traveling abroad (bootlegged imports), and add the quantity of cigarettes purchased by foreign citizens traveling in the home country (bootlegged exports). Since legal duty-free sales account for only a small portion of these sales, these are ignored in the subsequent analysis (see Joossens *et al.* (Chapter 16) for a more detailed discussion of duty-free sales). In symbolic language we write:

$$\text{sales} = f(P,Y,X) - \text{bootlegged imports} + \text{bootlegged exports.} \qquad (15.2)$$

We estimated eqn 15.2 using data on countries in Europe during the period 1989–95. We used the same price and income data used above in our analysis of experts' estimates of smuggling. Since the extent of bootlegging is not directly observed, we estimated it. We assumed that the incentive to bootleg for any particular traveler is proportional to the difference in price between the home and destination countries. We estimated the total number of cross-border travelers on the basis of data from the World Tourism Organization's *Yearbook of Tourism Statistics* from 1991 through 1995. The World Tourism Organization obtained the data primarily from a questionnaire sent to government offices, supplemented with data published by official sources. Using these data, we created variables that measure the aggregate incentive for bootlegged imports and bootlegged exports. Our procedures were similar to those used by Becker *et al.* (1994) in their study of the demand for cigarettes in the United States. Full details on the construction of these variables are contained in Appendix 15.2.

We also included a dummy variable for each year and a dummy variable for each country. These variables correct for any factors that are constant over time but vary by country (such as the cultural heritage of the country) or are constant across countries but vary over time (such as the state of knowledge about how smoking affects health.)

We do not have multiple estimates of the transparency index for each country. Even if we did have these data, we are skeptical that changes in long-distance smuggling mirror year-to-year changes in perceptions of corruption. To control for the average

Table 15.5 Cigarette consumption in Europe: alternative regression specifications* (t statistic in parens below coefficient)

Specification Sample	1 Europe	2 Europe	3 Europe	4 Europe	5 Europe
No. observations	146	146	101	101	101
No. countries	23	23	18	18	18
Mean of dependent variable	4.39	4.39	4.50	4.50	4.50
Mean price	1.51	1.51	1.14	1.14	1.14
Price-elasticity at the mean	−0.47	−0.24	−0.18	−0.14	−0.13
Adjusted r-square	0.5151	0.9757	0.9592	0.9606	0.9611
Aggregate incentive for bootlegged imports				−0.13 (1.88)	−0.14 (2.16)
Aggregate incentive for bootlegged exports				−0.02 (0.59)	−0.02 (0.67)
Price	−0.31 (9.93)	−0.16 (6.22)	−0.16 (4.19)	−0.12 (2.92)	−0.11 (2.95)
GDP per capita	1.12E-05 (1.03)	3.83E-05 (2.73)	2.83E-05 (1.71)	1.63E-05 (0.94)	1.09E-05 (1.38)
Square of GDP per capita	1.65E-10 (0.41)	−3.47E-10 (0.88)	−6.65E-10 (1.45)	−1.77E-10 (0.35)	
Year dummies	Yes	Yes	Yes	Yes	Yes
Country dummies	No	Yes	Yes	Yes	Yes

* All regression estimated by ordinary least squares.
Dependent variables is natural log of packs of 20 cigarettes per capita.

level of corruption in the country during the period of our study (1989–95) and large-scale organized wholesale smuggling, we used country dummies rather than the country's transparency index.

We obtained the regression results reported in Table 15.5. Specification 1 estimates a classic cigarette demand curve with data on 23 countries in Europe. Our empirical results are typical of empirical studies of cigarette demand. The adjusted r-squared was 0.515. The coefficient on price was negative and significant with an estimated price elasticity of demand of −0.47. The coefficients on GDP per capita and its square, while positive, were not significantly different from zero. As Kenkel and Chen explain (Chapter 8), this result may stem from the positive correlation between education and income. Higher education may lead to higher income but at the same time may discourage cigarette consumption.

In specification 2 of Table 15.5 we added country fixed effects to the specification in column 1. This resulted in a large increase in the adjusted r-squared and a large decline in the coefficient on price. The coefficient on GDP per capita increased and became statistically significant. The large decline in the coefficient on price suggests that countries with low cigarette prices tend to have other fixed characteristics that result in a relatively high level of smoking. Further research is necessary to investigate precisely which characteristics of these countries resulted in high levels of smoking.

Specification 3 replicated specification 2 with the smaller European sample for which we had sufficient information to construct measures of the incentives for bootlegging. This change in sample resulted in little change in the adjusted r-squared or the coefficients of the independent variables.

Specification 4 adds variables measuring the incentives for bootlegged imports and exports. These are the coefficients of primary interest to us. The estimated coefficient on incentives for bootlegged imports was negative and statistically significant, indicating that an increase in the incentive for home-country citizens to purchase cigarettes abroad lowered domestic sales. This is exactly the result that we would expect. Our variable indicating incentives for bootlegged exports is constructed so that it varies inversely with the incentive for bootlegged exports. Hence we also expect, and find, a negative coefficient on this variable. Although the coefficient on incentives for bootlegged exports was not significantly different from zero, the sum of the coefficients on incentives for bootlegged imports and exports were jointly significantly different from zero. We can be quite confident that a policy that raises incentives for bootlegging (such as a tax increase) will significantly reduce domestic sales. Finally, in specification 5, we dropped the insignificant variable for GDP per capita squared. This resulted in little change in our estimated coefficients.

We investigated many other regression specifications in the course of our research. The qualitative results reported here were generally maintained with alternative specifications. Thus, we have confidence that our findings would not be greatly altered by sensible but arbitrary changes in our statistical procedures. Some discussion of alternative estimates is presented in Appendix 15.2.

What percentage of European domestic sales do we estimate are bootlegged? Since the dependent variable in Table 15.5 is the natural logarithm of per capita sales, the coefficients on incentives for bootlegged imports and exports can be interpreted as the percentage change in sales from a one unit change in these variables. The mean value of the incentives for bootlegged imports in our European sample is 0.23. The estimated coefficient on this variable in specification 5 is (–0.14). If incentives for bootlegged imports fell from its mean level to zero, sales would fall by about 3% ($0.03 \cong 0.23*0.14$). Thus, we estimate that in a European country with the mean level of incentives for bootlegged imports, about 3% of sales are bootlegged cigarettes. On the other hand, the mean level of incentives for bootlegged exports is –0.53. We estimate that in a European country with the mean level of incentives for bootlegged exports a little more than 1% ($0.01 \cong 0.53*0.02$) of sales are bootlegged abroad. This is not necessarily inconsistent with our earlier estimates of the level of cigarette smuggling. In addition to European bootlegging we expect that some sales are the result of wholesale smuggling. While we control for the level of wholesale smuggling by including country-specific dummy variables we do not obtain quantitative estimates of wholesale smuggling in Europe.

The policy significance of our empirical results can be most easily understood by using the regression results to simulate the impact of specific policy changes. We present these simulations in Table 15.6. Columns 1–3 of the table present some of the

Table 15.6 Simulations of cigarette bootlegging in Europe

Country[a]	Population (in 000s)[b]	Observed price (nominal US dollars)[c]	Regression Predicted domestic sales[d]	Predicted domestic sales with no retail imports or exports[e]	Estimated Net bootlegging[f]	Predicted domestic sales with multilateral 10% price increase[g]	Estimated net bootlegging with multilateral 10% price increase[h]	Predicted domestic sales with unilateral 10% price increase[i]	Estimated net bootlegging with unilateral 10% price increase[j]	Predicted change in tax revenue with unilateral 10% tax increase[k]	Predicted change in tax revenue with multilateral 10% tax increase[l]
Austria	8054	$2.96	89	100	-11	86	-12	83	-14	2.9%	6.4%
Belgium-	10146	$3.32	79	88	-9	76	-10	74	-12	2.4%	6.1%
Bulgaria	8409	$0.31	99	99	0	99	0	99	0	9.7%	9.8%
CzeckRep	10332	$0.33	.	.	ne	ne	ne	ne	ne	ne	ne
Denmark	5220	$5.21	.	79	ne	ne	ne	ne	ne	ne	ne
France	58060	$2.90	75	79	-4	73	-5	72	-6	5.8%	7.0%
Finland	5110	$4.49	.	.	ne	ne	ne	ne	ne	ne	ne
Germany	81869	$3.38	80	101	-21	76	-22	74	-24	2.6%	4.7%
Greece	10467	$1.90	138	136	2	136	2	135	1	8.1%	8.6%
Hungary	10229	$0.52	120	116	3	120	4	119	3	9.5%	9.9%
Ireland	3586	$1.69	84	81	3	83	3	83	2	8.3%	9.0%
Italy	57204	$2.19	78	78	0	77	3	76	0	7.8%	8.2%
Netherla	15460	$2.99	55	57	-3	53	-3	52	-4	4.8%	7.1%
Norway	4354	$7.01			ne	ne	ne	ne	ne	ne	ne
Poland	38612	$0.37	125	118	7	125	8	124	7	9.6%	10.3%
Portugal	9927	$1.47	82	81	1	81	1	80	0	7.9%	8.9%
Romania	22692				ne	ne	ne	ne	ne	ne	ne
Slovakia	5369	$0.38	78	78	0	78	0	78	0	9.4%	9.7%
Spain	39199	$1.38	103	100	2	102	3	101	2	8.6%	9.1%
Sweden	8830	$4.58			ne	ne	ne	ne	ne	ne	ne
Switzerl	7039	$2.80	109	118	-8	106	-9	102	-13	2.6%	6.9%
Turkey	61058	$0.51	66	66	0	66	0	66	0	9.6%	9.6%
UK	58533	$4.58	75	80	-5	72	-6	71	-7	4.6%	5.9%
Median	10229	$2.50	82	88	0	81	0	80	0	7.9%	8.9%
Mean (unweighted)	23468	$2.51	90	93	-3	89	-3	88	-4	6.9%	8.2%

[a] Country name.
[b] Population.
[c] Observed price base on Market Facts data.
[d] Estimated sales using coefficients from Table 15.5 specification 5.
[e] Uses regression coefficients from Table 15.5 specification 5 and assumes no incentive for bootlegging.
[f] Column 5 − column 4.
[g] Uses regression coefficients from Table 15.5 specification 5 and assumes multilateral 10% price increase.
[h] Difference between column 7 and estimated sales when multilateral price increase of 10% and no incentive for bootlegging.
[i] Uses regression coefficients from Table 15.5 specification 5 and assumes unilateral 10% price increase.
[j] Difference between column 9 and estimated sales when unilateral price increase of 10% and no incentive for bootlegging.
[k] Ratio (1.10*column 9/column 4) minus 1.
[l] Ratio (1.10*column 7/column 4) minus 1.
ne = not estimated.
* Data are incomplete for some countries in some years.

observed data on key variables about each country in the sample. Observed prices vary from $0.31 per pack in Bulgaria to more than $7 per pack in Norway. We were unfortunately forced to exclude several countries from the complete analysis as a result of missing data.

Column 4 presents predicted sales on the basis of the regression results reported in Table 15.5, specification 5. Because the regression analyses closely tracked the data (the adjusted r-square was more than 96%) the estimates in column 4 are generally quite similar to the observed values. Predicted sales vary between 55 packs per capita in the Netherlands and 138 packs per capita in Greece.

Column 5 reports the predicted value of cigarette sales if there were no bootlegging (i.e. incentives for bootlegged imports and exports are set to zero), and column 6 reports the difference between column 4 and column 5. Thus, column 6 is our estimate of net bootlegging—the balance of trade in bootlegged cigarettes. Some countries have negative numbers in this column, indicating that they are, on balance, net importers of bootlegged cigarettes. Other countries have positive numbers, indicating that they are, on balance, net exporters of bootlegged cigarettes.[4] Net bootlegging varies from exports of 7 packs per capita in Poland to imports of 21 packs per capita in Germany. Importing countries tend to be those with relatively high prices and incomes, such as Austria, Germany and Switzerland. Exporting countries tend to have lower prices and incomes, such as Hungary and Poland.

We examined two policies to determine how they might affect domestic sales and net bootlegging. Policy one (reported on in columns 7 and 8), was a 10% tax increase which we assume is fully reflected in higher retail prices and is undertaken jointly by all countries in Europe. (See Merriman (1994) for some discussion of the assumption that increased taxes translate into increased retail prices). A 10% increase in price would require a price increase of $0.34 in Germany but only $0.04 in Poland. Because all countries raise their prices, domestic sales fall in every country (compare columns 7 and 4) with sales falling from 82 to 81 packs per capita in the median country.

Countries with relatively high prices experience a bigger absolute increase in price and so may experience a decline in net bootlegging (e.g. Germany and Austria). On the other hand, countries with relatively low prices may experience an increase in net bootlegged exports (e.g. Poland). In the median country there is zero net bootlegging in both the baseline case (column 6) and when we simulate a multilateral 10% tax increase (column 8). Because all countries simultaneously raise their prices, no country's net bootlegged exports fall precipitously (compare columns 8 and 6) and the net effect is that European cigarette consumption falls.

Compare this with the policy simulation presented in columns 9 and 10. Here we ask what happens if a single country (say Austria) increases its price by 10% while other countries do not change their price. In about half the countries, domestic sales drop by three packs per capita or more with median domestic sales dropping from 82 to 80 packs per capita (compare column 4 with column 9). However, in several cases, domestic consumption drops much less than sales because bootlegged exports drop substantially (compare column 10 with column 6). In Germany, for example, we

---

[4] Theoretically, the population-weighted average of net exports ought to be zero, since imports to one country have to come from another country. We have not econometrically imposed this restriction.

estimate that a unilateral 10% price increase would cause domestic sales to drop from 80 to 74 packs per capita, a drop in sales of 6 packs. However, we predict that net boot-legged imports would increase by 3 packs per capita from 21 to 24 packs per capita. Hence, the drop in domestic consumption would be only one-half the drop in domes-tic sales. With a multilateral price increase we predict that German domestic con-sumption would also drop by three packs per capita but domestic sales would drop only four, rather than six, packs per capita.

The simulations also suggest that there are a number of European countries that are relatively immune to bootlegging. According to our estimates a unilateral 10% price increase in Bulgaria, Hungary, Italy, Poland, Slovakia, Spain, and Turkey would have almost no effect on bootlegging in these countries. These relatively low-priced coun-tries need not fear increases in bootlegging from small to moderate increases in price.

Bootlegging may be a larger problem in relatively high-priced countries, such as Germany and France. In these countries, policies that emphasize coordinated increases in cigarettes taxes and prices will reduce consumption with the smallest increase in bootlegging.

Our simulation results may also be used to examine the relationship between ciga-rette tax increases and government revenues. Since governments can tax only domes-tic cigarette sales, bootlegged imports reduce tax revenue. On the other hand, boot-legged exports increase tax revenue.

If domestic demand was purely inelastic and bootlegged imports and exports were constant, a 10% tax increase would increase revenue by 10%. However, as shown in Table 15.5, specification 5, domestic sales fall, bootlegged exports decrease, and boot-legged imports increase, when price (or taxes) increase. Column 11 shows our predic-tion for each country's tax revenue as a result of a unilateral 10% tax increase. Our empirical results imply that increased revenues from a higher tax on remaining domes-tic sales are sufficiently high to offset losses in revenue due to declines in domestic sales. Thus, for every country in our sample, tax revenues would increase even from a unilateral tax increase. In some countries (Austria, Germany, and Switzerland) the revenue increase would be small because bootlegged imports would increase substan-tially. Countries with less vulnerability to bootlegged imports (such as Bulgaria or Hungary) would have larger revenue gains. The median country has an increase in tax revenue of 7.9% as a result of a unilateral 10% tax increase, even when we take into account increased bootlegging.

A multilateral tax increase would result in even greater revenue gains, as shown in Table 15.6, column 12. The reason for this is that neighboring countries' tax increases diminish the incentive for home-country bootlegged imports and increase the incen-tive for home-country bootlegged exports. Some countries (such as Austria, Belgium, Germany and Sweden) have much greater revenue gains with a multilateral tax than with a unilateral tax. Other countries (such as Bulgaria, Slovakia and Turkey) have nearly identical revenue gains. It is even possible that a country's total taxed sales increase as a result of a multilateral tax increase.

In conclusion, our simulation shows that moderate increases in cigarette tax rates for European countries will result in increases in revenue—even if the tax increases are undertaken unilaterally. Multilateral tax increases will lead to greater revenue gains.

15.5 Summary of empirical results

Because cigarette smuggling is an illegal and hidden activity it is notoriously difficult to study using econometric methodology. In view of the imperfect data at our disposal we undertook three separate, but limited, empirical exercises. Each analysis was designed to produce an independent estimate of the share of total cigarette consumption that is smuggled.

Table 15.7 summarizes the results. First, we compared aggregate recorded cigarette exports with imports for the period 1975–96. We found that exports exceeded imports by about 33% in recent years. A little less than one-fifth of cigarette production is exported in a given year. This suggests that roughly 6% of all cigarette consumption is smuggled. This methodology has several potential sources of error. Some cigarette imports are inadvertently misclassified. On the other hand, some cigarette exports may also be misclassified. Our analysis of United Nations data on imports and exports of a variety of goods suggests that the magnitude of disagreement between aggregate exports and imports is large for many goods. On the whole, we believe that this estimate has a downward bias because it does not measure smuggling of cigarettes that do not officially cross national boundaries and thus do not appear in the export statistics.

The population-weighted average of experts' estimates of smuggling in more than 30 countries was 8.5%. This estimate is in remarkably close agreement with the answer obtained from the analysis of cigarette import and export data. Cigarette industry

Table 15.7 Summary of empirical results

Exercise	Methodology	Estimate of smuggling as a percentage of worldwide domestic cigarette sales	Some possible sources of bias Direction of bias		
			Upward	Downward	Unknown
1	Compare recorded recorded exports and imports.	6%	Some imports misclassified.	Some exports misclassified. Smuggling that does not cross national boundaries is not identified.	
2	Population weighted average of experts' estimates.	8.5%	Tobacco industry experts may overstate the problem.	Police and anti-smoking sources may understate the problem.	
3	Correlation between recorded consumption and incentives for short-distance imports and exports in Europe.	Short distance imports about 3% in typical country. Short distance exports about 1% in typical country.		Wholesale smuggling is not investigated.	Price data refers to all brands but only higher priced brands are usually smuggled.

experts may have an incentive to exaggerate the smuggling problem (in order to lobby for reduced taxation of their product), while public health advocates may have an incentive to downplay smuggling. Police officials also may understate the problem to bolster public opinion about their job performance. Since we do not have precise information about which experts provided estimates of smuggling, we cannot completely evaluate the bias inherent in these estimates.

Our econometric analysis of experts' estimates of smuggling (see Table 15.4) was reassuring. Experts estimated lower levels of smuggling in countries generally viewed as having 'transparent' governments. We found no significant correlation between experts' estimates of smuggling and either the average price of cigarettes or the income in a country.

In our final analysis we used a more conventional methodology to measure bootlegging. We adapted procedures used in various studies of the United States (e.g. Thursby *et al.* 1991; Becker *et al.* 1994). Like these researchers, we reasoned that the lower the price in neighboring countries, the greater the incentive to smuggle into the home country. We measured neighbors by frequency of travel between countries rather than simple geographic proximity. We found that, consistent with our expectations, the greater the incentives for illegal importation, the lower were recorded sales. Similarly, the greater the incentives for illegal exportation, the higher were recorded sales. We estimated that, in a typical European country, bootlegged cigarettes accounted for about 3% of domestic consumption.

This analysis measured only bootlegging and not wholesale smuggling. As expected our estimates of smuggling using this method are less than our estimates using other methods. Our findings for Europe are similar to those obtained in studies of US states (Saba *et al.* 1995; Thursby and Thursby, 2000).

15.6 Conclusions and policy implications

Judging from the results of our three empirical analyses, a reasonable lower bound on the total amount of worldwide smuggling is 6% of all cigarettes consumed worldwide. In view of previous studies of bootlegging in the United States and our own study of bootlegging in Europe, we believe that the greatest part of worldwide smuggling is wholesale smuggling, i.e. smuggling in which cigarette taxes are never paid, even in the country of origin. Our best estimate of an upper bound on the amount of cigarette smuggling worldwide is 8.5%, although smuggling almost certainly exceeds this level in some countries.

Future research to confirm or challenge our estimates would certainly be worthwhile. Future studies should seek to explain discrepancies between reported cigarette exports and imports for particular pairs of countries. Explanations other than smuggling should also be carefully explored. Systematic surveys with carefully designed and documented procedures could provide better evidence about experts' judgments on the extent of cigarette smuggling in different countries. More complete data on cigarette prices, brands and retailing practices would facilitate better estimates of bootlegging between neighboring countries. Future research should also attempt to link specific types of corruption (such as lax border controls) with cigarette smuggling.

However, on the basis of the preliminary research we have done, some tentative conclusions may be drawn. Perhaps most importantly, we have learned that cigarette taxes that increase cigarette prices are only one, and probably not the most important, factor in cigarette smuggling. The perceived level of corruption statistically explains more of the variance in experts' estimates of cigarette smuggling than do cigarette prices. Other important determinants of the level of cigarette smuggling in a country include cigarette prices in nearby countries and the amount of travel between the home country and lower-priced countries.

Even when the potential for increased smuggling is taken into account, our simulations show that a unilateral increase in the cigarette tax rate results in an increase in tax revenue in all European countries. A multilateral tax increase would bring even greater increases in revenue.

Our results have important policy implications. Countries need not make a choice between higher cigarette tax revenues and lower cigarette consumption. Higher tax rates can achieve both objectives. Cigarette tax revenues can be enhanced still further by effective methods to reduce corruption that will result in diminished cigarette smuggling and increased tax collections. Lastly, cooperative multilateral efforts to increase cigarette tax rates on a regional basis are likely to be an effective way to combat smuggling.

Appendix 15.1 On the relationship between enforcement activity and smuggling

We generalize Norton's model by allowing μ (the probability of non-detection of smuggling) to depend on a parameter κ which represents the stringency of enforcement activity. We assume that enforcement activity increases with κ. We also assume that increases in κ do not influence the ability of firms to camouflage their bootlegging activity. In mathematical notation we assume:

$$\frac{\partial \mu(q^s, q^L | \kappa)}{\partial \kappa} = \mu_\kappa < 0 \quad \text{and}$$

$$\frac{\partial \mu(q^s, q^L | \kappa)}{\partial q^s \partial \kappa} = \mu_{s\kappa} = \frac{\partial \mu(q^s, q^L | \kappa)}{\partial q^L \partial \kappa} = \mu_{L\kappa} = 0.$$

The firm's objective function is given by:

$$
\begin{aligned}
\pi(d) = &\ \mu(q^s, q^L | \kappa)(p + pt + \theta)(1 - s)q^s \\
&- (1 - \mu)\alpha(1 - s)pq^s \\
&+ (p + \theta)(1 - L)q^L \\
&- p(q^s + q^L).
\end{aligned}
\tag{A1.1}
$$

As in Norton we set up the Lagrangean:

$$V = \pi + \lambda(\overline{q} - q^s - q^L) \tag{A1.2}$$

and derive the Kuhn–Tucker conditions (they are the same as Norton p. 111.)

$$\frac{\partial V}{\partial q^s} \leq 0 \Rightarrow (p + pt + p\alpha + \theta)(1 - s)(\mu + q^s\mu_s) - p - p\alpha(1 - s) \leq \lambda \qquad \text{(A1.3)}$$

$$\frac{\partial V}{\partial q^L} \leq 0 \Rightarrow (p + pt + p\alpha + \theta)(1 - s)(q^s\mu_L) + \theta - pL - \theta L \leq \lambda \qquad \text{(A1.4)}$$

$$\frac{\partial V}{\partial \lambda} \geq 0 \Rightarrow (\bar{q} - q^L - q^s) \geq 0. \qquad \text{(A1.5)}$$

To simplify the notation let:

$$(p + pt + p\alpha + \theta)(1{-}s) = A$$
$$B = -p - p\alpha (1{-}s)$$
$$C = \theta - pL - \theta L.$$

We consider interior solutions in which constraints in eqn A1.3 and A1.4 are both binding:

$$A(\mu + q^s\mu_s) + B = A(q^s\mu_L) + C, \qquad \text{(A1.6)}$$

solve for q^s:

$$q^s A(\mu_s - \mu_L) = C - B - A\mu, \qquad \text{(A1.7)}$$

divide through to get:

$$q^s = \frac{(C - B - A\mu)}{A(\mu_s - \mu_L)}. \qquad \text{(A1.8)}$$

Now differentiate with respect to the parameter κ:

$$\frac{\partial q^s}{\partial \kappa} = \frac{(-A\mu_\kappa)}{A(\mu_s - \mu_L)} - \frac{(C - B - A\mu)}{[A(\mu_s - \mu_L)]^2}[A(\mu_{s\kappa} - \mu_{L\kappa})] \qquad \text{(A1.9)}$$

Since $\mu_L > 0$ and $\mu_s < 0$ (p. 110 of Norton) and the cross-partials are zero by assumption (this is a parallel shift) equation (A1.9) reduces to:

$$\frac{\partial q^s}{\partial \kappa} = \frac{(-\mu_\kappa)}{(\mu_s - \mu_L)} < 0. \qquad \text{(A1.10)}$$

The optimal amount of bootlegging unambiguously falls with increased enforcement activity.

Appendix 15.2 Technical notes on econometric methodology

This appendix provides more complete details on the econometric analysis of links between recorded cigarette sales and prices in neighbouring European countries described in Section 15.4.

Basic methodology

Our basic econometric methodology is derived from Becker *et al.* (1994). Like them we estimate an aggregate cigarette demand function with price, income, country dummies, time dummies, and variables representing incentives to import and export as independent variables. Among other models, Becker *et al.* estimate a rational addiction model that allows current consumption to depend upon past and future consumption as well as the variables listed above. We focus on more conventional (static) functional forms for cigarette demand because our goal is to study smuggling rather than demand *per se.*

Construction of short-distance import and export variables

Construction of variables that represent consumption, price and income are relatively straightforward and are explained in the text. Construction of the variables for imports and exports are more complex and are explained below:

The basic logic behind Becker *et al.*'s short-distance import and exporting variables is that short-distance importing and exporting depends upon the relative prices and the amount of cross-border traffic among neighboring states. We generalize this idea to include countries that have frequent cross-border traffic, though they may not literally share a border (e.g. UK and France.)

If prices in country i are less than or equal to those in country j we assume that travelers from country i do not purchase cigarettes in country j. If cigarette prices in country i exceed those in j, we assume that each traveler from i makes a cigarette purchase in j. For each dollar that country i's price exceeds country j's price, each traveler from country i purchases b1% of his or her yearly cigarette consumption in country j.[5] The total share of country i's consumption purchased in country j is:

$$\left(b1 * (p_i - p_j) * \frac{trav_{ij}}{pop_i} \right) \text{ given that } (p_i > p_j), \tag{A2.1}$$

where $trav_{ij}$ is the number of travelers from country i to country j and pop_i is the population of country i. ($trav_{ij}/pop_i$) is the number of times the average resident of country i travels to country j in a year.

The total share of consumption purchased abroad by travelers from country i is:

$$b1 * \frac{1}{pop_i} \sum_{j=1}^{n} (p_i - p_j) \, trav_{ij} = b1 * sdimp_i. \tag{A2.2}$$

The summation in eqn A2.2 is taken over countries with lower priced cigarettes than country i; sdimp is our measure of the aggregate incentive for bootlegged imports. Note that by construction $sdimp_i > 0$.

---

[5] For example, suppose that b1 = 0.14 and country j's price exceeds country i's price by one-half dollar per pack. Then each traveler from country i to country j would buy 7% of his or her yearly consumption per trip to country j. Since there are a large number of travelers and we are only concerned with aggregate purchases we study a representative traveler and do not take variance in travelers' behavior into account.

Analogously, if cigarette prices in country j exceed those in i, we assume that each traveler from j buys cigarettes when he or she visits country i. For each dollar that country i's price is below j's, each traveler from j buys b2% of country i's yearly consumption.[6] The total share of country i's consumption sold to visitors from country j is:

$$\left(b2 * (p_i - p_j) * \frac{trav_{ji}}{pop_i} \right) \text{ given that } (p_i < p_j),$$
(A2.3)

where $trav_{ji}$ is the number of travelers from country j to country i

The total share of sales in country i purchased by travelers from abroad is:

$$b2 * \frac{1}{popi} \sum_{j=1}^{n} (p_i - p_j) trav_{ji} = b1 * sdexp_i.$$
(A2.4)

The summation in eqn A2.4 is taken over countries with higher priced cigarettes than country i; sdexp is our measure of the aggregate incentive for bootlegged exports. Note that by construction $sdexp_i < 0$.

Note on missing values

Because the summations in eqns A2.2 and A2.4 are taken over all countries in Europe, and since the origin–destination matrices for travelers are not always complete, missing values are a significant problem.

We have used the following procedure: $sdimp_i$ is coded as missing if we have data on travel from country i to less than three other countries for which we have price data. Analogously, $sdexp_i$ is coded as missing only if we have data on travel to country i from less than three other countries for which we have price data.

The logic for this coding is that we are most likely to have data on substantial tourist flows. Therefore, missing data is likely to be close to zero when we have some data on traffic flows.

Further comments on estimation of $Trav_{ij}$ and $Trav_{ji}$

We have two kinds of data on foreign visitors. In some countries we are told the total number of tourists from abroad in all accommodation establishments. We call this category 1 data. Countries for which we have category 1 data are Austria, Belgium–Luxembourg, Germany, Netherlands, and Switzerland. In other countries we are told the total number of tourists arriving at the frontier. We call this category 2 data. We have category 2 data for all other countries in our sample.

Category 2 data are necessary to estimate sdimp and sdexp as specified above. Therefore, we designate the number of travelers from country i arriving at the frontier of country j as $Trav_{ij}$. We assume that tourists staying in accommodations are a constant

---

[6] For example, suppose that b2 = 0.02 and country j's price exceeds country i's price by one-half dollar per pack. Then each traveler from country j to country i would buy 1% of the average yearly consumption in country i during each visit from country j.

Table A2.1 Primary travel partners of European countries, 1995

Country	Primary origin of travelers to country listed in column 1	Number of travelers from primary origin as a share of population of country listed in column 1	Primary destination of traveler from country listed in column 1	Number of travelers to primary destination as a share of population of country listed in column 1
Austria	Germany	124.33%	Italy	74.03%
Belgium–Lux	Netherlands	15.85%	France	72.02%
Bulgaria	Turkey	21.70%	Romania	8.49%
CzeckRep	na		Poland	146.17%
Denmark	na		Germany	12.28%
France	UK	19.24%	Spain	34.93%
Finland	na		Russia	24.98%
Germany	Netherlands	2.81%	Poland	57.62%
Greece	Germany	21.72%	Italy	5.70%
Hungary	Germany	33.36%	Romania	6.25%
Ireland	UK	80.17%	UK	55.44%
Italy	Switzerland	15.70%	France	8.82%
Netherlands	Germany	15.92%	France	34.84%
Norway	na		UK	9.94%
Poland	Germany	122.17%	Russia	1.73%
Portugal	Spain	45.80%	Spain	51.59%
Romania	Russia	9.28%	Hungary	14.53%
Slovakia	CzechRepulic	4.01%	Poland	81.04%
Spain	France	51.74%	Portugal	11.60%
Sweden	na		Germany	6.65%
Switzerland	Germany	29.99%	Italy	127.61%
Turkey	Germany	2.71%	Bulgaria	2.99%
UK	France	5.50%	France	19.09%
Russia	Finland	0.86%	Hungary	1.80%

fraction of those arriving at the frontier. We introduce a new variable called $Etrav_{ij}$ and define it as follows:

$$ETrav_{ij} = \begin{cases} (b3 * Trav_{ij}) & \text{in Austria, Belgium–Luxembourg, Germany, Netherlands and Switzerland} \\ Trav_{ij} & \text{otherwise} \end{cases}$$

We estimate versions of the model assuming b3 equal to 1, (1/2), and (1/3). We found that the estimated coefficients of the model were hardly altered by changing our assumption about b3. In the regression discussed in the text (Table 15.5), we adopted the assumption that b3 = (1/2).

Table A2.2 Cigarette consumption in Europe: sensitivity analysis (t statistic in parens below coefficient)

	1	2	3	4*	5
Method	OLS	OLS	OLS	OLS	OLS
Dependent variable	Lnc	Lnc	Lnc	Lnc	C
Sample	Europe	Europe	Europe	Europe	Europe
No. observations	101	101	101	101	101
No. countries	18	18	18	18	18
dep. mean	4.50	4.50	4.50	4.50	92.11
Mean price	1.14	1.14	1.14	1.14	1.14
Price elasticity at the mean	−0.13	−0.13	−0.13	−0.19	−0.09
Assumption about b3	1/2	1.00	1/3	1/2	1/2
Adjusted r-square	0.9611	0.9610	0.9611	0.9612	0.9611
Aggregate incentive for bootlegged imports	−0.14 (2.16)	−0.14 (2.11)	−0.14 (2.23)	−0.12 (1.76)	−11.93 (1.98)
Aggregate incentive for bootlegged exports	−0.02 (0.67)	−0.03 (0.81)	−0.02 (0.53)	−0.01 (0.29)	−2.87 (0.90)
Price	−0.11 (2.95)	−0.12 (3.04)	−0.11 (2.87)	−0.07 (1.17)	−7.49 (2.05)
Price times dummy for high income				−0.10 (1.11)	
GDP per capita	1.09E-05 (1.38)	1.12E-05 (1.41)	1.07E-05 (1.35)	1.14E-05 (1.44)	0.001 (1.01)
Year dummies	Yes	Yes	Yes	Yes	Yes
Country dummies	Yes	Yes	Yes	Yes	Yes

1 Aggregate incentives for bootlegged imports and exports are estimated assuming that incentive to cross-border shop for cigarettes depends on price differential and that amount of cross-border smuggling is proportional to number of cross-border travelers. See text of appendix for more details.
2 Price and GDP per capita are measured in real US dollars in 1982–84.
3 All specifications assume price is exogenously determined.
4 In column 4, price-elasticity is price elasticity for high income countries only.

We calculated short-distance importing and exporting variables using the World Tourism Organization data discussed in the text. Table A2.1 presents an extract of our data that may be useful in understanding the results. For each country in the sample we show the primary travel partners in 1995. For example, the country that sends the most travelers to Austria is Germany. The total number of Germans traveling in Austria is 124% of Austria's domestic population. The country that Austrians most travel to is Italy. The number of Austrians traveling to Italy is 74% of Austria's population. Of course, this does not mean that nearly three out of four Austrians visited Italy in 1995. It is quite possible for a single Austrian to make multiple trips to Italy. Analysis of this data shows that a country's primary travel partners are likely to be, but are not always, those with which they share a border.

Results from alternative regression specifications

Results from a number of alternative regression specifications are contained in Table A2.2. Column 1 simply reproduces some of the results reported in Table 15.5. Columns 2 and 3 test the sensitivity of these results to changes in the value used for b3. The empirical results are very similar regardless of which value of b3 is adopted. We use b3 equal to 1 (there are twice as many frontier arrivals as accommodation arrivals) in the text because this seems most reasonable to us.

Column 4 interacts price with a dummy variable equal to one for 'high-income' European countries since these countries may have a different responsiveness to price than low-income countries. The interacted variable is not significantly different from zero although including this variable raises the absolute value of the price elasticity in high-income countries and lowers the estimated price elasticity for low-income countries.

Finally, column 5 uses the un-transformed value rather than the natural log of consumption as the dependent variable. This is the dependent variable used by Becker *et al.* (1994). In the text we use the natural log of consumption as the dependent value since this restricts the predicted value of consumption to be a positive number. However, simply using the value of consumption as the dependent variable gives us similar qualitative results (coefficients on aggregate incentive for bootlegged imports and price are significant while other coefficients are not, estimated price elasticity of demand is quite low).

References

Baltagi, B. H. and Levin, D. (1986). Estimating dynamic demand for cigarettes using panel data: the effects of bootlegging, taxation and advertising reconsidered. *Review of Economics and Statistics*, **48**, 148–55.

Baltagi, B. H. and Levin, D. (1992). Cigarette taxation: raising revenue and reducing consumption. *Structural Change and Economic Dynamics*, **3**(2), 321–35.

Becker, G. S., Grossman, M., and Murphy, K. (1994). An empirical analysis of cigarette addiction. *American Economic Review*, **84**(3), 396–418.

Bhagwati, J. N. (1974a). Introduction. In *Illegal Transactions in International Trade* (ed. J. Bhagwati), pp. 1–6. North Holland Publishing Company, New York.

Bhagwati, J. (1974b). On the underinvoicing of imports. In *Illegal Transactions in International Trade* (ed. J. Bhagwati), pp. 138–47. North–Holland Publishing Company, Amsterdam.

Bhagwati, J. N. and Hansen, B. (1974). A theoretical analysis of smuggling. In *Illegal Transactions in International Trade* (ed. J. Bhagwati), pp. 9–22. North–Holland Publishing Company, New York.

Chaloupka, F. (1991). Rational addictive behavior and cigarette smoking. *Journal of Political Economy*, **99**(4), 722–42.

Chaloupka, F. and Corbett, M. (1998). Trade policy and tobacco: towards an optimal policy mix. In *The Economics of Tobacco Control* (ed. I. Abedian, R. van der Merwe, N. Wilkins, and P. Jha), Applied Fiscal Research Center, Cape Town, South Africa.

Chaloupka, F. J. and Warner, K. E. The Economics of Smoking. In *The Handbook of Health Economics* (ed. J. Newhouse and A. Culyer), North–Holland, Amsterdam.

Feenstra, R. C. *et al.* (1999). Discrepancies in international data: an application to China-Hong Kong entrepôt trade. *American Economic Review*, **89**(2), 338–43.

Galbraith, J. W. and Kaiserman, M. (1997). Smuggling and demand for cigarettes in Canada: evidence from time-series data. *Journal of Health Economics*, **16**(3), 287–301.

Joossens, L. (1998). Tobacco smuggling: an optimal policy approach. In *The Economics of Tobacco Control* (ed. I. Abedian, R. van der Merwe, N. Wilkins, and P. Jha), Applied Fiscal Research Center, Cape Town, South Africa.

Joossens, L. and Raw, M. (1998). Cigarette smuggling in Europe: who really benefits? *Tobacco Control*, **7**, 66–71.

Joossens, L., Chaloupka, F., Merriman, D., and Yurekli, A. (2000) Issues in smuggling of tobacco products. In *Tobacco Control in Developing Countries* (ed. P. Jha and F. J. Chaloupka), this volume (Chapter 16).

Market Tracking International Ltd (1997a). *World Tobacco File Emerging Asian Markets 1997.* Great Britain: Argus Business Media Ltd.

Market Tracking International Ltd (1997b). *World Tobacco File Emerging markets in Central and Eastern Europe 1997.* Great Britain: Argus Business Media Ltd.

Market Tracking International Ltd (1996). *World Tobacco File 1996.* London: International Trade Publications Ltd.

Merriman, D. (1994). Do cigarette excise tax rates maximize revenue? *Economic Inquiry*, **32**, 419–28.

Norton, D. A. (1988). On the economic theory of smuggling. *Economica*, **55**, 107–18.

Saba, R. P., Randolph Beard, T., Ekelund Jr., R. B., and Ressler, R. W. (1995). The demand for cigarette smuggling. *Economic Inquiry*, **33**, 189–202.

Simkin, C. G. F. (1974). Indonesia's unrecorded trade. In *Illegal Transactions in International Trade* (ed. J. Bhagwati), pp. 157–71. North–Holland Publishing Company, Amsterdam.

Thursby, M., Jensen, R., and Thursby, J. (1991). Smuggling, camouflaging, and market structure. *Quarterly Journal of Economics*, August, 789–814.

Thursby, J. G. and Thursby, M. C. (2000). Interstate cigarette bootlegging: extent, revenue losses and effects of Federal Intervention. *National Tax Journal.* March, 59–77.

Transparency International (1998). *1998 Corruption Perceptions Index.* Obtained from world-wide web site http://www.transparency.de/ on December 9.

United Nations Comtrade. Databank. Accessible at http://www.intracen.org/itc/infobase

US Department of Agriculture (1997). *Tobacco: World Markets and Trade.* Foreign Agriculture Service, US Department of Agriculture, Washington, D.C.

World Bank (1997). *World Development Report 1997.* New York: Oxford University Press.

World Tourism Organization (1989–1995) *Yearbook of Tourism Statistics.* World Tourism Organization, Madrid.

16
Issues in the smuggling of tobacco products

Luk Joossens, Frank J. Chaloupka, David Merriman,
and Ayda Yurekli

This chapter reviews several issues related to the smuggling of cigarettes and other tobacco products. First, the health and other consequences of cigarette smuggling are described, emphasizing the potential for cigarette smuggling to undermine tobacco-control efforts. This is followed by a description of the various legal, quasi-legal, and illegal activities that are broadly described as smuggling. The factors that create incentives for and/or facilitate these activities are reviewed, noting that non-price factors, such as the presence of corruption, organized crime, and widespread street-selling, can be as, or more, important than the levels of taxes and prices and the differentials between these in different jurisdictions. The impact of smuggling on tobacco tax revenues is then discussed, highlighting the experiences of Canada and Sweden, where cigarette taxes were reduced in response to the perception that cigarette smuggling was draining revenues. The role of the tobacco industry in smuggling is then discussed. Finally, a set of policy measures that can be used to counter cigarette smuggling is presented.

16.1 Introduction

The effects of cigarette price increases on cigarette consumption have been studied extensively and provide clear evidence that increases in cigarette taxes and prices lead to significant reductions in cigarette consumption (see Chapter 10). Some have argued, however, that higher cigarette and other tobacco taxes will contribute to increased smuggling and associated criminal activity. In jurisdictions that raise their tobacco taxes, sales will fall, they argue, but in nearby jurisdictions with lower taxes, sales of smuggled cigarettes and cross-border shopping will increase. Therefore, they argue, cigarette consumption will remain high and tax revenues will fall.

Several issues related to cigarette smuggling and cross-border shopping are described in this chapter; the previous chapter contains quantitative estimates on the magnitude of the cigarette smuggling problem and its determinants. This chapter begins with a discussion of the health concerns arising from smuggling. This is followed by definitions of the various types of smuggling, and a discussion of the incentives for, and factors that facilitate, each type. Next is a discussion of the effects of smuggling on sales and tax revenues that highlights the experiences of Canada and selected other countries. The role of multinational tobacco companies in smuggling is then described. Finally, recommendations for tackling the smuggling problem are presented.

16.2 Health, and other, consequences of cigarette smuggling

Cigarette smuggling raises several health-related concerns. First, because smuggled cigarettes compete with legal cigarettes, cigarette consumption in the face of smuggling can be higher and cigarette prices may be lower than they would be in the absence of smuggling. Similarly, the threat of smuggling can discourage governments from raising cigarette and other tobacco taxes, or can lead others to reduce their taxes, resulting in lower prices than would exist in the absence of smuggling. In Canada (1994) and Sweden (1998), for example, cigarette taxes were significantly reduced in response to what was perceived to be significant cigarette smuggling, while proposals for substantial tax increases in the United States (1998) were defeated, in part, by the threat that a black market would result. Given the evidence on the effects of price on tobacco use (see Chapter 10) and the well-documented health consequences associated with smoking (see Chapter 2), the resulting higher consumption will lead to greater smoking-related morbidity and mortality. Given the greater price sensitivity of youth and persons with lower incomes, the availability of lower-priced smuggled cigarettes will have the greatest impact on smoking and health among children and the poor.

Second, a black market in cigarettes can undermine efforts to limit youth access to tobacco products and other approaches to reducing overall availability of these products. While tobacco retailers may comply with national or local policies that prohibit the sale of tobacco products to underage persons and otherwise limit availability, it is much less likely that vendors of smuggled cigarettes will comply with these policies. Moreover, the presence of smuggled cigarettes can put legitimate retailers at a competitive disadvantage, leading some to be less compliant with tobacco-control laws than they would be in the absence of competition from a black market. The resulting increased availability of tobacco products to youth can lead to significant increases in youth smoking and its consequences. This is compounded by the fact that much of the black market in cigarettes consists of the multinationals' products that are likely to be favored by young people in low-income and middle-income countries, where Western products are regarded as sophisticated and stylish (Joossens and Raw 1998).

Third, contraband cigarettes generally avoid other restrictions and health regulations, such as requirements for health-warning labels in the local language, regulations on additives, and others. To the extent that health-warning labels and other policies reduce smoking by informing potential smokers about the health consequences of smoking, the lack of appropriate local warnings can lead to increased consumption and its consequences.

Finally, the potential profits associated with large-scale cigarette smuggling create incentives for organized crime networks to develop, bringing with them a number of problems (FIA International Research Ltd 1999a). Cigarette smuggling can be a relatively low-risk source of revenues for these networks, which can be used to help support their more high-risk activities. In addition, the growth of these networks can increase the general level of corruption in a country, both among its citizens who purchase cigarettes in the black market and among public officials who facilitate black-market activities. Finally, the presence of organized crime networks in black markets in cigarettes can place additional pressures on legitimate distributors and retailers, reducing their profitability and/or leading them to join in the black market.

16.3 Types and causes of cigarette smuggling and cross-border shopping

There are a wide variety of activities that fall into the broad categories of smuggling and cross-border shopping. To some extent, policies to reduce these activities are hindered by ambiguity about important concepts. The following definitions of these activities emphasize the distinctions between personal use versus commercial resale, legal versus illegal behavior, and small versus large quantities.

16.3.1 Legal circumvention

Legal cross-border shopping

This involves the purchase of cigarettes at a price that includes all relevant local taxes in neighboring lower-tax jurisdictions for an individual's personal consumption. For example, smokers living in Windsor, Ontario, during the time when Canadian taxes were relatively high, had a strong incentive to cross the border into Detroit to purchase cigarettes at prices that included all United States and Michigan excise and sales taxes. Similarly, cross-border shopping can take place within a country in response to significant differences in sub-national taxes. For example, in the United States, Californian smokers living near the border with Nevada have an incentive to purchase their cigarettes in Nevada where taxes are more than US$0.50 lower per pack.

The smoker's incentives for this type of cross-border shopping depend heavily on the differences in taxes and prices between neighboring countries or other taxing jurisdictions, the distance the individual lives from the lower cost area, and the costs of traveling between the two. Buck *et al.* (1994), for example, examined the incentives for cross-border shopping between France and Britain in 1994, concluding that the savings on 800 cigarettes bought in France for consumption in Britain would not have been sufficient to cover the costs of the trip. In practice, it is unlikely that smokers would be willing to travel long distances at high cost in order to save relatively modest amounts by doing so. Instead, it is more likely that much of the cross-border shopping in cigarettes occurs when smokers are already across the border for other reasons.

Estimates suggest that cigarette sales resulting from cross-border shopping can account for a significant share of total cigarette sales in some countries. For example, Luxembourg, because of its low taxes, has long been a source of lower-priced cigarettes for Belgian, French, and German smokers. Up to 85% of total cigarette sales in Luxembourg have been estimated to result from cross-border shopping (Joossens and Raw 1995).

Legal tourist shopping

This is similar to legal cross-border shopping, but involves purchases of tobacco products in non-neighboring jurisdictions in amounts that are allowable under customs regulations. The incentives for this type of legal activity depend on the magnitude of the differences in prices among countries and the extent of international travel among countries. Much lower cigarette prices in countries that are popular destinations for travelers can lead to much cigarette tax evasion of this type.

For most countries, this is a relatively minor problem. For example, Trackray (1998) estimated, based on survey data from over 48 000 international travelers to and from the United Kingdom, that legal tourist and cross-border shopping amounted to approximately 0.5% of cigarette sales and 3.0% of hand-rolling tobacco sales. In some countries, however, where prices are relatively high and international travel by residents is extensive, the scale of this problem can be larger. In Finland, for example, Piha (1998) estimated that legal cigarette imports by international travelers were approximately 12% of total domestic cigarette sales. Similarly high legal imports have been observed in Norway (Lund 1990).

Legal duty-free sales

These are related to legal tourist shopping, but involve tax-free purchases of tobacco products in amounts that are within specific allowances (200 cigarettes or 100 cigarillos or 50 cigars or 250 g of smoking tobacco). Most duty-free sales occur in airports and on airlines, with ferries the next largest source. As with the other forms of legal circumvention, differences in prices (in this case the net-of-tax price in the country visited and the price inclusive of taxes in the home country) and the extent of international travel are key determinants of the extent of duty-free cigarette and other tobacco-product sales.

Estimates indicate that more than 45 billion cigarettes per year were sold duty-free in recent years, with the absolute number rising over time as international travel increases even though tobacco's share of the duty-free market has fallen sharply over the past 15 years (Market Tracking International Ltd (MTI) 1998). While a significant number, total duty-free sales account for less than 1% of global cigarette consumption. This will probably be significantly reduced as a result of the elimination of duty-free shopping between European Union (EU) countries in July 1999. In recent years, the EU had accounted for nearly half of global duty-free sales (MTI 1998).

16.3.2 Quasi-legal circumvention

Internet sales

This is a relatively new phenomenon that, at least in some jurisdictions, may become a significant form of circumvention of cigarette and other tobacco taxes. In the United States, for example, Native American reservations are treated as sovereign nations and are not required to impose federal and state tobacco excise taxes on tobacco products sold on the reservations. In the past, this contributed to the type of cross-border shopping described above, with US smokers living near reservations avoiding taxes by purchasing cigarettes on these reservations. Moreover, many Indian tribes have set up sites on the Internet to sell tax-free cigarettes; the Seneca Indians, for example, have created more than three-dozen such sites (Beebe 1999). While US court rulings have held that tax-free sales to non-Indians are illegal, enforcement has been difficult. However, other sites created by private businesses in low-tax states that include federal and state taxes in their prices can legally sell cigarettes and other tobacco products over the Internet at a significant discount over retail prices in high-tax states. For example, given that state cigarette taxes range from US$0.025 per pack in Virginia to US$1.00 in Alaska and Hawaii, discounts of nearly US$10 per carton are possible. To date, little is known about the scale of legal and illegal Internet cigarette sales. Moreover, many governments are beginning to grapple with issues concerning the taxation of Internet sales. The growth of the Internet and increases in price differentials, however, suggest that this is an area that should be closely watched.

Gray-market cigarette sales

This is another relatively new phenomenon, which involves cigarettes that are produced domestically and exported to independent brokers, then re-imported into their country of origin for resale. Unlike the other forms of legal circumvention, these activities involve many more cigarettes and the resale of these cigarettes. The likelihood for a gray market to develop increases as the wholesale price differential for domestically produced cigarettes intended for domestic consumption and those intended for export increases. To date, this is something that is important only in the United States where the gray market in cigarettes has expanded rapidly over the past year (FIA International Research 1999b). This growth has largely resulted from wholesale cigarette price increases in the United States in late 1998 after the master settlement agreement (MSA) was reached between most US states and the tobacco industry. This price increase applied only to cigarettes produced for domestic consumption and raised prices by $4.50 per carton at the wholesale level. When combined with existing, quality-related price differentials between US-produced cigarettes intended for US smokers and those meant for export, wholesale price differences of as much as US$10 per carton result even after all relevant taxes have been paid (FIA International Research 1999b).

As noted by FIA International Research (1999b), the gray market in cigarettes raises a number of concerns, including its potential for manipulation by organized crime, its negative impact on industry payments to states under the MSA, and more. Currently, gray market cigarettes are legal in most states, as long as all relevant taxes are paid and other policies adhered to. A growing number of states, however, have adopted anti-gray market laws, and the US federal government recently adopted regulations that will make it illegal, beginning in 2000, to import and bring into domestic markets cigarettes that are intended for export only (FIA International Research 1999b). As with Internet sales, developments concerning gray markets in cigarettes should be observed closely.

16.3.2 Illegal circumvention

Bootlegging

This involves the purchase of cigarettes and other tobacco products in low-tax jurisdictions in amounts that exceed the limits set by customs regulations for resale in high-tax jurisdictions. While the number of cigarettes involved in this form of smuggling is large relative to those resulting from the legal circumvention activities described above, it is relatively small compared to that involved in other forms of illegal smuggling. In general, bootlegging involves transporting cigarettes over relatively short distances (e.g. between neighboring countries or other nearby jurisdictions). As with the legal activities, significant price differentials between jurisdictions create incentives for bootlegging. In addition, greater corruption reduces the risks associated with bootlegging.

Bootlegging is a relatively 'low-tech' type of cigarette smuggling. It requires relatively little investment and is often organized by small gangs. Bootleggers often use specially made delivery vans and trucks whose structures have been altered to include false walls, roofs, floors, and other hiding places. Profits from bootlegging cigarettes, however, can amount to thousands of dollars per day (Groom 1998). Nevertheless, given its small scale, bootlegging accounts for a relatively small share of illegal cigarette smuggling (Joossens *et al.* 1992).

Large-scale organized smuggling

In contrast, large-scale organized smuggling involves the illegal transportation, distribution, and sale of large consignments of cigarettes and other tobacco products, generally avoiding all taxes. This type of smuggling usually involves millions of cigarettes that are smuggled over long distances, often involving large organized crime networks and sophisticated systems for distributing smuggled cigarettes at the local level. Large-scale organized smuggling is likely to account for the vast majority of cigarettes smuggled globally. As demonstrated by Merriman *et al.* (Chapter 15), tax and price differentials among countries are not the only determinants of this type of smuggling, and may not be the most important. In European countries with some of the highest taxes, for example, there is little evidence of smuggling, while in Spain, Italy, and many Central and Eastern European countries where taxes and prices are much lower, a sizable black market in cigarettes exists (Joossens and Raw 1998). Other factors that make large-scale cigarette smuggling more likely include corruption, public tolerance, informal distribution networks, widespread street-selling, and the presence of organized crime.

While there are regional and market-level differences, several characteristics are common in large-scale smuggling operations. First, large-scale smuggling typically involves international brands produced by the large multinational tobacco companies given that the demand for these products in most markets allows them to be sold nearly everywhere (Barford 1993).

Second, large-scale smuggling generally takes advantage of the 'in transit' system that has been developed to facilitate international trade. This system allows for the temporary suspension of customs duties, excise taxes, and VATs payable on goods originating from and/or destined for a third country, while in transit across the territory of a defined customs area. For example, cigarettes exported from the United States that are destined for North Africa will enter Belgium while en route. Once in Belgium, the cigarettes are transported over the road through Spain, from where they will be shipped to North Africa. As long as the re-export of the goods is confirmed, no taxes would be paid while the cigarettes are in transit through the EU. However, less than adequate controls over the in-transit cigarettes result in substantial leakages, with many of the exported cigarettes failing to arrive at their intended destination. As described in the previous chapter, official trade statistics indicate that up to one-third of recorded cigarette exports do not reappear as recorded imports. Most of these are likely to be lost in transit, reappearing for sale in the black market. Godfrey (1997), for example, described how large shipping vessels would be loaded with cigarettes that had been imported into Hong Kong, with permits indicating that they were destined for SE Asian countries. When in international waters, however, small boats would meet the large vessels and cigarettes would be off-loaded and smuggled into China. Given that the cigarettes were officially exported, no import taxes, excise duties or VATs were paid while they were in Hong Kong.

Third, large-scale organized cigarette smuggling generally involves cigarettes that have passed through a wide range of owners (European Parliament 1997). The involvement of multiple separate buyers, usually over a short period of time, between the initial purchase of cigarettes and their eventual disappearance from legitimate circulation makes it much more difficult to identify where the leakages occur and who is responsible for them, hindering the enforcement of anti-smuggling policies.

Fourth, organized criminal networks play a significant role in large-scale cigarette smuggling. The European Commission (EC) (1998), for example, notes that over 50 criminal networks have been identified by investigations of large-scale smuggling of various products, including tobacco products. The EC goes on to note that these crime syndicates adapt quickly to smuggling counter-measures, and are very flexible when it comes to using different methods of transport, distribution, and money laundering. As described by Merriman *et al.* (Chapter 15), the corruption that often accompanies organized crime is a significant factor in explaining the extent of cigarette smuggling in many countries. As Transparency International (1997) describes, corruption is more pervasive in low-income and middle-income countries than in high-income countries, placing them at greater risk for large-scale smuggling activities.

Finally, large-scale smuggling requires a good local distribution network, most often involving extensive street-selling, through which the smuggled cigarettes can be easily and quickly sold. In Scandinavian countries where prices are high, street-selling is not widespread and cigarette smuggling is not a significant problem; in contrast, in Spain and Italy where prices are relatively low and street-selling is commonplace, smuggled cigarettes comprise a significant share of total consumption (Joossens and Raw 1998). Similarly, in Russia, a key feature of the retail system are the street sellers, typically older women, operating in front of transport stations and in markets; these 'Starushki-babushki' sell a limited selection of cigarettes, many of which are illegal imports (MTI 1997). In other countries, an informal distribution network in bars, pubs, and other outlets, also allows for the sale of contraband cigarettes. For example, Coleman (1998) concluded that most smuggled tobacco products consumed in the United Kingdom were sold in pubs. In general, however, unregulated street-selling is much more common in low-income and middle-income countries, implying that the potential for large-scale cigarette smuggling into these countries is greater than for high-income countries.

16.4 Cigarette smuggling and tax revenues

It has been argued, often by the tobacco industry, that higher cigarette taxes will not have their intended effect of raising revenues and, in some countries, discouraging cigarette consumption. This is largely based on the argument that higher taxes will lead to increases in all forms of legal and illegal circumvention in order to avoid the tax increases, thereby significantly reducing sales of the higher taxed cigarettes but not reducing overall consumption as legal and illegal substitutes are found. Some countries, most notably Canada and Sweden, have accepted these arguments, rolling back prior tax increases; others have foregone new increases given fears of increased cigarette smuggling. Others however, have increased tobacco taxes, achieving their goals of increasing revenues and/or reducing tobacco use.

While it is true that tax revenues are lower as a result of the presence of legal and illegal efforts to avoid taxes than they would be in their absence, this does not imply that cigarette tax revenues fall as a result of higher taxes. Additional discussions of the relationships between cigarette taxes and revenues are found elsewhere in this volume (Chapter 10, Chapter 15, and Chapter 17). This section provides additional descriptive evidence on the relationship between cigarette taxes and revenues based on the experiences in selected countries, most notably Canada and Sweden.

16.4.1 Canada

In 1980, cigarette prices in Canada were only slightly higher than prices in the neighboring United States. Between 1980 and 1984, this differential widened significantly as a result of a doubling of Canadian taxes. Subsequent provincial and federal tax increases further increased the differential, so that by 1994, average Canadian cigarette taxes per pack were more than five times the US average (Sweanor and Martial 1994). The large price differences that resulted led to significant smuggling of cigarettes from the US into Canada. Estimates suggest that the market share of smuggled cigarettes, which was low up to 1990, was nearly 30% at its peak in 1993 (Canadian Cancer Society *et al.* 1999). Several factors, including the long undefended border between the United States and Canada, relatively weak border controls, price differences along the border, the high concentration of the Canadian population near the US border, and the repeal of a Canadian tax on cigarette exports contributed to the magnitude of the smuggling problem (Sweanor and Martial 1994).

Much of the Canadian black market in cigarettes consisted of domestically produced cigarettes that had been exported to the United States and then illegally smuggled back into Canada. For example, cigarettes exported from Canada to the United States would end up on the Akwesasne reservation, parts of which were located in New York and the provinces of Ontario and Quebec, facilitating the 'round-tripping' of the cigarettes back into Canada, where the cigarettes would then be distributed throughout Canada for resale at significantly lower prices than cigarettes sold legitimately (O'Brien 1998).

The significant increases in Canadian cigarette taxes, coupled with other tobacco-control efforts, led to a more than 43% decline in per capita cigarette consumption from 1979 through 1993, after factoring-in the consumption of contraband cigarettes

(Canadian Cancer Society *et al.* 1999). Moreover, this decline continued even as smuggled cigarettes became increasingly important. Between 1990 and 1993, for example, while estimated contraband cigarette consumption rose from under 1.3 billion cigarettes to 14.5 billion cigarettes, per capita cigarette consumption declined by nearly 14%. In addition to the declines in per capita consumption, smoking prevalence also fell sharply as taxes were increased. This was particularly true for youth ages 15–19 years for whom smoking prevalence fell from 43% in 1981 to 23% in 1991 (Canadian Cancer Society *et al.* 1999). While total cigarette tax revenues fell somewhat from 1991 to 1993 as a result of the sharp upturn in cigarette smuggling, they were still well above tax revenues prior to the tax hikes of the late-1980s and early-1990s.

In response to an aggressive industry-sponsored campaign, the Canadian federal cigarette tax was reduced by CA$5.00 per carton on February 9, 1994; federal tax cuts of up to CA$10 per carton were added to match provincial tax cuts. In Quebec, for example, provincial taxes were cut by CA$11 per carton, which, combined with the federal tax cuts, reduced taxes by $26 per carton in Quebec. Several, but not all, provinces followed, leading to significantly lower cigarette prices in much of Canada. In addition, the roll-back of federal cigarette taxes was accompanied by the restoration of the tax on tobacco exports. As expected, average per capita cigarette consumption increased sharply in provinces where taxes were significantly reduced, with average per capita consumption over 27% higher in these provinces in 1998 than it was in 1993. In contrast, per capita consumption in the remaining provinces continued its downward trend, falling by 11% between 1993 and 1998. In addition, smoking prevalence among youth and adults has risen sharply since the tax roll-back, reversing the earlier downward trend associated with tax increases (Canadian Cancer Society *et al.* 1999). Finally, and somewhat surprisingly considering that several provinces continued to maintain high taxes and prices, the overall smuggling problem all but disappeared.

While the purpose of the tax cuts was to combat the smuggling problem and raise cigarette tax revenues, they have had the opposite impact, as more fully described by the Canadian Cancer Society *et al.* (1999). Federal tax revenues fell sharply after the tax cuts, from CA$2.98 billion in 1992–93, the last full fiscal year prior to the tax cuts, to CA$1.91 billion in 1994–95 the first full fiscal year after the tax cuts; revenues in the 1993–94 fiscal year were CA$2.7 billion (somewhat lower than they would have been had the higher taxes remained in place through the end of the fiscal year in March). This drop in revenues occurred despite a surge in tax paid cigarette sales, which rose from 30.2 billion cigarettes in 1993, to 45.6 billion cigarettes in 1994. Even sharper declines in tax revenues were observed in the provinces that cut their taxes. Over the same period (fiscal 1992–93 to fiscal 1994–95), cigarette tax revenues in these provinces fell from CA$1.55 billion to CA0.62 billion. In contrast, tax revenues remained relatively stable in the provinces where taxes remained high.

Interestingly, as noted by the Canadian Cancer Society *et al.* (1999), the direction of the flow of smuggled cigarettes has not been reversed as a result of the tax roll-backs. Cigarette prices in Quebec and Ontario are now well below cigarette prices in the United States, particularly those in bordering states. This is the result of the tax roll-backs in these provinces, and increases in industry prices and federal and state taxes in the United States. There is no evidence, however, that significant cigarette smuggling has taken place from Canada into the United States.

16.4.2 Sweden

Sweden had much the same experience as Canada following two significant tax increases and their subsequent roll-back in the mid-1990s. Unlike Canada, Sweden's cigarette taxes and prices have historically been higher than those of most countries in the EU. Despite this, cigarette smuggling was not considered a problem in Sweden. Persson and Andersson (1997), for example, estimated that untaxed cigarettes accounted for at most 2% of the Swedish cigarette market in 1996. Two significant tax increases, in December 1996 and August 1997 raised average cigarette prices by approximately 43%, to approximately US$6.00 per pack. The tax increases were effective in both increasing tax revenues and in reducing cigarette smoking in Sweden. Tobacco tax revenues rose by 9% in 1997 (Wendleby and Nordgren 1998). Smoking prevalence rates, based on annual survey data, fell sharply from 1996 to 1997, particularly among youth and young adults (Nordgren, personal communication).

At the same time, however, anecdotal reports and some very limited empirical evidence suggested that cigarette smuggling rose after the tax increases. Confiscations of cigarettes by customs authorities, for example, rose from 17 million cigarettes in 1996 to 39 million cigarettes in 1997 (Wendleby and Nordgren 1998). In response to the perception that smuggling was becoming a problem, as well as in response to the lack of public support for the tax increases, the August 1997 tax hike was repealed in August 1998. As a result, Swedish tax revenues from cigarettes decreased from SKE6313 in 1997 to SKE5770 in 1998, while tax paid sales per capita rose from 34 packs in 1997 to 51 packs in 1998 (Wicklin 1999).

16.4.3 Other countries

The experiences of many other countries mirror those of Canada and Sweden. That is, in country after country, with very rare exceptions, increases in cigarette and other tobacco excise taxes have led to increases in tax revenues and reductions in tobacco use. In South Africa, for example, cigarette excises were increased by 351% over the period from 1990 to 1997, increasing revenues by 177% and reducing tax paid sales by 22%. While smuggling increased from imperceptible levels to about 6% of the market, it fell far short of off-setting the impact of the tax increases (Salooje, personal communication). Similarly, estimates from the United Kingdom based on data from 1971 through 1993, imply a revenue elasticity for cigarette taxes of 0.6–0.9, indicating that a 10% increase in cigarette taxes raises cigarette tax revenues by between 6% and 9% (Townsend 1996). Likewise, France increased taxes and prices several times between September 1991 and December 1996, nearly doubling the nominal retail price of cigarettes. This led to a reduction of more than 14% in overall cigarette sales and reduced smoking prevalence by 15% (Baudier 1997). At the same time, tobacco tax revenues rose by nearly 80% while smuggling remained relatively unimportant.

16.5 The role of the tobacco industry

The tobacco industry could benefit from smuggling in several ways. First, cigarette smuggling is an effective way of introducing the industry's products into markets that would otherwise be closed by trade barriers and other restrictive practices (MTI 1996). In addition, the availability of lower-priced cigarettes via smuggling raises the overall consumption of cigarettes compared to consumption in the absence of smuggling, adding to the tobacco industry's sales. Furthermore, the threat of smuggling and the crime problems that accompany it can be effective in either discouraging governments from raising cigarette taxes or, as in the cases of Canada and Sweden, encouraging them to reduce taxes. The lower taxes that result keep prices lower and, consequently, tobacco industry sales are higher. A recent theoretical model by Thursby and Thursby (2000) provides additional support for this hypothesis, clearly indicating that some cigarette companies have an incentive to engage in 'commercial smuggling' in order to raise profitability. Their empirical application of this model to US state-level data for the period from 1972 through 1990 indicates that commercial smuggling accounted for a small, but statistically significant share of total US cigarette sales.

In addition, a number of recent criminal investigations and convictions in several countries provide evidence of tobacco companies' complicity in cigarette smuggling. For example, several criminal investigations arose from the smuggling between the United States and Canada in the early 1990s (Canadian Cancer Society et al. 1999). These investigations led to the convictions of former executives of several tobacco companies. Further investigations of a number of companies continue. Similarly, in Hong Kong, China, a former tobacco industry executive was found guilty in court for his role in an operation that smuggled cigarettes into China. Other investigations continue, spurred on, in part, by internal industry documents released in various lawsuits brought against tobacco companies.

16.6 Discussion

Theoretical, empirical, and descriptive evidence indicates that a number of factors contribute to cigarette smuggling. While tax levels and tax and price differentials are important factors, the evidence suggests that others, including the presence of informal distribution networks, organized crime, industry participation, and corruption, may be as, or more, important. In general, many of the factors that facilitate smuggling are more common in low-income and middle-income countries. Nevertheless, the magnitude of the cigarette-smuggling problem is generally overstated, particularly when it comes to the impact of smuggling on the changes in cigarette smoking and tax revenues that result from increases in cigarette excise taxes. The experiences from numerous countries clearly indicate that increases in cigarette taxes will lead to reductions in cigarette smoking and increases in cigarette tax revenues, even when they are accompanied by increases in cigarette smuggling, while reductions in taxes that are aimed at reducing the smuggling problem will lead to reductions in tax revenues and greater smoking.

While cigarette smuggling and the crime that generally accompanies it can be significant problems, governments need not forego cigarette tax increases because of fears over them. Instead, the appropriate response to smuggling is to adopt policies that make it less profitable, more difficult, and more costly to engage in smuggling. Several options are available to accomplish these objectives.

Cigarette packs can be marked in several different ways to make it easier to detect smuggled cigarettes. Prominent tax stamps that are difficult to counterfeit can be placed on all packages under the cellophane (see Chapter 17 for further discussion of the use of tax stamps). Similarly, to the extent that duty-free sales are permitted, all relevant packages could require special markings to indicate tax-exempt status, making it easier to distinguish them from sales on which taxes are to be paid. For cigarettes that are destined for export, packages could be labeled to indicate the country of final destination and could include appropriate, country-specific health-warning labels. Manufacturers could be required to print a unique serial number on all packages of tobacco products, making it easier to identify the manufacturer of each. Similarly, a chain of custody mark could be attached to all packages at each step in the distribution chain, making it less difficult to identify the source of cigarettes that disappear while in transit.

In addition, more extensive computerized record keeping and tracking systems could be required in order to facilitate the monitoring of cigarette exports and imports from their original source to their final destination. Combined with labeling the country of final destination, and the serial numbers and chain of custody markings described above, this would make enforcement of anti-smuggling policies and the identification of those involved in smuggling much simpler. In addition, exporters could be required to post bonds on cigarette shipments that could only be released after all of the cigarettes reach their intended destinations. Similarly, all manufacturers, importers, exporters, wholesalers, transporters, warehouses, and retailers could be required to have a license for their tobacco-related activities. These licenses would help identify and monitor the different players in the tobacco-distribution network, and the suspension or revocation of these licenses for participation in smuggling could deter some would-be smugglers. Moreover, additional resources could be devoted to enforcing new and existing policies aimed at reducing smuggling. These could be combined with stronger penalties, so as to significantly raise the expected costs associated with engaging in smuggling. Furthermore, mass-media campaigns and other efforts could be used to raise public awareness concerning the problems associated with cigarette smuggling, something that is often viewed as a 'victimless crime'. Finally, efforts could be undertaken to coordinate tax rates among neighboring countries, so as to minimize the incentives for many of the legal and illegal circumvention activities described above.

Several governments have begun to adopt many of these strategies. Many countries, for example, require prominent tax stamps on tobacco products sold within their borders. Some, such as France and Singapore, require licenses for at least some of those involved in the cigarette manufacturing and distribution chain. Others, such as Hong Kong, employ sophisticated computer-tracking systems to monitor the movement of cigarettes through the distribution chain. Germany engaged in an effective mass-media campaign to combat the view that cigarette smuggling was relatively harmless. Regional agreements, such as that governing the EU, set floors on tobacco taxes for member countries. Proposed agreements, such as the World Health Organization's Framework Convention on Tobacco Control, would further coordinate tobacco-control efforts across countries, including tobacco taxes and efforts to combat smuggling.

References

Barford, M. F. (1993). New dimensions boost cigarette smuggling. *Tobacco Journal International*, **3**, 16–8.

Baudier, F. (1997). Le tabagisme en 1997: etat des lieux. *La Sante de L'Homme*, **331**, 14.

Beebe, M. (1999). Tobacco's new road. *Buffalo News*, December 12.

Buck, D., Godfrey, C., and Richardson, G. (1994). *Should Cross Border Shopping Affect Tax Policy?* York: Centre for Health Economics.

Canadian Cancer Society, Non-Smokers' Rights Association, Physicians for a Smoke-Free Canada, Quebec Coalition for Tobacco Control (1999). *Surveying the Damage: Cut-Rate Tobacco Products and Public Health in the 1990s*. Canadian Cancer Society, the Non-Smokers' Rights Association and Physicians for a Smoke-Free Canada, Ottawa.

Coleman, T. (1998). Stuck in the middle. *Tobacco International*, March 26–28.

European Commission (1998). *Fight Against Fraud*. COM(98) 276 Final. CEC, Brussels.

European Parliament (1997). *Committee of Inquiry into the Community Transit System*. European Parliament, Brussels

FIA International Research Ltd (1999a). *Organized Crime and the Smuggling of Cigarettes in the United States – The 1999 Update*. FIA International Research Ltd, Washington D.C.

FIA International Research Ltd (1999b). *The Gray Market in Cigarettes in the United States: A Primer*. FIA International Research Ltd, Washington D.C.

Godfrey, A. A. (1997). *Investigation and Prosecution of Smuggling*. Presentation at the 10th World Conference on Tobacco or Health, Beijing, August 1997.

Groom, B. (1998). Battling bootleggers disturb Dover's calm. *Financial Times*, March 18.

Joossens, L. and Raw, M. (1995). Smuggling and cross border trade of tobacco in Europe. *British Medical Journal*, **3**, 1393–7.

Joossens, L. and Raw, M. (1998). Cigarette smuggling in Europe: who really benefits? *Tobacco Control*, **7**(1), 66–71.

Joossens, L., Naett, C., and Howie, C. (1992). *Taxes on Tobacco Products: a Health Issue*. European Bureau for Action on Smoking Prevention, Brussels.

Piha, T. (1998). *Conclusions and proposals for future measures*. Presentation at: Tourist Imports and Smuggling of Cigarettes: an International Seminar on Health Policy, Helsinki, January 1998.

Lund, K. E. (1990). *A Note on the Changes in Tobacco Use Since 1970*. National Council on Tobacco and Health, Oslo.

Market Tracking International (1996). *World Tobacco File 1996*. DMG Business Media, London.

Market Tracking International (1997). *World Tobacco File 1996: Emerging Markets in Central and Eastern Europe*. DMG Business Media, London.

Market Tracking International (1998). *World Tobacco File 1998*. DMG Business Media, London.

O'Brien, J. (1998). Indians say they had help at front end; Akwesasne case could topple industry arguments against proposed cigarette tax. *Herald American*, June 7.

Persson, L. G. W. and Andersson, J. (1997). *Cigarette Smuggling*. Swedish National Police College, Stockholm.

Sweanor, D. T. and Martial, L. R. (1994). *The Smuggling of Tobacco Products: Lessons from Canada*. Ottawa: Non-Smokers' Rights Association/Smoking and Health Action Foundation. Ontario, Canada.

Thursby, J. G. and Thursby, M. C. (2000). Interstate cigarette bootlegging: extent, revenue losses, and effects of federal intervention. *National Tax Journal*, **53**(1), 59–78.

Townsend, J. (1996). Price and consumption. *British Medical Bulletin*, **52**(1), 134–42.

Trackray, M. (1998). Customs and excise estimates of revenue losses and smuggling. Presentation at Tourist Imports and Smuggling of Cigarettes: An International Seminar on Health Policy, Helsinki, January 1998.

Transparency International (1997). *1997 Corruption Perception Index*. Transparency International, Berlin.

Wendleby, M. and Nordgren, P. (1998). Balancing the price: Sweden. Presentation at Tourist Imports and Smuggling of Cigarettes: An International Seminar on Health Policy, Helsinki, January 1998.

Wicklin, B. (1999). *Tobacco Statistics*. Statistical Bureau VECA, Stockholm.

Section V
Policy directions

17

The design, administration, and potential revenue of tobacco excises

Emil M. Sunley, Ayda Yurekli, and Frank J. Chaloupka

This chapter discusses the design and administration of tobacco excise taxes. With respect to design, the issues reviewed here include the choice of tobacco products to excise, the treatment of imports, and the choice of specific taxes (based on quantity) versus *ad valorem* taxes (based on value). We also briefly discuss the impact of smuggling on tax revenues. With respect to tax administration, the issues discussed here include the use of registration and licensing to facilitate administration, bonding, physical control of tobacco products, and the use of tax stamps. Finally, the revenue-generating potential of higher cigarette taxes is examined. Using data on tax revenues, tax rates, and prices, we calculate that an increase in cigarette taxes of 10% globally would raise cigarette tax revenues by nearly 7%, with relatively larger increases in revenues in high-income countries and smaller, but sizable, increases in revenues in low-income and middle-income countries.

17.1 Introduction

The aim of this chapter is to provide brief information on the design and administration of tobacco excise taxes and to examine the likely outcome, for revenue generation, of an increase in cigarette taxes applied globally. The impact of tobacco taxes on tobacco consumption is not discussed in this chapter (see Chapter 10 for a detailed discussion of this issue).

17.2 The design of tobacco excises[1]

17.2.1 Which tobacco products to excise?

Most governments impose tobacco excises primarily to raise revenue, although some have recently increased their taxes to discourage tobacco consumption and promote public health. Tobacco excises, and excises on alcoholic beverages and petroleum products, are a significant revenue source in most countries. Among the OECD countries in 1994, for example, excises raised amounts varying from 3% of total revenues (in the United States) to 23% (in Greece), with the majority of countries raising sums in the range between 6% and 11% of total revenues. Some low-income and middle-income countries raise more than 20% of their total revenues by excises, particularly those

---

[1] For further discussion and sources, see Terra (1996), McCarten and Stotsky (1995), and Ferron (1984).

countries that have not adopted a broad-based value-added tax (VAT) through the retail stage. The share of all excise taxes attributable to tobacco excise is substantial in most countries. A clear advantage of tobacco excises is that they are easier to administer than broad-based consumption taxes or direct taxes on income.

Cigarettes are the primary tobacco product and generally account for more than 90% of the revenue from tobacco excises. It is customary, however, for countries to tax all types of tobacco—cigarettes, cigars, pipe tobacco, snuff, or chewing tobacco—although the tax rates on tobacco products other than cigarettes are typically lower. All tobacco products compete with each other and all have health effects that warrant a tax. Many countries excise hand-rolling tobacco to eliminate any tax incentive to 'roll your own'. A system that imposes differential taxes and, consequently, results in significant differences in prices, can lead consumers to substitute away from relatively highly priced products towards those with lower prices. For example, when Egypt increased its tax on manufactured cigarettes but not on *shisha* tobacco (a type of pipe tobacco), *shisha* smoking increased while cigarette smoking declined (Townsend 1998).

17.2.2 Treatment of imports

The best international practice is to impose excises on the destination basis, under which imports are taxed and exports are freed of tax. Moreover, excises should apply equally to goods that are imported or domestically produced. This ensures that the excises apply uniformly to all domestic consumption of the excisable goods. Under the General Agreement on Tariffs and Trade, countries may impose compensatory taxes on imports and may exempt, or remit, taxes on exports, but they are not required to do so. Discrimination is also forbidden: imported products shall 'not be subject, directly or indirectly, to internal taxes or internal charges of any kind in excess of those applied directly or indirectly to like domestic products' (Terra 1996). In general, the principle of non-discrimination requires that a country levy an identical excise on domestic products and the same or similar products imported from other member countries.

Most countries follow the practice of excising imports and not taxing exports, although a few countries (Pakistan, for example) follow the old Commonwealth tradition that excises are levied on domestic production alone. Though in theory import duties can be coordinated with excises that apply only to domestic products, there can be difficulties in doing so, particularly when import prices are subject to change.

Most countries impose both a customs duty and an excise tax on excisable imports specifying the excise base for *ad valorem* excises as the price plus the customs duty. Although following this procedure appears to result in a tax on a tax, it ensures that a customs duty of, say, 10% will raise the cost of an imported good by 10% even when the imported good is subject to the excise tax. Consider this illustration. If the customs value is 100, a customs duty of 10% increases the cost to 110. If the customs duty is included in the base of the excise tax, a 20% excise tax will increase the cost further to 132. This cost is 10% higher than if the import were subject only to the excise tax (i.e. 132 is 10% higher than 120). Similarly, most countries that impose value-added taxes impose them on a base that includes any excise tax and customs duty. A VAT of 10% will raise the cost of the good by 10%, even when the good is subject to an excise tax (or a customs duty).

17.2.3 Specific taxes versus *ad valorem* tax rates

Excises can be either specific taxes (based on quantity) or *ad valorem* (based on value). Many countries impose specific rates on certain excisable goods and *ad valorem* rates on other excisable goods, particularly for goods varying widely in quality, such as jewellery or fur coats, that would be difficult to assess under specific rates. The United States, for example, excises cigarettes and small cigars using specific rates but excises large cigars using *ad valorem* rates. Some countries impose specific minimum rates with *ad valorem* supplements on some excisable goods.

In the European Union (EU), the excise duty of each member country on cigarettes must consist of two parts: one *ad valorem* and one specific. The specific element must represent between 5% and 55% of the total tax burden (excise duty plus VAT) of the most popular price category (MPPC) sold in that country (usually, king-size filter brands). The combination of specific and *ad valorem* rates reflects a political compromise that 'blessed' the then-current tax regime for cigarettes in most EU countries. The minimum rates for other manufactured tobacco—cigars and cigarillos, hand-rolling tobacco, and other smoking tobacco—are expressed in *ad valorem* terms. Some countries, (Armenia, for example) impose a specific excise that serves as a floor under the general *ad valorem* tax. The taxpayer pays either the *ad valorem* tax or the specific excise, whichever is greater.

In general, tobacco taxes in low-income and middle-income countries are well below taxes in high-income countries; consequently, cigarette prices in low-income and middle-income countries are well below prices in high-income countries. Cigarette taxes, for example, account for two-thirds or more of the pack price in most high-income countries (with the notable exception of the United States), compared to half or less of the pack price in low-income and middle-income countries (see Table 17.1).

Ad valorem taxation has a multiplier effect as part of any increase in the consumer price goes to the government as tax revenue (Keen 1998). In contrast, specific excises protect the revenues from price wars or reductions. With an *ad valorem* tax, the government, in effect, 'subsidizes' the price reduction. Specific excises can facilitate revenue forecasts inasmuch as external influences may significantly change the buying patterns in regard to 'high-' or 'low-quality' products, even though the overall demand is relatively inelastic. The multiplier effect creates a disincentive to the manufacturer to improve a product's quality, while specific taxation encourages upgrading when variants of the product differ in quality. For example, specific excises may lead to greater consumption of the high-quality brands. Thus, when quality and variety are considered important in a type of product, economic theory points to specific taxation.

If a primary purpose of the excise is to discourage consumption of cigarettes, a strong case can be made for specific excises that would impose the same tax per cigarette. There are exceptions, however, since the tobacco industry is likely to seek ways to minimize the impact of these taxes on consumption. Townsend (1998), for example, describes how in the United Kingdom, the switch from a system where taxes were based on the weight of tobacco to a system in which they were imposed per cigarette led tobacco companies to market 'king-sized' and 'super king-sized' cigarettes, actually lowering the total tax per amount of tobacco smoked. Similarly, Evans and Farrelly (1998) found that increases in cigarette excise taxes, while significantly reducing smoking prevalence, led some continuing smokers to switch to longer cigarettes or

Table 17.1 Cigarette prices and taxes, selected countries, by income group

	Tax (US$)	Tax as % of price
High-income		
Australia	3.15	65
Austria	2.16	73
Belgium	2.49	75
Canada	2.04	51
Denmark	4.38	84
Finland	3.28	73
France	2.17	75
Germany	2.43	72
Ireland	1.27	75
Italy	1.60	73
Japan	1.46	60
Korea, Republic of	0.46	60
Netherlands	2.15	72
New Zealand	3.19	68
Norway	5.47	78
Portugal	1.19	81
Spain	0.99	72
Sweden	3.16	69
Switzerland	1.45	52
United Kingdom	3.24	78
United States	0.58	30
Upper middle-income		
Argentina	0.97	70
Brazil	0.79	75
Chile	0.62	70
Czech Republic	0.0003	0.1
Greece	1.39	73
Hungary	0.22	42
Malaysia	0.23	33
Mexico	0.38	60
Poland	0.20	39
Slovak Republic	0.20	34
Slovenia	0.68	63
South Africa	0.44	33
Lower middle-income		
Bolivia	0.20	61
Bulgaria	0.25	42
Colombia	0.03	45
El Salvador	0.28	42
Indonesia	0.0001	30
Jamaica	0.16	42
Philippines	0.14	63
Thailand	0.37	62
Turkey	0.22	42
Venezuela	0.04	50
Low-income		
Albania	0.20	70
Armenia	0.10	50
Bangladesh	0.03	30
Cambodia	0.01	20
China	0.08	38
India (cigarettes)	0.28	75
Pakistan	0.21	73
Sri Lanka	0.25	24
Vietnam	0.04	36
Zambia	0.20	30
Zimbabwe	0.34	80

Source: Marketfile and World Bank Tobacco Survey 1989–1995.

brands with a higher yield of nicotine and tar. This has been interpreted by some as an increase in the quality of the average cigarette consumed (Barzel 1976; British American Tobacco 1994; Sobel and Garrett, 1997).

Some countries may favor *ad valorem* excises (or specific excises with several quality bands) if the cheaper brands of cigarettes are domestic products and the prestige brands are imported (or produced locally by foreign-controlled companies). *Ad valorem* excises in this situation will give greater protection to domestic producers. When there are large quality differentials between domestic and imported excisable products, import duties can be imposed on the imported product to offset the inherent effect that a specific excise is 'bad' for low-priced (lower quality) domestic production. When customs duties are imposed for protection, specific excises can be imposed on both domestic production and imports.

Specific excises have another advantage. They are easier to administer because it is necessary only to determine the physical quantity of the product taxed, and not to determine its value. An exception to this general rule would be situations where the government controls the retail price of the excised good and the price is changed only a few times a year. These taxes are generally collected at the manufacturing, wholesaling, or importing stage. Specific taxation, however, does require a precise definition of what constitutes 'one unit' of quantity. International experience suggests, for example, that it is easier to administer a cigarette excise if the unit of quantity is 1000 cigarettes than if the unit of quantity is a kilogram of fine cut tobacco.

Under *ad valorem* taxation, determining the value is particularly difficult when taxpayers use abusive transfer prices to reduce their tax liabilities. For example, if the *ad valorem* cigarette excise is a percentage of the manufacturer's price, the manufacturer may sell cigarettes to a related marketing company at an artificially low price, thus reducing its excise liability. It is just this problem that led the Philippines in 1996 to abandon *ad valorem* taxes on cigarettes in favor of specific excises. Similarly, as part of its 1996 tax reforms, the Russian Federation unified the excises on imported and domestic products, and adopted specific excises for cigarettes. Until then, specific excises had been imposed on the domestic production of cigarettes but imports had been subject to *ad valorem* excises.

The valuation problem of *ad valorem* taxation should not be overstated, however. The tax administration can be given the authority to make price adjustments in situations where under-pricing of excisable goods has reduced the excise tax base, and, for some products, the value is fairly readily determinable. For example, a solution to the valuation problem is to impose the *ad valorem* cigarette excises, which are collected from the manufacturer or importer, on the maximum retail price that is specified by the manufacturer and printed on the package. Penalties are imposed on any sales of cigarettes at prices in excess of the maximum retail price. This approach to *ad valorem* taxation may be cumbersome or unworkable if prices are changing rapidly as it creates a problem regarding the inventory of packaging materials pre-printed with the retail price. Another possible solution would be to impose the excise at the retail stage where most sales would be to final consumers. However, this solution would create serious problems for tax administration, as there are many more retailers than there are manufacturers and importers.

International experience indicates that *ad valorem* taxes keep pace with inflation better than specific taxes. For example, in the United States, the federal specific tax on cigarettes remained unchanged (at 8 cents a pack) for 30 years, although states were regularly increasing their rates. *Ad valorem* taxes, however, are no guarantee that tax revenues will keep pace with inflation. Governments can adjust *ad valorem* rates to out-pace or lag inflation.

Specific taxes can keep pace with inflation if they are automatically adjusted by reference to the consumer price index (CPI). The CPI is the preferred index because once issued it is not revised, unlike some other price indicators such as the GDP deflator. Moreover, the concept of the CPI adjustment is judged to be understood by the public. Alternatively, specific excises could be adjusted to changes in the dollar or ECU exchange rate. However, it should be recognized that domestic currencies can appreciate relative to the dollar or the ECU, and when this occurs, excise rates, expressed in the domestic currency, would be reduced.

Ad valorem tax rates can be specified on a tax-exclusive basis (that is, net of tax) or a tax-inclusive basis (i.e. gross of tax). At one level it does not matter which way the *ad valorem* rates are specified as it easy to translate a tax-exclusive rate into a tax-inclusive rate or vice versa. For example, a 100% tax-exclusive rate is exactly equivalent to a 50% tax-inclusive rate.[2] However, in countries other than the former Soviet Union, excise rates usually are specified on a tax-exclusive basis because these rates are more transparent than tax-inclusive ones, especially when considering excise rates in conjunction with rates for the VAT and trade taxes that are normally expressed in tax-exclusive terms. Some countries collect excises from manufacturers and importers but impose them on the retail price. The retail price may be fixed by the government or it could be the manufacturers' suggested price of the maximum retail price set by the manufacturer. When the tax is imposed on the retail price, the tax may be expressed in tax-inclusive terms. The use of tax inclusive rates in the former Soviet Union may have reflected the old view that the final price is given and the excise tax should capture a share of the margin. In contrast, an excise tax in a market economy is treated as a cost added onto the sales price, which is easier for consumers to grasp if the excises are specified on a tax-exclusive basis.

On balance, given the weak tax administrations in most developing and transition countries, specific excises on cigarettes automatically adjusted for inflation should be preferred to *ad valorem* excises. These specific taxes could be adjusted *automatically* whenever the CPI has increased by more than, say, 5% since the previous adjustment. It is critical that the inflation adjustment be automatic: that is, it should be made by administrative order, and should not require a decision by an executive agency or approval by a legislative body.

Finally, in countries where the production and sale of tobacco products is monopolized by the state, the taxation of these products may be less obvious, but nonetheless important. Rather than levying a specific or *ad valorem* tax, the government collects revenues by increasing the prices of the tobacco products it produces and/or distributes. The indirect taxation resulting from a state monopoly on tobacco products can generate substantial government revenues from tobacco. For example, in Taiwan, the

---

[2] If t_n is the tax inclusive rate and t_e is the tax exclusive tax rate, both expressed in percentage terms, then $t_n = 100t_e/(100 + t_e)$ and $t_e = 100t_n/(100 - t_n)$.

government historically used its monopoly on opium, salt, camphor, wine, and tobacco products to generate significant revenues. Hsieh and Lin (1998) compared the profits earned by the Taiwan Tobacco and Wine Monopoly Bureau (TTWMB) to the average return on assets for the top 1000 firms in Taiwan (their measure of normal economic profit), to get an estimate of the excess profits earned by the state monopoly. For the period 1985–96, they estimate that the TTWMB's excess profit rate, a measure of the indirect tax associated with the government monopoly, was in the range between 28% and 51%.

17.2.4 Smuggling

If raising revenue is the sole justification for tobacco excises, one must recognize that some balance is required, at least in some low-income and middle-income countries where demand for tobacco products is relatively less inelastic and where smuggling may be more problematic. In general, the revenue-generating potential of cigarette and other tobacco taxes will be highest where the demands for these products is more inelastic and/or where taxes as percentages of prices are relatively low. Consider Zimbabwe, for example, where cigarette demand has been estimated to be relatively more elastic than in high-income countries (although still inelastic), with a price elasticity of demand of -0.85. For most of the past two decades, tobacco taxes as a percentage of price and tobacco tax revenues generally moved in the same direction. The exception to this was in 1984 when a sharp increase in cigarette taxes led to a significant decline in tax revenues. Part of this decline in revenue almost certainly reflects the substantial smuggling of cigarettes into Zimbabwe after the tax increase.

If the excise rates are set at very high levels, there may be a negative impact on revenues from other taxes such as income taxes and value-added taxes. Additionally, organized crime benefits from excise taxes that are higher than the government is willing and able to enforce and than the public is willing to support. What constitutes 'high' is difficult to determine, but taxes that account for 80% or more of cigarette pack price in some countries have not resulted in significant problems from smuggling. Overall, the evidence suggests that, when setting tobacco excise tax rates, key factors that must be considered in reducing the risk of smuggling include the purchasing power of local consumers, tax rates in neighboring markets, and the effectiveness of the tax authority to enforce compliance. For more detailed discussions of smuggling, see Merriman *et al.* (Chapter 15) and Joossens *et al.* (Chapter 16). In general, the more appropriate response to the threat of smuggling is the adoption and implementation of strong measures to counteract the smuggling itself.

17.3 Tax administration[3]

Tobacco excises are generally administered similarly to customs duties. If collected at the border, then the customs procedures apply directly. However, even the tax on domestic producers follows procedures analogous to customs, with the producer's facility being analogous to a customs warehouse. To ensure that all tobacco products are

---

[3] This section draws heavily on technical assistance reports and notes prepared by James Walsh and Katherine Baer of the Fiscal Affairs Department of the IMF.

covered by the excise schedule, countries may choose to define the various excises by reference to the numbers of the Harmonized System that has been adopted for tariff classification purposes and that is used by most of the trading nations of the world (Hussey and Lubick 1996).

The control of excise tax collections should be comparatively easy in relation to other taxes, particularly where there are only a small number of large excise taxpayers. Nevertheless, the administration of excises, like other taxes, requires an integrated strategy for taxpayer registration, filing and payment, collection of overdue taxes, audit, appeals, and taxpayer services. In high-income countries, excises can be administered by relying on the taxpayer to submit tax returns and then auditing the taxpayer's books of account. In low-income and middle-income countries, however, the effective enforcement of excises on tobacco products will require much greater physical control over the products.

The high degree of compliance with excise taxes that is experienced in many high-income countries is based, at least in part, on the maintenance of a professional relationship between the taxing authority and the taxpayer. Development of such professional relationships should be part of the overall strategy to strengthen tax administration and tax compliance.

17.3.1 Registration and licensing

Given the importance of tobacco excises for a country's revenues, all importers on a commercial basis and all producers of these excisable goods should be required to register with the tax authority and obtain a license. In conformity with international trade practices, the licensing of importers of excisable goods should not discriminate against imports or be excessive.

Effective enforcement begins with a stringent licensing system to screen out individuals and businesses that are not likely to pay their taxes or conduct their operations in strict conformity with all laws and regulations. Before licenses are given, background checks on owners and operators may be appropriate if there is any suspicion of a criminal background or involvement with smuggling. Penalties for not obtaining a license should be relatively severe, thereby facilitating administration of the tax. The licensing system may be extended to wholesalers. In addition, retailers may be required to purchase products only from licensed importers, wholesalers, or producers.

17.3.2 Timing of tax liability and tax payment

Excises on tobacco products are usually levies imposed on the production or importation of these goods; they are not levies imposed on the final sale of the goods. With appropriate physical controls (discussed below), it is much easier to determine when goods were produced or shipped than when they were sold or paid for. Although the tax liability is fixed when the goods are imported or produced, countries may permit deferment of the payment of the tax, with suitable guarantees that the tax will be paid. A deferment can allow the timing of the tax payment to coincide roughly with the time that the consumer buys the product.

17.3.3 Bonding

It is recognized that producers may experience cash-flow problems if they are required to maintain inventories of excisable goods on a tax-paid basis. This problem can be alleviated if producers can purchase a bond or similar security to ensure that all tax liabilities are paid. When there are bonded production facilities, the tax liability can be imposed when the excisable goods are removed from the bonded facility (i.e. released for consumption) and not when they are produced. Thus a cigarette producer could manufacture cigarettes and place them in a bonded warehouse. Tax would be due when the production is removed from the bonded warehouse unless it is withdrawn under a transfer bond for transfer to another bonded production center for further processing or it is withdrawn under an export bond for export.

17.3.4 Physical controls

Governments that have effective tax administration systems ensure that shipments into and out of tobacco production facilities are controlled. The producer should make records available for inspection by the tax authority on a regular basis, either weekly or monthly. Periodically, the tax authorities must take stock of the products at hand and check against the taxpayer's production and shipment records. Control may also include checking inventory by counting cigarette packs. An employee of the company may perform the actual measuring under the supervision of a tax official. To help ensure integrity, the control officials should be rotated frequently among different locations and the supervisor should make surprise visits.

High-income countries have, in the past, adopted intensive physical controls on excisable goods. For example, whisky distilleries in Scotland once had official locks on their entrances, exits, and key areas of the production process that were vulnerable to unlawful extraction. Each distillery had a resident excise officer who lived in a provided house next door to the distillery, and no activity could take place without the officer being present to unlock the locks. Similarly, in the United Kingdom, each bonded warehouse used to have a resident officer who had to unlock and lock the warehouse. Now, the United Kingdom relies on the warehouse keeper to exercise day-to-day control with official control based on spot checks and systems of audit. Some developing countries might need to consider similarly intensive controls on tobacco products. As in all such systems, however, the potential for fraud by the excise officer would have to be considered.

17.3.5 Use of stamps

Excise stamps are another method of ensuring payment of excise tax and ensuring that goods for which the tax appropriate for one jurisdiction has been paid do not get shipped to another. These stamps can be sold to the taxpayer, allowing the government to collect its money in advance. Alternatively, the stamps can be provided to bonded producers, with payment delayed until the excise would otherwise be payable. Stamps that represent the full payment of the excise are particularly effective for the payment of specific excises. If the price of the stamps does not represent the full payment of the excise, as in the Russian Federation, the stamps can still be used to represent payment of excises. However, the tax authority, by requiring excise taxpayers to account accurately for the storage and use of stamps, must ensure that the full excise tax is paid on products bearing stamps. In this situation, stamps can serve to complement other administrative programs to help determine the tax liabilities of producers. In the case of *ad valorem* excises, different stamps are needed for each value of the excised good. In the case of cigarettes, manufacturers can apply the excise stamp directly to the pack as part of the manufacturing process. It can then be applied under the cellophane.

The introduction of stamps involves some costs for the producers of the excised goods, both in terms of the labor and equipment needed to apply the stamps, and the slower production lines that result from the application of the stamps. Stamping machines, for example, may cost in the region of US$40 000 each and some large taxpayers may require as many as 100 stamping machines. Stamps impose an additional cost on producers in that they lose flexibility: once stamped for one national market the product cannot than be shipped instead to another.

If a country is going to adopt excise stamps, then it must control both the excisable good and the stamps. In many countries, the excise stamps are re-used. In some countries, stamps have been easy to counterfeit. To limit counterfeiting, stamps should be of high quality, difficult to duplicate, serially numbered, and adhere to the package so that they will be broken when the package is opened. Stamps will serve little purpose in control unless their utilization is monitored at the retail level and retailers believe that the stamp program is being strictly enforced. There must be strong penalties or criminal sanctions for producing or possessing counterfeit stamps and for persons who deal in illicit products. Similarly, it should be an offence for a retailer or wholesaler to possess tobacco products that do not bear authentic stamps. Governments need to have the authority to revoke the operating licenses for retailers and wholesalers who are repeat offenders.

17.3.6 Refunds and credits

The excise law should provide for a refund or credit of excise tax previously paid on a product that is destroyed prior to being marketed or that is returned to the manufacturer. In addition, if excise stamps are used, stamps destroyed or damaged in transit or in the manufacturing process should be fully credited to the manufacturer. In these instances, there is no excisable sale or use of the product.

17.3.7 Floor stocks tax

To limit the opportunities for evasion and to ease administration, tobacco excises, as discussed earlier, should be levied at the manufacturing stage. However, whenever excise rates are increased, a tax can be imposed on the 'floor stocks', of the excised goods held by distributors and retailers on the date of the tax increase. This 'floor-stocks tax' limits the downstream windfalls that can result from tax increases that take effect on price immediately, even when distributors and retailers are holding inventory that was taxed at the previous lower rate. A floor-stocks tax is not needed every time an excise rate is increased, only when the rate increase is significant. Also, any floor-stocks tax should exempt a *de minimis* holding of inventory.

17.4 Tax rates and revenues

We turn now to the discussion of the revenue-generating potential of tobacco taxes. A key question is the level at which tobacco tax rates should be set. If tobacco excises are viewed as an internalization of the social costs of smoking (see Chapter 4 and Chapter 6), one could attempt to measure this cost and to set the tax rates accordingly. If the purpose of the excise is to deter the consumption of tobacco, one could estimate the effect of higher prices on the demand for tobacco, and set the tax rate to reduce consumption to target levels in the short and longer term. As discussed elsewhere, however, the factors that govern the determination of optimal taxes are quite complex and will vary, depending on what the taxes are intended to accomplish (see Chapter 10 for a lengthier discussion of these issues). Historically, however, taxes on cigarettes and other tobacco products have been seen more simply as an efficient source of revenues, and their design has been driven primarily by this motive.

17.4.1 European Union tax rates and transition economies

The tax rates levied on tobacco products in the European Union (EU) may provide a benchmark for certain transition economies in Central and Eastern Europe, and the former Soviet Union for the following reasons:

(1) the EU is the largest trade partner of these economies, and is likely to become increasingly so;
(2) the EU raises substantial tax revenue from excises; and
(3) the EU rates are a demonstration of what can be supported and accepted by market economies within a European culture.

The EU requires member countries to impose minimum rates, subject to certain agreed derogations (Table 17.2). The EU originally proposed, in its White Paper on *Completing the Internal Market*, that the excise rates on alcohol, tobacco, and petroleum products within the EU should be fully harmonized (Commission on the European Communities, COM(85)). When agreement could not be reached on harmonized rates, the EU in 1992 adopted minimum rates that were set sufficiently low that most countries did not have to increase their excise rates. At the end of 1998, excises on cigarettes in the EU countries ranged from 34 ECU/1000 cigarettes in Spain to 156 ECU/1000 cigarettes in the United Kingdom (Table 17.3)

17.4.2 Tobacco excise tax revenues

Tobacco tax revenues have accounted for more than 10% of total excise tax revenues and more than 1% of total tax revenues in many countries (Table 17.4). The share of tobacco taxes in total tax revenues and excise tax revenues strongly depends on the proportion of the cigarette pack price that is due to excise tax, the amount of cigarette

Table 17.2 Minimum tobacco excise duty rates in the European Union

Tobacco products	Amount or rate (in ECU)
Cigarettes	57% of retail sales price
Fine cut smoking tobacco	30% of retail selling price of ECU 20/kg
Cigars and cigarillos	5% of retail selling price of ECU 7/1000 items or ECU 7/kg
Other smoking tobacco	20% of retail selling price or ECU 15/kg

Source: Commission of the European Communities, COM(95) 285 final, September 13, 1995. Rate consists of specific plus ad valorem rates, excluding VAT. Retail sale price includes all taxes and refers to cigarettes of the most popular price category. Each member State's excise duty on cigarettes must consist of two parts; one *ad valorem*, and one specific, with the specific element representing between 5% and 55% of the total tax burden (excise plus VAT) of the most popular category of cigarettes sold in that member State.

Table 17.3 Cigarette excise yield in EU Countries, January 1, 1995

Member States	Excise yield/1000 cigarettes (in ECU)
Austria	66.35
Belgium	74.48
Denmark	123.59
Finland	108.74
France	85.62
Germany	76.29
Greece	55.52
Ireland	120.11
Italy	55.65
Luxembourg	52.53
Netherlands	68.98
Portugal	56.86
Spain	33.90
Sweden	107.55
United Kingdom	155.99

Source: European Commission, *Excise Duty Tables* (December 1998).

expenditures, and the other taxes paid for goods and services as a proportion of income.[4] As the data in Table 17.4 illustrate, taxes that account for a significant share of price can be supported and accepted by market economies and can generate significant revenues.

[4] TER/TTR = (TER/CSC) * (CSC/GDP) * (GDP/TTR) (*denotes 'multiplied by')
Where: TER (Tobacco Excise Revenue) = number of cigarettes consumed * tax rate, and TTR (Total Tax Revenue) = tax revenues from excise taxes (including tobacco excises), and other goods and services. CSC (Consumer Spending on Cigarettes) = number of cigarettes consumed * cigarette price, and GDP = Gross Domestic Product. Similarly the percentage share of cigarette excise tax revenue in excise tax revenue is equal to:

TER/ER = (TER/CSC) * (CSC/GDP) * (GDP/TTR)* (TTR/ ER), where ER = Excise Revenue.

Table 17.4 Tobacco excise tax rates and revenues as % of total tax and excise tax revenues for countries by income group, 1994–95

	Cigarette excise as a percentage of	Tobacco excise tax revenues as a percentage of:	
	price	Total tax revenues	Excise tax revenues
High-income			
Australia	65	3.38	28.00
Austria	73	0.16	2.58
Denmark	84	2.03	18.84
Finland	73	2.03	12.26
France	75	0.37	5.18
Germany	72	1.38	11.89
Japan	60	0.02	0.34
Korea, Rep.	60	3.46	27.54
Netherlands	72	1.44	21.30
Norway	78	1.76	10.37
Spain	72	2.37	24.69
Sweden	69	1.63	12.23
Switzerland	52	1.69	73.61
UK	78	3.23	25.38
US	30	0.44	12.50
Upper-middle			
Argentina	70	4.34	36.89
Brazil	75	7.37	66.23
Chile	70	4.10	40.82
Croatia		0.82	6.76
Greece	73	8.69	35.31
Hungary	42	0.02	0.21
Mexico	60	1.41	13.10
San Marino		3.35	10.58
Poland	39	3.26	28.27
Seychelles	44	3.71	
South Africa	33	1.15	22.38
Uruguay	60	2.64	23.27
Lower middle-income			
Bulgaria	42	3.63	36.58
Colombia	45	0.91	17.73
Costa Rica	75	1.58	12.67
Egypt Rep.	57	1.34	6.58
Estonia	70	1.29	14.87
Indonesia	30	3.38	68.57
Lithuania		0.16	1.42
Romania		0.20	4.73
Turkey	42	0.21	1.90
Venezuela	50	2.30	56.93
Low-income			
China	40	2.79	15.22
India	75	2.43	6.53
Kenya		0.09	0.63
Nepal	73	6.37	75.68
Pakistan	73	0.11	0.43
Zambia	30	0.04	0.23
Zimbabwe	80	1.17	22.81

Source: unpublished data, IMF, WHO, and the World Bank Tobacco Survey.

17.4.3 Potential revenue from cigarette excises

When forecasting excise revenues, it is necessary to consider whether the excises are *ad valorem* or specific, and, if specific, whether they are indexed for inflation. To estimate the revenue effect of changes in excise rates, the following reasonably straightforward calculation is required: multiply the tax base by the increase in the tax rate and adjust this for changes in the tax base. To illustrate, assume initially that a specific excise tax of 10 rupees per pack represents 50% of the retail price of cigarettes (i.e. 20 rupees per pack). If sales were 10 million packs per year, excise revenue would be 100 million rupees. If the excise is increased by 10% to 11 rupees per pack, the price of cigarettes will rise by 5% to 21 rupees per pack. If the demand elasticity for cigarettes is –0.8, the 5% increase in the price of cigarettes will reduce the demand for cigarettes by 4% to 9.6 million packs per year. Thus tax revenue will increase by 5.6 million rupees (11 × 9.6 million – 10 × 10 million), or by 5.6%.

The estimates from a similar exercise conducted for 70 countries are presented in Table 17.5. These estimates were obtained using data obtained from the World Health Organization (WHO 1997) and a commercial database (Market Tracking International 1999) on cigarette prices, taxes as a percentage of price, and current cigarette consumption. Based on these data, the impact of a 10% increase in cigarette taxes on cigarette consumption and cigarette tax revenues is estimated. Based on the literature on cigarette demand (see Chapter 10), the short-run price-elasticity of demand for cigarettes is assumed to be –0.8 in low-income and middle-income countries and –0.4 in high-income countries. In addition, the tax increase is assumed to be fully passed on to smokers; that is, the 10% increase in the tax is assumed to lead to an x% increase in price, where x is equal to one-tenth of the percentage of cigarette price accounted for by taxes.

These estimates imply that a modest 10% increase in cigarette taxes would lead to a reduction of just over 3% in total cigarette consumption in these 70 countries. Moreover, total cigarette tax revenues would rise by nearly 7% as a result of this tax increase. Given the relatively more elastic demand in low-income and middle-income countries, cigarette consumption would fall by more in these countries (3.45%) than it would in high-income countries (2.24%). While cigarette tax revenues would rise significantly in all countries, the percentage in low-income and middle-income countries would be somewhat smaller (4.8%) than that in high-income countries (7.2%), due to the relatively larger decline in consumption in these countries and the lower share of cigarette price accounted for by excises. In general, the reduction in cigarette consumption is smaller and the rise in revenues larger when tax accounts for a relatively smaller share of price, all else being equal. Larger tax increases would lead to larger reductions in consumption but continue to generate significant increases in tax revenues.

A few caveats should be noted concerning the revenue-generating potential of tax increases on cigarettes and other tobacco products. First, in the exercise presented above, the price-elasticity of demand was assumed to be constant. Changes in this assumption would produce different estimates for the effects of changes in tobacco taxes on demand and tax revenues. If a linear demand curve is assumed, then the price-elasticity of demand will rise as taxes and prices rise, implying more rapid reductions in demand and smaller increases in tax revenues than estimated when the price-

Table 17.5 Estimated impact of a 10% increase in cigarette taxes on cigarette consumption and cigarette tax revenues, various countries

Country	Change in cigarette consumption (%)	Change in cigarette tax revenues (%)
Lower middle-income		
Belize	−2.24	7.54
Bolivia	−4.88	4.63
Bulgaria	3.33	6.33
Colombia	−3.60	6.04
Costa Rica	−6.00	3.40
Dominican Rep.	−1.07	8.82
Egypt	−4.56	4.98
El Salvador	−3.40	6.26
Estonia	−5.60	3.84
Jamaica	−3.36	6.30
Moldova	−1.49	8.36
Panama	−4.80	4.72
Paraguay	−0.80	9.12
Philippines	−5.06	4.44
Slovak Rep.	−2.76	6.97
Thailand	−4.96	4.54
Turkey	−3.36	6.30
Low-income		
Albania	−5.60	3.84
Armenia	−4.00	5.60
Bangladesh	−2.40	7.36
Cambodia	−1.60	8.24
China	−3.23	6.45
Honduras	−0.80	9.12
India	−6.00	3.40
Indonesia	−2.40	7.36
Nepal	−5.86	3.56
Pakistan	−5.84	3.58
Sri Lanka	−1.91	7.90
Vietnam	−2.88	6.83
Zambia	−2.40	7.36
Zimbabwe	−6.40	2.96
High-income		
Australia	−2.60	7.14
Austria	2.92	6.97
Belgium	−3.00	6.70
Canada	−2.05	7.74
Denmark	−3.36	6.30
Finland	−2.92	6.79
France	−3.00	6.70
Germany	−2.88	6.83

Table 17.5 (*cont.*)

Country	Change in cigarette consumption (%)	Change in cigarette tax revenues (%)
Ireland	−3.00	6.70
Italy	−2.92	6.79
Japan	−2.40	7.36
Korea, Republic	−2.40	7.36
Netherlands	−2.88	6.83
New Zealand	−2.72	7.01
Norway	−3.12	6.57
Portugal	−3.24	6.44
Singapore	−2.92	6.79
Spain	−2.88	6.83
Sweden	−2.76	6.96
Switzerland	−2.08	7.71
Taiwan	−0.15	9.84
United Kingdom	−3.12	6.57
United States	−1.20	8.68
Upper middle-income		
Argentina	−5.60	3.84
Brazil	−6.00	3.40
Chile	−5.60	3.84
Czech Republic	−0.01	9.99
Greece	−2.92	6.79
Hungary	−3.39	6.27
Malaysia	−2.67	7.06
Mexico	−4.83	4.69
Slovenia	−5.04	4.46
South Africa	−2.66	7.07
Uruguay	−4.80	4.72
Poland	−3.14	6.55

Source: authors' calculations.

elasticity of demand is assumed to be constant. Indeed, this linear demand curve and the resulting rising elasticity would imply an inverted U-shaped relationship between tobacco taxes and tobacco revenues, where initial increases in taxes would lead to increased revenues but beyond some point, additional increases would lead to disproportionately large reductions in demand, thereby causing revenues to fall. In contrast, given that most studies conclude that the demands for cigarettes and other tobacco products are inelastic, assuming a constant elasticity of demand based on these estimates would imply that even very large increases in tobacco taxes would always generate increases in tax revenues. Either assumption could be questioned and, in reality, the revenue effects of a tax increase are likely to fall somewhere between the predictions obtained from the two. The impact of the assumption about the shape of the demand curve, however, is relatively small for the modest tax increase discussed above.

A second caveat is that, in the exercise presented above, and consistent with much of the empirical literature, it was assumed that an increase in tobacco taxes was fully passed on to consumers. The impact of tobacco tax increases on tax revenues will depend on how the tobacco industry responds to the tax increase. To some extent, given the monopoly power of firms in the industry, tobacco companies can adjust their pricing so that the resulting tax revenues fall short of their expected levels. As noted earlier, Townsend (1998) suggested that one disadvantage of an *ad valorem* tax system is that the tobacco industry might keep prices, and consequently tax revenues, below where they would otherwise be. Similarly, if tobacco companies use a scheduled tax increase as an opportunity for an oligopolistic price increase that is greater than the tax increase (as suggested by Harris 1987), then the greater-than-expected decline in demand would lead to a smaller-than-expected increase in tax revenues.

17.5 Conclusion

Countries that need to generate additional tax revenue often adopt increases in tobacco excise rates. In addition to the increased revenues, however, there are also health benefits from reduced tobacco consumption. In setting tobacco tax rates, governments need to take into account several factors, including the impact of smuggling, cross-border shopping, and duty-free purchases. It is in the interest of governments to reduce tobacco smuggling, not only to increase excise revenues but also to limit the loss of revenues from other taxes, including income taxes and value-added taxes, as underground transactions replace legal ones. Ultimately, tobacco excise tax rates should consider the purchasing power of the local consumers, rates in neighboring countries, and, above all, the ability and willingness of the tax authority to enforce compliance. As the exercise in this chapter demonstrates, increases in tobacco excise taxes can generate significant increases in tobacco tax revenues.

With respect to the structure of tobacco excises, countries should tax all types of tobacco—cigarettes, cigars, pipe tobacco, snuff or chewing tobacco, and hand-rolling tobacco. The best international practice is to impose excises on the destination basis under which imports are taxed and exports are freed of tax. Excises can be either specific taxes (based on quantity) or *ad valorem* (based on value). If a primary purpose of the excise is to discourage tobacco consumption, a strong case can be made for specific excises that would impose the same tax per cigarette. Specific taxes also are easier to administer, because it is necessary only to determine the physical quantity of the product taxed, and not its value. *Ad valorem* taxes, however, may keep pace with inflation better than specific taxes, even specific taxes that are adjusted fairly frequently.

The administration of domestic tobacco excises requires an integrated strategy for taxpayer registration, filing and payment, collection of overdue taxes, audit, and taxpayer services. Low-income and middle-income countries may need to treat tobacco production facilities as extra-territorial, and administer excises similar to customs duties. The tax authority is required to control shipments into and out of the production facility. Excise stamps can assist in ensuring the payment of excises and ensuring that goods that have paid the tax appropriate for one jurisdiction are not shipped to another. The introduction of stamps, however, involves some costs for producers of excised goods. Stamps will serve little purpose in control unless their utilization is monitored at the retail level.

References

Barzel, Y. (1976). An alternative approach to the analysis of taxation. *Journal of Political Economy*, **84**(1), 1177–97.

British American Tobacco (1994). *Tobacco Taxation Guide: A Guide to Alternative Methods of Taxing Cigarettes and Other Tobacco Products.* Optichrome The Printing Group, Woking (England).

European Commission (1986). *Completing the Internal Market: White Paper from the Commission to the European Council (Milan, 28–29 June 1985). COM/85/310 Final.* European Commission, Brussels.

European Commission (1995). *Commission Report to the Courcil and European Parliament on the Rates of Duty Laid Down In Council Directive 92/79/EEC of 19 October 1992 on the Approximation of Taxes on Cigarettes, Council Directive 92/80/EEC of 19 October 1992 on the Approximation of Taxes on Manufactured Tobacco Other Than Cigarettes, Council Directive 92/84/EEC of 19 October 1992 on the Approximation of the Rates of Excise Duty on Alcohol and Alcoholic Beverages and Council Directive 92/92/EE of 19 October 1992 on the Approximation of the Rates of Excise Duties on Mineral Oils. COM/95/285 Final.* European Commission, Brussels.

European Commission (1998). *Excise Duty Rates.* Taxation and Customs Union, Directorate Geneva, European Commission, Brussels.

Evans, W. N. and Farrelly, M. C. (1998). The compensating behavior of smokers: taxes, tar, and nicotine. *RAND Journal of Economics*, **29**(3), 578–95.

Ferron, M. J. (1984). *Excise Taxation: Theory and Practice in Developed and Developing Countries.* IMF, FAD/84/2.

Harris, J. E. (1987). The 1983 Increase in the Federal Cigarette Tax. In *Tax Policy and the Economy*, vol. 1 (ed. L. H. Summers), pp. 87–111. MIT Press, Cambridge (MA).

Hsieh, C. R. and Lin, Y. S. (1998). The economics of tobacco control in Taiwan. In the Economics of Tobacco Control: Towards An Optimal Policy Mix (ed. I. Abedian, R. van der Merwe, N. Wilkins and P. Jha), pp. 306–29. Applied Fiscal Research Centre, University of Cape Town, Cape Town.

Hussey, W. M. and Lubick, D. C. (ed.) (1996). *Basic World Tax Code and Commentary.* Tax Analysts, Arlington, Va.

Keen, M. (1998). The balance between specific and *ad valorem* taxation. *Fiscal Studies*, **19**(1), 1–37.

Market Tracking International (1999). Tobacco Marketfile; http://www.marketfile.com/market/tobacco. Market Tracking International Ltd, London.

McCarten, W. J. and Stotsky, J. (1995). Excise taxes. In *Tax Policy Handbook* (ed. S. Parthasarathi), pp. 100–3. Tax Policy Division, Fiscal Affairs Department, International Monetary Fund, Washington D.C.

Sobel, R. S. and Garrett, T. A. (1997). Taxation and product quality: new evidence from generic cigarettes. *Journal of Political Economy*, **105**(4), 880–7.

Terra, B. (1996). Excises. In *Tax Law Design and Drafting* (ed. V. Thuronyi), pp. 246–63. International Monetary Fund, Washington D.C.

Townsend, J. L. (1998). The role of taxation policy in tobacco control. In *The Economics of Tobacco Control: Towards an Optimal Policy Mix* (ed. I. Abedian, R. van der Merwe, N. Wilkins, and P. Jha), pp. 85–101. Applied Fiscal Research Centre, University of Capetown, Cape Town (South Africa).

World Health Organization (1997). *Tobacco or Health: a Global Status Report.* World Health Organization, Geneva.

18

The effectiveness and cost-effectiveness of price increases and other tobacco-control policies

Kent Ranson, Prabhat Jha, Frank J. Chaloupka, and Son Nguyen

This chapter provides conservative estimates of the effectiveness and cost-effectiveness of tobacco-control policies. Using a model of the cohort of smokers alive in 1995, we find that tax increases that would raise the real price of cigarettes by 10% worldwide would cause about 42 million of these smokers to quit. This price increase would prevent a minimum of 10 million tobacco-related deaths. A combined set of non-price measures (such as comprehensive bans on advertising and promotion, bans on smoking in public places, prominent warning labels, and mass information) would cause some 23 million smokers alive in 1995 to quit and would prevent 5 million deaths. The non-price measures are assumed to have an effectiveness of 2%—a conservative assumption. Increased use of nicotine-replacement therapies (NRTs), with an assumed effectiveness of 0.5%, would enable some 6 million smokers alive in 1995 to quit and would avert 1 million deaths.

The cost-effectiveness of these interventions in low-income and middle-income countries has also been estimated. By weighing the public-sector costs of implementing and running tobacco-control programs against the years of healthy life saved, measured in disability-adjusted life years, or DALYs, we find that price increases on tobacco would be cost-effective in many circumstances. Depending on various assumptions, price increases could cost between US $4 and $34 per DALY in low-income and middle-income countries. Non-price measures are also cost-effective, ranging from $34 to $685 per DALY in low-income and middle-income countries. NRTs with public provision are also cost-effective in low-income and middle-income countries, ranging from $276 to $851 per DALY. Given that, in practice, there is substantial local variation in the likely effectiveness and costs of these interventions, local assessments are required to guide policy.

18.1 Introduction

Governments considering intervention in the tobacco market need to weigh the costs versus the benefits. In previous chapters, we have discussed the economic costs of control policies (Chapter 7, Chapter 10 and Chapter 13). We now ask whether tobacco control is cost-effective relative to other health interventions. For governments considering intervention, such information may be a further important factor in deciding how to proceed.

The cost-effectiveness of different health interventions can be evaluated by estimating the expected gain in years of healthy life that each will achieve in return for the requisite public costs needed to implement that intervention. According to the World Bank's World Development Report, *Investing in Health* (1993), interventions are considered to be cost-effective if they save a year of healthy life for less than the average gross domestic product per capita of the country. That same report found tobacco-control policies to be cost-effective and worthy of inclusion in a minimal package of healthcare. Existing studies (summarized in Jha *et al.* (1998)) suggest that policy-based programs cost about US$20 to $80 per discounted year of healthy life saved. (For a full explanation of the disability-adjusted life year, or DALY, the reader is referred to Murray and Lopez (1996).)

The purpose of this analysis is to estimate the effectiveness and cost-effectiveness of tobacco-control policies. We examine price increases, nicotine-replacement therapy (NRT), and non-price interventions other than NRT, separately. Effectiveness is measured in terms of the decrease in the number of smokers and decrease in tobacco-attributable deaths. The estimated costs of these interventions are entered into the model so as to generate broad estimates of cost-effectiveness. As with many cost-effectiveness analyses, this analysis is subject to considerable measurement error (Over 1991). Thus, we have ensured that assumptions err on the conservative side, so that the potential impact of the proposed package of interventions is, if anything, underestimated.

18.2 Methods

We have created a simple static model of the impact of tobacco-control policies using the 1995 baseline cohort of *current* smokers. This analysis is restricted to current smokers and is not a dynamic forecast model that includes cohorts of *future* smokers. There are several reasons for our choice of model. First, restricting analyses to current smokers provides results that are conservative, given that future smokers (mostly children) would be expected to be even more responsive to control policies than current smokers (see, for example, Chapter 10, for a discussion of how children are more price-responsive than adults). Second, most of the tobacco-attributable deaths that will occur over the next 50 years will be among current smokers (see Figure 19.1 in Chapter 19). Avoidance of death among this group is, therefore, the most pressing public policy question in tobacco control. Third, a model that incorporates future cohorts of non-smokers becoming smokers and then some of these smokers going on to death is more complex. Changes in future life expectancy, competing mortality, types of tobacco products used in the future, and variation in delay between exposure and disease are some of the factors that might affect whether a non-smoker takes up smoking and whether he or she eventually dies from it. It would be expected that our model would be sensitive to variation in age-specific responsiveness to control policies (Mendez *et al.* 1998). In response, we use conservative values wherever possible. We also limit the total variation in responsiveness to control policies to a certain value, even if age-specific variation is considerable. For example, the total price-elasticity for any region is the age-weighted average of the age-specific elasticities, and does not exceed –0.4 for high-income countries and –0.8 for low-income and middle-income countries. Finally, we present analyses of impact for mortality only, since the addition of disability results introduces further complexities, such as variation in disability weights across regions. However, in order to compare cost-effectiveness results with other studies, we convert these mortality estimates into DALYs, so that the cost in US dollars per healthy year of life saved can be seen.

We used smoking prevalence data for 89 countries from the World Health Organization (WHO 1997) and from the literature to derive estimates by age, region, and gender of smoking prevalence and the number of cigarettes smoked per day (see details in Chapter 2). From these numbers we took the following steps to estimate the global impact of price and non-price interventions.

18.2.1 Baseline numbers of smoking-attributable deaths by region, gender, and age

Using the total number of smokers alive in 1995 we made conservative assumptions about the numbers of deaths among these smokers. Recent studies in high-income countries, and in China and India (Chapter 1; Peto *et al.* 1994), suggest that at least one in two regular smokers who begin smoking during adolescence will eventually be killed by tobacco. The vast majority of smokers live in developing countries, where the prevalence of smoking has been rising in recent decades. Compared to populations in developed countries, these populations have higher death rates associated with causes other than tobacco, and fewer smokers have been smoking since early adult life. Thus, for a conservative analysis, the assumption of a mortality risk of one in two may be too high. The US Centers for Disease Control and Prevention (CDC) estimated how many children and adolescents aged 0–17 would become regular smokers as adults, and, recognizing that not all of them would stay as regular smokers, estimated that 32% of this smoking population would die prematurely from smoking-related diseases (CDC 1996). However, the applicability of these findings worldwide is uncertain. Quitting is rare in low-income and middle-income countries, where most smokers live, and thus the 1995 cohort of smokers probably represents long-term regular smokers (Chapter 2). Therefore, a one-in-three mortality risk may be too low. To be conservative, however, we assumed that 'only' one-third of current smokers would ultimately die of a smoking-attributable cause in all regions. The one-third risk is assumed to be true for males and females and for smokers of all ages. Further we assume that *bidis*, a type of hand-rolled cigarette common in South Asia, confer the same risk of premature death as cigarettes, based on epidemiological studies from India (Gajalakshmi and Peto 1997; Gupta and Mehta, in press). As noted below, we assume that men and women respond equally to interventions. Thus, the differences in results reflect underlying differences in smoking prevalence and age structure in 1995.

18.2.2 The potential impact of price increases

Step 1: Price-elasticity for low- and medium-income, and high-income regions

We assume a price-elasticity of –0.8 in low-income countries and –0.4 in high-income countries, based on an overall review of all available price-elasticity studies (Chapter 10). We reached similar values when we used alternative methods, such as relying on the most recent studies or averaging results across countries. To be conservative, we used short-run elasticities because they indicate a smaller response to a price increase than do long-term estimates. The price-elasticity of *bidis* in South Asia is assumed to be equal to the price-elasticity of cigarettes in low-income and middle-income regions. We base this assumption on the data from Finland (Pekurinen 1989) suggesting that price-responsiveness for hand-rolled cigarettes is approximately equal to that for cigarettes. It is assumed that price-elasticity is the same for males and females; while one study found that women were more responsive to price than men, other studies have suggested the opposite (Chaloupka and Warner, in press).

Step 2: Price-elasticity by age category

Most recent studies in high-income countries that have used nationally representative surveys have found that youth are more responsive to price changes than adults. This finding is consistent with economic theory. Based on several reviews (Warner 1986; Chaloupka 1998), we assume in this analysis that price-elasticity is three times higher amongst 15–19-year-olds, and 1.5 times higher amongst 20–29-year-olds, than amongst those 30 years of age and older. The total price-elasticity for any region is the age-weighted average of the age-specific elasticities, and does not exceed –0.4 for high-income countries and –0.8 for low- and middle-income countries.

Step 3: Impact of a price increase on the number of smokers and the number of smoking-attributable deaths

Price-elasticity expresses the *net* impact of a price change on the quantity demanded for cigarettes (or *bidis*). A price change can either impact on the *fact* of smoking (or prevalence) or the *rate* of smoking (conditional demand) by continuing smokers (CDC 1998). The relative impact of price on prevalence and on conditional demand varies across studies in OECD countries. For these analyses, we used a value of 50% for impact on prevalence. These come from various studies suggesting that slightly more than half of the price effect is on prevalence and just less than half is on average consumption by continuing smokers. Farrelly, for example, found that price-elasticity in the United States was –0.25, with a prevalence elasticity of –0.15 and conditional demand of –0.10 (CDC 1998). Chaloupka and Grossman (1996) and Chaloupka and Wechsler (1997) found that the effect on prevalence for youth and young adults, respectively, is about half of the overall effect. The effect of price on the prevalence of smoking may vary by age group, but for simplicity we assume constant effects on prevalence across age groups.

Calculations are performed for price increases of 10% and 100%. The results of the

100% price increase are more uncertain. Thus, we present these largely as illustrative, and focus the discussion on the smaller price increase. Change in the number of smokers is the product of:

(1) percentage change in the price of cigarettes;
(2) price-elasticity;
(3) impact of 50% on prevalence (see above); and
(4) total number of smokers.

Change in the number of smoking-attributable deaths is the product of:

(1) percentage change in the price of cigarettes;
(2) price-elasticity;
(3) prevalence impact of 50%;
(4) number of tobacco-attributable deaths prior to the price increase; and
(5) a 'mortality adjustment factor'.

Mortality adjustment is intended to account for the fact that not all smokers will be able to avoid a premature, tobacco-related death by quitting. As of yet, there are few large epidemiological studies that provide reliable studies of the age- and sex-specific benefits of cessation. The likelihood of avoiding such a death depends on several factors, including the number of years of smoking, the number of cigarettes smoked per day, and the presence or absence of disease at the time of quitting. Several studies suggest that the reduction in risk with cessation is not linear with age. The results of the American Cancer Society's Cancer Prevention Study II show that although the benefits of cessation extend to quitting at older ages, the relative reduction in risk of dying is greatest for younger quitters (USDHHS 1990). Doll *et al.* (1994) found that doctors in the United Kingdom who quit before age 35 returned to life-table estimates of mortality very close to those of people who had never smoked. Smokers who quit at ages 35–44, 45–54, 55–64, and 65 or older, were also found to have reduced risks of tobacco-related death, but these risks appeared not have a linear relationship with the age of quitting. Earlier work by Peto (1986) suggests that, at least for lung cancers, a three-fold increase in the duration of exposure would increase lung-cancer risk by 100-fold, whereas a three-fold increase in the number of cigarettes smoked daily would increase the risk by only three-fold. Based on data from these studies, we make the following conservative assumptions: 95% of quitters aged 15–29 years will avoid tobacco-related death, while only 75% of quitters aged 30–39, 70% of quitters aged 40–49, 50% of quitters aged 50–59, and 10% of quitters aged 60 or older will avoid tobacco-related death. In keeping with the conservative nature of this analysis, we assume that a decrease in the rate of smoking by those who continue smoking has no impact on mortality.

18.2.3 The potential impact of NRT

The aim of NRT is to provide smokers with modest doses of nicotine in an attempt to suppress the craving for cigarettes. NRT in its various forms (chewing gum, transdermal patches, nasal spray, and inhalers) has repeatedly been shown to increase smokers' chances of quitting (Chapter 12; Raw *et al.* 1998; Silagy *et al.* 1998). A recent meta-analysis found that rates of cessation after at least 6 months are 1.73 times higher with NRT than in controls (Silagy *et al.* 1998). A previous meta-analysis by the same authors found that the pooled abstinence rates (at the longest duration of follow-up available) were 19% among those allocated to NRT and 11% among controls (Silagy *et al.* 1994). Despite this evidence for the efficacy of NRT (most of it from high-income countries), it is difficult to estimate the effectiveness of NRT in real-world settings. Even if NRT could be made widely available at low cost (or even for free), it is difficult to know how many people would choose to access it and use it as indicated.

We estimate that NRTs have an overall effectiveness of 0.5–2.5%. This effectiveness range was derived from reviews of NRT use in the United States (Shiffman *et al.* 1997, 1998), which found that about 40–50% of smokers want to quit and that, of these, between 5% and 35% would wish to use NRTs. We assume that adults of ages 30–59 years will be more willing and able to use this intervention than individuals of ages 15–29 years, and 60 years and older, given they have more disposable income, and are more likely to be aware of the risks of smoking and the benefits of cessation (USDHHS 1990). Hence, NRT is assumed to be 1.5 times as effective among adults aged 30–59 as among other adults.

18.2.4 Potential impact of non-price interventions other than NRT

Non-price interventions other than NRT include the following: complete bans on advertising and promotion of all tobacco products, related logos or trademarks; dissemination of information on the health consequences of smoking (including new research findings); and restrictions on smoking in public places and work places. Complete bans on advertising and promotion may have a modest impact on prevalence (see Chapter 9). As discussed in detail by Kenkel and Chen (Chapter 8), information 'shocks' and new research in the United States in the 1960s are judged to have been responsible for reducing the prevalence of smoking by 5–10% (USDHHS 1989). Workplace bans on smoking in the United States are judged to have reduced total smoking prevalence by approximately 4–10% (Chapter 11). Specific attempts to quantify the aggregate impact of non-price interventions have not yet been made. Thus, in this analysis, it is assumed that a package including all of the non-price interventions would reduce prevalence by between 2% and 10%. Given research that youths are more sensitive to advertising and promotion, at least in the United States (DiFranza *et al.* 1991), we assume that a complete ban on advertising and promotion would more likely effect adolescents. On the other hand, clean-air laws and mass information are more likely to reduce adult smoking. Low-income and middle-income countries can more easily enforce advertising and promotion bans than they can clean-air laws (see Table 11.1 in Chapter 11). For these reasons, we assume constant effectiveness of a package of these interventions across age groups.

18.2.5 Cost-effectiveness of anti-smoking interventions

Many tobacco-control policies cost very little. Tax increases can often be done by legislation alone, if a strong tax-collection system is in place. To be conservative, we estimate that interventions, such as research dissemination and mass counter-advertising campaigns, incur administrative costs, and that tax increases incur enforcement costs to collect taxes. We further assume that one-time costs for NRTs would be required to help some of the 1995 cohort of smokers to quit. We use the same annual, public-sector costs for both price increases and the set of non-price interventions other than NRT. Based on costing estimates in the World Bank Review of Disease Control Priorities (Barnum and Greenberg 1993), and an unpublished review of costs for mass information campaigns in World Bank projects, we assume that the annual costs of *each* are 0.005–0.02% of current Gross National Product (GNP). The low end of this range approximates actual levels of spending on tobacco control in North America. For example, expenditure on tobacco research and education in Canada totalled 0.009% of GNP in 1996 and 0.002% in 1997. In the United States, an average of 0.003% of GNP was spent on tobacco research and education from 1994 to 1996 (Pechman *et al.* 1998). The US Centers for Disease Control and Prevention (CDC 1999) recommends that American states spend 0.026–0.036% of GNP on tobacco research and education. This level slightly exceeds the high end of the range used in this analysis. World Bank estimates of GNP for each of the regions are used (in 1997 US dollars). The assumed cost of the NRT intervention can be broken down into two components. The first is the 'non-drug' costs of the intervention (e.g. administrative and education costs). These costs are assumed to be the same as the cost of a price increase and the cost of non-price interventions other than NRT (i.e. 0.005–0.02% of GNP per person per year). The second component is the cost of the drugs themselves (i.e. the cost of nicotine gum, patches, etc.). Based on industrial marketing data (IMS 1998) we assume that each individual who attempts to quit in low-income or middle-income countries will spend $50 for short-term use of NRT. In high-income countries we assume that the amount spent will be $100. Further, based on data from Silagy *et al.* (1998), we calculate NRT costs to include the fact that for every person who is successful at quitting, ten others will use NRT unsuccessfully. The costs of a price increase and of NRT are assumed to occur only for the year of implementation. Non-price interventions, in contrast, comprise ongoing costs for counter-advertising and research, so these costs are assumed to recur each year for a period of 30 years. Costs of interventions are discounted by between 3% and 10% per annum.

The effectiveness of the interventions is measured by the numbers of deaths averted, calculated as described above. Future deaths among the cohort of smokers alive in 1995 are converted into DALYs using the region-specific ratios of tobacco-attributable deaths from a study by Murray and Lopez (1996; WHO 1996). Murray and Lopez estimate that DALYs lost will be at a steady rate over the next 30 years. The exact trend in deaths or DALYs is uncertain. A linear trend seems reasonable, given projections from China (Liu *et al.* 1998). Like costs, DALYs lost in the future are discounted by between 3% and 10%.

18.3 Results

18.3.1 Baseline estimates of smoking-attributable deaths

Of the estimated 1.1 billion smokers in 1995, it is estimated that one-third, or about 377 million, will ultimately die of a smoking-related illness (Table 18.1). Low-income

Table 18.1 Estimated number of smokers alive in 1995 who will ultimately die of smoking-attributable causes, by region

Region	Smoking-attributable deaths	
	Number (millions)	Percentage of total
East Asia and Pacific	136	36
Europe and Central Asia	48	13
Latin America and Caribbean	31	8
Middle East and North Africa	13	4
South Asia (cigarettes)	29	8
South Asia (bidis)	33	9
Sub-Saharan Africa	19	5
Low-income and middle-income	310	82
High-income	68	18
World	377	100

Source: authors' calculations. Note: numbers have been rounded.

and middle-income countries account for 82% (or 310 million) smoking-attributable deaths, and an equivalent percentage of the world's population aged 15 years and older. East Asia and the Pacific, which includes China, accounts for 36% (136 million) of smoking-attributable deaths, but only 32% of the population aged 15 years and over.

18.3.2 Potential impact of price increases

With a price increase of 10%, it is predicted that more than 40 million people will quit smoking worldwide (4% of all smokers in 1995, Table 18.2). This same price increase will result in 10 million smoking-attributable deaths being averted (3% of all smoking-attributable deaths expected amongst those who smoke in 1995). A price increase of 100% results in proportional increases in these outcome variables. Low-income and middle-income countries account for about 90% of quitters and averted deaths. East Asia and the Pacific alone account for roughly 40% of quitters and averted deaths.

Of the tobacco-related deaths that would be averted by a price increase, 80% would be male, reflecting the higher overall prevalence of smoking in men (Table 18.3). The greatest relative impact of a price increase on deaths averted is among younger age-cohorts. With a price increase of 100%, more than 80% of smoking-attributable deaths amongst smokers who are 15–19 years of age in 1995 would be averted, and about 40% of deaths amongst smokers aged 20–29 in 1995 would be averted. A significant portion

Table 18.2 Change in number of smokers and smoking-attributable deaths with price increases of 10% and 100%, by World Bank region, for smokers alive in 1995

Region	Change in number of smokers in millions (and % of all smokers) with price increases of			Change in number of deaths in millions (and % of all smoking deaths expected) with price increases of		
	10%	100%	% Total	10%	100%	% Total
East Asia and Pacific	−16.5 −(4.0)	−165.2 −(40.0)	39.7	−4.3 −(3.1)	−42.8 −(31.4)	41.3
Europe and Central Asia	−5.8 −(4.0)	−57.9 −(40.0)	13.9	−1.4 −(3.0)	−14.2 −(29.8)	13.8
Latin America and Caribbean	−3.8 −(4.0)	−38.1 −(40.0)	9.1	−1.0 −(3.3)	−10.4 −(33.3)	10.1
Middle East and North Africa	−1.6 −(4.0)	−16.1 −(40.0)	3.9	−0.4 −(3.0)	−4.0 −(29.9)	3.8
South Asia (cigarettes)	−3.5 −(4.0)	−35.3 −(40.0)	8.5	−0.7 −(2.5)	−7.3 −(25.0)	7.0
South Asia (bidis)	−4.0 −(4.0)	−39.5 −(40.0)	9.5	−0.8 −(2.5)	−8.1 −(24.8)	7.8
Sub-Saharan Africa	−2.4 −(4.0)	−23.6 −(40.0)	5.7	−0.7 −(3.4)	−6.6 −(33.8)	6.3
Low-income and middle-income	−37.6 −(4.0)	−375.7 −(40.0)	90.2	−9.3 −(3.0)	−93.4 −(30.1)	90.2
High-income	−4.1 −(2.0)	−40.9 −(20.0)	9.8	−1.0 −(1.5)	−10.1 −(15.0)	9.8
World	−41.7 −(3.6)	−416.6 −(36.4)	100.0	−10.3 −(2.7)	−103.5 −(27.4)	100.0

Source: authors' calculations.

(40%) of deaths averted will occur among smokers who are aged 30 years and older at the time of cessation.

18.3.3 Potential impact of NRT

Provision of NRTs with an effectiveness of 0.5% is predicted to result in about 6 million people giving up smoking and 1 million smoking-attributable deaths being averted (Table 18.4). NRT of 2.5% effectiveness is predicted to have five times the impact. Low-income and middle-income countries account for roughly 80% of quitters and averted deaths, and more than 70% of the global decrease in tobacco consumption.

Table 18.3 Worldwide change in number of smoking-attributable deaths, with a price increase of 100%, by age and gender, for smokers alive in 1995

Age categories	Males		Females		Males and Females	
	Number in millions (and % of all male smoking deaths in each category)	% of all averted male smoking deaths	Number in millions (and % of all female smoking deaths in each category)	% of all averted female smoking deaths	Number in millions (and % of all smoking deaths in each category)	% of all averted smoking deaths
15–19	−23.2 −(81.8)	27.0	−3.1 −(75.9)	17.6	−26.3 −(81.1)	25.4
20–29	−27.7 −(39.5)	32.2	−6.7 −(37.0)	38.2	−34.4 −(39.0)	33.2
30–39	−16.8 −(21.6)	19.5	−3.8 −(19.7)	21.6	−20.6 −(21.2)	19.9
40–49	−12.1 −(20.1)	14.1	−2.6 −(18.4)	15.2	−14.7 −(19.8)	14.2
50–59	−5.2 −(14.7)	6.1	−1.0 −(13.9)	5.9	−6.3 −(14.5)	6.1
60+	−1.0 −(2.9)	1.1	−0.3 −(3.0)	1.6	−1.3 −(3.0)	1.2
TOTAL	−86.0 −(28.2)	100.0	−17.4 −(24.2)	100.0	−103.5 −(27.4)	100.0
% Total	83.1		16.9		100.0	

Source: authors' calculations.

Males account for about 80% of tobacco-attributable deaths averted as a result of NRT (Table 18.5). The relative impact of NRT on deaths averted is 1.4–2.2% amongst individuals aged 15–59 years, and lower amongst those 60 years and older. The cohort aged 30–59 in 1995 will account for 65% of deaths averted.

18.3.4 Potential impact of non-price interventions other than NRT

A package of non-price interventions, other than NRT, that decreases the prevalence of smoking by 2% is predicted to cause about 23 million people to quit smoking world-wide (2% of all smokers in 1995, Table 18.6). This same package of interventions would result in about 5 million smoking-attributable deaths being averted (1% of all smoking-attributable deaths amongst those who smoke in 1995). A package of interventions that decreases the prevalence of smoking by 10% would have an impact five times greater. As with NRT, low-income and middle-income countries account for approximately three-quarters of quitters and averted deaths.

Of all tobacco-attributable deaths averted as a result of non-price interventions, 80% would be male (Table 18.7). The greatest relative impact of non-price interventions on deaths averted would be among younger age cohorts. A package that results in a 10%

Table 18.4 Change in number of smokers and smoking-attributable deaths with NRT of 0.5% and 2.5% effectiveness, by World Bank region, for smokers alive in 1995

Region	Change in number of smokers in millions (and % of all smokers) with effectiveness of			Change in number of deaths in millions (and % of all smoking deaths expected) with effectiveness of		
	0.5%	2.5%	% Total	0.5%	2.5%	% Total
East Asia and Pacific	−2.1 −(0.5)	−10.3 −(2.5)	36	−0.5 −(0.4)	−2.4 −(1.8)	37
Europe and Central Asia	−0.7 −(0.5)	−3.6 −(2.5)	13	−0.2 −(0.3)	−0.8 −(1.7)	13
Latin America and Caribbean	−0.5 −(0.5)	−2.4 −(2.5)	8	−0.1 −(0.4)	−0.6 −(1.9)	9
Middle East and North Africa	−0.2 −(0.5)	−1.0 −(2.5)	4	−0.05 −(0.3)	−0.2 −(1.7)	3
South Asia (cigarettes)	−0.4 −(0.5)	−2.2 −(2.5)	8	−0.1 −(0.3)	−0.4 −(1.5)	7
South Asia (bidis)	−0.5 −(0.5)	−2.5 −(2.5)	9	−0.1 −(0.3)	−0.5 −(1.5)	7
Sub-Saharan Africa	−0.3 −(0.5)	−1.5 −(2.5)	5	−0.1 −(0.4)	−0.4 −(1.9)	6
Low-income and middle-income	−4.7 −(0.5)	−23.5 −(2.5)	82	−1.1 −(0.3)	−5.4 −(1.7)	82
High-income	−1.0 −(0.5)	−5.1 −(2.5)	18	−0.2 −(0.3)	−1.2 −(1.7)	18
World	−5.7 −(0.5)	−28.6 −(2.5)	100	−1.3 −(0.3)	−6.6 −(1.7)	100

Source: authors' calculations.

decrease in smoking prevalence would avert roughly 10% of smoking deaths amongst smokers aged 15–29 in 1995, and 5–9% of deaths amongst smokers aged 30–59 in 1995. The cohort aged 20–29 in 1995 will account for the greatest percentage (about 32%) of deaths averted.

18.3.5 Cost-effectiveness of anti-smoking interventions

Price increases are found to be the most cost-effective anti-smoking intervention. These could be achieved for a cost of US$18–151 per DALY saved globally. Wider access to NRT could be achieved for between $353 and $1869 per DALY saved, depending on a wide range of conditions. Non-price interventions other than NRT

Table 18.5 Worldwide change in number of smoking-attributable deaths, with NRT of 2.5% effectiveness, by age and gender, for smokers alive in 1995

Age categories	Males		Females		Males and Females	
	Number in millions (and % of all male smoking deaths in each category)	% of all averted male smoking deaths	Number in millions (and % of all female smoking deaths in each category)	% of all averted female smoking deaths	Number in millions (and % of all smoking deaths in each category)	% of all averted smoking deaths
15–19	−0.5 −(1.9)	9.9	−0.1 −(1.9)	6.0	−0.6 −(1.9)	9.2
20–29	−1.3 −(1.9)	24.5	−0.3 −(1.9)	26.8	−1.6 −(1.9)	24.9
30–39	−1.7 −(2.2)	31.9	−0.4 −(2.2)	33.6	−2.1 −(2.2)	32.2
40–49	−1.2 −(2.0)	22.9	−0.3 −(2.0)	23.5	−1.5 −(2.0)	23.0
50–59	−0.5 −(1.4)	9.7	−0.1 −(1.5)	8.7	−0.6 −(1.5)	9.5
60+	−0.1 −(0.2)	1.2	0.0 −(0.2)	1.5	−0.1 −(0.2)	1.3
TOTAL	−5.3 −(1.8)	100.0	−1.2 −(1.7)	100.0	−6.6 −(1.7)	100.0
% Total	81.1		18.9		100.0	

Source: authors' calculations.

could be implemented for between $140 and $2805 per DALY saved, again, with a wide range of conditions (Table 18.8). Thus, NRT and other non-price measures are slightly less cost-effective than price increases, but remain cost-effective in many settings.

For a given set of assumptions, the variation in the cost-effectiveness of each intervention between low-income and middle-income regions is relatively small. All three interventions are most cost-effective in South Asia and Sub-Saharan Africa, and least cost-effective in Latin America and the Caribbean. The difference between low-income and middle-income countries, and high-income countries is more pronounced. For NRT, the cost per year of healthy life gained is three to eight times higher in high-income countries than elsewhere. For non-price interventions other than NRT, the cost in high-income countries is 20 times higher; and for price increases, almost 40 times higher.

The estimates of cost-effectiveness are subject to wide ranges. For price increases, the high-end estimates are roughly eight times the low-end estimates, and this difference is consistent among the regions. For NRT, the high-end estimates are 2.5–10 times the low-end estimates, varying among the regions. Finally, for non-price interventions

Table 18.6 Change in number of smokers and smoking-attributable deaths, with non-price interventions (other than NRT) of 2% and 10% effectiveness, by World Bank region, for smokers alive in 1995

Region	Change in number of smokers in millions (and % of all smokers) with effectiveness of			Change in number of deaths in millions (and % of all smoking deaths expected) with effectiveness of		
	2%	10%	% Total	2%	10%	% Total
East Asia and Pacific	−8.3 −(2.0)	−41.3 −(10.0)	36.1	−2.0 −(1.4)	−9.9 −(7.2)	37.2
Europe and Central Asia	−2.8 −(2.0)	−14.5 −(10.0)	12.7	−0.7 −(1.4)	−3.3 −(7.0)	12.6
Latin America and Caribbean	−1.8 −(1.9)	−9.5 −(10.0)	8.3	−0.5 −(1.6)	−2.5 −(7.9)	9.3
Middle East and North Africa	−0.8 −(2.0)	−4.0 −(10.0)	3.5	−0.2 −(1.4)	−0.9 −(6.9)	3.5
South Asia (cigarettes)	−1.8 −(2.0)	−8.8 −(10.0)	7.7	−0.3 −(1.2)	−1.7 −(5.9)	6.5
South Asia (bidis)	−2.0 −(2.0)	−9.9 −(10.0)	8.6	−0.4 −(1.2)	−1.9 −(5.9)	7.2
Sub-Saharan Africa	−1.1 −(1.9)	−5.9 −(10.0)	5.1	−0.3 −(1.6)	−1.5 −(7.9)	5.8
Low-income and middle-income	−18.6 −(2.0)	−93.9 −(10.0)	82.1	−4.4 −(1.4)	−21.8 −(7.0)	82.1
High-income	−4.0 −(2.0)	−20.5 −(10.0)	17.9	−0.9 −(1.4)	−4.7 −(7.0)	17.9
World	−22.6 −(2.0)	−114.4 −(10.0)	100.0	−5.3 −(1.4)	−26.5 −(7.0)	100.0

Source: authors' calculations.

other than NRT, the high-end estimates are 20 times the low-end estimates, and this difference is consistent among the regions.

18.4 Discussion

Our analyses suggest that price increases of 10% would be the most effective and cost-effective of the three interventions examined. Accepting that the results in this study represent very conservative estimates, the reductions in mortality are still quite impressive. Price increases as low as 10%, NRT use that enables 0.5% of smokers to quit, and

Table 18.7 Worldwide change in number of smoking-attributable deaths, with non-price interventions (other than NRT) of 10% effectiveness, by age and gender, for smokers alive in 1995

Age categories	Males		Females		Males and Females	
	Number in millions (and % of all male smoking deaths in each category)	% of all averted male smoking deaths	Number in millions (and % of all female smoking deaths in each category)	% of all averted female smoking deaths	Number in millions (and % of all smoking deaths in each category)	% of all averted smoking deaths
15–19	–2.7 –(9.5)	13	–0.4 –(9.5)	8	–3.1 –(9.5)	12
20–29	–6.7 –(9.5)	31	–1.7 –(9.5)	34	–8.4 –(9.5)	32
30–39	–5.8 –(7.5)	27	–1.4 –(7.5)	29	–7.3 –(7.5)	27
40–49	–4.2 –(7.0)	20	–1.0 –(7.0)	20	–5.2 –(7.0)	20
50–59	–1.8 –(5.0)	8	–0.4 –(5.0)	7	–2.2 –(5.0)	8
60+	–0.3 –(1.0)	2	–0.1 –(1.0)	2	–0.4 –(1.0)	2
TOTAL	–21.5 –(7.0)	100	–5.0 –(6.9)	100	–26.5 –(7.0)	100
% Total	81.1		18.9		100.0	

Source: authors' caculations.

non-price interventions that reduce smoking prevalence by 2%, could save many lives if applied to large populations. Table 18.9 summarizes these results.

8.4.1 Comparison with existing estimates

We can compare our results against existing studies only for high-income countries, given the lack of studies in low-income countries. Moore (1996) has conducted the only direct study of the deaths avoided by tax increases on tobacco. Using data from the United States on tobacco-related death rates for the period from 1954 through 1988, he estimated the impact of an increase of 10% in the cigarette tax. Assuming that taxes are 25% of price, a 10% tax increase results in a price increase of 2.5%. The higher price resulted in a 1.5% decrease in the annual number of deaths from respiratory cancers and a 0.5% decrease in the annual number of deaths from cardiovascular disease. Based on mortality data from Peto *et al.* (1994), this represents a short-run decrease in tobacco-related deaths of more than 1.5%. Other studies using an indirect methodology similar to ours have generally found greater reductions in smoking or smoking-attributable mortality with smaller price increases (Harris 1983; Warner 1986;

Table 18.8 Range of cost-effectiveness values for price, NRT and non-price interventions (US dollars/DALY saved), by region

Region	Price increase of 10%		NRT effectiveness of 0.5–2.5%		Non-price other than NRT effectiveness of 2–10%	
	Low-end Estimate[1]	High-end Estimate[2]	Low-end Estimate[3]	High-end Estimate[4]	Low-end Estimate[5]	High-end Estimate[6]
East Asia and Pacific	3	26	335	911	26	527
Europe and Central Asia	4	33	227	739	33	658
Latin America and Caribbean	10	87	241	1213	86	1726
Middle East and North Africa	7	58	223	944	60	1192
South Asia	2	16	289	722	15	309
Sub-Saharan Africa	2	19	196	566	19	386
Low-income and middle-income	4	34	276	851	34	685
High-income	165	1370	749	7142	689	13775
World	18	151	353	1869	140	2805

[1] Calculations based on: intevention cost of 0.005% of GNP, benefits (DALYs saved) distributed over 30 years, and discounted at 3%.
[2] Calculations based on: intervention cost of 0.02% of GNP, benefits distributed over 30 years and discounted at 10%.
[3] Calculations based on: effectiveness of 2.5%, intervention cost of 0.005% of GNP (plus drug costs), benefits distributed over 30 years, and discounted at 3%.
[4] Calculations based on: effectiveness of 0.5%, intervention cost of 0.02% of GNP (plus drug costs), benefits distributed over 30 years, and discounted at 10%.
[5] Calculations based on: effectiveness of 10%, intervention cost of 0.005% of GNP and repeated annually over 30 years, and discounted at 3%, benefits distributed over 30 years and discounted at 3%.
[6] Calculations based on: effectiveness of 2%, intervention cost of 0.02% of GNP and repeated annually over 30 years, and discounted at 10%, benefits distributed over 30 years and discounted at 10%.

Source: authors' calculations.

Chaloupka 1998). For example, Warner (1986) estimated that an increase of 8% in cigarette prices in the United States would avoid about 450 000 deaths, or about 3% of the tobacco-attributable deaths. In contrast, we find that in high-income countries, a 10% price increase would decrease tobacco-attributable premature deaths by 1.5%. This suggests our analyses are conservative.

Our cost-effectiveness results for high-income countries appear to be conservative compared with those of other studies in high-income countries. A 1997 study from the United Kingdom found that the cost per life-year gained using community-wide interventions varied from £107 to £3622 (approximately US$171–5800). Brief advice from a physician was found to cost £469 ($750) per life-year saved, while the addition of nicotine gum cost £2370 ($3800) per life-year saved (Buck *et al.* 1997). In general,

Table 18.9 Summary of effectiveness of tobacco-control policies, by region

Region	Change in the number of smokers (million)			Change in the number of deaths (million)		
	10% price increase	NRT that enables 0.5% of smokers to quit	Non-price measures that reduce smoking prevalence by 2%	10% price increase	NRT that enables 0.5% of smokers to quit	Non-price measures that reduce smoking prevalence by 2%
Low-income and middle income	−37.6	−4.7	−18.6	−9.3	−1.1	−4.4
High-income	−4.1	−1.0	−4.0	−1.0	−0.2	−0.9
World	−41.7	−5.7	−22.6	−10.3	−1.3	−5.3

Source: authors' calculations.

these results fall within the lower half of our range of estimates of cost-effectiveness for high-income countries. A separate study of nicotine gum found that, as an adjunct to counseling, it would cost between $4113 and $6465 per year of life saved for males, and between $6880 and $9473 per year of life saved for females (Oster *et al.* 1986). Another study found the cost-effectiveness of nicotine patch therapy matched with brief physical counselling to range from $4390 for 35–39-year-old males to $10 943 for 65–69-year-old males (Fiscella and Franks 1996). These values overlap with the higher end of the range of estimates of cost-effectiveness of NRT for high-income countries calculated above. An evaluation of a proposed mass television campaign for the United Kingdom suggested that one year of life could be saved for US$10–20 (Reid 1996). This value falls far below the range of cost-effectiveness values for non-price interventions other than NRT calculated in the present analysis. Reid assumed lower costs (US$18 million per year, or 0.0015% of GNP), and a quit rate of 2.5%.

8.4.2 Comparing cost-effectiveness to other health interventions

Our findings suggest that these interventions are also cost-effective relative to other health interventions (Table 18.8). The cost-effectiveness of tax increases compares favorably with many health interventions. Depending on the assumptions made about the administrative costs of raising and monitoring higher tobacco taxes, the cost of implementing a price increase of 10% ranges from $4 to $34 per DALY in low-income and middle-income countries Table 18.10 summarizes these results.

Countries that implement these interventions may experience much wider ranges (see Table 18.8, where for the low-income and middle-income countries, the values for price increases of 10% range from 2 to 87). Overall, tax increases represent cost-effectiveness values comparable to many health interventions financed by governments, such as child immunization (cost per DALY of about $25; World Bank 1993). Non-price measures may also be highly cost-effective for low-income and middle-

Table 18.10 Summary of cost-effectiveness of tobacco control policies, by region, in US$ per DALY

Region	Price increases of 10%	Non-price measures with effectiveness of 2–10%	NRTs with effectiveness of 0.5–2.5%
Low-income and middle income	4–34	276–851	34–685
High-income	165–1370	749–7142	689–13775
World	18–151	353–1869	140–2805

Source: authors' calculations.

income countries. Depending on the assumptions on which the estimates are based, a package could be delivered for as little as $34 per DALY. This level of cost-effectiveness compares reasonably with several established interventions in public health, such as the package for the integrated management of the sick child, which has been estimated to cost between $30 and $50 per DALY in low-income countries and between $50 and $100 in middle-income countries (WHO 1996). NRT and other non-price interventions are also likely to be good investments, but the extent to which they should be utilized should be determined with country-specific cost-effectiveness analyses.

8.4.3 Effectiveness by region and with combined interventions

In this analysis, the effectiveness of non-price interventions is assumed to be the same in all regions. It may be possible, however, that effectiveness of these interventions differs between countries. For example, information campaigns may be much more effective in developing countries, given the relative novelty of the information (Chapter 8), and thus their impact might be similar to the impact of the health reports of the 1960s in the United States and the United Kingdom. One could similarly argue that advertising and promotion bans would also be relatively more effective in these countries. In contrast, clean-air laws are less likely to have an effect in low-income countries (Chapter 11).

No attempt has been made in this analysis to examine the impact of combining the various packages of interventions (e.g. price increases with NRT, or NRT and other non-price interventions). Although a number of studies have compared the impact of price and non-price interventions, few empirical attempts have been made to assess how these interventions might interact (CDC 1996b). It might be expected that the marginal impact of one policy could be lower or higher in the presence of another. For example, if price increases and NRT both facilitate cessation amongst the small population that is 'least addicted', then the impact of these two interventions combined might be less than the sum of their impacts if implemented independently. Alternatively, if these interventions act on different segments of the smoking population, then it is possible that the two interventions would interact in an additive fashion. It is also quite possible that interventions interact synergistically. For example, a mass-media campaign might potentiate the impact of NRT by making more people aware of the availability and benefits of this intervention.

8.4.4 Conservative assumptions on effectiveness and cost-effectiveness

Several features of our analyses suggest that our results are appropriately conservative. First, we use only the 1995 cohort of smokers, and ignore effects on future cohorts. Second, we estimate that 'only' one in three of current smokers are killed by their addiction. Third, we estimate that the reduced rate of smoking has no impact on mortality. Fourth, in estimating effectiveness, we do not calculate the additional benefits expected from reductions in morbidity over and above the benefits of preventing deaths (USDHHS 1990). Finally, our analysis is also conservative in estimating the public-sector costs of intervening. Some of the interventions, such as raising taxes or banning advertising and promotion, have zero or minimal costs, as these are 'stroke-of-the pen' interventions. To be conservative, we have assigned substantial implementation and administrative costs, along with drug costs for NRT.

Our assumptions on price elasticities merit further elaboration. We use short-run price-elasticities. In high-income countries, it appears that long-run elasticities may be two-fold higher. The long-run elasticity in low-income and middle-income countries may not be double the short-run elasticities in these countries, however. This is partly because the reasons that lower-income countries are more price-sensitive will have some impact on the ratio of short- to long-run elasticities, but would still be expected to be greater (Chapter 10). As such, our estimated reductions in mortality are likely to be smaller than the real number. In addition, we assume that price responsiveness for younger age groups is high and similar across regions. Economic theory would suggest that part of the greater price sensitivity in lower-income countries is for the same reasons as the greater price sensitivity of youth (Chapter 10). Thus, we might have over-estimated the impact of price changes on the prevalence of smoking in young people. Of course, for these same reasons, we might have under-estimated the impact on adult smoking in low-income countries, given that the overall price-responsiveness was fixed in our model not to exceed –0.8 for all age groups in those countries. Finally, we use a constant price-elasticity. An alternative is to assume linear demand, implying that elasticity rises as price rises, and that larger price increases produce disproportionately larger reductions in smoking. There is no reliable evidence population-based studies to verify a linear demand curve. However, some behavioral economics studies suggest that elasticity does rise with price (Bickel and Madden 1999).

It is important to point out that the costs assessed in our cost-effectiveness analyses do not include those borne by individuals. The omission of these costs from similar earlier analyses has led some experts to criticize them (Warner 1997). For example, it is difficult to describe the personal (or individual) costs of being prevented from smoking in certain places. As discussed in earlier chapters (e.g. Chapter 7), the biggest costs of tax increases are likely to be those borne by individuals. The welfare impact is difficult to estimate, given that welfare losses would differ for current smokers versus future smokers, and because of information and addiction issues. Moreover, the inclusion of such costs would force us to enter the more complex area of cost–benefit analyses, which require the analyst to impose a dollar value on a year or human life, which many are unwilling to do, and also to include non-health burdens, such as lost income from disease. For the purposes of the health sector, cost-effectiveness analyses are assumed to be a better choice. Private costs are, as a rule, not included in cost-effectiveness analyses of health interventions (Over 1991; Jamison 1993) and many health interventions do impose such costs. For example, child immunization imposes costs of parents taking time off work, travel to the clinic etc. Tobacco-control interventions are not, in principle, different from these other interventions.

18.5 Conclusions

Existing instruments of tax increases, a set of non-price information measures, and NRT policies, are all highly effective, and make small but quite worthwhile reductions in mortality. Several millions of premature deaths could be avoided with a combination of these interventions.

Tobacco control is cost-effective relative to other health interventions. Our analyses suggest that tax increases would be cost-effective. Non-price measures are also cost-effective in many settings. Measures to liberalize access to NRT, e.g. by changing the conditions for its sale, are likely to be cost-effective in most settings. However, individual countries would need to make careful assessments before deciding to provide subsidies for NRT and other cessation interventions for poor smokers. As with all cost-effectiveness analyses, our estimates are subject to considerable variation in actual settings, notably in costs. Thus, local cost-effectiveness studies are required to guide local policy.

References

Barnum, H. and Greenberg, R. E. (1993). Cancers. In *Disease Control Priorities in Developing Countries* (ed. D. T. Jamison, H. W Mosley, A. R. Measham, and J. L. Bobadilla), pp. 529–60. Oxford Medical Publications, New York.

Bickel, W. K. and Madden, G. J. (1997). *The Behavioral Economics of Smoking*. Presented at the National Bureau of Economic Research Conference on The Economic Analysis of Substance Use and Abuse: An Integration of Econometric and Behavioral Economic Research, Boston.

Buck, D., Godfrey, C., Parrott, S., and Raw, M. (1997). *Cost-effectiveness of Smoking Cessation Interventions*. Centre for Health Economics, University of York and Health Education Authority, York.

Centers for Disease Control and Prevention (1996a). Cigarette smoking before and after an excise tax increase and an antismoking campaign—Massachusetts, 1990–1996. *Morbidity and Mortality Weekly Report*, **45**(44), 996–70.

Centers for Disease Control and Prevention (1996b). Projected smoking-related deaths among youth—United States. *Morbidity and Mortality Weekly Report*, **45**(44), 966–70.

Centers for Disease Control and Prevention (1998). Response to increases in cigarette prices by race/ethnicity, income, and age groups—United States, 1976–1993. *Morbidity and Mortality Weekly Report*, **47**(29), 605–9.

Centers for Disease Control and Prevention (1999). *Best practices for Comprehensive Tobacco Control Programs–August 1999*. US Department of Health and Human Services, Centers for Disease Control and Prevention, National Center for Chronic Disease Prevention and Health Promotion, Office on Smoking and health, Atlanta GA.

Chaloupka, F. J. (1998). *The Impact of Proposed Cigarette Price Increases*. Policy Analysis No. 9, Health Science Analysis Project, Advocacy Institute, Washington D.C.

Chaloupka, F. J. and Grossman, M. (1996). *Price, Tobacco-control policies and Youth Tobacco Use*. National Bureau of Economic Research Working Paper number 5740.

Chaloupka, F. J. and Warner, K. E. The economics of smoking. In *The Handbook of Health Economics* (ed. J. Newhouse and A. Culyer). New York: North-Holland. (In press.)

Chaloupka, F. J. and Wechsler, H. (1997). Price, tobacco-control policies and smoking among young adults. *Journal of Health Economics*, **16**(3), 359–73.

DiFranza, J. R., Richards, J. W., Paulman, P. M., Wolf-Gillespie, N., Fletcher, C., Jaffe, R. D. *et al.* (1991). RJR Nabisco's cartoon camel promotes camel cigarettes to children. *JAMA*, **266**(22), 3149–53.

Doll, R., Peto, R., Wheatley, K., Gray, R., and Sutherland, I. (1994). Mortality in relation to smoking: 40 years' observations on male British doctors. *BMJ*, **309**, 901–11.

Fiscella, K. and Franks, P. (1996). Cost-effectiveness of the transdermal nicotine patch as an adjunct to physicians' smoking cessation counselling. *Journal of the American Medical Association*, **275**(16), 1247–51.

Gajalakshmi, C. K. and Peto, R. (1997). *Studies on Tobacco in Chennai, India*. Presented at the 10th World Conference on Tobacco or Health, Chinese Medical Association, Beijing.

Gupta, P. C. and Mehta, H. C. A cohort study of all-cause mortality among tobacco users in Mumbai, India. *The International Journal of Public Health*. (In press.)

Harris, J. E. (1987). The 1983 increase in the federal cigarette excise tax. In *Tax Policy and the Economy*, vol. 1 (ed. : L. H. Summers), pp. 87–111. MIT Press, Cambridge (MA).

IMS Global Services (1998). *Medical Information Database (MIDAS)*. Plymouth Meeting, PA, USA.

Jamison, D. T. (1993). Disease control priorities in developing countries: an overview. In *Disease Control Priorities in Developing Countries* (ed. D. T. Jamison, H. W. Mosley, A. R. Measham, and J. L. Bobadilla), pp. 3–34. Oxford Medical Publications, New York.

Jha, P., Novotny, T. E., and Feachem, R. (1998). The role of governments in global tobacco control. In *The Economics of Tobacco Control: Towards an Optimal Policy Mix* (ed. I. Abedian, R. van der Merwe, N. Wilkins, and P. Jha), pp. 38–56. Applied Fiscal Research Centre, University of Cape Town, South Africa.

Leu, R. E. and Schaub, T. (1983). Does smoking increase medical expenditures? *Social Science & Medicine*, **17**(23), 1907–14.

Liu, B. Q., Peto, R., Chen, Z. M., Boreham, J., Wu, Y. P., Li, J. Y. *et al.* (1998). Emerging tobacco hazards in China. I. Retrospective proportional mortality study of one million deaths. *BMJ*, **317**(7170), 1411–22.

Mendez, D., Warner, K. E., and Courant, P. N. (1998). Has smoking cessation ceased? Expected trends in the prevalence of smoking in the United States. *Am. J. Epidemiol.*, **148**(3), 249–58.

Moore, M. J. (1996). Death and tobacco taxes. *RAND Journal of Economics*, **27**(2), 415–28.

Murray, C. J. and Lopez, A. D. (ed.) (1996). *The Global Burden of Disease*. Harvard University Press, Boston.

Oster, G., Huse, D. M., Delea, T. E., and Colditz, G. A. (1986). Cost-effectiveness of nicotine gum as an adjunct to physician's advice against cigarette smoking. *JAMA*, **256**, 1315–18.

Over, M. (1991). *Economics for Health Sector Analyses: Concepts and Cases*. Economic Development Institute. Technical Materials. Washington. DC World Bank.

Pechman, C., Dixon, P., and Layne, N. (1998). An assessment of US and Canadian smoking reduction objectives for the year 2000. *Am. J. Public Health*, **88**(9), 1362–7.

Pekurinen, M. (1989). The demand for tobacco products in Finland. *British Journal of Addiction*, **84**, 1183–92.

Peto, R. (1986). Influence of dose and duration of smoking on lung cancer rates. In *Tobacco: a Major International Health Hazard* (ed. R. Peto and D. Zaridze), pp. 23–34. International Agency for Research on Cancer, Lyon. IARC Scientific Publications, no.74.

Peto, R., Lopez, A. D., Boreham, J., Thun, M., and Clark Jr, H. (1994). *Mortality from Smoking In Developing Countries 1950–2000*. New York: Oxford University Press.

Raw, M., McNeill, A., and West, R. (1998). Smoking cessation guidelines for health professionals. A guide to effective smoking cessation interventions for the health care system. Health Education Authority. *Thorax*, **53**(Supplement 5)(1), S1–19.

Reid, D. (1996). Tobacco control: overview. *British Medical Bulletin*, **52**(1), 108–20.

Shiffman, S., Gitchell, J., Pinney, J. M., Burton, S. L., Kemper, K. E., and Lara, E. A. (1997). The public health benefit of over-the-counter nicotine medications. *Tobacco Control*, **6**, 306–10.

Shiffman, S., Mason,, M. K., and Henningfield, J. E. (1998). Tobacco dependence treatments: review and prospectus. *Annual Review of Public Health*, **19**, 335–58.

Silagy, C., Mant, D., Fowler, G., and Lodge, M. (1994). Meta-analysis on efficacy of nicotine replacement therapies in smoking cessation. *The Lancet*, **343**, 139–142.

Silagy, C., Mant, D., Fowler, G., and Lancaster. T. (1998). Nicotine replacement therapy for smoking cessation (Cochrane Review). In *The Cochrane Library, Issue 4*. Oxford: Update Software.

US Department of Health and Human Services (1989). *Reducing the Health Consequences of Smoking: 25 Years of Progress. A Report of the Surgeon General*. Rockville, Maryland: US Department of Health and Human Services, Public Health Service, Centers for Disease Control, Center for Chronic Disease Prevention and Health Promotion, Office on Smoking and Health. DHHS Publication No. (CDC)89–8411.

US Department of Health and Human Services. (1990). *The health benefits of smoking cessation*. US Department of health and Human Services, Public Health Service, Centers for Disease Control, Center for Chronic Disease Prevention and Health Promotion, Office on Smoking and Health. DHHS Publication No. (CDC) 90–8416, 1990.

Warner, K. E. (1986). Smoking and health implications of a change in the federal cigarette excise tax. *JAMA*, **255**(8), 1028–32.

Warner, K. E. (1997). Cost-effectiveness of smoking cessation therapies: interpretation of the evidence and implications for coverage. *Pharmaco.Economics*, **11**, 538–49.

World Bank (1993). *World Development Report 1993: Investing in Health*. New York: Oxford University Press.

World Health Organization (WHO) (1996). *Investing in Health Research and Development*. Report of the Ad Hoc Committee on Health Research Relating to Future Intervention Options (Document TDR/Gen/96.1.), Geneva, Switzerland.

World Health Organization (WHO) (1997). *Tobacco or Health: a Global Status Report*. Geneva: World Health Organisation.

19

Strategic priorities in tobacco control for governments and international agencies

Prabhat Jha, Fred Paccaud, and Son Nguyen

Any review of strategic priorities in tobacco control will tend to be simplistic, given the variation in factors affecting policy at the local level. The key goal of comprehensive tobacco-control programs is to improve health, but correcting market failures and reducing inequality are other important goals. For short-term progress in reducing mortality, programs need to be focused both on reducing the uptake of smoking by children and on helping adults to quit. Most tobacco-control programs will be a combination of price, information, and regulation interventions, but the relative importance of each of these three components will vary across countries by income level and administrative capacity. Where such combined control programs have been evaluated, they appear to be effective, and they can be implemented at low per capita costs. We examine some responsibilities of the international agencies reviewing their own policies and programs, acting regionally on specific control instruments, and sponsoring research. Finally, the political economy of tobacco control is discussed.

19.1 Introduction

While the health arguments for acting against tobacco are largely beyond dispute, there is substantial debate on the economics of tobacco control. Many believe that smoking is a sovereign choice made by informed adults, and that, as such, the state has no business intervening (*The Economist* 1995, 1997). The tobacco industry has argued that measures to reduce tobacco demand would reduce tax revenues, cause massive and sudden unemployment, and increase smuggling. Finally, some in the public health community have doubted the efficacy of price interventions (Pierce *et al.* 1998).

The preceding chapters of this volume address some of these economic questions. While much more research is required, several clear conclusions emerge. First, in addition to health reasons, governments are justified in intervening to correct the evident failures in the tobacco market. These failures, which result in inefficient allocation of resources, are: a lack of information about the health consequences of tobacco use; a lack of information about the risks of addiction; and the costs imposed on non-smokers. Government intervention is also justified to reduce inequalities between rich and poor. A second key conclusion is that if tobacco taxes were increased, tax revenues would not fall in the short- to medium-term but rather would rise. A third conclusion is that measures to reduce tobacco demand would cause few, if any, net job losses in most economies around the world. Fourth, tobacco smuggling, although a serious and growing concern for some countries, is best addressed by tackling crime and not by lowering tax rates. Fifth, there are several effective and cost-effective interventions including price increases, information measures and greater access to nicotine replacement therapies (NRT).

This chapter describes key issues faced by countries and international developmental agencies in applying these interventions. Societies take into account many factors, and not only economics, in deciding on and implementing policies. The determination of suitable tobacco-control policies is a complex matter and policies must be tailored to each country. We do not aim to provide a blueprint for action at country level, but rather to provide a general framework, which various governments and international agencies may consider when reviewing their tobacco control policies.

We first discuss comprehensive national tobacco-control programs, focusing on their goals, targets, and instruments, relevance to different countries, effectiveness, and costs. Next, we outline some major challenges that require international action. Third, we suggest an agenda for research and development (R&D) in tobacco control. Finally, we discuss the political economy of implementing control programs.

19.2 National, comprehensive tobacco-control programs

Comprehensive control programs need to be based on multiple interventions, and they should include coordination and evaluation functions. The goals, targets, and instruments of such programs are briefly reviewed, as well as their costs and outcomes. We also ask how well such programs transfer between countries.

19.2.1 Goals, targets and instruments

The chief goal of a tobacco-control program is to improve health. In addition, such programs can address market failures by deterring children from smoking, protecting non-smokers, and providing all smokers with information about the effects of tobacco. As governments increasingly turn their attention to health inequalities (World Bank 1993), the reduction of inequalities in tobacco-attributable deaths between poor and non-poor groups becomes an additional goal. Table 19.1 shows the degree to which each of the three goals is met by a range of effective instruments.

Many societies might consider that the strongest reason for acting to control tobacco is to deter children and adolescents from smoking. The public health community has often focused on reducing the uptake of smoking by children (see, for example, Institute of Medicine (1994)). A group of economists also concluded that the strongest rationale for increasing tobacco taxes was to deter children from smoking (Warner *et al.* 1995).

However, interventions that specifically target only children and adolescents, such as youth information or restrictions on sales to young people, are unlikely to have the desired effect, especially if done in isolation (Chapter 7, Chapter 8, and Chapter 11). Interventions that *are* effective in dissuading children from smoking, chiefly tax increases, also reduce adult consumption.

In any case, tobacco-control policies with the sole effect of deterring children from

Table 19.1 Goals for tobacco control: policy and instruments

Policy instrument		Improve health	Correct market failures			Reduce inequalities in health outcomes
			Protect children	Protect non-smokers	Inform adults	
Demand side						
Taxation	Raise tax.	3	3	1	1	3
Information	Research causes, consequences and costs.	2	1	2	3	1
	Mass information, prominent warning labels.	2	2	2	2	2
Regulation	Ban advertising and promotion.	2	3	1	2	2
	Restrict public and workplace smoking.	2	1	3	1	1
	De-regulate nicotine replacement products.	1	0	1	2	2
Supply side						
	Control smuggling.	1	2	0	0	1

Source: authors' calculations, based on a survey of 23 economists and tobacco-control experts during a technical review meeting for this volume held in Lausanne, Switzerland, in November 1998.
3 = highly relevant, 2 = relevant, 1 = somewhat relevant, 0 = not relevant.

starting to smoke would have minimal impact on global smoking deaths for many decades, since most of the projected deaths for the first-half of the next century are those of existing smokers (see Fig. 19.1). There are, therefore, as we have seen, strong practical reasons for adopting control measures that affect adults as well as children.

Next, we discuss the optimal levels of control interventions. These levels will, of course, depend on each society's particular goals and willingness to accept the different control instruments. Take the complex question of the optimal tax on tobacco products. As Chaloupka *et al.* discussed in Chapter 10, any attempt to determine the optimal tax on cigarettes depends on empirical facts that are often difficult to measure, such as the scale of the costs to non-smokers, and the differing costs to smokers of different income levels. It also depends on varying societal values, such as the extent to which children should be protected, and the specific goal that the tax seeks to achieve, such as a specific gain in revenue or a specific reduction in disease burden. Townsend (1993), for example, suggests that a 64% increase in cigarette price by the year 2000 in the United Kingdom would have reduced cigarette use per adult by about 34%.

The optimal level of another major tobacco-control intervention, the provision of information to consumers, is equally dependent on each society's specific goals. If the

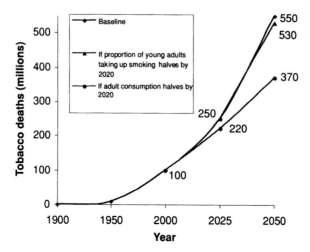

Fig. 19.1 Unless current smokers quit, tobacco deaths will rise steeply in the next 50 years. Estimated cumulative tobacco deaths 1900–2050 with different intervention strategies.

Note: Peto and others estimate that there were 60 million smoking-related deaths between 1950 and 2000 in the high-income countries and former socialist economies. Based on recent data from China and India, it appears likely that there were between 15 and 30 million deaths from tobacco use over the same time period in developing countries. We estimate an additional 5–15 million deaths worldwide between 1900 and 1950. Projections for deaths from 2000–2050 are based on Peto and Lopez (in press).

Source: Peto *et al.* (1994) and Peto and Lopez (in press).

goal is to ensure widespread awareness of the health risks of smoking then, as a minimum, local studies of the health consequences of tobacco are required. As Kenkel and Chen have discussed in Chapter 8, independent scientific reviews, such as reports by the United States Surgeon General and the United Kingdom Royal College of Physicians, were milestones in declines in consumption in high-income countries. Two major studies have recently published data on tobacco mortality in China (Liu *et al.* 1998; Niu *et al.* 1998) and smoking trends there will be carefully watched to see whether a comparable effect is seen.

In the high-income countries, research on the causes, the consequences, and the costs of tobacco use has contributed to a social climate where effective tobacco control can occur. The lack of such information in most low-income and middle-income countries may hinder control efforts. For example, in many of the countries where tobacco-attributable mortality will be highest in absolute numbers in the next few decades, there is a lack of direct evidence on the absolute and relative health risks from tobacco use in those regions (Chapter 2; Jha *et al.* 1998). Awareness of the health consequences of smoking appears to be a key determinant of the success of some other interventions. For example, high awareness of the consequences of environmental tobacco smoke helps to make clean-air laws 'self-enforcing', and awareness of the benefits of smoking cessation is likely to increase demand for NRTs.

There is widespread evidence that total bans on tobacco advertising and promotion are effective. Partial restrictions on advertising, in contrast, allow the tobacco industry to exploit other media and alternative promotional tactics (Chapter 9). Thus, unlike other interventions, the optimal level is always going to be the same: a total ban. In 1983, cigarette companies spent about $1.4 billion (in 1993 US dollars) on promotion and an equal amount on advertising in the United States. By 1993, they spent $5.5 billion on promotion and only $0.8 billion on advertising (Federal Trade Commission 1995). The European Union is moving towards a complete ban on tobacco advertising and promotion by 2006.

19.2.2 Policy instruments and their relevance in different countries

While current smoking patterns in low-income and middle-income countries are expected to cause unprecedented loss of life, it is clear from the analyses presented in the preceding chapters that mortality and disability can be substantially reduced with effective action. The experience of the industrialized countries shows that rising incomes in the earlier decades of the twentieth century initially led to increased consumption of tobacco, but that with increased information and education about the hazards of smoking, consumption is now in steady overall decline. Similar patterns might be expected to emerge in low-income and middle-income countries as information is made more widely available (Jha *et al.* 1998). Consumers in low-income and middle-income countries appear to be particularly responsive to price (Chapter 10). Table 19.2 assesses the relevance of the various policy instruments we have discussed to countries of different income levels. Clearly, this table has an heuristic value only, and individual countries would need to make their own assessments in the light of the evidence.

Many low-income countries could gain health benefits and higher revenues from taxing tobacco more heavily, particularly with modest investments in improved tax administration and with overall tax reform (Chapter 17; Stotsky 1995). World Bank data reveal that in high-income countries, the average percentage of all government revenue derived from tobacco tax is 0.63%, whereas in middle-income countries the average is 0.51%, and in low-income countries it is 0.42%.

Table 19.2 Relevance of tobacco control policies to countries of different income levels

Policy instrument	Low-income	Middle-income	High-income
Raise tax	3	3	3
Research causes, consequences and costs	2	2	2
Mass information, prominent warning labels	3	3	2
Ban advertising and promotion	3	3	3
Restrict public and workplace smoking	2	2	3
De-regulate nicotine replacement products	1	2	3
Control smuggling	3	3	2

Source: authors' calculations, based on a survey of 23 economists and tobacco control experts during a technical review meeting for this volume held in Lausanne, Switzerland, in November 1998.
3 = highly relevant, 2 = relevant, 1= somewhat relevant, 0= not relevant.

In order to conduct local research on the consequences of tobacco use, and then disseminate the results of that research, some countries would require increased capacity in R&D. Many would also require improved record-keeping in their health systems, e.g. in making systematic ascertainment of the cause of each death. Because such vital statistics provide information on tobacco-attributable diseases, as well as other diseases, they are a strategic priority for low-income and middle-income countries (Lopez 1998). Mass information campaigns would probably need to be integrated with other health promotion efforts, although this might lessen the specificity and effectiveness of tobacco control messages (Goldman and Glantz 1998). In the immediate term complete bans on advertising and promotion could be relatively attractive measures in low-income countries, as they would be comparatively easy to enforce. Smoking restrictions in public and working places are likely to be more difficult to enforce, partly because of a smaller formal labor sector.

Middle-income countries, whose tax infrastructure tends to be more robust, and for which there are often better processes for monitoring restrictions and a stronger R&D capacity, could introduce a wider range of instruments. For example, middle-income countries may also be in a stronger position to deregulate NRTs. They might also be able to control smuggling more effectively, given stronger customs infrastructure.

In all countries, successful programs are likely to have certain common features. One is enabling policy makers to gain 'ownership' of the chosen interventions by providing them with the research findings on which the interventions are based. As for other disease-control programs, clear objectives, management plans, sound information, and regular review, are also essential. Programs would need to be sensitive to cultural values and the historical experiences of the country. For example, bans on smoking in public places may currently be unacceptable in some of the former socialist economies of Europe, simply because the memory of totalitarian governments is too fresh (Makara 1994).

Finally, a critical feature of a successful tobacco-control program is its ability to engage many different sectors of government. Table 19.3 illustrates some of the links between government ministries that would facilitate effective action. Effective tobacco control involves several disciplines, and the staffing and skill mix is likely to be determined by each country's specific needs at the time.

19.2.3 Effectiveness of tobacco-control programs

There have been few attempts to evaluate tobacco-control programs. As shown by Ranson *et al.* (Chapter 18), individual interventions are capable of preventing millions of deaths globally, but whether a package of measures would save even more lives than the sum of each individual intervention is as yet unknown.

A limited number of evaluations of comprehensive tobacco-control programs in high-income countries suggest that they can be successful. In the United States, the States of California and Massachusetts have been funding their comprehensive tobacco programs using state excise taxes since 1989 and 1993, respectively. The key components of both programs were excise tax increases between 25 and 50 cents per

Table 19.3 Inter-ministerial action required for tobacco control

Issue	Agency or ministry
Taxation	Finance, Trade, Customs, Social Security
Research on causes, consequences and costs of tobacco use	National Statistics Offices (for smoking on death certificates) Industry, Commerce, Trade, Agriculture, Health
Mass information	Education, Telecommunication, Health
Ban advertising and promotion	Commerce, Finance, Telecommunication
Deregulate nicotine replacement markets	Commerce, Trade, Drug Controller, Health
Restrict public and workplace smoking	Commerce, Tourism, Hotels
Control smuggling	Trade, Customs, Finance
Employment and agricultural issues	Agricultural, Labor, Commerce

Source: authors.

pack, a proportion of which was used for counter-advertising, and local community programs to increase cessation, promote smoke-free workplaces, and educate young people (CDC 1999a).

From 1989 to 1993, Californian's decline in per capita annual cigarette consumption was 52% greater than for the rest of the United States, i.e. a decline of 0.64 packs per person per year in California versus 0.42 packs per person per year in other states (Pierce *et al.* 1998). An econometric analysis estimates that 78% of the reduction in Californian cigarette sales from 1990 to 1992 was attributable to tax increases, and that the remaining 22% was attributable to information campaigns (Hu *et al.* 1995). Pierce *et al.* (1998) suggest that from 1994 to 1996 California continued to have greater declines in per capita consumption than the rest of the United States, but that declines in smoking prevalence were no greater. The authors attribute this to the industry's pricing and political activities. Industry spending on advertising and promotion increased markedly during this time. In addition, it should be noted that the tax increase occurred only in 1989, while real disposable incomes have increased substantially in California over the period. An independent evaluation of the Massachusetts program found that per capita consumption declined by 31% in that state and by 8% in the rest of the United States from 1992 to 1997 (Abt Associates 1998). In Massachusetts, the decline in per capita consumption was more consistent than that in California (CDC 1996). At the time of writing, there were no data available on the impact of the 1996 excise tax increase in Massachusetts.

Other econometric studies have examined changes in consumption in countries, and not specific programs. The United Kingdom experienced a 23% decline in cigarettes consumed per adult from 1976 to 1988. Regression analysis suggest that real price increases lowered consumption by about 17%, while rising income increased consumption by about 12%; the residual reduction of 18% (i.e. 23 − 17 + 12) has been attributed to increased health promotion campaigns and lower advertising and tobacco promotion (Townsend 1993). A retrospective analysis of 22 high-income countries from 1960 to 1986 suggests that if tobacco advertising and promotion had been banned and if real prices had been raised by 36%, then consumption would have fallen by 13.5% by 1986 (Laugesen and Meads 1991).

19.2.4 Costs and financing of comprehensive tobacco-control programs

There are only rudimentary estimates of the costs of implementing a comprehensive tobacco-control program. The evidence from high-income countries suggests that such comprehensive programs can be delivered for a relatively small sum of money. Currently, for different states in the United States, annual funding for tobacco-control programs ranges from $2.5 to $10 per capita. The US Centers for Disease Control and Prevention (1999a) recommends $6–16 per capita for the US. This is equal to spending between 0.3% and 0.9% of US public spending per capita on health. In 1996, Canada spent US$1.65 per capita on tobacco-control activities, the equivalent of 0.1% of its public spending per capita on health (Pechmann *et al.* 1998).

In this context, tobacco control in middle-income and low-income countries is likely to be affordable, even in countries where per capita public expenditure is extremely low. The World Bank's 1993 *World Development Report 1993: Investing in Health* estimated that to deliver an essential package of public interventions that includes tobacco control, governments would need to spend $4 per capita in low-income countries and $7 in middle-income countries (World Bank 1993). As a fraction of the total, the cost of tobacco control would be small.

19.3 Strategic priorities for international agencies

Certain activities for tobacco control may be beyond the reach of national governments. For example, strong international law to establish the legal framework for tobacco control cannot be achieved by single countries. In such cases, there is likely to be a role for international agencies, such as the World Health Organization (WHO), the World Bank, and the International Monetary Fund (IMF), as well as for regional political entities, such as the European Union. A key to effective international action is vigorous leadership on tobacco control. The WHO has recently launched its Tobacco Free Initiative (TFI). A detailed description of the TFI can be found on the WHO website (*http://www.who.int/toh*). One of the chief goals of the TFI is to implement the Framework Convention on Tobacco Control—a new international legal instrument that aims to address issues as diverse as tobacco advertising and promotion, smuggling, taxes, and subsidies.

International activities could be classified in three broad categories: review of programs and policies; regional or international action on specific control instruments; and research. We briefly discuss the first two. A more detailed discussion on research follows.

19.3.1 Review of international programs and policies

Most international bodies lack clear policies and effective instruments for tobacco control. On the supply side, the World Bank adopted a policy in 1991 of not lending directly for, investing in, or guaranteeing investment or loans for tobacco production, processing, or marketing. More recently, the United States Agency for International Development has adopted a similar position of not supporting tobacco production. In contrast, the European Union continues to subsidize its tobacco farmers to the extent of about $1.2 billion a year through its Common Agricultural Policy (Joossens and Raw 1996). As discussed in Chapter 13, such supply-side policies are important politically, but are likely to have a minimal impact on consumption.

Where demand-side policies have been adopted, they have sometimes been implemented with the least effective instruments. For example, in the past, the World Bank has supported some school education programs against tobacco, but their effectiveness is questionable. Equally, while public funds can be used in a relatively straightforward way to control certain diseases, such as infectious vaccine-preventable diseases of childhood, it is more difficult to develop public policy instruments against tobacco, since its control depends more heavily on regulation and information than on the direct treatment of individuals. Thus, for development agencies that lend or grant funds to low-income and middle-income countries, new lending tools, such as loans or credits that disburse against specific monitorable polices, are required.

Table 19.4 describes some ways in which the international agencies might provide external support for countries' tobacco-control activities. To some extent, adjustment lending by multilateral agencies offers this possibility, particularly when short-term revenue collection and stabilization are important (Chapter 17). Yet most structural

Table 19.4 Objectives and modalities for external support for tobacco control

Objectives and modalities	Program implementation	Capacity building
Service delivery	Generally limited (mass information campaigns or NRT finance for the poor are possibilities).	Improve capacity in counter-advertising, mass information, smuggling control, and NRT regulation. Analyze possible subsidies for NRTs for the poor.
Policy implementation	Conditionality as part of financial package (e.g. tax increases or advertising and promotion bans). Policy advice.	Analytic units within public sectors (e.g. investing in Ministries of Finance to build tobacco taxation policies).
Research on causes, consequences and costs of tobacco use	Analyses, including policy-based lending/aid instruments	Economic and health policy research within countries to inform and guide control programs (e.g. University of Cape Town project supported by Canada's International Development and Research Centre).

Source: authors.

lending efforts have not consistently examined tobacco tax increases. Similarly, there has been little consideration of how to integrate tobacco-control policies within 'sector-wide approaches' (Cassels and Janovsky 1998). Beyond program implementation, all agencies could adopt policies to strengthen capacity within countries in service delivery, policy analysis, and research, often using existing loans or grants.

19.3.2 Regional or international action on specific control instruments

Beyond reviewing their own programs and policies, there is much more that the international agencies could do. They could help governments to achieve regional and multilateral agreements on smuggling controls and taxation, for example. Price differentials between countries represent a clear incentive for smuggling and legal cross-border shopping. Smuggling reduces government revenue and, in the long term, may increase cigarette consumption, because illegal cigarettes are usually cheap and the availability of such cigarettes in a country is often used as an argument in favor of lower tax rates. Policy responses to tobacco smuggling have been the subject of insufficient methodological work or field testing. However, in addition to measures to reduce demand, common customs programs, strict enforcement, active research, and new measures, such as warning labels in local language and tax stamps inside plastic wrappings, can help to reduce smuggling.

With the globalization of broadcasting, telecommunications, and Internet media, it is also increasingly likely that international agencies will be needed to play a role in banning advertising and promotion. International agencies may also have a role to play in devising and monitoring very limited crop-diversification programs for farmers in the small minority of countries that are heavily dependent on tobacco, such as Zimbabwe and Malawi. The World Bank has a policy of supporting diversification in agrarian countries that are heavily dependent on tobacco as a source of income and of foreign exchange earnings.

19.4 Strategic priorities in research and development

While a detailed discussion of the enormously wide-ranging interdisciplinary research agenda required on tobacco control is beyond the scope of this chapter, we mention a few key principles.

19.4.1 The current situation

Currently, investment in tobacco research is relatively modest compared with investment in research on other health problems of a comparable scale. In recent years, for every death due to tobacco (based on 1990 estimates), governments and public agencies spent about $50 on tobacco research (a total in the range of $148–164 million). In comparison, they spent $3000 for every HIV death in the same year (a total of $919–985 million) (WHO 1996). The vast majority of research and development in tobacco control, as for HIV/AIDS, has been taking place in high-income countries. For example, more than 80% of the papers presented at the 9th World Conference on Tobacco and Health in Paris in 1994 were studies done in high-income countries (Slama 1995). Detailed biological and physiopathological research findings are likely to be transferable from high-income, to low-income and middle-income countries. But epidemiological research and applied research may be less transferable.

A key problem is the overall lack of standardized and comparable data. The WHO, the US Centers for Disease Control and Prevention, the World Bank, and the International Union Against Cancer are actively developing a global surveillance system that will improve standardization (CDC 1999b). The World Bank has commissioned a series of price-elasticity studies. With new international interest in tobacco control, it is likely that there will be improvements in the quality of research data (Samet *et al.* 1998; Baris 1999). The International Research and Development Centre in Canada has launched an initiative called Research for International Tobacco Control (http://www.idrc.ca/ritc/Aboutus.htm). More recently, more than 35 million tobacco industry documents have become available as a result of litigation in the United States (http://www.cdc.gov/tobacco/industrydocs/index.htm), but have not yet been fully researched.

19.4.2 Future options

Research in tobacco control aims mainly to spur the application of existing effective instruments to control tobacco use. The Institute of Medicine (1998) suggested five criteria could help to set priorities for broader research in control of cardiovascular disease. These apply also to tobacco control. First, the research should have a large-scale population impact. Second, it should use methods and processes (but not necessarily provide results) that are broadly transferable to other low-income and middle-income countries. Third, investments should yield results within a reasonable timeframe: say, up to 10 years. Fourth, research should be clearly linked to potential action plans, programs, and policies. Fifth, investments should focus on studies that produce measurable data and, for the most part, use established methodologies in epidemiology, health policy, economics, and social behavioral sciences.

Table 19.5 provides a matrix of research on the causes, consequences and costs of tobacco use, in relation to key demand-side instruments of price rises (through tax increases), information, and regulation and to the supply-side instrument of smuggling control. Research on causes refers to understanding the determinants of smoking uptake and persistence. Consequences refer to the health and non-health impacts of tobacco use and of tobacco-control policies. Cost refers to the costs of consumption borne by smokers and non-smokers or costs of control policies imposed on individuals. The grouping is by no means watertight. Research findings, such as price-elasticity, will influence all types of research as well as instruments. Obviously the table is simplistic and needs to be tailored to individual countries. For an expanded discussion of research priorities, see Baris (1999) and Samet *et al.* (1998). This table suggests that a key research priority is to continue monitoring and analyzing information on the health consequences of smoking. Other priorities include refinement of the data on price-elasticities for tobacco, especially in low-income countries, and more detailed analyses of how different forms of health information are used by different consumers.

Table 19.5 Priorities for research on tobacco control policies in low-income and middle-income countries

Intervention or R&D type	Causes	Consequences	Costs
Price	• Price elasticities, including by age group, income status. • Substitutability of different tobacco products (e.g. *bidis*).	• Price effects of switching to cheaper cigarettes or decreased amounts, and on mortality and morbidity.	• Tax burden on poor and non-poor. • Health care and pension costs of smokers.
Information	• Poor, non-poor differences in uptake. • Degree to which information is internalized by smokers. • Peer influences on smoking uptake.	• Estimates of tobacco-attributable mortality and disability from different tobacco products, and amounts. • Health effects of environmental tobacco smoke.	• Information search costs with advertising and promotion bans.
Regulation	• NRT impact on tobacco demand. • Advertising and promotion expenditures. • NRT product research (e.g. nicotine/tar content, delivery system, additives, taste, size, etc.).	• Impact of lower-tar and lower-nicotine cigarettes on health risk.	• Health insurance and government subsidies of NRTs. • Local cost-effectiveness and incidence-subsidy studies about use of NRTs by poor and non-poor groups.
Supply	• Determinants of smuggling, including influence of corruption, border and customs policy and product tracking. • Industry influences on control policies and political process.	• Impact on tax revenue from smuggling. • Research on trade policy, impact of new trade agreements.	• Dynamic and static models of employment impacts of reduced consumption.

Source: authors.

The table does not mention the tracking of tobacco-related deaths, which obviously are critical in monitoring the impact of control efforts. Thus, at the level of individual countries, the key long-term indicator of tobacco control is mortality reduction. Shorter-term indicators are likely to include total cigarette sales (to capture initiation), and ex-smoking rates (to capture quitting). Thus, for example, in the United Kingdom, annual tobacco deaths at ages 35–69 fell from 80 000 to 40 000 over the past three decades (Peto *et al.* 1994), and total cigarette sales fell from 130 billion to 80 billion. Over the same period, the 'ex-smoker' proportion of the population has roughly doubled (Wald and Nicolaides-Bouman 1988). In contrast, there have been recent increases in smoking rates among younger British age groups (UK Department of Health 1998).

Research and development efforts cannot be implemented without building the appropriate capacity. Effective tobacco control needs competent and well-informed personnel working in settings aimed to support their efforts. Therefore, investments must be made in both institutional and human capacity development. Key areas of work include enhancing local capacity, including identifying a focal point within a government agency, assessing research capacity, education efforts for physicians and academics on tobacco, and networking and communications.

As discussed in more detail elsewhere, much of the information generated from research is an international public good (WHO 1996). Thus, there is a strong argument for international finance for this research.

19.5 Political-economy issues in tobacco control

To be effective, any government that decides to implement tobacco controls must do so in a context in which the decision has broad popular support. Governments alone cannot achieve success without the involvement of civil society, the private sector, and interest groups. Programs are more likely to succeed if there is collective agreement on, and ownership of, them across a broad coalition of social interests with the power to implement and sustain change. There are few useful methodologies on how to work with such other agencies. Historically, in the United States, tobacco control started as a medical issue, moved into advocacy, and has now proceeded toward a focus on legal and policy issues (Gorovitz *et al.* 1998).

Governments contemplating action to control tobacco face major political obstacles to change. Yet, by identifying the key stakeholders on both the supply and demand sides in each country, policy-makers can assess the size of each constituency, whether it is dispersed or concentrated, and other factors that may affect the constituency's response to change. Careful planning and political mapping would be essential to achieve a smooth transition from reliance on tobacco to independence from it, whatever the nature of the economy and the national political framework. Such mapping exercises have been conducted, for example, in Vietnam (Efroymson *et al.* 1996).

In low-income countries, opposition to tobacco control from the supply side would tend to come from farmers. However, as Jacobs *et al.* discuss (Chapter 13), only a handful of countries are highly dependent on tobacco for foreign exchange earnings.

World Bank data suggest that the average foreign exchange earnings from tobacco (as a percentage of GDP) are 0.16% in low-income countries, 0.06–0.10% in middle-income countries, and 0.06% in high-income countries. Supply-side objections in middle-income countries are more likely to come from arguments about tax revenue and the size of the tobacco industry than they are from arguments about farming.

One intervention that has received widespread support from advocates of tobacco control is the earmarked tobacco tax: that is, a proportion of tax revenue collected from cigarettes that must be devoted to a specific activity, such as health education or healthcare. Earmarking introduces clear restrictions and inefficiencies on public finance (Stotsky 1995). For this reason alone, most macro-economists do not favor earmarking, no matter how worthy the cause. Analysis does suggest, however, that the efficiency or dead-weight losses from earmarking tobacco taxes are minimal (Hu *et al.* 1998). Earmarking could be justified if governments used these funds for services that would not have been otherwise used. However, earmarked taxes also have a political function, in that they help to concentrate political winners of tobacco control, and thus influence policy. Earmarked funds that support broad health and social services (such as other disease programs) broaden the political and civil-society support base for tobacco control. In Australia, broad political support among Ministries of Sports and Education helped to convince the Ministry of Finance that raising tobacco taxes was possible. Indeed, once an earmarked tax was passed, the Ministry of Finance went on to raise tobacco taxes further without earmarking them (Galbally 1997).

In theory, there may be efficiency gains with combinations of earmarking and government finance for services targeted at the poorest socio-economic groups (World Bank 1993). This would provide double health gains—reducing tobacco consumption and improving access to core public health and clinical services. In China, for example, conservative estimates suggest that a 10% increase in cigarette tax would decrease consumption by 5%, increase revenue by 5%, and that the increase would be sufficient to finance a package of essential health services for one-third of China's poorest 100 million citizens (Saxenian and McGreevey 1996).

19.6 Conclusion

There is convincing evidence that, even on conservative assumptions, millions of deaths could be prevented over the next few decades by implementing modest, cost-effective tobacco-control policies. These policies include higher taxes, comprehensive bans on the promotion and advertising of tobacco, better and more widely publicized research into the consequences of smoking, prominent warning labels, de-regulated access to NRTs, and tight controls on smuggling. Investing in these policies represents an unprecedented opportunity for governments to improve their nations' health. It is likely that the optimal mix of strategic priorities for tobacco control will differ for different countries, depending on their economic, cultural, and political circumstances. Ultimately, globalization requires that international agencies such as WHO, the World Bank and the IMF play a role in enabling countries to achieve effective tobacco control. Decisive, collaborative, and focused action over the next few years will be critical in curbing a global epidemic that will otherwise claim one billion lives in the twenty-first century.

References

Abt Associates Inc. (1998). *Independent Evaluation of the Massachusetts Tobacco Control Program*. 4th annual report, January 1994–June 1997. Abt Associates Inc., Cambridge, MA.

Baris, E. (1999). *Confronting the Epidemic: a Global Agenda for Tobacco Control Research*. World Health Organization and Research for International Tobacco Control, Geneva.

Cassels, A. and Janovsky, K. (1998). Better health in developing countries: are sector-wide approaches the way of the future? *Lancet*, **352**(9142), 1777–9.

Centers for Disease Control and Prevention (1996). Cigarette smoking before and after an excise tax increase and an antismoking campaign—Massachusetts, 1990–1996. *Morbidity and Mortality Weekly Report*, **45**(44), 966–70.

Centers for Disease Control and Prevention (1999a). *Best Practices for Comprehensive Tobacco-Control Programs*. US Department of Health and Human Services, Centers for Disease Control and Prevention, National Center for Chronic Disease Prevention and Health Promotion, Office on Smoking and Health, Atlanta GA.

Centers for Disease Control and Prevention (1999b). *Global Tobacco Surveillance System: a Multi-partner Project*. Proceedings of the workshop on 'Regional Surveillance Systems for Tobacco Control', June 28–29, 1999, Atlanta, GA.

The Economist (1995). An anti-smoking wheeze: Washington needs a sensible all-drugs policy, not a 'war' on teenage smoking. 19 August, pp. 14–15.

The Economist (1997). Tobacco and tolerance. 20 December, pp. 59–61.

Efroymson D., Phuong, D. T., Huong, T. T., Tuan, T., Trang, N. Q., Thanh, V. P. N. *et al.* (1996). *Decision-mapping for Tobacco Control in Vietnam*. Report to the international tobacco initiative. PATH Canada. Project 94–0200–01/02214.

Federal Trade Commission (1995). Cigarette advertising and promotion in the United Sates, 1993: a report of the Federal Trade Commission. *Tobacco Control*, **4**, 310–3.

Galbally, R. L. (1997). Health-promoting environments: who will miss out? *Aust N Z J Public Health*, **21**, 429–30.

Goldman, L. K. and Glantz, S. A. (1998). Evaluation of antismoking advertising campaigns. *Journal of the American Medical Association*, **279**(10), 772–7.

Gorovitz, E., Mosher, J., and Pertschuk, M. (1998). Preemption or prevention?: lessons from efforts to control firearms, alcohol, and tobacco. *Journal of Public Health Policy*, **19**(1), 36–50.

Hu, T. W., Sung, H. Y., and Keeler, T. E. (1995). Reducing cigarette consumption in California: tobacco taxes vs an anti-smoking media campaign. *American Journal of Public Health*, **85**(9), 1218–22.

Hu, T. W., Xu, X., and Keeler, T. (1998). Earmarked tobacco taxes: lessons learned. In *The Economics of Tobacco Control* (ed. I. Abedian *et al.*), pp. 102–18. Applied Fiscal Research Centre, University of Cape Town, Cape Town, South Africa:

Institute of Medicine (1994). *Growing Up Tobacco Free: Preventing Nicotine Addiction in Children and Youths*. National Academy Press, Washington DC.

Institute of Medicine (1998). *Control of Cardiovascular Diseases in Developing Countries*. Research, Development and Institutional Strengthening. National Academy Press, Washington DC.

Jha, P., Novotny, T. E., and Feachem, R. (1998). The role of governments in global tobacco control In *The Economics of Tobacco Control* (ed. I. Abedian *et al.*), pp. 38–56. Applied Fiscal Research Centre, University of Cape Town, Cape Town, South Africa:

Joossens, L. and Raw, M. (1996). Are tobacco subsidies a misuse of public funds? *BMJ*, **312**(7034), 832–5.

Laugesen, M. and Meads, C. (1991). Tobacco advertising restrictions, price, income and tobacco consumption in OECD countries, 1960–1986. *British Journal of Addiction*, **86**(10), 1343–54.

Liu, B. Q., Peto, R., Chen, Z. M., Boreham, J., Wu, Y. P., Li, J.Y. *et al.* (1998). Emerging tobacco hazards in China. I. Retrospective proportional mortality study of one million deaths. *BMJ*, **317**(7170), 1411–22.

Lopez, A. D. (1998). Counting the dead in China. Measuring tobacco's impact in the developing world. *BMJ*, **317**(7170), 1399–400.

Makara, P. (1994). Policy implications of differential health status in East and West Europe. The case of Hungary. *Social Science and Medicine*, **39**(9), 1295–302.

Niu, S. R., Yang, G. H., Chen, Z. M., Wang, J. L., Wang, G. H., He, X. Z. *et al.* (1998). Emerging tobacco hazards in China 2. Early mortality results from a prospective study. *BMJ*, **317**(7170), 1423–4.

Pechmann, C., Dixon, P., and Layne, N. (1998). An assessment of US and Canadian smoking reduction objectives for the year 2000. *American Journal of Public Health*, **88**(9), 1362–7.

Peto, R., Lopez, A. D., Boreham, J., Thun, M., and Clark Jr, H. (1994). *Mortality from Smoking in Developed Countries 1950–2000*. New York: Oxford University Press.

Peto, R. and Lopez, A. D. (in press). The future worldwide health effects of current smoking patterns. In *Global Health in the 21st Century* (ed. E. C. Koop, C. E. Pearson, and R. M. Schwarz. Jossey-Bass, New York, 2000.

Pierce, J. P., Gilpin, E. A., Emery, S. L., White, M. M., Rosbrook, B., Berry, C. C. *et al.* (1998). Has the California tobacco control program reduced smoking? *Journal of the American Medical Association*, **280**(10), 893–9.

Samet, J. M., Taylor, C. E., Becker, K. M., and Yach, D. (1998). Research in support of tobacco control. *BMJ*, **316**(7128), 321.

Saxenian, H. and McGreevey, B. (1996). *China: Issues and Options in Health Financing*. World Bank Report No. 15278-CHA, Washington, D.C.

Slama, K. (ed.) (1995). *Tobacco and Health*. Plenum Press, New York.

Stotsky, J. G. (1995). Summary of IMF tax policy advice. In *Hand Book of Tax Policy* (ed. P. Shome), pp. 79–84. International Monetary Fund, Washington DC.

Townsend, J. (1993). Policies to halve smoking deaths. *Addiction*, **88**(1), 37–46.

UK Department of Health (1998). *Smoking Kills*. A white paper on tobacco. The Stationery Office, London.

Wald, N., and Nicolaides-Bouman, A. (ed.) (1998). *UK Smoking Statistics*. Oxford University Press, Oxford.

Warner, K. E., Chaloupka, F. J., Cook, P. J. *et al.* (1995). Criteria for determining an optimal cigarette tax: the economist's perspective. *Tobacco Control*, **4**, 380–86.

World Bank (1993). *The World Development Report 1993: Investing in Health*. Oxford University Press, New York, NY.

World Health Organization (1996). *Investing in Health Research and Development*. Report of the Ad Hoc Committee on Health Research Relating to Future Intervention Options (Document TDR/Gen/96.1). World Health Organization, Geneva.

Appendixes

Appendix 1

This appendix provides the definitions and characteristics of the country-level data used in various analyses in this volume. Data on the economics of tobacco control, once scarce, especially for low-income and middle-income countries, are improving in both quantity and quality due to better data collection efforts by governments, international agencies, and commercial entities. As the data are continuously updated, this appendix does not provide actual numbers, but refers to the sources where such data are available.

General socio-economic indicators

General country-level socio-economic indicators relevant to various discussions in this book include population (by age and gender), national economic performance (Gross Domestic Product and Gross National Product), and employment. For the purposes of consistency and comparability, all these indicators were extracted from the World Bank's World Development Indicators (WDI) 1998 database. Data on total revenues, revenues from excise taxes and all taxes are obtained from the Government Finance Database of the International Monetary Fund (IMF).

Smoking prevalence

Smoking prevalence is the percentage of current smokers in the total population. The World Health Organization (WHO) defines a current smoker as a person who has smoked daily for at least six month during his or her life and smokes at the time of the survey (WHO 1998). In this volume, unless otherwise indicated, smoking prevalence means the prevalence of current adult smokers (aged 15 years and above). Smoking prevalence is estimated by prevalence-surveys. Many countries report smoking prevalence by different age and gender groups. Definitions of current smoking and adult smokers sometimes vary across different studies and may lead to incomparability of data. For example, a current adult smoker was defined by a survey in Ireland as a person aged 18 years and older who smoked at the time of the survey or quitted within the month prior to the survey (Shelley *et al.* 1996). On the other hand, in a study in India, this definition was a person above 25 years of age who was currently smoking and who had smoked more than 100 cigarettes or bidis in his or her lifetime (Narayan *et al.* 1996).

The sources for most of the smoking prevalence data by country used in this book are from studies compiled in a WHO publication (1997). These studies were judged to be 'methodologically sound and to provide reasonably reliable and comparable results'. Other sources were found from literature searches (see Appendix 2).

Cigarette consumption

The number of cigarettes sold annually in a country is considered as its total cigarette consumption (often in million sticks). This is often estimated as: Total Cigarette Consumption = Cigarette Production + Cigarette Imports − Cigarette Exports. 'Per adult' cigarette consumption is calculated by dividing total cigarette consumption by the total population of those who are 15 years old and older. In some countries, where cigarette smuggling is a significant problem, consumption estimated by this method is less reliable.

Data for total cigarette consumption for most countries were obtained from the Economic Research Service (ERS) of the United States Department of Agriculture (USDA). These can be found in an ERS Statistical Bulletin entitled *US Tobacco Statistics, SB-869, April 1994*, or online at http://www.econ.ag.gov/briefing/tobacco/. Other data were from WHO (1997) and the MarketFile (1998), a commercial online tobacco database (http://www.marketfile.com).

Smoking-attributable burden of disease

Peto *et al.* (1994) have provided indirect estimates of smoking-attributable mortality by different causes for 46 developed countries (which include the former Socialist economies of Europe) in a publication titled *Mortality from Smoking in Developed Countries 1950–2000*. For each developed country, the authors compared the national lung cancer death rate with the rate that has been seen in the main epidemiological studies of US non-smokers, and to attribute the excess to tobacco. This absolute excess mortality from lung cancer was then used indirectly as a guide to the proportions of the deaths from other causes that should be ascribed to smoking. Direct estimates of smoking-attributable mortality in China are available with two recent studies (Lie *et al.* 1998; Niu *et al.* 1998).

Disability-adjusted life years (DALYs) are the sum of life years lost due to premature mortality and years lived with disability, adjusted for severity. Estimates for smoking-attributable DALYs for different regions, including 1990–2020 projections, can be obtained from WHO (1996, 1999). Smoking-attributable DALYs refer only to disease among smokers, and exclude the effects of smoking on non-smokers. Murray and Lopez (1996, 1997) used the above-mentioned method by Peto *et al.* to calculate the smoking-attributable burden of disease by region for 1900–2020, employing a smoking impact ratio, which is defined as:

$$\text{Smoking impact ratio} = (C - N)/(S - N),$$

where C is the observed lung cancer rate in a given age group of a population; S is the smoker lung-cancer rate in the US Cancer Prevention Study; N is the non-smoker lung-cancer rate in the US Cancer Prevention Study.

This ratio was used as a surrogate for the prevalence of cumulative exposure to calculate the smoking-attributable fraction of the disease burden. Because non-smoker lung-cancer rates are higher in China and Asia, than in the United States, alternative non-smokers lung-cancer rates were used for these two regions. Preliminary results from a large-scale case-control study in China were used to estimate the attributable fractions reported for China and Asia. Deaths from tobacco-chewing among women in India were also estimated with attributable fractions reported by a local study (Murray and Lopez 1997).

Tobacco production, trade, and employment

Tobacco production
Tobacco leaves production (in metric tons) refers to the actual harvested tobacco leaves producted from the field, excluding harvesting and threshing losses and that part of tobacco crop not harvested for any reason. Tobacco harvest area (or tobacco acreage) refers to the area from which tobacco leaves are gathered. Cigarette production is the number of cigarettes (usually in million sticks) manufactured in a year.

Tobacco leaves production and harvest areas were obtained from the statistical database of the Food and Agriculture Organization (FAO), Agricultural Production subset. This database can be found online at http://apps.fao.org/cgi-bin/nph-db.pl?subset=agriculture. Data on cigarette production were gathered from the US Department of Agriculture (http://www.econ.ag.gov/briefing/tobacco/) and MarketFile (http://www.marketfile.com).

Tobacco trade
Tobacco leaves (or cigarette) exports (or imports) by volume refers to total tobacco leaves (or manufactured cigarettes) exported (or imported) in metric tons (or million sticks). These indicators are also available by value in millions of current US dollars. They were all obtained from the FAO statistical database (Agriculture and Food Trade subset) at the above-mentioned internet address.

Employment in tobacco manufacturing
Tobacco-manufacturing employment refers to the number of persons engaged in tobacco manufacturing. While data for tobacco-agricultural employment (the number of persons engaged in tobacco farming activities) are only available for a few country through literature searches, data for tobacco-manufacturing employment for several countries are available in the database maintained by the United Nations Industrial Development Organization (UNIDO) (http://www.unido.org).

Tobacco price

Producer price of tobacco leaves refers to the producer price of a metric ton on tobacco leaves in local currency. This indicator were obtained from the statistical database of FAO (Producer prices subset) at the internet address mentioned above.

Retail cigarette price is the average retail price for a pack of 20 cigarettes. It is obtained by two methods:

(1) through the World Bank's Economic Survey of Tobacco Use, which collects information on the retail price (including all taxes) for a pack of the most popular brand of cigarettes in a country;

(2) using the formula: Average retail cigarette price per pack of 20 sticks = [Total value of domestic sale of cigarettes/Total number of domestic sale of cigarettes (sticks)] × 20.

The source of country-level data on total value of domestic cigarette sale is MarketFile. The total number of domestic sales of cigarettes (expressed in sticks) for selected countries is available from USDA and MarketFile.

Tobacco taxation and revenues

Tobacco excise taxes can be specific (i.e. a fixed amount of duty per 1000 cigarettes or per 1000 g of tobacco) or ad valorem (i.e. a percentage of the retail selling price) or a combination of both. Total tobacco tax revenue refers to the total revenue that the central government earns annually from tobacco taxes. This includes not only revenue generated from tobacco excise taxes but also from value-added taxes (VAT), where the latter are applicable. Data on tobacco excise tax structure and tobacco tax revenue were obtained through the World Bank Economic Survey of Tobacco Use and through literature searches.

Non-price tobacco control measures

Non-price tobacco control measures, which many countries have adopted, include health-warning labels and tar and nicotine information on packages of cigarettes or tobacco products, restrictions or bans on advertising and promotion of tobacco products, restriction on smoking in public places, and bans of cigarette sales to minors (defined as under 16–21 years old in different countries).

Data on non-price tobacco control measures were obtained from different sources. The main sources are two WHO publications:

(1) the *International Digest of Health Legislation, 1970–1995*; and
(2) *Tobacco or Health: A Global Status Report 1997*.

The other source is the MarketFile commercial database.

Summary of key data sources

- Food and Agriculture Organization (FAO) *Statistical Database* (http://apps.fao.org/cgi-bin/nph-db.pl?subset=agriculture). Data on tobacco leaves production and harvest area, producer prices for tobacco leaves, tobacco leaves and cigarette trade (export–import) by volume and value.
- International Monetary Fund (IMF) (1999). *Government Financial Statistics*. Washington DC. Data on total revenues, revenues from excise taxes and all taxes.
- MarketFile (http://www.marketfile.com). A commercial online tobacco database. Data on cigarette consumption, production, price and tobacco control measures.
- Peto, R., Lopez, A. D., Boreham, J., Thun, M., and Heath Jr, C. (1994). *Mortality*

from Smoking in Developed Countries 1950–2000. Oxford University Press. Oxford, Data on smoking-attributable mortality for 46 developed and former Soviet economies.

- United Nations Industrial Development Organization (UNIDO) (http://www.unido.org) Tobacco manufacturing employment.
- United States Department of Agriculture (USDA), Economic Research Service (ERS) (http://www.econ.ag.gov/briefing/tobacco/). Data on cigarette sales, cigarette and tobacco leaves production.
- US Centers For Disease Control and Prevention (CDC), Office on Smoking and Health (OSH) (http://www.cdc.gov/tobacco/index.htm). Current and historical state-level data on the prevalence of tobacco use, the health impact and costs associated with tobacco use, tobacco agriculture and manufacturing, and tobacco control laws in the United States.
- World Bank (1998). *World Bank Economic Survey of Tobacco Use.* Data on average retail price for most popular domestic and foreign cigarettes, cigarette excise tax, tobacco tax revenue. (The results of this survey, along with other data on the economics of tobacco collected by the World Bank, is available online at http://www.worldbank.org/tobacco).
- World Bank (1998). *World Development Indicators.* Washington DC. General socio-economic, population, and health indicators for 148 countries and 14 country groups. Parts of the content of the database are available at http://www.worldbank.org/data/wdi/home.html.
- World Health Organization (1996). *Investing in Health Research and Development.* Report of the Ad Hoc Committee on Health Research Relating to Future Intervention Options. Geneva:, Switzerland. Estimates of tobacco-attributable burden of disease by region, 1990–2020.
- World Health Organization (1997). *Tobacco or Health: a Global Status Report.* Geneva, Switzerland. Country-level data on smoking prevalence, cigarette consumption, tobacco production, trade, industry, health impact and tobacco control legislation. The content of this book is also available online at http://www.cdc.gov/tobacco/who/whofirst.htm.
- World Health Organization (1999). *The World Health Report 1999: Making a Difference.* Geneva, Switzerland. Estimates of tobacco-attributable burden of disease by region, 1998.

References

Liu, B. Q., Peto, R., Chen, Z. M., Boreham, J., Wu, Y. P., Li, J. Y., *et al.* (1998). Emerging tobacco hazards in China. I. Retrospective proportional mortality study of one million deaths. *BMJ,* **317**(7170), 1411–22.
Murray, C. J. and Lopez, A. D. (ed.) (1996). *The Global Burden of Disease: a Comprehensive Assessment of Mortality and Disability from Disease, Injuries, and Risk Factors in 1990 and projected to 2020.* Harvard School of Public Health, Cambridge, Mass.
Murray, C. J. and Lopez, A. D. (1997). Global mortality, disability, and the contribution of risk factors: global burden of disease study. *Lancet,* **349**(9063), 1436–42.

Narayan, K. M., Chadha, S. L., Hanson, R. L., Tandon, R., Shekhawat, S., Fernandes, R. J. *et al.* (1996). Prevalence and patterns of smoking in Delhi: cross-sectional study. *BMJ*, **312**(7046), 1576–9.

Niu, S. R., Yang, G. H., Chen, Z. M., Wang, J. L., Wang, G. H., He, X. Z. *et al.* (1998). Emerging tobacco hazards in China 2. Early mortality results from a prospective study. *BMJ*, **317**(7170), 1423–4.

Peto, R., Lopez, A. D., Boreham, J., Thun, M., and Heath Jr, C. (1994). *Mortality from Smoking in Developed Countries 1950–2000*. Oxford: Oxford University Press.

Shelley, E., Collins, C., and Daly, L. (1996). Trends in smoking prevalence: the Kilkenny Health Project Population Surveys 1985 to 1991. *Irish Medical Journal*, **89**(5), 182–5.

WHO (World Health Organization) (1996). *Investing in Health Research and Development*. Report of the Ad Hoc Committee on Health Research Relating to Future Intervention Options. Geneva, Switzerland.

WHO (1997). *Tobacco or Health: a Global Status Report*. Geneva, Switzerland.

WHO (1998). *Guidelines for Controlling and Monitoring the Tobacco Epidemic*. Geneva, Switzerland.

WHO (1999). *The World Health Report 1999: Making a Difference*. Geneva, Switzerland.

Appendix 2

Studies of smoking prevalence, by World Bank region

Country	Population aged 15 and over ('000)	Year of study	Adult smoking prevalence (%) (aged 15 and above)		Source (Unless stated otherwise, all data are from WHO (1997))
			Men	Women	
East Asia and the Pacific					
1 China	885 686	1996	63%	4%	Chinese Academy of Preventive Medicine (1997)
2 Fiji	506	1988	59%	31%	
3 Indonesia	128 750	1986	53%	4%	
4 Malaysia	12 469	1986	41%	4%	
5 Mongolia	1496	1990	40%	7%	
6 Papua New Guinea	2614	1990	46%	28%	
7 Philippines	42 132	1987	43%	8%	
8 Samoa	103	1994	53%	19%	
9 Thailand	42 104	1996	45%	3%	ASH Thailand (1999)
10 Tonga	69	1991	65%	14%	
11 Viet Nam	46 392	1997	73%	4%	Jenkins *et al.* (1997)
Weighted average			61%	4%	
Europe and Central Asia					
12 Albania	2221	1990	50%	8%	
13 Bulgaria	6875	1997	38%	17%	Balabanova *et al.* (1998)
14 Czech Republic	8386	1994	43%	31%	
15 Estonia	1179	1997	54%	24%	Pudule *et al.* (1999)
16 Hungary	8368	1989	40%	27%	
17 Latvia	2009	1997	56%	11%	Pudule *et al.* (1999)
18 Lithuania	2918	1997	53%	8%	Pudule *et al.* (1999)

Appendix 2 (*cont.*)

Country	Population aged 15 and over ('000)	Year of study	Adult smoking prevalence (%) (aged 15 and above)		Source (Unless stated otherwise, all data are from WHO (1997))
			Men	Women	
19 Malta	288	1992	40%	18%	
20 Poland	29729	1993	51%	29%	
21 Russian Federation	115514	1996	63% (a)	30% (b)	(a) Bobak *et al.* (1998); (b) WHO (1997)
22 Slovakia	4144	1992	43%	26%	
23 Slovenia	1630	1994	35%	23%	
24 Turkey	40946	1988	63%	24%	
25 Turkmenistan	2760	1992	27%	1%	
26 Uzbekistan	13583	1989	40%	1%	
Weighted average			57%	26%	
Middle East and North Africa					
27 Algeria	17239	1980	53%	10%	
28 Bahrain	364	1991	24%	6%	
29 Egypt	36096	1986	40%	1%	
30 Iraq	11645	1990	40%	5%	
31 Morocco	17209	1990	40%	9%	
32 Saudi Arabia	10470	1990	53% (a)	1% (b)	(a) WHO (1997) (b) Jarallah *et al.* (1999)
Weighted average			44%	5%	
Latin America and the Caribbean					
33 Argentina	24664	1992	40%	23%	
34 Bolivia	4411	1992	50%	21%	
35 Brazil	109387	1989	40%	25%	
36 Chile	9974	1990	38%	25%	
37 Colombia	24166	1992	35%	19%	
38 Costa Rica	2211	1988	35%	20%	
39 Cuba	8524	1990	49%	25%	
40 Dominican Republic	5085	1990	66%	14%	
41 El Salvador	3408	1988	38%	12%	
42 Guatemala	5896	1989	38%	18%	
43 Honduras	3339	1988	36%	11%	
44 Jamaica	1707	1990	43%	13%	
45 Mexico	58688	1990	38%	14%	
46 Paraguay	2959	1990	24%	6%	
47 Peru	15326	1989	41%	13%	
48 Uruguay	2409	1990	41%	27%	
Weighted average			40%	21%	
South Asia					
49 Bangladesh	67811	1990	60%	15%	
50 India	607504	1980	40%	3%	
51 Pakistan	73237	1990–94	36%	9%	Alam (1998)
52 Sri Lanka	12682	1988	55%	1%	
Weighted average			42%	5%	

Appendix 2 (cont.)

Country	Population aged 15 years and over ('000)	Year of study	Adult smoking prevalence (%) (aged 15 and above)		Source (Unless stated otherwise, all data are from WHO (1997))
			Men	Women	
Sub-Saharan Africa					
53 Lesotho	1144	1989	38%	1%	
54 Mauritius	833	1992	47%	4%	
55 Nigeria	60977	1990	24%	7%	
56 Seychelles	52	1989	51%	10%	
57 South Africa	25911	1996	50%	19%	Medical Research Council of South Africa (1999) (unpublished data)
58 Sudan	19281	1995	12%	1%	Idris et al. (1998)
Weighted average			29%	9%	
High-income countries					
59 Australia	14152	1995	27%	23%	Hill et al. (1998)
60 Austria	6632	1995	39%	24%	Haidinger et al. (1998)
61 Bahamas	202	1989	19%	4%	
62 Belgium	8313	1993	31%	19%	
63 Canada	23381	1991	31%	29%	
64 Cook Islands	15	1988	44%	26%	
65 Cyprus	542	1990	43%	7%	
66 Denmark	4315	1994	54%	46%	Osler et al. (1998)
67 Finland	4129	1994	27%	19%	
68 France	46682	1993	40%	27%	
69 Germany	68375	1995	31%	18%	Microcensus (1995) cited in Helmert (1999)
70 Greece	8672	1994	46%	28%	
71 Iceland	206	1994	31%	28%	
72 Ireland	2741	1993	30%	28%	Irish Department of Health (1993) cited in Shelley et al. (1996)
73 Israel	3915	1989	45%	30%	
74 Italy	48646	1995	34%	17%	Pagano et al. (1998)
75 Japan	104663	1994	59%	15%	
76 Korea, Rep.	34296	1989	68%	7%	
77 Kuwait	1087	1991	52%	12%	
78 Luxembourg	336	1993	32%	26%	
79 Netherlands	12709	1994	36%	29%	
80 New Zealand	2723	1992	24%	22%	
81 Norway	3516	1994	36%	36%	
82 Portugal	8081	1994	38%	15%	
83 Singapore	2277	1995	32%	3%	
84 Spain	32581	1993	48%	25%	
85 Sweden	7182	1994	22%	24%	
86 Switzerland	5835	1992	36%	26%	
87 United Kingdom	47157	1999	29%	28%	ASH UK (1999)
88 United States	205413	1993	28%	23%	
Weighted average			38%	21%	

References

Action on Smoking and Health (ASH) (1999), Thailand. http://www.ash.or.th/situation/situation.htm.

Action on Smoking and Health (ASH) (1999). The Untied Kingdom. http://www.ash.org.uk/.

Alam, S. E. (1998). Prevalence and pattern of smoking in Pakistan. *Journal of the Paskistani Medical Association*, 48(3), 64–6.

Balabanova, D., Bobak, M., and McKee, M. (1998). Patterns of smoking in Bulgaria. *Tobacco Control*, 7(4), 383–5.

Bobak, M., Pikhart, H., Hertzman, C., Rose, R., and Marmot, M. (1998). Socioeconomic factors, perceived control and self-reported health in Russia. A cross-sectional survey. *Social Science and Medicine*, 47(2), 269–79.

Chinese Academy of Preventive Medicine (1997). *Smoking in China: 1996 National Prevalence Survey of Smoking Pattern.* Beijing: China Science and Technology Press.

Haidinger, G., Waldhoer, T., and Vutuc, C. (1998). The prevalence of smoking in Austria. *Preventive Medicine*, 27(1), 50–5.

Helmert, U. (1999). Income and smoking behavior in Germany—a secondary analysis of data from the 1995 microcensus. *Gesundheitswesen*, 61(1), 31–7. (In German.)

Hill, D. J., White, V. M., and Scollo, M. M. (1998). Smoking behaviours of Australian adults in 1995: trends and concerns. *Medical Journal of Australia*, 168(5), 209–13.

Idris, A. M., Ibrahim, Y. E., Warnakulasuriya, K. A., Cooper, D. J., Johnson, N. W., and Nilsen, L. R. (1998). Toombak use and cigarette smoking in the Sudan: estimates of prevalence in the Nile state. *Preventive Medicine*, 27(4), 597–603.

Jarallah, J. S., al-Rubeaan, K. A., al-Nuaim, A. R., al-Ruhaily, A. A., and Kalantan, K. A. (1999). Prevalence and determinants of smoking in three regions of Saudi Arabia. *Tobacco Control* 8(1), 53–6.

Jenkins, C. N., Dai, P. X., Ngoc, D. H., Kinh, H. V., Hoang, T. T., Bales, S. *et al.* (1997). Tobacco use in Vietnam: prevalence, predictors, and the role of the transnational tobacco corporations. *Journal of the American Medical Association*, 277(21), 1726–31.

Osler, M., Prescott, E., Gottschau, A., Bjerg, A., Hein, H. O., Sjol, A. *et al.* (1998). Trends in smoking prevalence in Danish adults, 1964–1994: the influence of gender, age, and education. *Scandinavian Journal of Social Medicine*, 26(4), 293–8.

Pagano, R., La Vecchia, C., and Decarli, A. (1998). Smoking in Italy, 1995. *Tumori*, 84(4), 456–9.

Pudule, I., Grinberga, D., Kadziauskiene, K., Abaravicius, A., Vaask, S., Robertson, A. *et al.* (1999). Patterns of smoking in the Baltic Republics. *Journal of Epidemiology and Community Health*, 53(5), 277–82.

Shelley, E., Collins, C., and Daly, L. (1996). Trends in smoking prevalence: the Kilkenny Health Project Population Surveys 1985 to 1991. *Irish Medical Journal*, 89(5), 182–5.

WHO (World Health Organization) (1997). *Tobacco or Health: a Global Status Report.* Geneva, Switzerland.

Appendix 3

Countries of the world by income and region (World Bank's classification)

	East Asia and Pacific	Europe and Central Asia	Latin America and the Caribbean	Middle East and North Africa	South Asia	Sub-Saharan Africa	High-income OECD	Other high-income
Low-income	Cambodia	Armenia	Guyana	Yemen, Rep.	Afghanistan	Angola		
	China	Azerbaijan	Haiti		Bangladesh	Benin		
	Lao PDR	Bosnia and Herzegovina	Honduras		Bhutan	Burkina Faso		
	Mongolia	Kyrgyz Republic	Nicaragua		India	Burundi		
	Myanmar	Moldova			Nepal	Cameroon		
	Vietnam	Tajikistan			Pakistan	Central African Republic		
					Sri Lanka	Chad		
						Comoros		
						Congo, Democratic Republic		
						Congo, Republic		
						Côte d'Ivoire		
						Equatorial Guinea		
						Eritrea		
						Ethiopia		
						Gambia, the		
						Ghana		
						Guinea		
						Guinea-Bissau		
						Kenya		
						Lesotho		
						Liberia		
						Madagascar		
						Malawi		
						Mali		
						Mauritania		
						Mozambique		
						Niger		
						Nigeria		
						Rwanda		
						São Tomé and Principe		
						Senegal		
						Sierra Leone		
						Somalia		
						Sudan		
						Tanzania		
						Togo		
						Uganda		
						Zambia		
						Zimbabwe		
Lower-middle income	Fiji	Albania	Belize	Algeria	Maldives	Botswana		
	Indonesia	Belarus	Bolivia	Egypt, Arab Rep. of		Cape Verde		
	Kiribati	Bulgaria	Colombia	Iran, Islamic Republic		Djibouti		
	Korea, Dem. Rep	Estonia	Costa Rica	Iraq		Namibia		
	Marshall Islands	Georgia	Cuba			Swaziland		
	Micronesia Fed. Sts.	Kazakstan	Dominica					
	Papua New	Latvia	Dominican	Jordan				

Guinea Philippines Samoa Solomon Islands Thailand Tonga Vanuatu Lithuania Macedonia, FYR Romania Russian Fed. Turkey Turkmenistan Ukraine Uzbekistan Yugoslavia, FR.	Republic Ecuador El Salvador Grenada Guatemala Jamaica Panama Paraguay Peru St. Vincent & the Grenadines Suriname Venezuela	Lebanon Morocco Syrian Arab Republic Tunisia West Bank and Gaza		
Upper-middle income American Samoa Malaysia Palau Croatia Czech Rep. Hungary Isle of Man Malta Poland Slovak Rep. Slovenia	Antigua and Barbuda Argentina Barbados Brazil Chile Guadeloupe Mexcio Puerto Rico St. Kitts and Nevis St. Lucia Trinidad and Tobago Uruguay	Bahrain Libya Oman Saudi Arabia	Gabon Mauritius Mayotte Seychelles South Africa	
High-income				
Australia Austria	Japan Korea, Rep.	Andorra Aruba	Guam Hong Kong, China	

Appendix 3 (cont.)

East Asia and Pacific	Europe and Central Asia	Latin America and the Caribbean	Middle East and North Africa	South Asia	Sub-Saharan Africa	High-income OECD		Other high-income	
						Belgium	Luxembourg	Bahamas,	The Israel
						Canada	Netherlands	Bermuda	Kuwait
						Denmark	New Zealand	Brunei	Liechtenstein
						Finland	Norway	Cayman Is.	Macao
						France	Portugal	Channel	Martinique
						Germany	Spain	Islands	Monaco
						Greece	Sweden	Cyprus	Netherlands
									Antilles
						Iceland	Switzerland	Faeroe	New Caledonia
						Ireland	United	Islands	Northern Mariana
							Kingdom		Islands
						Italy	United	French	Qatar
							States	Guyana	Reunion
								French	Singapore
								Polynesia	United Arab
									Emirates
								Greenland	Virgin Islands
									(US)

Source: The World Bank (1999). *World Development Indicators 1999*. The World Bank, Washington DC.

Index

Printed in the United Kingdom
by Lightning Source UK Ltd.
127119UK00001B/5/A

9 780192 632463